Atlas of Oral Implantology

Atlas of Oral Implantology

A. Norman Cranin, DDS, D. Eng
FAAID, FADSA, FICD, FAAHD, FADM, FACD, FBSE

The Dr. Samuel Cranin Dental Center
The Brookdale University Hospital and Medical Center
Brooklyn, New York

Chairman, Department of Dental and Oral Surgery and the Dental Implant Group
The Brookdale University Hospital and Medical Center

Clinical Professor, Oral and Maxillofacial Surgery and Implantology
New York University College of Dentistry

Clinical Professor, Oral and Maxillofacial Surgery, Prosthodontics and Biomaterials
University of Medicine and Dentistry of New Jersey

Adjunct Clinical Professor of Oral and Maxillofacial Surgery
University of Pennsylvania School of Dental Medicine

Associate Clinical Professor of Dentistry
The Mount Sinai School of Medicine
City University of New York

Consultant, Oral and Maxillofacial Surgeon
Brooklyn Developmental Center

Consultants

Michael Klein, DDS

Clinical Associate Professor
Department of Implant Dentistry
New York University
New York, New York

Clinical Assistant Professor
Department of Prosthodontics
University of Medicine and Dentistry of New Jersey
New Jersey Dental School
Newark, New Jersey

Private Practice
Cedarhurst, New York

Alan Simons, DDS

Private Practice
Farmington Hills, Michigan

Formerly, Associate Professor
Department of Diagnostics and Surgical Sciences
University of Detroit Mercy
School of Dentistry
Detroit, Michigan

Second Edition

with 1300 *illustrations*

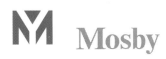

Mosby

St. Louis Baltimore Boston Carlsbad Chicago Minneapolis New York Philadelphia Portland
London Milan Sydney Tokyo Toronto

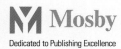

Mosby
Dedicated to Publishing Excellence

Publisher: John Schrefer
Editor: Penny Rudolph
Developmental Editor: Angela Reiner
Project Manager: Linda McKinley
Production Editor: Rich Barber
Designer: John C. Ritland
Design Manager: Renée Duenow
Cover Illustration: Teri McDermott

Composition by Top Graphics, Inc.
Printing/binding by Walsworth Press, Inc.

Mosby, Inc.
11830 Westline Industrial Drive
St. Louis, Missouri 64146

International Standard Book Number: 1-55664-552-X

99 00 01 02 03 / 9 8 7 6 5 4 3 2 1

This Atlas is dedicated to my grandchildren

Olivia and Joshua Cranin
Jesse and Sophie Cranin
Emily and Rebecca Cooperstein

from whom I receive much delight and gratification

May they enjoy long, happy, healthy lives
and never have need for the benefits described in this book.

And to their indomitable grandma, Dr. Marilyn Sunners Cranin, who started it all.

Foreword

Dental implant history dates back thousands of years and includes civilizations such as the ancient Chinese, who 4000 years ago inserted bamboo into the jaw bone for fixed tooth replacements. The Egyptians and, later, physicians from Europe used ferrous and precious metals for implants over 2000 years ago, and the Incas used pieces of sea shells, inserted into the jaw bones to replace missing teeth. The United States began its involvement in implant dentistry with Greenfield and his iridioplatinum cage in 1909.

Today, oral implantology has changed the entire discipline of dentistry. Most every specialty incorporates this field into its clinical and research activities, but oral surgery, periodontics, and prosthodontics have taken a major role. Approximately 40 to 50 years ago, a handful of men helped mold and shape the discipline as we know it today. Gershkoff (the subperiosteal implant), Tatum (bone grafting specifically for implants), Linkow (the blade and self-tapping root form), and Brånemark (the predictable method to create a direct bone interface), to name a few, made major contributions during that time, which benefit us to this day. However, very few of the early pioneers who had directed implantology over the last four decades are prepared to lead us into the new millennium.

One of the few men who is so prepared is Dr. A. Norman Cranin. He has been the "orthodontic appliance" to oral implantology. For 50 years he has placed the correct amount of *pressure* in the right *areas* in order to help *move* the profession toward an intellectual and a predictable method to incorporate implants into clinical practice.

Dr. Cranin is a pioneer in clinical implantology, an implant researcher, an editor, an implant educator, and an author. He is the only oral surgeon to insert and restore dental implants for more than 40 years. He developed a blade implant design and modified the subperiosteal implant more than 25 years ago. His research has extended from the basic sciences of implant biomaterials and metallurgy to wound healing and bone grafting. He has performed many clinical trials to evaluate root form designs. Yet one of the most important contributions to implant dentistry has been his dedication to organized implant education. Thirty years ago, A. Norman Cranin developed the first structured implant program in the United States. This program has permitted him to focus on the profession in a unique way. Many of his implant fellows have continued his undying commitment to implant dentistry as clinicians, researchers, and professors of implantology at dental schools and hospitals both in the United States and abroad.

Dr. Cranin has also contributed widely to the literature of implant dentistry. His publications have extended over many decades and have helped pave the way for others in this discipline to understand and also help improve the field. He has been the editor of two major referred journals, the prestigious *Journal of Biomedical Materials Research,* which he steered for more than 10 years, and *Oral Implantology,* which has been and continues to be under his direction for the last 8 years. As with all things in his life, he has been committed to make these entities reliable and guiding lights to the profession.

A. Norman Cranin is also an author; this is the second edition of the *Atlas of Oral Implantology.* The first edition was published only 7 years ago during a period in which the discipline exploded. He is not only a mentor: he is the consummate student, which has allowed him to update his Atlas and to remain in the forefront of this dynamic discipline in the form of this brilliant contribution. He is a role model to me and to the profession, giving leadership, knowledge, and experience. I strongly recommend this Atlas to every practicing dentist. No dental office in the next millennium can escape the need to know more about implant dentistry. This book will be a study guide for the experienced practitioner and a reference source for those who are less involved.

I am honored to have been given the privilege of writing the foreword to such a needed contribution to oral implantology.

Carl E. Misch, BS, DDS, MDS
Clinical Associate Professor
University of Pittsburgh
School of Dental Medicine

Director
Misch Implant Institute

Clinical Associate Professor
University of Michigan
School of Dentistry

Adjunct Professor
University of Alabama at Birmingham
School of Engineering

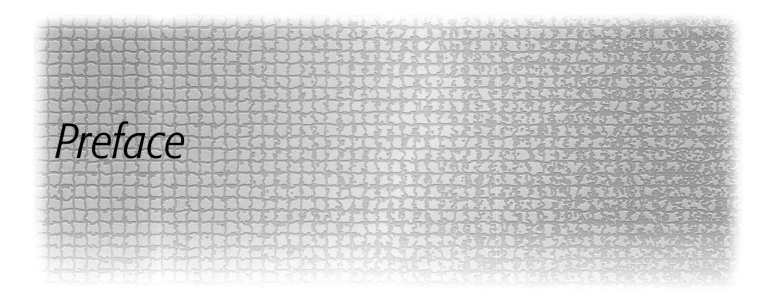

Preface

When the editors at Mosby invited me to provide them with a second edition to this Atlas, not only was I pleased and flattered to be an author for the outstanding medical publisher in the world, I also believed that I had been granted a sinecure.

The assignment would probably be completed in a short time, correcting a paragraph here, inserting a photograph there, and updating the chapter on abutments. (Oh, those abutments!)

I'd been teaching and operating regularly and did not realize the radical changes to which our specialty has been exposed.

I asked my fellows to update the root form implant charts, to review the latest information on membranes (GTRMs), and to call for all the details on the newest abutments, and frankly, I thought that with a few hours at the computer, the revision would be completed.

As my more sophisticated readers know, this discipline of ours, from imaging to implant designs and textures, from abutments to methods of overdenture fixation, has grown exponentially over the past decade.

As the realization of the great quantity of new material became clear, enthusiasm turned to panic. The book grew in size and content, and a review demonstrated that our references had quintupled in number and expanded enormously in content. Surgical and grafting techniques had been found to be limited only by the capabilities and imagination of the surgeons. Restorative dentists were producing lifelike results that defied nature.

With each new idea, each catalog and each publication, my avarice became greater for leaving no stone unturned in making this an encyclopedic effort. As a personal learning experience for my colleagues and me, there could have no greater exercise than updating and supplementing 10-year-old information in an area of practice so vital and dynamic.

It is my consummate desire that the information found in the pages of this Atlas will contribute to the comprehension, capabilities, and skills of its readers and to the improvement of the health, well-being, and quality of life of their patients.

ACKNOWLEDGMENTS

Although producing this second edition was essentially a singular effort, I need to acknowledge the efforts of a great number of friends and colleagues. I want to tender gratitude to my senior fellow, John Ley, for assembling the chapter on abutments and for spending hours collecting, selecting, and labeling hundreds of new photographs; to Michael Katzap, my junior fellow, who totally revised the reading lists, updated the many charts, virtually reconstituted Chapters 10 and 11 (the new proprietaries), and spent hours with me on the improvement of illustrations; and to Edmund Demirdjan, my new fellow, who wrote and rewrote many of the legends and spent hours reading proof.

Monica Grant typed this manuscript from the first page to the last, with skill, patience, and humor, and never so much as frowned when yet another revision was put before her.

My secretary and good friend, Ethel Bruck-Leibowitz, and her daughter, Rachel, spent hours typing the seemingly endless lists of references and reading materials selected for inclusion in this Atlas and offered me the continuing encouragement so important in the dark days when the task seemed almost insurmountable.

Michael Klein outlined three of the prosthetic chapters and was kind enough to have contributed some illustrations, which improved their content. Alan Simons organized several of the introductory chapters, read proof, and assisted in the compilation of the materials in Chapters 10, 11, and 28.

Marc Kaufman, a member of the Brookdale Dental Implant Group, rendered advice in regard to the prosthetic chapters and contributed a novel technique to Chapter 24. Aram Sirakian sent the spark erosion photographs; Robert Sumners supplied the information and illustrations on sub-antral osteotomies; Manuel Chanavaz contributed the first half of Chapter 3 on health care screening; and Carol Cave-Davis, Chief Medical Librarian of the Brookdale University Hospital and Medical Center, served as an endless source of reprints and references.

Joel Herring suffered resiliently with my many corrections and produced some lovely new artwork for Chapters 10 and 11.

The cooperation of the representatives of numerous implant companies made the cataloging of products simpler and allowed us to codify them into readily comprehensible charts and tables. Among them were Carl Misch of BioHorizons; Jim Iannaccone of Steri-Oss; Brian Banton of Paragon; Jack Wimmer of Park Dental Research; Marc McAllister of Innova Stereolithography; Rick Hayse of 3i; Jay Huggins of Innova Implants; and the representatives of Sulzer-Calcitek, Straumann, Lifecore, NobelBiocare, Bicon, Kyocera, Pacific Bone Bank, and the Cal Ceram Dental Laboratory.

This second edition would not have come to fruition were it not for the confidence expressed in me by the senior editors of my publisher, Mosby, Inc. of St. Louis. Particularly important are Linda Duncan, formerly in charge of dental publications; Penny Rudolph, the current dental editor; and Angela Reiner, who listened to my every complaint.

The Brookdale University Hospital and Medical Center, my professional home for over three decades, believed in formal dental implant training since 1970, when my program and fellowship were established, and continues to support it to this day.

An effort of this magnitude could not have been completed without the support and understanding of a wonderful and patient wife. Marilyn Cranin made many pots of late night coffee and offered support and advice for which I am very grateful.

Dr. Bob James of Loma Linda University served as my dear friend and counsel until his untimely death. Many of the techniques described in this book were generated by his innovative skills and fertile imagination.

Finally, my inspiration and dedication to dentistry were initiated by my dad, Dr. Sam Cranin, whose spirit, still tangible and vibrant, remains constantly with me.

A. Norman Cranin
Brooklyn, New York

Contents

Atlas of Oral Implantology

1

Introduction to the Atlas of Oral Implantology

W e welcome the reader to the second edition of *Atlas of Oral Implantology*. This book is an instructional manual on how to choose patients, evaluate host sites, select implant types (however, no preferences are given for specific proprietary products), place implants step by step, observe patients, diagnose incipient problems, institute remedial techniques ("troubleshooting"), perform a wide variety of restorative modalities, and maintain and follow patients during the postoperative period.

This atlas is arranged in a unique manner. It is suggested that it be read in its entirety before any future workups are performed or patient care is rendered. There are chapters, or portions of chapters, in which the reader may have no interest. However, in order to harvest the optimal benefits from the book, an understanding of its design and the material described should be acquired in their entirety.

Chapters 2, 3, 4, 5, and parts of the Appendixes explain the values and applications of implants in general, how to choose the appropriate design for each condition presented, which patients should be treated with implants and why, the tests that should be performed to assess the eligibility of patients, what the anatomic characteristics of potential host sites may be, how the basic implant designs differ, and, in these differences, how they may serve doctor and patient best. Read these chapters first before proceeding to any later chapters on specific techniques.

Chapter 6 explains the armamentarium an implant surgeon is expected to have before undertaking any procedure. In addition, the beginning of each implant technique chapter gives a list of special or additional instruments peculiar to the specific modality being described. As added information, most chapters start with "caveats" for each described technique. To be forewarned is to be forearmed. Chapter 6 suggests a classic operatory design as well, and although it is not mandatory that a specific room be dedicated to implant surgery, it is necessary to have all the requisite instruments and supplies available that will permit the implantologist to perform the surgery or change a treatment plan during the procedure. For example, a blade might be indicated instead of a planned root form because the

ridge is too narrow, or a larger diameter implant may be required if the osteotomy becomes too wide. Chapters 9, 10, and 11 concern root form surgery and offer this information because not all companies have implants of larger diameters that can serve this purpose. In fact, the decision to do a subperiosteal implant should be a viable one if endosteals are not suitable. The supplies and facilities for such a procedure must be immediately available as well. It is hoped that the reader will become a "complete" implantologist, that is, one who acquires the capabilities to manage any situation in which implants of any design may be used or substituted for the type that had been selected at the time of treatment planning.

Incidentally, it is suggested that a practitioner ought not attempt to insert implants if the necessary experience obtained from having taken hands-on courses is lacking or if the requisite surgical skills gained from previous training and clinical involvement are absent. In addition, the information given in these chapters is not etched in stone. There are often specific problems, deviations from the expected, and the occurrence of unpredictable events that must be anticipated as one proceeds with planning and operative efforts.

Chapter 5 is important because it offers advice on the prosthetic options available. The method of reconstruction should be selected before the implants have been placed. A decision as to the choice of an overdenture, a single tooth replacement, a fixed-detachable prosthesis, or a cemented bridge should be made with the assistance of the patient. Patient preference, local conditions, costs, and the doctor's skills and philosophies all play a role in governing these selections.

After a prosthetic technique has been chosen, the reader will find in Chapters 2, 5, 9, 10, and 11 the specific implant types that lend themselves to the prosthetic options that best suit the patient's needs.

In Chapter 4, relatively noninvasive techniques that serve as guides to "sound" the bone, that is, measure its height and its width, are offered so that the kind of implant that is simplest to use and offers the best chances for success will be chosen. The principles of surgery and anesthesia are of paramount importance. Chapters 6, 7, and 8 offer instruction in incision making; techniques of dissection and reflection; methods of retraction; use of coolants; handling of drills, burs, and handpieces; management of osteotomies; soft and hard tissue manipulations; bone grafting; oral plastic surgery; and the types of and ways to use available sutures. These fundamentals may seem rudimentary, but it is suggested that they be read because they apply to all implant techniques. In addition, Chapter 6 and all other basic or introductory chapters (such as Chapter 9 on the generic root form implant) have been written and illustrated to make the use of this atlas simple and efficient. They contain basic principles that apply to all techniques and methods and allow the reader to proceed as being guided by a personal tutor on how to incise, reflect, cut bone, and suture because these topics are logically arranged chapter after chapter.

Once the appropriate implant design has been chosen, the reader should proceed as follows:

If it is to be a root form implant, review Chapter 9. Here one may find, regardless of which root form design has been chosen (threaded, self-tapping or non-self-tapping, press-fit, one-piece, or two-stage submergible), instructions on how to perform the initial steps of placement, such as bur and drill sizes, number-by-number, up to the requisite diameter. By following these instructions, the surgeon can supply himself with a generic drill set (i.e., Brasseler) that is not only economical in cost and time, but may also be used for all of the steps except the final one needed to seat every type of root form implant. In addition, the names, addresses, and telephone numbers of the manufacturers whose products are described in this atlas are listed in the Appendixes.

After completing Chapter 9, the reader may proceed to Chapters 10 and 11 and choose a specific implant among those described. In these chapters, there are step-by-step reviews of the surgery for virtually every implant system, from the first to the final proprietary maneuver, by name or number, including counter-sinks, bone taps, try-ins, and the seating of the implant. Logically, the healing screws, caps, or inserts that are available are described next. Closure is covered in Chapter 6, along with suture types, materials, and techniques. Of primary importance to the reader is the new section that follows in Chapters 20 to 27: "Prosthodontics." This is the next logical step in completing implant-borne reconstruction, and the chapters have been organized so that each of the numerous alternatives are available to the restorative dentist, from single tooth implants to the complexities of abutment selection and fixed-detachable, full arch rehabilitation.

If a blade implant, a ramus frame, a subperiosteal, or even an intramucosal insert is selected, there are specific chapters to guide the reader through each of the relevant procedures.

Not to be forgotten are endodontic implants, ridge maintenance, and augmentation procedures using autogenous bone and bone substitute grafting materials (hydroxyapatite, tricalcium phosphate [TCP], demineralized freeze-dried bone [DFDB], irradiated bone, and others); membranes, both absorbable and nonabsorbable; and for the oral and maxillofacial surgeon, jaw augmentation, skeletal reconstruction with biomaterials, and transosteal implant procedures that are described in detail in Chapters 8 and 18.

If, during implant surgery, the practitioner runs into a problem, or if, during the postoperative period, difficulties or unexpected sequelae arise, help is available in Chapter 28.

The Appendixes offer product and manufacturers' information; methods of metal passivation, defatting, and sterilization; suggestions for postoperative management; and one reasonable example of an implant surgery consent form. A glossary of implant terminology and newly expanded suggested reading lists are also included within this atlas.

It is hoped that this book will meet many of the needs of the practitioner in clinical implant activities.

Suggested Readings

Adell R: A 15 year study of osseointegrated implants in the treatment of the edentulous jaw, *Int J Oral Surg* 6:387, 1981.

Bahat O: Treatment planning and placement of implants in the posterior maxilla: report of 732 consecutive Nobelpharma implants, *Int J Oral Maxillofac Implants* 8:151, 1993.

Bain CA, Moy PK: The association between the failure of dental implants and cigarette smoking, *Int J Oral Maxillofac Implants* 8:609, 1993.

Balkin BE: Implant dentistry: historical overview with current perspective, *J Dent Ed* 52:683-685, 1988.

Branemark PI: Osseointegration and its experimental background, *J Prosthet Dent* 50:399-410, 1983.

Devge C, Tjellstrom A, Nellstrom H: Magnetic resonance imaging in patients with dental implants: a clinical report, *Int J Oral Maxillofac Implants* 12:354-359, 1997.

Dharmar S: Locating the mandibular canal in panoramic radiographs, *Int J Oral Maxillofac Implants* 12:113-117, 1997.

Fernandez RJ, Azarbal M, Ismail YH: A cephalometric tomographic technique to visualize the buccolingual and vertical dimensions of the mandible, *J Prosthet Dent* 58:446-470, 1987.

Gilbert GH, Minaker KL: Principles of surgical risk assessment of the elderly patient, *J Oral Maxillofac Surg* 48:972-979, 1990.

Higginbottom F, Wilson T: Three-dimensional templates for placement of root form dental implants: a technical note, *Int J Oral Maxillofac Implants* 11:787-793, 1996.

Hobo S, Ichida E, Garcia LT: Osseointegration and occlusal rehabilitation, *Quintessence* 153-162, 1990.

Jaffin RA, Berman CL: The excessive loss of Branemark fixtures in type IV bone: a 5 year analysis, *J Periodont* 1991.

Lekholm U, Zarb GA: Patient selection and preparation. In Branemark P-I, Zarb GA, Albrekisson T (eds): Tissue-integrated prostheses: osseointegration in clinical dentistry, *Quintessence* 199-209, 1985.

Misch CE: *Bone density and root form implants (manual),* Dearborn, Mich, 1984, Quest Implant.

Misch CE: Density of bone: effect on treatment plans, surgical approach, healing and progressive bone loading, *Int J Oral Maxillofac Implants* 6:23-31, 1990.

Misch CE: Medical evaluation of the implant candidate, *Int J Oral Maxillofac Implants* 9:556-570, 1981.

Misch CE, Crawford EA: Predictable mandibular nerve location—a clinical zone of safety, *Int J Oral Implant* 7:37-40, 1990.

National Institutes of Health: National Institutes of Health consensus development conference statement: dental implants, *J Am Dent Assoc* 117:509, 1988.

Parfitt AM: Investigation of the normal variations in alveolar bone trabeculation, *Oral Surg Oral Med Oral Pathol* 15:1453-1463, 1962.

Petrowski CG, Pharoah MJ: Presurgical radiographic assessment of implants, *J Prosthet Dent* 61:59-64, 1989.

Sones S, Fazio R, Fang L (eds): *Principles and practice of oral medicine,* Philadelphia, 1984, WB Saunders.

Tulasne JF: Implant treatment of missing posterior dentition. In Zarb G, Albrektsson T (eds): The Branemark implant, *Quintessence,* 1989.

Verstreken K, Van Marchal G, Naert I: Computer assisted planning of oral implant surgery: a three-dimensional approach, *Int J Oral Maxillofac Implants* 11:806-810, 1996.

Youse T, Brooks SL: The appearance of mental foramina on panoramic and periapical radiographs, *Oral Surg Oral Med Oral Pathol* 68:488-492, 1989.

Zabalegui J, Gil JA, Zabalegui B: Magnetic resonance imaging as an adjunctive diagnostic aid in patient selection for endosseous implants: preliminary study, *Int J Oral Maxillofac Implants* 5:283-288, 1991.

Zarb G, Leckholm U: Tissue integrated prostheses, *Quintessence* 199-209, 1985.

2

Implant Types and Their Uses

Implant Types

Endosteal Implants

*W*e begin with a general introduction to the implant types that are available and the physical conditions required for their placement. Although their basic characteristics are listed in this chapter, the reader should refer to Chapter 5 for optimal prosthetic use; it would be best to read Chapter 5 after completing this chapter, since one of the key guides to implant selection is the patient's prosthetic requirements.

Root Form Implants

Given sufficient width and height of the bone available, root forms (submergible, two-stage and single-stage, one-piece) are the first choice in selecting an implant. The following types are available:

Press-fit (unthreaded but covered with a roughened hydroxyapatite [HA] or titanium plasma spray coating [TPS]) (Fig. 2-1)
Self-tapping (threaded) (Fig. 2-2)
Pre-tapping (threaded) (Fig. 2-3)

Prosthetic options: Prostheses may be supported by fixed, fixed-detachable, overdenture, and single tooth purposes (antirotational design required).
Required bone:

>8-mm vertical bone height
>5.25-mm bone width (buccal to lingual)
>6.5-mm bone breadth (mesial to distal) per implant, including the interproximal spaces mesially and distally

Crête Mince (Thin Ridge) and Other Mini Implants

Crête Mince implants are threaded, self-tapping, titanium spirals (Fig. 2-4, *A*).

Prosthetic options: These Crête Mince, thin-ridge implants add retention to long-term fixed bridge prostheses by pinning them through their pontics to the underlying bone, or they may be used to support transitional prostheses (Fig. 2-4, *B*, *C*).

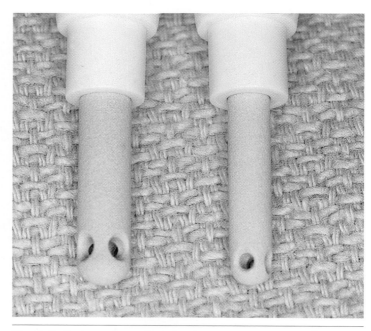

Fig. 2-1 Endosteal root form implants, 3.25- to 4-mm diameters, press-fit, both hydroxyapatite coated.

When placed into confined areas between teeth or implants, they add long-term additional buttressing to superstructures.

Blade Implants

Blade implants are available as submergible, two-stage and single-stage, one-piece devices (Fig. 2-5) as follows:

Prefabricated
Custom-cast
Alterable (by cutting, bending, and shaping at chairside)

Prosthetic options: Single or multiple abutments. The suggested use for blade implants is for fixed bridge prostheses in combination with natural tooth abutments, although they may be used in multiples for full arch edentulous reconstructions. If there is adequate height but inadequate width of available bone for root forms and osteoplasty is not an option, these are the second choice in implant selection. The design of the blade that is chosen should follow that of the anchor philoso-

phy in which the shoulder does not meet the cervix at right angles but rather dips in a semicircular configuration at the site of the neck.

Suitable arch: Maxillary or mandibular, completely or partially edentulous.

Required bone:

>8-mm vertical bone height
>3-mm bone width (buccal to lingual)
>10-mm bone breadth (mesial to distal except for single tooth designs, which require less)

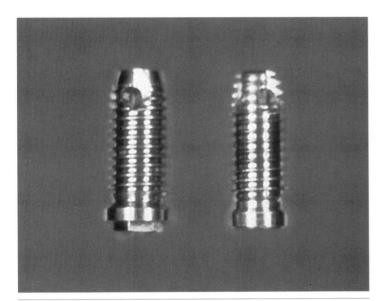

Fig. 2-2 Commercially pure (CP) titanium, self-tapping implants are of the Brånemark style.

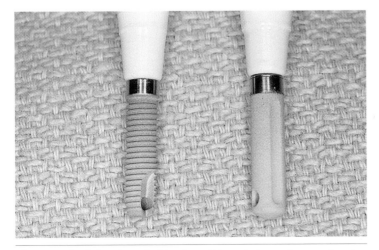

Fig. 2-3 Steri-Oss threaded implant, HA coated, requires pre-tapping of bone. Adjacent is a coordinated HA-coated press-fit design of the same diameter.

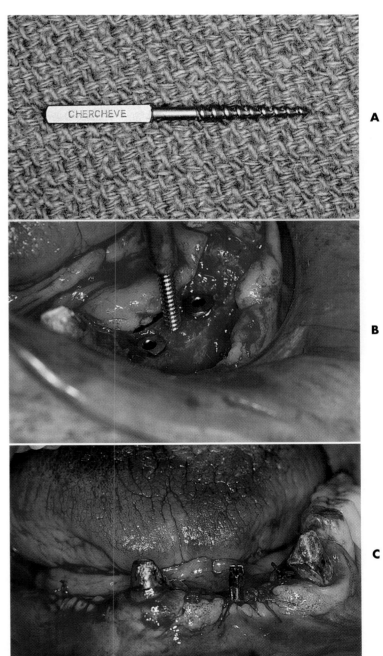

Fig. 2-4 **A,** Crête Mince (M. Chérchève) titanium-threaded implant for thin ridges. **B** and **C,** Dentatus implants of small dimensions can be placed in strategic sites for the support of interim prostheses during the periods of osseointegration of the conventional implants at sites No. 24 and 25.

Ramus Blade and Ramus Frame

The ramus implant is a one-piece blade made for use in the posterior mandible when insufficient bone exists in the body of this jaw (Fig. 2-6). The ramus frame is a three-blade, one-piece device designed for relatively atrophied mandibles for which the subperiosteal implant, because of cost or operator preference, is not desirable.

Prosthetic option: overdentures
Suitable arch: mandibular, completely edentulous
Required bone:

>6-mm vertical bone height (symphysis, rami)
>3-mm bone width (buccal to lingual)

Transosteal Implants

Transosteal implants are one-piece, transmandibular complex implants or are available as individual abutments. A submental skin incision is required under operating room conditions when this modality has been selected. One advantage of using the transosteal implant is predictable longevity. Several designs are available:

Single component (Fig. 2-7)
Multiple component, staple designs (several varieties) (Fig. 2-8)
Prosthetic options: The usual application for these implants is to support an overdenture. Fixed bridges are rarely made as alternatives.
Suitable arch: Mandible, anterior region, completely or partially edentulous (single component may be used in the presence of adjacent teeth).
Required bone:
>6-mm vertical bone height
>5-mm bone width (labial to lingual)

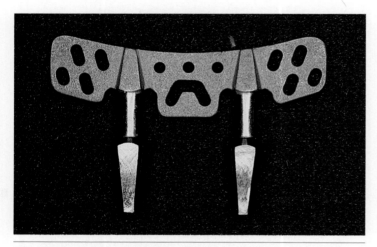

Fig. 2-5 Titanium, submergible blade implant with its abutments attached (Park/Startanius). The anchor configuration is embodied in the shoulder design.

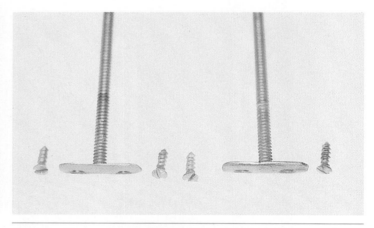

Fig. 2-7 Chrome alloy, threaded transosteal implants (Cranin/Vitallium).

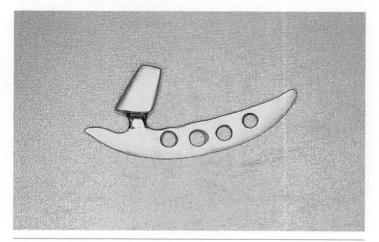

Fig. 2-6 Ramus blade, a plate form implant designed for the mandibular ramus in instances when insufficient bone exists in the body of the mandible.

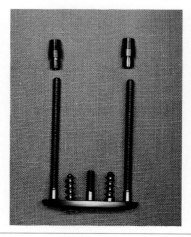

Fig. 2-8 Titanium, two-component staple implant (I. Small/Zimmer).

Subperiosteal Implants

Complete, Universal, and Unilateral

Use subperiosteal implants, which generally are quite reliable, when sufficient bone is unavailable for the use of end-osteal varieties. However, when extreme mandibular atrophy exists, mandibular augmentation (see Chapter 8) further improves the prognosis (Fig. 2-9).

Subperiosteal implants are always custom made. They may be fabricated either by making a direct bone impression (see Chapter 14) or by using stereolithographic technology. They may be used in any part of either jaw, and will serve as abutments for a variety of prosthetic configurations, although the overdenture is the most widely used to complement the complete subperiosteal implant (Figs. 2-10 and 2-11).

Prosthetic options: overdentures, fixed bridges

Suitable arch: maxillary or mandibular, completely or partially edentulous

Required bone: >5 mm or mandibular augmentation is required

Extremely thin (pencil-like) mandibles and maxillae may permit subperiosteal implants to settle through them. Therefore, seek a moderate amount of vertical bone height (at least 5 mm), or make plans to augment the inferior mandibular border or elevate the antral floor on a preventive basis.

Other Implants

Endodontic Stabilizers

Endodontic stabilizers are highly successful, tooth root–lengthening implants. One reason for their success is that they have no site of permucosal penetration because they are placed into bone through the apices of natural teeth (Fig. 2-12).

This implant offers a one-stage treatment for the stabilization of teeth that suffer from inadequate crown-root ratios. Their percentage of success when periodontal problems have been treated approaches that of conventional endodontic therapy.

Prosthetic options: Crown and fixed bridge abutments

Suitable arch: maxillary or mandibular; any tooth may be treated.

Required bone: 8 mm of lesion-free bone in direct proximity to the apex—within the long axis of the recipient root canal.

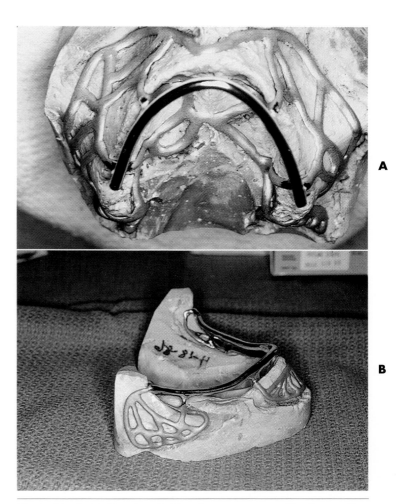

Fig. 2-10 **A,** Additional cortical-bearing areas are used by the maxillary pterygohamular subperiosteal implant. **B,** The mandibular subperiosteal implant has undergone many design changes.

Fig. 2-9 Titanium mortise mesh form, filled with autogenous bone harvested from the anterior iliac crest, materially alters the shape of the atrophied mandible.

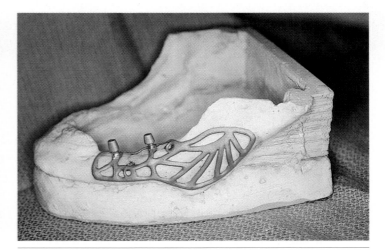

Fig. 2-11 Unilateral mandibular subperiosteal implant employs the same design principles as the complete device.

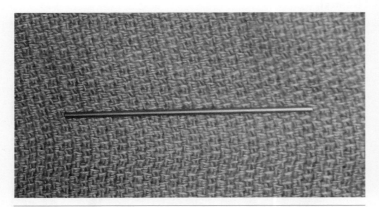

Fig. 2-12   Smooth-surfaced, matte-finished Co-Chro-Mo alloy endodontic implant (Howmedica/Vitallium).

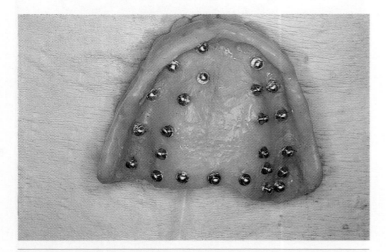

Fig. 2-13   Intramucosal inserts (stainless steel) processed into a denture (Jermyn/Densert).

Intramucosal Inserts

Intramucosal inserts are buttonlike, nonimplanted retention devices that can be used to stabilize full and partial maxillary and mandibular removable denture prostheses (Fig. 2-13). Because of the simple and relatively noninvasive nature of the procedure placement, they are of particular value for patients who are poor medical risks.

Prosthetic options: removable dentures, full or partial

Suitable arch: maxillary, completely or partially edentulous; mandibular, partial only

Required bone: none; required mucosa, 2.2 mm thick (bone beneath thinner mucosa may be deepened in nonantral areas)

Bone Augmentation Materials, Including Guided Tissue Regeneration Membranes

Use bone augmentation materials for ridge maintenance after dental extractions, for ridge augmentation, for periodontal and periimplant repair and support, and for maxillofacial surgical onlay and inlay purposes when bone replacement is required

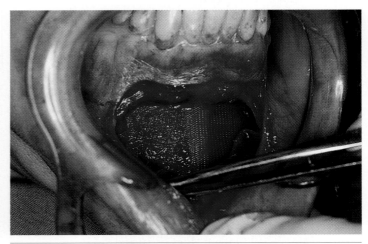

Fig. 2-14   Classical donor site for autogenous bone is the parasymphyseal area. Repair of the area is done with demineralized freeze-dried bone (DFDB) mixed with HA and covered with a resorbable Vicryl mesh membrane.

(Fig. 2-14). None but autogenous bone and possibly bone morphogenic protein (BMP) is osteogenic. Demineralized freeze-dried bone (DFDB) is said to be osteoinductive.

CERAMIC

Resorbable, tricalcium phosphate (TCP)
Nonresorbable: hydroxyapatite
Porous particulate and block forms
Nonporous particulate and block forms
Blocks are available as particles held together in resorbable collagen media, strung like beads with polyglycolic acid suture or supported in a matrix of calcium sulfate (plaster of Paris-Hapset).

POLYMERIC

Hard tissue replacement (HTR) particulate and porous block forms

BIOLOGIC

Autogenous bone
Irradiated bone
DFDB
Bovine (i.e., BioOss)
Membranes: Resorbable and nonresorbable

Suggested Readings

Abouzgia MB, James DF: Temperature rise during drilling through bone, *Int J Oral Maxillofac Implants* 12:342-353, 1997.

Albrektsson T et al: Osseointegrated oral implants: a Swedish multicenter study of 8,139 consecutively inserted Nobelpharma implants, *J Periodont* 59:287-296, 1988.

Babbush CA: *Dental implants: principles and practice,* Philadelphia, 1991, WB Saunders.

Babbush CA: ITI endosteal hollow cylinder implant systems, *Dent Clin North Am* 30:133-149, 1986.

Balkin BE: Implant dentistry: historical overview with current perspective, *J Dent Educ* 52:683-685, 1988.

Becker W et al: One-step surgical placement of Branemark implants: a prospective multicenter clinical study, *Int J Oral Maxillofac Implants* 12:454-462, 1997.

Casino AJ et al: Influence of type of incision on the success rate of implant integration at stage II uncovering surgery, *Int J Oral Maxillofac Surg* 55:31, 1997.

Cranin AN et al: Comparison of incisions made for the placement of dental implants, *J Dent Res* 70:279, 1991 (abstract 109).

Cranin AN et al: Evolution of dental implants in the twentieth century, *Alpha Omegan Scientific* 1:24-31, 1987.

Crossetti H et al: Experience with multiple endosseous implant systems in private practice, *Int J Oral Maxillofac Implants* 9(suppl):10, 1994.

David TS et al: A histologic comparison of the bone-implant interface utilizing the Integral and three surface variations of the Micro-Vent implant (in press).

Donovan TE, Chee WWL: ADA acceptance program for endosseous implants, *J Calif Dent Assoc* 20:60, 1992.

English CE: An overview of implant hardware, *J Am Dent Assoc* 121:360, 1990.

English CE: Cylindrical implants, *J Calif Dent Assoc* 16:17-20, 834-838, 1988.

Eriksson RA, Albrektsson T: Temperature threshold levels for heat-induced bone tissue injury, *J Prosthet Dent* 50:101-107, 1983.

Finger IM, Guerra LR: Integral implant-prosthodontic considerations, *Dent Clin North Am* 33:793-819, 1989.

Fonseca RJ, Davis W: *Reconstructive preprosthodontic oral and maxillofacial surgery,* Philadelphia, 1986, WB Saunders.

Friberg B, Grondahl K, Lekholm U: A new self-tapping Branemark implant: clinical and radiographic evaluation, *Int J Oral Maxillofac Implants* 7:80, 1992.

Hahn JA: The Steri-Oss implant system. In *Endosteal dental implants,* St Louis, 1991, Mosby.

Ismael JYH: A comparison of current root form implants: biomechanical design and prosthodontic applications, *NY State Dent J* 55:34, 1989.

Johansson C, Albrektsson T: Integration of screw implants in the rabbit: a 1 year follow-up of removal torque of titanium implants, *Int J Oral Maxillofac Surg* 2:69, 1987.

Kirsch A: The two-phase implantation method using IMZ intramobile cylinder implants, *J Oral Implant* 11:197-210, 1983.

Kirsch A, Ackerman KL: The IMZ osteointegrated implant system, *Dent Clin North Am* 33:733-791, 1989.

Kirsch A, Mentag P: The IMZ endosseous two phase implant system, *J Oral Implant* 12:494-498, 1986.

Kiyak HA et al: The psychological impact of osseointegrated dental implants, JOMI on CD-ROM, *Quintessence* 5(1):61-69, 1990.

Lambert P et al: Relationship between implant surgical experience and second-stage failures: DICRG interim report, No 2, *Implant Dent* 3:97, 1994.

Langer B, Langer L: The overlapped flap: a surgical modification for implant fixture installation, *Int J Periodont Rest Dent* 10:209, 1990.

Lekholm U, Jemt T: Principles for single tooth replacement. In Albrektsson T, Zarb GA (eds): The Branemark osseointegrated implants, *Quintessence* 117-126, 1989.

Linkow L: *Implant dentistry today: a multidisciplinary approach,* Piccin.

Lozada JL: Eight-year clinical evaluation of HA-coated implants: clinical performance of HA-coated titanium screws in type IV bone, *J Dent Symp* 1:67, 1993.

Malmquist JP, Sennerby L: Clinical report on the success of 47 consecutively placed Core-Vent implants followed from 3 months to 4 years, *Int J Oral Maxillofac Implants* 5:53, 1990.

McKinney R: *Endosteal dental implants,* St Louis, 1990, Mosby.

Misch CE: The Core-Vent implant system. In *Endosteal dental implants,* St Louis, 1991, Mosby.

Niznick G, Misch CE: The Core-Vent system of osseointegrated implants. In Clark JW (ed): *Clinical dentistry,* Philadelphia, 1987, Harper & Row.

Olive J, Aparicio C: The Periotest method as a measure of osseointegrated oral implant stability, *Int J Oral Maxillofac Implants* 5:390, 1990.

Ring ME: *Dentistry: an illustrated history,* St Louis, 1990, Mosby.

Rosenquist B: A comparison of various methods of soft tissue management following the immediate placement of implants into extraction sockets, *Int J Oral Maxillofac Implants* 12:43-51, 1997.

Rosenquist B: Immediate placement of implants into extraction sockets: implant survival, *Int J Oral Maxillofac Implants* 11:205-209, 1996.

Saadoun AP, LeGall ML: Clinical results and guidelines on Steri-Oss endosseous implants, *Int J Periodont Rest Dent* 12:487, 1992.

Sabiston DC (ed): *Textbook of surgery,* ed 14, Philadelphia, 1991, WB Saunders.

Scharf DR, Tarnow DP: The effect of crestal versus mucobuccal incisions on the success rate of implant osseointegration, *Int J Oral Maxillofac Implants* 8:187, 1993.

Spiekermann H, Jansen VK, Richter EJ: A 10-year follow-up study of IMZ and TPS implants in the edentulous mandible using bar-retained overdentures, *Int J Oral Maxillofac Implants* 10:231, 1995.

Stultz ER et al: A multicenter 5 year retrospective survival analysis of 6200 Integral implants, *Compend Contin Ed Dent* 14:478, 1993.

Sullivan D et al: The reverse torque test: a clinical report, *Int J Oral Maxillofac Implants* 11:179-185, 1996.

Symposium on Implants, *Dent Clin North Am* 24:399-592, 1980.

Valeron JF, Velasquez JF: Placement of screw-type implants in the pterygomaxillary-pyramidal region: surgical procedure and preliminary results, *Int J Oral Maxillofac Implants* 12:814-819, 1997.

Walker L et al: Periotest values of dental implants in the first 2 years after second-stage surgery: DICRG interim report, No 8, *Implant Dent* 6:207, 1997.

Weber SP: A mucobuccal fold extension for implant and other surgical procedures, *J Prosthet Dent* 27:423, 1972.

3

Evaluation and Selection of the Implant Patient

Patient Screening and Medical Evaluation for Implant and Preprosthetic Surgery

Manuel Chanavaz

mplant and preprosthetic surgeries aim to restore normal anatomic contours, function, comfort, esthetics and oral health. As such they are not lifesaving procedures. The prime concern must therefore be not to undermine the patient's overall health and safety. Take every step to select the appropriate treatment plan and maximize the longevity of the implanted system, including the overlying prostheses.

One important category into which a number of possible complications may fall is the inadequate systemic screening of patients before implant and biomaterial insertion. Without wishing to enter into the whole human pathology, it is no longer appropriate to limit the general contraindications of implantology to the traditionally considered malfunctions of the pancreas, liver, or hematopoietic system and to ignore the devastating long-term effects of smoking or inadequate dietary habits. There are, in fact, a number of systemic problems that may occur to create major risk factors. On the other hand, modern standards of care should not systematically exclude the use of implant surgery on patients with relative or marginal health conditions without exploring the possibilities of improving and stabilizing those conditions. As newer techniques of general anesthesia and intravenous sedation are more frequently used on an ambulatory basis, allowing implant surgeons to take their patients into various degrees of conscious or deep sedation, the patient screening should also take into consideration factors related to this form of management.

An arbitrary guideline for patient selection may be based on the classification of the American Society of Anesthesiology. This guideline restricts (with very few exceptions) intraosseous implants and implant-related graft surgeries to patients who fall into ASA1 or ASA2 categories of the classification.

In the domain of subperiosteal implants for treatment of advanced atrophy of the mandible, the body response seems to be much less dramatic than to endosseous devices. The cortical histoarchitecture and metabolism are, by far, less affected by organ disorders than the deeper endosseous structures.

This chapter presents a number of *absolute contraindications* and analyzes a series of *relative contraindications* for which the doctor's judgment remains the decisive factor. In this latter case, it proposes treatment patterns that could optimize certain marginal heath conditions or stabilize unbalanced biological functions before or at the time of surgery. As life expectancy in the industrial countries is continually increasing, a greater number of elderly patients are equipped with implant-supported prosthetics. The effort must therefore be focused on keeping a regular and watchful eye on their general health and screening for possible geriatric conditions responsible for long-term implant failure.

An optimal knowledge of internal medicine must be a prerequisite for the future academic implant education.

Introduction to Patient Screening and Medical Evaluation*

Technically speaking, contemporary implant surgery is a relatively innocuous procedure. It is also conceivable to recognize that a stable, well-integrated implant is as "clean" as a healthy tooth. However, whereas the management of complications in patients with minor systemic disorders is usually straightforward and successful, this may not be the case with patients

---

*Reprinted from the *Journal of Oral Implantology* 24:220-227, 1998.

who are systemically compromised. For example, the surgeon should not make a treatment plan for a heart valve patient without fully considering the gravity of potential immediate or delayed complications when unexpected problems arise. It is not only the implant that may become compromised.

Occasionally there are patients with marginal health conditions who are, in addition, "oral invalids" and urgently need comprehensive dental treatment. The natural inclination for many implantologists in such cases is to put the functional oral rehabilitation in the same priority list as the actual treatment of the critical health condition. They do not easily consider the deferral of the implant treatments. Until the patient's general health is stabilized, supply him or her with only provisional conventional prostheses not requiring surgery. When a proper state of health has been achieved, undertake definitive implant surgery.

Implant dentistry on the whole has made vast progress during the past 20 years. Every aspect of it, whether scientific or clinical, is taught in academic institutions around the world with an intensity equal to all other surgical disciplines. As the life expectancy in the industrial countries is continually increasing and greater numbers of elderly patients are supplied with implant-supported prostheses, one underutilized domain is the meticulous physical evaluation of patients before, at the time of, and after implant treatments. Most patient follow-ups are restricted to the local oral evaluation of the implanted sites. These evaluations seldom extend beyond 10 years. The long-term implant complications arising from ailing health are often neglected. A total of 25 years of clinical experience in implant and preprosthetic surgery has brought us into contact with a significant number of long-term complications (beyond 15 to 20 years) that were totally independent of the oral environment. That is why the effort must focus on keeping a regular and watchful eye on patients' general health and screening for possible geriatric systemic conditions that might be responsible for long-term implant failure.

An arbitrary but practical method of patient selection may be based on the American Society of Anesthesiology's classification (ASA). This classification defines the limits of risk factors on five categories of patients. Because both implant and preprosthetic procedures are elective surgeries aimed at restoring function and comfort of patients, restrict them to ASA1 (patients with no health problems) and ASA2 (patients with minor health problems who respond well to treatments). Any patient, whose health condition places him or her in Category ASA3 (major health problems with partial correction) or higher should be carefully screened for *Relative Contraindications* or possibly *Absolute Contraindications*.

Absolute Contraindications

Absolute contraindications relate to health conditions that have the potential to jeopardize the patient's overall health and safety and seriously compromise the survival of implanted systems causing residual chronic complications (Table 3-1). It is therefore essential that they be well comprehended and methodically sought when examining the patient.

1. *Recent myocardial infarction:* Contemporary cardiology including nonsurgical intervention procedures, has greatly improved the care and the treatment of patients suffering from myocardial infarction. This has led to a much reduced use of potent anticoagulants on a permanent basis, while the cardiovasoprotectors, beta-adrenergic blocking agents, hypotensive drugs and mild anticoagulants (aspirin) are extensively used. A stable condition for these patients is usually reached between 6 to 12 months after the primary care. However, it is important to avoid any surgical stress that could trigger uncontrolled vasoconstriction with possible tachyarrhythmia until the stable condition remains unchanged for at least 3 to 6 months. Furthermore, if anticoagulants are prescribed, their interruption in the early stages of the disease may prove extremely dangerous.

Table 3-1 Systemic Absolute Contraindications to Implant Surgery and Their Impact on Predictability

HEALTH CONDITION	RISKS FOR PATIENT'S GENERAL HEALTH	SEVERITY OF IMMEDIATE IMPLANT COMPLICATIONS	LONG-TERM PREDICTABILITY OF IMPLANT SYSTEM
1. Recent myocardial infarction	++++	+	++
2. Valvular prosthesis	++++	+	++
3. Severe renal disorder	++++	++++	0
4. Treatment-resistant diabetes	+++	++++	0
5. Generalized secondary osteoporosis	++	++++	+
6. Chronic or severe alcoholism	+++	++++	0
7. Treatment-resistant osteomalacia	+	+++	+
8. Radiotherapy in progress	+++	++++	0
9. Severe hormone deficiency	+++	++++	+
10. Drug addiction	++	++	+
11. Heavy smoking habits	++	++	+

The number of + relates to the degree of gravity of the complications associated with implant and graft surgery. One + is the least complicated (least predictable), and four ++++ is the most complicated (most predictable). Zero corresponds to total unpredictability.

2. *Valvular prosthesis:* The onset of bacteremia in patients fitted with valvular prostheses constitutes a major threat to the longevity of the cardiac valve. The oral cavity has traditionally been recognized as the principal gateway to such infections. It is therefore important not to plan any implant surgery until the patient's stable condition is reached, usually between 15 to 18 months after cardiac surgery. According to the type of valve used, the patients may be on permanent, potent anticoagulants (for mechanical valves) and mild plasma volume elevators (for porcine valves). Any planned procedure must take into consideration the occurrence of the surgical stress, anticoagulant imbalance, and infection risk, which may in extreme cases lead to acute malignant endocarditis and loss of the artificial valve.

3. *Severe renal disorder:* The severe renal disorder is probably the most important single contraindication to any form of implant or bone graft surgery. This can occur from a number of possible causes, of which the most common are recurrent kidney infections (nephritis), malignant or voluminous benign tumors (or multiple cystic kidneys), uncontrolled diabetes and/or complications arising from kidney stones. Most recently in Europe and other industrial countries, the reappearance of tuberculosis of the

kidneys has further expanded the list of potential complications. In all events, damage to the nephrons may cause bone destruction by urinary calcium loss and interruption in the production of the active metabolite of vitamin D. In fact, the lack of reabsorption of Ca^{++} together with the malfunction of parathyroid hormone (PTH) in the secondary loop of Henle could lead rapidly to metabolic osteopenia and retention of plasmatic endotoxins with major infection risks.

Figure 3-1 illustrates the daily calcium metabolism. The kidneys initially filter some 10g of calcium per day into the primary urine.

4. *Treatment-resistant diabetes:* This refers to confirmed, severe diabetes, which does not respond to proper treatment. The complications are related to the serum hyperosmolarity (sugar, urea, ions, etc.), metabolite disorders (Cl^-, Na^+, Mg^{++}, etc.), dehydration, and micro/macro angiopathia. The latter may in turn predispose the patient to tissue degeneration and compromised healing with increased risk of infection.

5. *Generalized secondary osteoporosis:* This is an anatomic and structural syndrome with significant loss of bone mass and volume leading to rarefaction of cancellous bone and

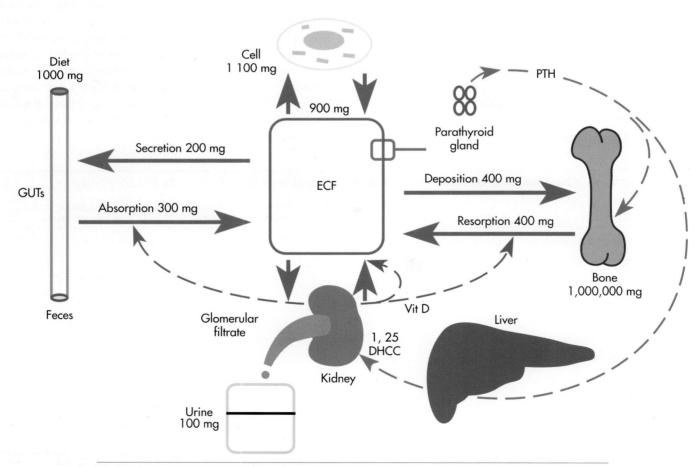

Fig. 3-1 The complex mechanisms governing calcium metabolism. *ECF,* extracellular fluid.

thinning of the cortical plates. Bone becomes devoid of osteoid, and presents osteoclasia and medullary fibrosis. It results in nonintegration of endosseous implants. One practical and useful screening tool to evaluate the extent of osteoporosis is bone densitometry (Dual Photon Absortiometry). Use it regularly on all patients who have clinical signs of bone fragility.

6. *Chronic or severe alcoholism:* This is a major condition leading frequently to liver disorder, cirrhosis and medullary aplasia with a cascade of possible complications such as platelet diseases, distress infarction, aneurysm and risk of insidious hemorrhage. Patients suffering from severe alcoholism often present retarded healing aggravated by malnutrition, psychologic disorder, inadequate hygiene, and major infection risk. The most common tests for hepatic disorders by the implant surgeon focus on measuring the following:
   - γ-Glutamyl-transpeptidase: (γ-GT) (<25 mU/ml), elevations in alcoholic cirrhoses to 50, hepatitis to 100, jaundice to 200 to 300, and pancreatic cancer to 1000.
   - Transaminases: *serum glutamo-oxalic transaminase* (SGOT) (5 to 35 IU) and *serum glutamopyruvic transaminase* (SGPT) (5 to 25 IU), which are increased in hepatic cytolysis, infectious and toxic hepatitis and prolonged salicylic treatment. In myocardial infarction, SGOT alone is increased.
   - Bilirubin: (total <10 IU or 6 mg ±2), which is increased in cases of hemolysis, cholestasis, and jaundice.
   - Alkaline phosphatases: with a pH 9.2 (13 to 39 IU or 0.22 to 0.65 m mol/s/l), which are increased in hyperparathyroidism, Paget's disease, hepatic disorders, and bone metastases.
   - KAPTTT *kephalin-activated partial thromboplastin time test* or prothrombin-activated kephalin test, which is a coagulation indicator. Vitamin K participates in coagulation with factors II, V, VII, IX, and X.

7. *Treatment-resistant osteomalacia:* Rickets is a rare disease in the industrial countries, seldom found in adults. This mineralization deficit (hypophosphocalcic bone with osteoidosis), which leads to demineralized osteopathy (soft bone), responds favorably, in more than 95% of the cases, to vitamin D therapy in conjunction with the intake of a calcium supplement. However, when the treatment fails, osteomalacia may lead to nonintegration of an implant and increased infection risk.

8. *Radiotherapy in progress:* Disruption of defense mechanisms, a compromised endosseous vascular system and inhibition of osteoinduction are the main insults to the body while radiotherapy is in progress. However the periosteum is the principal "organ" of which physiologic activities are virtually entirely disrupted. This may lead, depending on the proximity of the irradiated zone, to soft and hard tissue necrosis, major infection risk, and disruption of osteoconduction.

9. *Severe hormone deficiency:* This refers to patients with more than two different families of hormone disorders. The endocrine systems most affected that may be screened are thyroid and parathyroid, pancreas, adrenal, pituitary, and gonads.

10. *Drug addiction:* Most drug addicts suffer from the loss of sense of priorities, low resistance to disease, predisposition to infection, malnutrition, psychologic disorder, lack of hygiene, and difficulty with follow-up.

11. *Heavy smoking habits (more than 20 cigarettes per day):* This factor was added to the list of absolute contraindications in 1996 because of the occurrence of a number of long-term implant complications in heavy smokers who had no other systemic disorder. The main problems, other than early stage poor healing, arose from relatively accelerated bone loss (possibly due to altered vascularity) and disorders related to poor oral hygiene.

Relative Contraindications

These contraindications are related directly to the nature and severity of the systemic disorders and whether they can be satisfactorily corrected before surgery. They require a meticulous screening of the patient's medical records. In reality, patient selection in relation to relative contraindications is much more subtle, where among other criteria, the doctor's judgment remains the critical factor. For a dental practitioner who is not medically oriented, it may mean referral to other specialists. If the disorder is adequately corrected, carry out the treatment plan; otherwise, postpone the procedure until optimal conditions prevail. Table 3-2 shows the impact of implant and bone graft surgery on patients with relative contraindications. The number of + relates successively to the degree of the gravity of the complications, patients' responses to treatment, and predictability of the implanted system. One + is the least complicated or least favorable, and four + + + + is the most complicated or most predictable. Zero corresponds to total unpredictability. A question mark (?) represents variable and uncertain responses.

1. *AIDS and other seropositive diseases:* A seropositive (HIV-positive) patient may be considered normal, since current statistic life expectancy after primary infection is about 15 to 20 years. On the other hand, the implant indication for a confirmed AIDS patient is evaluated in accordance with the Atlanta CDC classification. The stage of development of the disease, life expectancy, and patient's wishes are very important considerations. A careful assessment of possible systemic complications arising from the disease may entirely contraindicate any form of surgery or may dictate a pragmatic treatment plan with more realistic objectives based on function, comfort, and relief.

2. *Prolonged use of corticosteroids:* This scenario is often associated with retarded healing, disorders of phosphocalcic metabolism (osteoporosis), and medullary aplasia. A number of authors have also reported bone fragility, renal and adrenal deficiency, metabolic disorders, including blood glucose metabolism, and water retention. Furthermore, the prolonged use of corticosteroids may inhibit bone formation. It is therefore important to determine why such

Table 3-2   Systemic Relative Contraindications to Implant Surgery and Their Impact on Predictability

HEALTH CONDITION	RISKS FOR PATIENT'S GENERAL HEALTH	LONG-TERM IMPLANT PREDICTABILITY IN ABSENCE OF PROPER DIAGNOSIS OR TREATMENT	PATIENT'S POSSIBLE RESPONSE TO MEDICAL TREATMENT BEFORE IMPLANT SURGERY	LONG-TERM IMPLANT PREDICTABILITY AFTER PROPER DIAGNOSIS AND TREATMENT
1. AIDS (1) and other seropositive diseases (2)	++++ (1) ++ (2)	0 ++	++ ++	0 +++
2. Prolonged use of corticosteroids	+++	++	++	+++
3. Disorders of P-Ca metabolism	+++	+	++	+++
4. Hematopoietic disorder	+++	++	++	++++
5. Buccopharyngeal tumors	+++	0	++	+++
6. Chemotherapy in progress	+++	0	++	+++
7. Mild renal disorder	+	0	++	+++
8. Hepatopancreatic disorder	+++	0	++	+++
9. Multiple endocrine disorder	+++	0	++	+++
10. Psychologic disorder, psychosis	+	+	++?	+++
11. Unhealthy life-style	++	+	+++	+++
12. Smoking habits	++	+	++?	+++
13. Lack of understanding and motivation	0	+	++	++
14. Unrealistic treatment plan	0	?	?	++

treatment is being administered and to evaluate the patient's response to it. If corticosteroids are used exclusively for their antiinflammatory properties, reversal of this contraindication may be as simple as changing the medication to one of the many newer nonsteroidal antiinflammatory drugs.

3. *Disorders of phosphocalcic metabolism:* An imbalanced diet (excessive protein, inadequate Ca^{++}, and/or vitamin D) may frequently lead to such disorders. However, minor hormone deficiencies, especially during menopause, in conjunction with systemic disorders and an unhealthy life-style may combine to bring about a phosphocalcic (P:Ca) imbalance. One typical example is a disorder of the gastrointestinal tract such as repeated colitis, chronic diarrhea, or Crohn's disease, which may be corrected or contained by carefully planned long-term treatment. In patients for whom such problems are not managed effectively, daily calcium and phosphorus absorption may be completely disrupted, leading to metabolic bone disease (phosphocalcic imbalance) and poor quality of mineralized bone.

4. *Hematopoietic disorder:* The possible complications arising from hematopoietic disorders in the short- and medium-terms are not as dramatic as those encountered in other forms of frank bone pathology and osteoporosis. However, satisfactory functioning of the hematopoietic system remains an essential factor for the long-term success of implant and reconstructive surgery. In a suspected bone marrow disorder, in addition to exploring the maturation cycle of the megakaryocytes, which are precursors of platelets, it is important to screen the transformation of the premonocyte lineage to macrophages, osteoclasts, and circulating monocytes. The same attention must be paid to the lymphocyte cycle.

5. *Buccopharyngeal tumors:* Analyze these tumors in regard to their malignancy or nonmalignancy, their proximity to the proposed implant site, and the oncologic treatment being carried out. Obviously if radiotherapy has been used very close to the planned surgical site, the contraindication becomes absolute. However, discourage routine rejection grafts or implants after resective surgery. If there is no obvious reason to suspect short- and medium-term metastases or extension of the tumor in a patient with otherwise satisfactory systemic screening, he or she may be offered improved oral health rather than the observation of an indefinite period of waiting until a possible recurrence of the tumor is excluded.

6. *Chemotherapy in progress:* The administration of anticancer drugs has rarely been a subject of study by implant and bone graft surgeons, who have frequently followed a restrictive general guideline with some ambiguity. In fact many of the drugs used in contemporary anticancer regimens have a very limited or unknown direct destructive role relative to implantology. For instance, methotrexate, a common chemotherapeutic agent, is extensively used (in smaller dosage) in contemporary rheumatology. However, it may produce severe thrombopenia and a disturbed osteogenic cycle when used in massive doses in oncology. The contraindication of chemotherapy is essentially related to the damage caused to the vital organs, which may also be involved in calcium metabolism. Furthermore, when chemotherapy is used for bone metastases, patient screening should preferably take into account the extension of the metastasis rather than the actual drugs used to contain it. One additional factor to analyze before implant surgery is the patient's degree of tolerance to the administered drugs. In any event, a close collaboration between the implant surgeon and the oncologist is mandatory.

Table 3-3   The Roles of Chemotherapeutics in Affecting Critical Metabolic Functions

TYPE OF ANTICANCER DRUG OR AGENT	DRUG FAMILY	COMMERCIAL BRAND	PRINCIPAL COMPLICATIONS, DISORDERS, OR AFFECTED ORGANS
1. Antimetabolic	•Antifolic	Methotrexate	Thrombopenia, osteogenesis
2. Alkylating	•Nitrogen-mustards (III)	Ifosfamide	Blood, bone (osteogenesis)
	•Nitrogen-urea (IV)	Streptozocin	Renal, hepatic, blood
	•Mitomycine	Ametycin	Renal, hepatic, blood
3. Spindle poisons	•Vinca alkaloids (III)	Vincristine	Renal, hepatic, blood
4. Interpolating	N/A	N/A	N/A
5. Splitting	•Bleomycin	Bleomycin	Pulmonary fibrosis
6. Cytolytic	•Plicamycin	Mithramycin	Renal, hepatic, blood, $(Ca)^{++}$
7. Steroids	•Progestates	Medroxyprogesterone Ethynodiol Norethisterone	Renal, hepatic
	•Estrogens	DES Fosfestrol	Breast, uterine malignancies
8. Interferons (Int-F)	•Int-F alfa-2a	Intron-A	Dehydration, thyroid, parathyroid
	•Int-F alfa-2b	Roferon-A	
9. Interleukin-2	•Aldesleukin-2	Proleukin	Cardio-nephro-hepato-myelo-toxic

Modern chemotherapy uses a wide range of drugs belonging to 10 to 12 pharmacologic families. The treatment for each patient may include a complex combination of these drugs. Table 3-3 shows the principal cancer treatments that may present absolute contraindications to implantology at the time of their administration or for up to a minimum of 6 months thereafter. Table 3-2 also shows a proportionately limited number of drugs that are incompatible with the simultaneous insertion of implant devices. The interpolating agents on the whole, seem to be devoid of adverse effects on implantology. The interferons and interleukins prescribed in advanced stages of pathology, however, are particularly contraindicated.

7. *Mild renal disorder:* These common disorders (uremia and creatinemia) are frequently revealed by an initial blood test after the first physical examination. However, such disorders may be predictors of the onset of major renal disorders or other systemic conditions, which will then become absolute contraindications to implant and preprosthetic surgery (absolute contraindications). It is therefore wise to investigate all renal problems and ascertain that they are no more than mild disorders, responding to treatment and not compromising calcium metabolism.

8. *Hepatopancreatic disorder:* Gall stones and infectious and viral hepatitis (except the severe B, C and E family) are among liver disorders that have very little destructive effect on the long-term success rate of implant surgery. Nevertheless, further hepatic tests, after a thorough physical examination, may reveal the onset of more serious liver or pancreatic conditions, which would be detrimental to the outcome of implant treatment.

9. *Multiple endocrine disorder:* This is a complex syndrome, ranging from metabolic loss of calcium (PTH) to secondary osteoporosis induced by hyperadrenocortism, or

glucocorticosteroid disorders (Cushing's syndrome, Addison's disease), mineralocorticosteroid syndrome (Conn's syndrome), or hyperandrogenism, any of which may lead to failure of the implanted material.

One arbitrary but practical method of screening a suspected hormone deficiency for an implant candidate may be the preoperative evaluation of the hormones involved in bone remodeling. These hormones can be classified into two categories according to their dependence levels on calcium homeostasis (Ca-H): *1-Ca-H dependent, 2-non-Ca-H dependent.*

Ca-H-dependent hormones are essentially: parathormone, which stimulates bone resorption (SBR), vitamin D or 1-25-dihydroxycholecalciferol (SBR) and calcitonin, which inhibits bone resorption (IBR).

Parathormone (PTH) is a monocatenary, hormonal polypeptide secreted by the parathyroid glands. It has four principal functions which are of interest to implant and bone graft surgeons:

• It is hypercalcemic (or less accurately referred to as *osteoporotic*) by removing the calcium ions from bone and transferring them to the circulating blood.
• It increases the urinary elimination of phosphates by reducing their tubular reabsorption.
• It contributes to maintaining an optimal calcemia by intervening in physiologic kidneys' tubular reabsorption of calcium.
• It plays an important role in the intestinal absorption of calcium in synergy with vitamin D.

Vitamin D_3 (1-25-dihydroxycholecalciferol) is renal metabolite intimately linked with PTH activity. Principal functions include active absorption of calcium in the proximal intestine, *in vitro* increases in the number and the activity of osteoclasts and the production of collagen, GLA bone proteins, and alkaline phosphatases, and direct action on PTH secretion, which however, has not been shown.

Calcitonin is a 32 amino-acid peptide synthesized by the C cells of the thyroid. Its principal functions are related to inhibiting bone resorption (antiosteoclastic and hypocalcemic).

Non-Ca-H-dependent hormones: thyroid hormones (SBR), estrogens (IBR and SBR), glucagon (IBR), insulin (stimulates bone formation [SBF]), growth hormones (SBF), and corticosteroids (inhibit bone formation [IBF]).

Thyroid hormones: Thyroglobulin (Iodoprotein)
>Iodothyronines
> Iodotyrosines
T_3: Triiodothyronin (70 to 190 ng/100 ml)
T_4: Thyroxine or tetraiodothyronin (4 to 12 μg/100 ml)
TSH: Thyroid-stimulating hormone (adenohypophysis hormone) (0.5 to 3.5μ U/ml)

Thyroid pathology and treatment: Table 3-4 shows the two possible origins of thyroid disorders and the standard treatment regimens before implant surgery.

10. *Psychologic disorders, psychoses:* This is one of the most difficult contraindications to evaluate and implement. It depends essentially on the severity of the disorder and the patient's response to psychotherapeutic medication. A number of the psychoactive drugs severely alter the oral environment and cause dryness of the mouth, mucosal irritation, or polyaphthosis. All of these conditions can potentially cause damage to peri-implant tissues. In all events, analyze these conditions in collaboration with the treating psychiatrist considering the patient's priorities, function, comfort, and esthetics. Make the patient aware of the decisions involved. Avoid implant surgery in psychotic patients who are not under strict surveillance and therapy.

11. *Unhealthy life-style:* Poor nutrition, chronic dieting, lack of exercise, inadequate hygiene, and excessive use of drugs, alcohol, and tobacco contribute to an unhealthy life-style. Irregular eating habits, repeatedly identical or unvaried menus, fast foods (imbalanced diet), and inadequate time allocated to consuming each meal are common problems in modern society. Chronic or "yo-yo" dieting, especially in the female population and in patients with anorexia or bulimia, may cause serious health and bone disorders. These contraindications are further aggravated by a lack of regular physical exercise. If the patient is amenable to correcting these habits, implant and preprosthetic surgeries are viable forms of therapy; otherwise a markedly unhealthy life-style becomes an absolute contraindication.

12. *Smoking habits:* Tobacco is one of the most severe limitations because it damages the angiogenic mechanisms for forming and maintaining bone, peri-implant and periodontal soft tissues. Depending on the daily consumption of cigarettes, the patient's awareness of the dangers of smoking and his or her willingness to drastically reduce or completely stop the habit, this particular contraindication

Table 3-4 Thyroid Pathology and Therapeutics

THYROID HORMONES AND DRUGS	NATURE OF DISORDER	ANTITHYROID DRUGS
a) Inferior origin (lower) Thyroid gland disorder		
T_3: Liothyronine		T_3: Propythiouracil Benzythiouracil-BASDENE
T_4: L-Thyroxine L-thyroxin Levothyrox	**Hyperthyroidism** **Hypothyroidism**	T_4: Carbimazol (Imidazole) Neo-Mercazole
b) Superior origin (upper) Adenohypophysis disorder		
TSH: Thyroid extracts		

may be reconsidered. If not, smoking remains an absolute contraindication for the long-term success of implant systems.

13. *Lack of understanding and motivation:* Patients who do not have a clear understanding of the implant techniques in spite of repeated explanations or who remain entirely passive to any form of motivation may constitute a category for whom extensive implant treatment should be avoided. On the other hand, if they respond positively to motivation, comprehend the explanation of the proposed treatment, understand the necessity of a close collaboration with the implantologist, and recognize the importance of regular follow-up sessions, they may become satisfactory candidates for implant surgery. Attempting to treat an ignorant, unmotivated patient is a disaster for all concerned.

14. *Unrealistic treatment plan:* This contraindication can be lifted if an in-depth analysis both from the clinical and economic standpoints is carried out. This analysis should consider whether there is a gross disproportion among the proposed treatment plan and the patient's chief complaint, cultural predisposition, life-style, social environment, and finances. The assessment of the physical and psychological status of a patient must be realistic in relationship to the proposed treatment.*

In all events, implant surgery will have to be considered as are all medical disciplines for which efforts must be focused on meticulous patient selection and on keeping a regular and watchful eye over patients' general health to treat possible geriatric conditions possibly responsible for long-term implant failure. The reader should now proceed to the next section, which presents additional specific information of great clinical value designed to complement the observations just made.

*This section appeared originally in the *Journal of Oral Implantology* 24: 222-229, 1998.

Indications and Contraindications for Treatment

Aram Sirakian
Marcia Cahn-Geller

If one is thorough in the evaluation of an implant patient, complications and the possibilities of failure are minimized. It is important to determine whether the patient can successfully undergo implant therapy or whether existing medical or psychologic conditions contraindicate treatment. The guidelines already introduced in this chapter offer an excellent overview. Specifically, the mechanics of evaluation employ the health history as the most important step (see Appendix A). This allows assessment of the patient's existing systemic conditions. Follow any positive responses with specific questions to elicit details of the past medical history.

Take vital signs as part of the routine screening process.

These establish a baseline for each candidate. Record pulse, blood pressure, respiration, and temperature. Verify and resolve any significant variations from normal.

Along with the health history, record vital signs, proper medical consultations, routine chemistries, blood counts, and urinalysis before surgery. Tables of normal values are found in Appendix B. These offer suggestions of the presence of some of the listed diseases. Note any discrepancies and make proper referrals for evaluation and treatment.

In-office blood sugar hematocrit, bleeding and clotting time examinations are of value.

Laboratory Tests-In Office

Hematocrit Examination

After preparation of a fingertip on the patient's nondominant hand, pierce the skin with a disposable stylet, blot the alcohol dry, squeeze the fingertip to obtain a fresh drop of blood, and lay the open end of a capillary tube alongside the drop. Draw the blood into the tube by capillary attraction, and after about 60% to 70% has been filled, remove it, swab the fingertip with alcohol, and use a dry sponge for tamponade. Plug each end of the tube with clay and place it into a slot in the microhematocrit centrifuge. Place a second tube across from it for balance, close the top, and rotate the tubes for 3 minutes. On retrieval of the tube, examination reveals that the cells have been spun to the bottom and the percentage of serum to cells may be determined by inserting the tube into a reader.

Blood Sugar Examination

To establish a reasonably accurate serum glucose level, obtain a second drop of blood from the same finger stick, and follow the instructions on the label of the bottle of reagent strips. Select a strip, cover the chemically treated end with blood and, after 60 seconds, wash it under cool running water for 60 seconds.

Compare the color of the strip at the blood site with a chart of standards that is printed on the bottle label, which reveals the result. Acetone levels should be given as well.

The practitioner should be sure to note at the time that these values are recorded if and when the patient had eaten, when insulin or other antihyperglycemic medication had been taken, and whether these are part of a regular regimen. This history plays an important role in assessing the levels of glucose and acetone.

Clotting Time

This test is performed easily with simple supplies. They include a finger-stick stylet, and 10-cm long, fine, glass capillary tubes.

After fingertip sterilization, pierce the skin, lay down the glass tube with one open end obliquely against the bleeding site. Capillary attraction will draw the blood into the tube. At 30-second intervals, break off a small length of tube and lay it aside. Do this until the blood strings out with a fibrinous thread. At that juncture, count the glass segments and divide by two. The result presents clotting time in minutes (normal 4 to 6 minutes) (Figs. 3-2, 3-3).

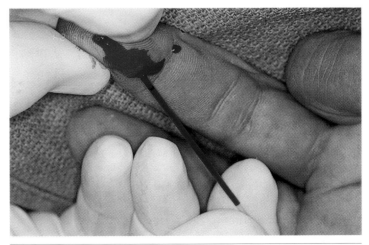

Fig. 3-2 A glass tube, when placed obliquely against the blood drop from a finger stick, fills by capillary attraction.

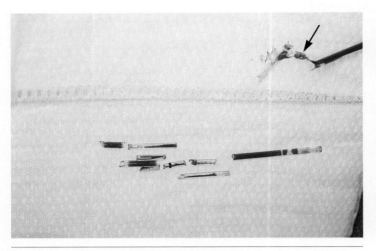

Fig. 3-3 Every 30 seconds a segment of capillary tube is broken until the blood threads out as a result of fibrin *(arrow)*. Counting the glass segments and dividing by two gives the clotting time in minutes.

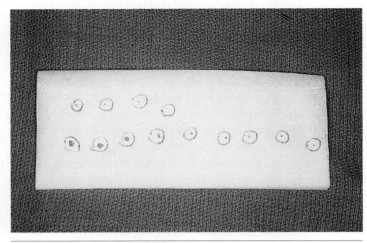

Fig. 3-4 Ascertain bleeding time using the same finger stick. Touch the bleeding spot to a clean piece of blotting paper until no blood stain appears, count the marks, and divide by two to give the bleeding time in minutes.

Bleeding Time

This test is performed simultaneously with clotting time and requires a clean piece of white filter paper. Use the same fingertip puncture for this simple evaluation. After each capillary tube segment is broken off (30-second intervals), touch the untreated fingertip (i.e., no gauze, no pressure, no alcohol) to the filter paper. After cessation of blood transfer marks, count the red dots and divide by two. The result is bleeding time in minutes (normal 5 to 8 minutes) (Fig. 3-4).

Absolute Systemic Contraindications

Some conditions should be considered as absolute contraindications for implant treatment. These include:

- Uncontrolled diabetes mellitus
- Long-term immunosuppressant drug therapy
- Diseases of connective tissue (e.g., disseminated lupus erythematosus)
- Blood dyscrasias and coagulopathies (e.g., leukemia, hemophilia)
- Regional malignancy (e.g., oral, perioral)
- Metastatic disease
- Previous radiation to the jaws that might lead to post-surgical osteoradionecrosis
- Alcohol or drug addiction
- Severe psychologic disorders

In addition, there are many relative contraindications to treatment. If these are managed properly, however, a patient may undergo implant surgery with very good chances for success. Consultations with a patient's physician may be required so that patient acceptability is clarified and the requisite details of surveillance and support therapy are instituted throughout and after the procedure. Some of the more important relative systemic contraindications are found in tabular form in the following sections.

Relative Systemic Contraindications

Abbreviations

ACE	= angiotensin-covering enzyme	LH	= luteinizing hormone
ACTH	= adrenocorticotropic hormone	MCHC	= mean corpuscular hemoglobin concentration
ANA	= antinuclear antibody	MCV	= mean corpuscular volume
BP	= blood pressure	PCP	= *pneumocystis carinii* pneumonia
BUN	= blood urea nitrogen	PT	= prothrombin time
CPK	= creatine phosphokinase	PTA	= plasma thromboplastin antecedent
CVA	= costovertebral angle	PTC	= plasma thromboplastin component
CXR	= chest x-ray	PTH	= parathormone
ECHO	= echocardiogram	PTT	= partial thromboplastin time
EKG	= electrocardiogram	RBC	= red blood cell
ESR	= erythrocyte sedimentation rate	RF	= rheumatoid factor
FSH	= follicle-stimulating hormone	SPEP	= serum protein electrophoresis
GH	= growth hormone	T_3	= triiodothyronine
Hgb	= hemoglobin	T_4	= thyroxine
LDH	= Lactic dehydrogenase	TIBC	= total iron binding capacity
LDL	= low density lipoprotein	TSH	= thyroid-stimulating hormone
LFT	= liver function tests	WBC	= white blood cell count

Endocrinopathies

At the clinical level, endocrinopathy can result from hormone deficiency, hormone excess, or resistance to hormone action.

Hormone Deficiencies

Diabetes mellitus, pituitary and adrenal insufficiency, hypothyroidism

HORMONE EXCESS

Overproduction by the usual site of its production (endocrine gland) thyrotoxicosis, acromegaly, Cushing's disease.

Hormone produced by a tissue (usually malignant) that ordinarily is not an endocrine organ (e.g., ACTH production in oat-cell carcinoma).

Overproduction of hormones in peripheral tissues from circulating prohormones.

Iatrogenic causes (e.g., overadministration of glucocorticoids).

HORMONE RESISTANCE

Universal feature: presence of a normal or elevated level of the hormone in the circulation in a patient with evidence of deficient hormone action; frequently secondary to hereditary causes (e.g., pseudohypoparathyroidism).

While evaluating the patient, certain symptoms either subjective or objective may become apparent. The following list presents them. If they are present, further in-depth investigation is warranted. Most of the pathoses included in this chapter do not constitute absolute contraindications to implant surgery.

DIABETES MELLITUS

Type I: Insulin Dependent

Clinical Findings	Laboratory Findings/Studies
Polyuria and thirst	Glucosuria
Weakness and fatigue	Ketonuria
Polyphagia and weight loss	High fasting glucose level,
Recurrent blurred vision	>140 ml/dl
Vulvovaginitis or pruritus	
Peripheral neuropathy	
Nocturnal enuresis	

Type II: Non-insulin Dependent (Adult Onset)

Clinical Findings	Laboratory Findings/Studies
Polyuria	Same as for type I
Weakness and fatigue	
Recurrent blurred vision	
Vulvovaginitis	
Peripheral neuropathy	
Often asymptomatic	

PITUITARY INSUFFICIENCY

Clinical Findings	Laboratory Findings/Studies
Weakness and fatigability	Fasting blood glucose may be low
Lack of resistance to stress, cold, and fasting	Marked insulin sensitivity (measured by insulin tolerance test)
Axillary and pubic hair loss	Mild anemia
Sexual dysfunction	
	Dilutional hyponatremia
	Decreased growth hormone
	Low T_4 (thyroid hormone)
	Thyroid-stimulating hormone
	Decreased ACTH
	Low plasma cortisol
	Decreased testosterone
	Decreased estradiol

ACUTE ADRENAL INSUFFICIENCY (WATERHOUSE FRIDERICHSEN SYNDROME)

Clinical Findings	*Laboratory Findings/Studies*
Headache	Eosinophilia
Lassitude	Decreased blood glucose and
Nausea and vomiting	sodium
Abdominal pain	Hypercalcemia
Diarrhea	Decreased blood and urinary cortisol
Fever >40.6° C (105° F)	Increased plasma ACTH if primary
Confusion or coma	adrenal disease (>200 pg/ml)
Dehydration	Positive blood cultures (usually
Hypotension	meningococci)
Cyanosis, petechiae	
Abnormal skin pigmentation	
with sparse axillary hair	
Lymphadenopathy	

CHRONIC ADRENAL INSUFFICIENCY (ADDISON'S DISEASE)

Clinical Findings	*Laboratory Findings/Studies*
Weakness and fatigability	Moderate neutropenia
Anorexia	(5000/ml)
Nausea and vomiting	Lymphocytosis
Diarrhea	Eosinophilia
Nervous and mental irritability	Hemoconcentration
Fainting, especially after	Increased BUN
missing meals	Increased K$^+$
Diffuse bronzing of the skin	Decreased fasting blood glucose
Pigmentation of mucous	Hypercalcemia
membrane and gingivae	Low AM cortisol accompanied by
Pigmentation around lips	simultaneous increase in ACTH
Vitiligo (7 to 15%)	
Hyperplasia of lymphoid tissue	
Scant to absent axillary	
and pubic hair	
Absense of sweating	
CVA tenderness	

HYPOTHYROIDISM

Clinical Findings	*Laboratory Findings/Studies*
Weakness and fatigue	T_4 <3.5 mg/dl
Cold intolerance	Free T_4 <0.8 ng/dl
Constipation	Radioiodine uptake decreased
Menorrhagia	T_3 resin uptake decreased
Hoarseness	TSH increased in first-degree
Thin brittle nails	hypothyroidism and decreased in
Dry, cold, yellow puffy skin	second degree (pituitary) hypothy-
Scant eyebrows	roidism
Enlargement of tongue (could	Anemia (macrocytic)
lead to malocclusion)	Antithyroid antibodies (increased
Bradycardia	in Hashimoto's thyroiditis)
Delayed return of deep	
tendon reflexes	

HYPERTHYROIDISM (THYROTOXICOSIS)

Clinical Findings	*Laboratory Findings/Studies*
Restlessness, nervousness,	T_4, radioiodine, and T_3 resin uptake
easy fatigability	Low TSH
Unexplained weight loss in	
spite of increased appetite	
Excessive sweating and heat	
intolerance	
Tremors	
Diarrhea	

Clinical Findings

Rapid irregular heartbeat
Wasting of muscle and bone
Alveolar atrophy and eruption
of permanent teeth is
greatly accelerated

ACROMEGALY (ADULT-ONSET HYPERPITUITARISM)

Clinical Findings	*Laboratory Findings/Studies*
Extreme growth of hands,	GH increased >7 ng/ml in active
feet and jaw	phase
Protrusion of mandible	Inorganic phosphate >4.5 mg/dl
Excessive sweating	Gonadotropins normal or low
Enlarged tongue, tipping of	Glucosuria and hyperglycemia
teeth to buccal or labial sides	Insulin resistance
Temporal headaches	T_4 normal or low
Photophobia and reduction	
in vision	

CUSHING'S SYNDROME (HYPERADRENAL CORTICAL SYNDROME)

Clinical Findings	*Laboratory Findings/Studies*
Moonface	Glucose tolerance low, often with
Buffalo hump	glucosuria
Obesity with protuberant	Insulin resistance
abdomen and thin extremities	Absence of diurnal variation of
Osteoporosis	cortisol
Oligomenorrhea or amenorrhea	Increased WBC or low eosinophils
Weakness	Lymphocytes under 20%
Headache	Increased RBC
Hypertension	
Mild acne	
Hirsutism	
Purple striae	
Bruises easily	

HYPOPARATHYROIDISM

Clinical Findings	*Laboratory Findings/Studies*
Muscular fatigue and weakness	Hypocalcemia
Numbness and tingling	Hyperphosphatemia
in extremities	Decreased PTH
Hypoplasia of teeth (when	
condition develops before	
tooth formation), chronic	
candidiasis	

HYPERPARATHYROIDISM

Clinical Findings	*Laboratory Findings/Studies*
Bone pain	Hypercalcemia
Joint stiffness	Hypophosphatemia
Pathologic fractures	Hyperparathormone
Urinary tract stones	Hypercalcuria
Giant cell tumor or cyst	Radiographic, general radiolucency
of the jaw	of affected bone, oval lobulated
Generalized osteoporosis	lesions in the jaws, a "ground glass"
Malocclusion	appearance

Granulomatous Diseases

TUBERCULOSIS

Clinical Findings	*Laboratory Findings/Studies*
Fatigue	*Mycobacterium tuberculosis* in sputum
Weight loss	culture

Clinical Findings	Laboratory Findings/Studies
Fever	Positive tuberculin skin test
Night sweats	Classic CXR
Cough	
Hemoptysis	

SARCOIDOSIS

Clinical Findings	Laboratory Findings/Studies
Fever	Elevated ESR
Malaise	Leukopenia
Dyspnea	Eosinophilia
Skin rash	Elevated ACE
Parotid gland enlargement	Hypercalcemia (10%), CXR
Hepatosplenomegaly	

Cardiovascular Diseases

ATHEROSCLEROSIS

Clinical Findings	Laboratory Findings/Studies
Intermittent claudication	Angiography
Weakness in legs	Elevated cholesterol and LDL
Distal pulses absent	
Atrophic skin changes	
Dependent rubor	

ARTERIOSCLEROSIS (ARTERIOSCLEROTIC CORONARY HEART DISEASE)

Clinical Findings	Laboratory Findings/Studies
Chest pain	ECG

HYPERTENSIVE VASCULAR DISEASE

Clinical Findings	Laboratory Findings/Studies
Elevated BP >140/90 mmHg,	Increased BUN
headaches	Increased creatinine
Lightheadedness	Proteinuria
Tinnitus	Granular casts in aldosteronism
Palpitation	Low serum K^+
Often asymptomatic	Increased Na^+ and HCO_3
presentation	ECG, stain pattern of ST segment
	CXR that shows aortic dilation or calcification

ORTHOSTATIC HYPOTENSION

Clinical Findings

Syncope
Dizziness
Lightheadedness on standing
Increased heart rate
Lowered BP on standing
Disease of the aorta (see also Endocarditis)

Peripheral Vascular Diseases

TEMPORAL ARTERITIS

Clinical Findings	Laboratory Findings/Studies
Headache	Increased ESR
Often associated with myalgia	
Malaise	
Anorexia	
Weight loss	
Loss of vision	
Tenderness of scalp	

THROMBOANGIITIS OBLITERANS (BUERGER'S DISEASE)

Clinical Findings	Laboratory Findings/Studies
Intense rubor of feet	No pathognomonic diagnostic studies
Superficial migratory thrombophlebitis	
Absent foot pulses	
Decreased ulnar or radial pulse	

ARTERIOVENOUS FISTULAE

Clinical Findings	Laboratory Findings/Studies
Headaches	CT scan, electroencephalogram,
Hemorrhage	arteriography to localize site of lesion
Seizures	
Auscultative bruit	

CONGESTIVE HEART FAILURE

Clinical Findings	Laboratory Findings/Studies
Dyspnea	Diagnostic tests
Orthopnea	Chest x-ray
Dry, hacking cough	Electrocardiogram
Paroxysmal nocturnal dyspnea	Echocardiogram
Chest pain	Radionucleotide angiography "gated blood pool scan"
Nocturia	
Increased heart size	Cardiac catheterization and myocardial biopsy
Sinus tachycardia	
Ventricular gallop	Stress testing
Rales	Systolic versus diastolic dysfunction
Neck vein distention	
Peripheral pitting edema	

ENDOCARDITIS/VALVULAR DISEASE (REQUIRES ANTIBIOTIC PROPHYLAXIS)

MITRAL STENOSIS

Clinical Findings	Laboratory Findings/Studies
Orthopnea	ECHO, shows thickened valve that
Dyspnea	opens and closes slowly
Paroxysmal nocturnal dyspnea	
Pulmonary edema hemoptysis	
Middiastolic murmur	

MITRAL REGURGITATION (INSUFFICIENCY)

Clinical Findings	Laboratory Findings/Studies
Pansystolic murmur	Enlargement of left atrium on CXR
Orthopnea	ECHO
Exertional dyspnea	Cardiac catheterization to assess left
Paroxysmal nocturnal dyspnea	ventricular function and pulmonary
Right heart failure	artery pressure

MITRAL VALVE PROLAPSE

Clinical Findings	Laboratory Findings/Studies
Mostly asymptomatic presentation	ECHO
Chest pain	
Fatigue	
Palpitation	
Late systolic murmur	
Midsystolic click	

AORTIC INSUFFICIENCY

Clinical Findings

Soft diastolic murmur
Exertional dyspnea
Chest pain
Heart failure

Laboratory Findings/Studies

ECHO shows diastolic flattening of
  anterior mitral valve leaflet or
  septum produced by regurgitant jet

TRICUSPID STENOSIS

Clinical Findings

Right heart failure
Hepatomegaly
Ascites
Dependent edema
Cyanosis
Jaundice
Diastolic rumble
Liver pulsation

Laboratory Findings/Studies

ECHO demonstrates the lesion
Right heart catheterization
  is diagnostic

TRICUSPID INSUFFICIENCY

Clinical Findings

Harsh systolic murmur along
  left sternal border
Regurgitant systolic V waves
Presence of an inspiratory S_3

Laboratory Findings/Studies

ECHO

Hypersensitivity Reactions

ATOPIC DISEASES (HAY FEVER, ATOPIC DERMATITIS, ALLERGIC ASTHMA, ALLERGIC ECZEMA, ANAPHYLACTIC REACTION)

Clinical Findings

Eczema; itching rash on face,
  trunk, extremities
History of asthma
Atopic spontaneous allergy

Laboratory Findings/Studies

Delayed blanch reaction to
  methacholine, eosinophilia
Positive skin test to multiple antigens, increased IgE binding to
  Staphylococcus aureus

ANAPHYLAXIS

Clinical Findings

Apprehension
Paresthesia
Generalized urticaria
Edema
Choking
Cyanosis
Wheezing
Incontinence
Shock
Fever
Dilation of pupils
Loss of consciousness
Convulsions

Laboratory Findings/Studies

URTICARIA

Clinical Findings

Wheals
Hives
Itching
Swelling

Laboratory Findings/Studies

Skin testing
Eosinophilia

ANGIONEUROTIC EDEMA

Clinical Findings

Edema commonly of the lips
  or another part of the face

Laboratory Findings/Studies

Drug Hypersensitivity

Clinical Findings

Rash
Fever
Wheezing
Cough
Cyanosis
Abdominal pain
Loss of consciousness
Convulsions

Eosinophilia
Increased ESR

DERMATOMUCOSITIDES

PEMPHIGUS VULGARIS

Clinical Findings

Relapsing crops of bullae
Superficial detachment of
  skin after pressure
  (Nikolsky's sign)
Tender oral lesions

Laboratory Findings/Studies

Tzanck test shows acantholysis
  on biopsy
Increased ESR, anemia
Eosinophilia
Leukocytosis

BULLOUS EROSIVE LICHEN PLANUS

Clinical Findings

Pruritic papules
Koebner's phenomenon
Erosive papules
Predilection for flexor surfaces
  and trunk and in the oral cavity

Laboratory Findings/Studies

Histopathology

METABOLIC/OTHER DISEASES OF BONE
HISTIOCYTOSIS X (LANGERHAN'S CELL GRANULOMATOSIS)
HAND-SCHÜLLER-CHRISTIAN DISEASE (MULTIFOCAL EOSINOPHILIC GRANULOMA)

Clinical Findings

Single or multiple areas of
  "punched-out bone"
Bone destruction in skull
Unilateral or bilateral
  exophthalmos
Diabetes insipidus in young adults
Tissue tenderness and swelling,
  facial asymmetry
Otitis media
Nodular lesions of skin
Sore mouth, gingivitis
Loose teeth
Failure of healing following
  extractions
Loss of alveolar bone

Laboratory Findings/Studies

Anemia
Leukopenia
Thrombocytopenia
Histologic confirmation

EOSINOPHILIC GRANULOMA

Clinical Findings

Local pain and swelling, skull
  and mandible common sites
General malaise and fever

Laboratory Findings/Studies

Radiographic, irregular radiolucencies of jaws and other bones
Pancytopenia, histologic confirmation

ORGANOMEGALY
LETTERER-SIWE DISEASE (CHILDREN AND TEENAGERS)

Clinical Findings	*Laboratory Findings/Studies*
Skin rash involving trunk, scalp, and extremities	Progressive anemia
Low-grade, spiking fever with malaise and irritability (in infants)	Leukopenia Thrombocytopenia
Splenomegaly, hepatomegaly	
Lymphadenopathy	
Oral ulcerative lesions	
Gingival hypertrophy	
Diffuse destruction of bone in jaw	
Premature eruption of teeth ectopically placed	

PAGET DISEASE (OSTEITIS DEFORMANS)

Clinical Findings	*Laboratory Findings/Studies*
Bone pain	Radiographic, initial deossification followed by osteoblastic phase giving a "cotton wool" appearance
Headaches	
Skeletal deformity	
Deformities of spine, femur, and tibia	Increased serum alkaline phosphatase
Progressive enlargement of skull, spacing of teeth, pathologic fractures	Increased urinary hydroxyproline Normal calcium and phosphorus

POLYOSTOTIC FIBROUS DYSPLASIA (ALBRIGHT'S DISEASE)

Clinical Findings	*Laboratory Findings/Studies*
Painless swelling of bone	Calcium and phosphorus normal
Bones lesions and cysts	Alkaline phosphatase and urinary hydroxyproline increased
Traumatic fractures	
Café au lait spots on skin usually directly over bone lesions	Radiograph reveals rarefaction and expansion of bones with multi-locular cystic appearance
Precocious puberty	
Hypogonadism	
Hyperthyroidism	
Enlarged jaw	

Blood Dyscrasias and Hematologic Disorders
MEGALOBLASTIC ANEMIA

Clinical Findings	*Laboratory Findings/Studies*
Anorexia	Increased MCV (large red cells)
Fatigue	Megaloblasts
Diarrhea	
Paresthesias in peripheral nerves	
Decreased vibration and position senses	
Glossitis	
Deficiency state of folate and vitamin B_{12}	

ALLERGIC PURPURA (HENOCH-SCHÖNLEIN DISEASE)

Clinical Findings	*Laboratory Findings/Studies*
Purpuric rash on extensor surfaces of arms, legs, buttocks	Increased anemia
	Increased ESR
Colicky abdominal pain	Increased alpha-globulin and fibrinogen
Polyarthralgia	Normal muscle enzyme levels

Clinical Findings	*Laboratory Findings/Studies*
Polyarthritis	X-rays shows narrowing of joint spaces
Hematuria	Osteophyte formation
	Bone cysts
	Increased density of subchondral bone

HEREDITARY HEMORRHAGIC TELANGIECTASIA (OSLER-WEBER-RENDU SYNDROME)

Clinical Findings	*Laboratory Findings/Studies*
Epistaxis	Anemia
Murmur of arteriovenous malformation over lung fields	
Multiple telangiectasia (readily seen on skin and in mouth) (may also be internal)	

IDIOPATHIC THROMBOCYTOPENIC PURPURA

Clinical Findings	*Laboratory Findings/Studies*
Purpura	Decreased platelet count
Mucosal, gingival, and skin bleeding	Increased normal morphology bleeding time
Epistaxis	Some large platelets
Menorrhagia	Mild anemia
Petechiae	Positive tourniquet (Rumple-Leeds test (>3 petechiae in a 2.5-cm circle below inflated BP cuff-systolic after 1 minute)

SECONDARY TO HYPERSPLENISM

Clinical Findings	*Laboratory Findings/Studies*
Purpura	Decreased platelet count
Enlarged spleen	

Hereditary Coagulation Disorders
HEMOPHILIAS (FACTOR VIII DEFICIENCY)

Clinical Findings	*Laboratory Findings/Studies*
Bleeding into joints, muscles and gastrointestinal tract	Anemia
	Normal PT
Fever	Increased PTT
Anemia	Low Factor VIII
Massive gingival hemorrhage	Normal Factor VIII antigenic activity
Only males affects	Normal von Willebrand factor

VON WILLEBRAND'S DISEASE (PSEUDOHEMOPHILIA)

Clinical Findings	*Laboratory Findings/Studies*
Epistaxis	Prolonged bleeding time
Bruises easily	Low Factor VIII coagulation activity
Menorrhagia	Defective in vitro platelet aggregation in response to ristocetin
Gingival bleeding	
Troublesome bleeding after a mild laceration or dental extraction	Platelet number and morphology normal
Either sex may be affected	Low Factor VIII antigenic activity

Factor Deficiencies

Factor IX, Christmas Factor (PTC deficient)

Clinical Findings	Laboratory Findings/Studies
Bleeding	Low Factor IX
	Increased PTT

Factor X, Stuart Factor

Clinical Findings	Laboratory Findings/Studies
Bleeding	Abnormal PT and PTT
	Low Factor X

Factor XII (PTA deficient)

Clinical Findings	Laboratory Findings/Studies
Bleeding	Increased PTT
	Low Factor XII

Acquired Coagulation Disorders

Deficiency of the Vitamin K-Dependent Coagulation Factors

Clinical Findings	Laboratory Findings/Studies
Bleeding	Increased PT, corrected by giving vitamin K (Hykinone)
	Normal fibrinogen, prothrombin time, and platelet count

Disseminated intravascular coagulopathy (DIC)

Clinical Findings	Laboratory Findings/Studies
Bleeding (especially if from multiple sites) (frequently posttraumatic)	Decrease in plasma fibrinogen
Purpura	
Ecchymoses	Increased fibrin degradation products
Digital ischemia and gangrene	Increased PT
	Increased PTT
	Thrombocytopenia
	Depleted antithrombin III levels
	Decreased hematocrit

Granulocytopenia

Clinical Findings	Laboratory Findings/Studies
Opportunistic infections	Decreased WBCs

Cyclical neutropenia

Clinical Findings	Laboratory Findings/Studies
Fever	Cylical fluctuations of WBCs, platelets, and RBCs
Malaise	
Mouth ulcers	(Have patient keep diary of oral lesions and attempt to match
Cervical adenopathy	them with laboratory findings.)

Lymphocytopenia

Clinical Findings	Laboratory Findings/Studies
Recurrent viral infections	Decreased lymphocytes

Leukemias

Acute myeloid leukemia

Clinical Findings	Laboratory Findings/Studies
High fever	Anemia
Bleeding	Thrombocytopenia
Severe prostration	Neutropenia
Infection	Increased LDH
Gingival hypertrophy	Hyperuricemia
Bone and joint pain	Hypokalemia
Enlargement of liver, spleen, and lymph nodes	Auer red inclusions

Chronic Myeloid Leukemia

Clinical Findings	Laboratory Findings/Studies
Palpable splenomegaly	Presence of Philadelphia chromosome
Anemia	
Weight loss	Platelets normal or elevated
Night sweats	Hypercellular bone marrow with left-shifted myelopoiesis
Fever	
Severe bleeding	Decreased leukocyte alkaline phosphatase
Infection during blast crisis	

Acute Lymphocytic Leukemia

Clinical Findings	Laboratory Findings/Studies
Fatigue	Pancytopenia
Bleeding	Positive surface markers of primitive lymphoid cells
Infection	Positive terminal deoxynucleotide transferase in 95%, positive rosette formation with sheep erythrocytes
Enlargement of liver, spleen, and lymph nodes	Identification of cell markers by monoclonal antibodies in T cell leukemias

Chronic Lymphocytic Leukemia

Clinical Findings	Laboratory Findings/Studies
Fatigue	Lymphocytosis
Lymphadenopathy	WBC >20,000/ul
Enlargement of liver and spleen	Bone marrow infiltration with small lymphocytes
	Hypogammaglobulinemia

Lymphomas

Hodgkin's Disease

Clinical Findings	Laboratory Findings/Studies
Painless, enlarged mass in neck, axilla, or groin	Increased ESR
Fever	Thrombocytosis
Night sweats	Leukocytosis
Fatigue	Decreased iron and iron-binding capacity
Weight loss	Increased leukocyte alkaline phosphatase
Generalized pruritus	

Non-Hodgkin's Disease (lymphosarcoma, reticulum cell sarcoma)

Clinical Findings	Laboratory Findings/Studies
Painless adenopathy in lymph nodes or extranodal sites	Peripheral blood usually normal
Night sweats	Bone marrow with paratrabecular lymphoid aggregates
Weight loss	CXR, mediastinal mass

BURKITT'S LYMPHOMA

Clinical Findings	*Laboratory Findings/Studies*
Extralymphatic tumor in bones of jaws	Presence of Epstein-Barr virus
Abdominal viscera	
Ovaries, meninges, breasts	

PLASMA CELL DYSCRASIA AND MULTIPLE MYELOMA

Clinical Findings	*Laboratory Findings/Studies*
Frequent or recurrent infections, especially pneumonias	Increased ERS
	Anemia
Chronic renal dysfunction	Rouleau formation on blood smear
Painful fractures and bony lesions	Increased uric acid
	Hypercalcemia
Back pain	Bence-Jones protein in urine
	Finding of paraprotein on SPEP (monoclonal spike in beta- or gamma-globulin region)
	Radiographic: lytic lesions or generalized osteoporosis

COLLAGEN (CONNECTIVE TISSUE) DISEASES

RHEUMATOID ARTHRITIS (SEVERE)

Clinical Findings	*Laboratory Findings/Studies*
Fatigue	Rheumatoid factor
Joint stiffness	Increased ESR
Myalgia	Anemia
Symmetrical joint swelling, proximal interphalangeal and metacarpophalangeal joints of fingers as well as wrists, knees, ankles, and toes	Radiographic soft tissue swelling, osteoporosis, erosion of peripheral bare space of bone surface not covered by cartilage, joint space narrowing
Subcutaneous nodules over bony prominences	

SJÖGREN'S SYNDROME

Clinical Findings	*Laboratory Findings/Studies*
Keratoconjunctivitis	Mild anemia
Xerostomia	Hypergammaglobulinemia
Xerophthalmia	Special antibody from salivary duct
Chronic arthritis	Positive RF in 70%
Parotid enlargement	Eosinophilia
Severe dental caries	Leukopenia
Dysphagia	Schirmer's test to measure volume of tears and saliva secreted
Pancreatitis	
Pleuritis	
Vasculitis	

SYSTEMIC LUPUS ERYTHEMATOSUS

Clinical Findings	*Laboratory Findings/Studies*
Arthritis	Positive lupus erythematosus cells
Myalgia	ANA positive
Butterfly rash (nose)	Increased ESR
Nephritis	Anemia
Fever	Leukopenia
Weight loss	Thrombocytopenia
Raynaud's phenomenon	Decreased serum complement
Splinter hemorrhage	Mildly abnormal LFTs
Nail-fold infarcts	

SCLERODERMA (PROGRESSIVE SYSTEMIC SCLEROSIS)

Clinical Findings	*Laboratory Findings/Studies*
Diffuse thickening of skin	Anemia
Subcutaneous edema	Increased ESR
Telangiectasia	ANA positive
Polyarthralgia	RF and lupus erythematosus cells
Raynaud's phenomenon	Anticentromere
Dysphagia	Scleroderma antibody (SCL-70) positive in 35% of patients
Hypomotility of gastro-intestinal tract	
Pigmentation, depigmentation	
Limited oral opening	

POLYMYOSITIS

Clinical Findings	*Laboratory Findings/Studies*
Bilateral proximal muscle weakness	Increased CPK
Papules over knuckles	On electromyography, polyphasic potentials
Periorbital edema	Fibrillation and high frequency action potentials
Raynaud's phenomenon	

DERMATOMYOSITIS

Clinical Findings	*Laboratory Findings/Studies*
Polymyositis symptoms: skin rash	Increased CPK

VASCULITIS
POLYARTERITIS NODOSUM

Clinical Findings	*Laboratory Findings/Studies*
Fever	Leukocytosis
Chills	Anemia
Tachycardia	Proteinuria
Arthralgia and myositis with muscle reticularis	Cylinduria
Hypertension	Hematuria
Abdominal pain	ESR
Mononeuritis multiplex	RF
	ANA
	Serum complement normal or increased

Immunodeficiency Diseases
ACQUIRED IMMUNODEFICIENCY SYNDROME (AIDS)

Clinical Findings	*Laboratory Findings/Studies*
Fever	Decreased in T4
Weight loss	Increased in T8
Lymphadenopathy	Leukopenia
Diarrhea	
Frequent infections	
Oral candidiasis	

SEVERE COMBINED IMMUNODEFICIENCY DISEASE

Clinical Findings	*Laboratory Findings/Studies*
Increased susceptibility to infections at 3 to 6 months	Immunoglobulin G <1%, lymphocytes <2000/ml
Diarrhea from *Salmonella* or *Escherichia coli*	Decreased delayed hypersensitivity reaction
Pneumonia with PCP and *Pseudomonas*	
Candidiasis in oral cavity	

Local and Regional Problems

Besides these systemic conditions, certain local problems also exist that will need to be evaluated before undertaking implant treatment. These include the following:

Root tips
Cysts
Infections
Neoplasms
Fibro-osseous disease

Once it has been ascertained that the patient does not present a medical or psychologic risk or that the risks can be adequately controlled, a specific oral reconstructive approach may be initiated.

Dr. Manuel Chanavaz is professor and chairman of the department of Oral and Maxillofacial Implants at the Lille University School of Medicine in Lille, France.

Dr. Aram Sirakian was a Fellow in Biomaterials and Dental Implants at the Brookdale Hospital Medical Center and is now in the private practice of dental implantology in Boston, Massachusetts.

Ms. Marcia Cahn-Geller is a Certified Physicians Assistant and a student of metabolic diseases.

Suggested Readings

Bain CA, Moy PK: The association between the failure of dental implants and cigarette smoking, *Int J Oral Maxillofac Implant* 8:609, 1993.

Boot AM et al: Bone mineral density and bone metabolism of prepubertal children with asthma after long-term treatment with inhaled corticosteroids, *Pediatr Pulmonol* 24(6):379-384, 1997.

Bot ta Fridlund D: Acute diarrhea, *La Rev du Praticien* 113-120, Jan 1995.

Braunwald et al: *Harrison's principles of internal medicine,* ed 11, New York, 1987, McGraw-Hill.

Chomienne C, Da Silva N: Hematopoietic growth factors, receptors, intracellular signals, *Pathologie Science* 15-28, 1996.

Civitelli R et al: Bone turnover in post menopausal osteoporosis: effect of calcitonin treatment, *J Clin Invest* 82:1268-1274, 1988.

Cline JL et al: Effect of increasing dietary vitamin A on bone density in adult dogs, *Anim Sci.* 75(11): 2980-2985, 1997.

Consensus Development Conference: Diagnosis, prophylaxis and treatment of osteoporosis, *Am J Med* 94:646-650, 1993.

Coquard R: Late effects of ionizing radiations on the bone marrow, *Cancer Radiother* 1(6):792-800, 1997.

Cranin AN: Endosteal implants in a patient with corticosteroid dependence, *J Oral Implantol* 17:414-417, 1991.

Cranin AN: Physical evaluation of the surgical implant patient, *Oral Implantol,* Springfield, Ill., 1970, Charles C. Thomas.

Crowley S et al: Collagen metabolism and growth in prepubertal children with asthma treated with inhaled steroids, *J Pediatr* 132 (3 Pt 1):409-413, 1998.

Desombere I, Willems A, Leroux-Roels G: Response to hepatitis B vaccine: multiple HLA genes are involved, *Tissue Antigens* 51(6):593-604, 1998.

Dombret H: Intensive chemotherapy in myelodysplastic syndromes, *Pathol Biol* (Paris) 45(8):627-635, 1997.

Foa P et al: Long-term therapeutic efficacy and toxicity of recombinant interferon-alpha 2a in polycythaemia vera, *Eur J Haematol* 60(5):273-277, 1998.

Gagnon L et al: Influence of inhaled corticosteroids and dietary intake on bone density and metabolism in patients with moderate to severe asthma, *J Am Diet Assoc* 97(12):1401-1406, 1997.

Harris ST et al: Four-year study of intermittent cyclic etiodronate treatment of postmenoposal osteoporosis: three years of blinded therapy followed by one year of open therapy, *Am J Med* 95:557-567, 1993.

Hellstrom-Lindberg E et al: Treatment of anemia in myelodysplastic syndromes with granulocyte colony-stimulating factor plus erythropoietin: results from a randomized phase II study and long-term follow-up of 71 patients, *Blood* 1:92(1): 68-75, 1998.

Juturi JV, Hopkins T, Farhangi M: Severe leukocytosis with neutrophilia (leukemoid reaction) in alcoholic steatohepatitis, *Am J Gastroenterol* 93(6):1013, 1998.

Krouse DS et al: CD34 : structure, biology, and clinical utility, *Blood* 87: 1-13, 1996.

Leroy J et al: H'mostase et thrombose, *La Simarre* 1-179, 1988.

Marolleau JP: L'hématopoéise, *Pathologie Science JL* 1-13, 1996.

Matson MA, Cohen EP: Acquired cystic kidney disease: occurrence, prevalence, and renal cancers, *Medicine* (Baltimore) 69(4): 217-226, 1990.

Meunier PJ: Les osteoporeuses, *La Rev du Praticien* 1059-1135, May 1995.

Mini Book 3: *Endocrinologie-métabolisme-nutrition,* pp 9-76, 1991.

Nguyen QH et al: Interleukin (IL)-15 enhances antibody-dependent cellular cytotoxicity and natural killer activity in neonatal cells, *Cell Immunol* 185(2):83-92, 1998.

Pasanen M et al: Hepatitis A impairs the function of human hepatic CYP2A6 in vivo, *Toxicology* 5(3):177-184, 1997.

Pouillés JM: Apport de l'ostéodensitometrie á la définition et au diagnostic des ostéoporoses, *La Revue du Praticien* 1096-1101, 1995.

Richardson ML: Bone marrow abnormalities revealed by MR imaging, AJR, *Am J Roentgenol* 171(1):261-262, 1998.

Saitz R: Patients with alcohol problems, *N Engl J Med* 19:339(2): 130-131, 1997.

Sanchez-Perez J et al: Lichen planus and hepatitis C virus infection: a clinical and virologic study, *Acta Derm Venereol* 78(4):305-306, 1998.

Spikkelman A, de Wolf JT, Vellenga E: The application of hematopoietic growth factor in drug induced agranulocytosis. a review of 70 cases, *Leukemia* 8:2031,

Vallespi T et al: Diagnosis, classification, and cytogenetics of myelodysplastic syndromes, *Haematologica* 83(3):258-275, 1998.

WHO Study Group: Assessment of fracture risk and its application to screening for postmenopausal osteoporosis. In Who Technical Report Series 843, Geneva World Health Organization, pp 1-129, 1994.

Woodcock A: Effects of inhaled corticosteroids on bone density and metabolism, *J Allergy Clin Immunol* 101:4(2):S456-S459, 1998.

4

How to Choose the Proper Implant

Diagnostic Methods

Examination

*O*nce *a decision* has been made to perform implant therapy and the patient has been found to be physically and medically acceptable, complete a thorough diagnostic evaluation and treatment plan to choose the proper approach. A visual examination should be the first step. View the edentulous areas and conceptualize the height, width, and length of the proposed operative sites. Also, note the amount of attached and/or keratinized gingivae. In addition, note the level of the lip line and exposed gingivae along with any muscle attachments. If natural teeth remain, they should be free of decay, and the periodontal tissues should be healthy. Neither infections nor localized areas of pathologic change can be permitted.

The next step in the diagnostic sequence is manual palpation. With thumb and index finger, palpate the edentulous ridges (Fig. 4-1). Assess the firmness and thickness of the soft tissues. A determination of the uniformity of thickness over the entire height and length of the underlying bone is important. Concavities and convexities may exist that might not be evident on visual or digital examination. To clarify and define the presence and extent of such irregularities, prepare to sound the bone (or delineate the shape by closed examination). Use a 30-gauge needle to deposit a small amount of local anesthetic along the labial and lingual aspects of the edentulous areas that are being considered as potential implant sites. Then, use a sharpened periodontal probe to make soft tissue thickness measurements. These and all other calibrations should be recorded on a diagnostic chart. Next, use a sterilized Boley gauge with sharpened beaks to puncture the soft tissues by squeezing the calipers directly through tissue to bone (Figs. 4-2, 4-3). The beaks should oppose one another so that an accurate reading will result. This presents a measurement of bone width at varying ridge sites. By doing this repeatedly from superior to inferior and from medial to distal at 5-mm intervals, the clinician develops a topographic map of the soft and hard tissue dimensions of the areas into which implant placement is intended. Record these measurements on the chart. When these measurements are used, an accurate three-dimensional representation of the operative site can be sketched (Fig. 4-4).

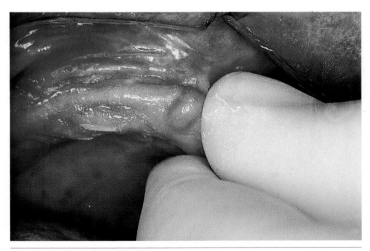

Fig. 4-1 Digital palpation of the planned host site reveals undercuts, irregularities, and defects of the bone. Zones of attached gingivae may be ascertained as well.

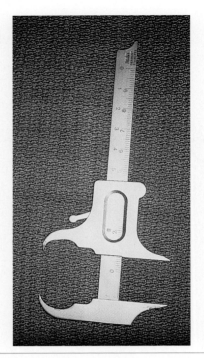

Fig. 4-2 A standardized Boley gauge can be sharpened and sterilized for purposes of sounding. Such a device also is available commercially.

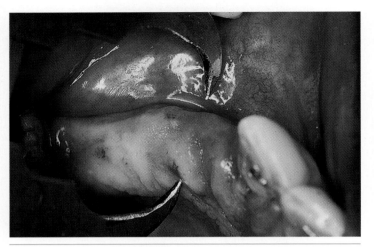

Fig. 4-3 After anesthetization, the sharpened Boley gauge tips penetrate the soft tissues so that accurate direct bone dimensions may be recorded.

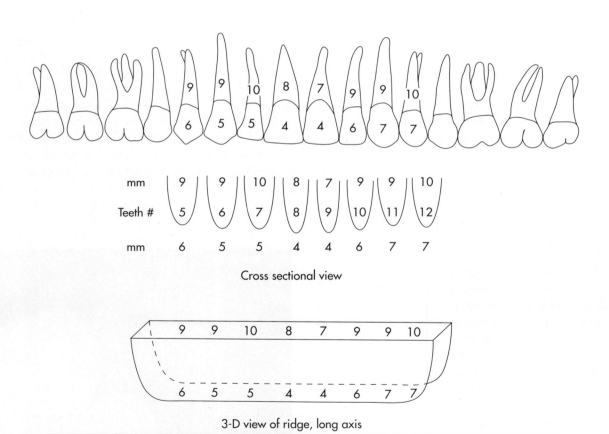

Cross sectional view

3-D view of ridge, long axis

Fig. 4-4 The Boley gauge measurements of bone are transferred to a dental chart. From these numbers, cross-sectional and three-dimensional views can be plotted to serve as dimensional guides in millimeters during surgery.

(Courtesy Dr. Sylvia Seu.)

Study Casts

At this point, make full arch alginate impressions of both arches so that the dimensions may be transferred to the casts made from them. Pour the impressions immediately with dental stone, and make a second (surgical planning) cast of the arch that is to be restored with implants. A centric recording in the material of choice is needed to allow the casts to be mounted on a semiadjustable articulator (Whip Mix, Hanau). Proper articulation of casts is an essential part of every restorative procedure. By correctly reproducing the patient's occlusal relationships on an articulator, proper planning may be accomplished and a great deal of time that is usually wasted adjusting prostheses may be eliminated. If the casts are not related to the condylar axis of the patient before articulator mounting, the accuracy of the bite record may not be valid.

The face-bow is a relatively simple device to use. Its purpose is to relate the maxilla to the same location on the articulator that is found in the patient's skull. The face-bow consists of three components: the bite fork, the bow, and the locator rods. To place the device properly, locate the patient's condyles. Palpation of these important structures while the patient repeatedly opens and closes the mouth reveals their locations with accuracy. Mark these points on the skin with an indelible pencil so that the axis locator rods of the face-bow may be placed against them. In addition to the palpation method for locating the condyles, the external auditory meatus may be used. They are related consistently to the condylar head axes. Several systems provide earpieces on the face-bow for this purpose.

Next, affix a U-shaped, softened sheet of wax to the bite fork. The patient's mouth should be closed in centric relationship lightly into the wax so that indentations are made by the cusp tips of the teeth. For edentulous patients, use stable base plates. Attach the maxillary wax rim to the fork. Guide the patient into a centric closure of the proper vertical dimension. With the bite fork held in place by the patient's teeth, assemble the face-bow. The axis locators should be allowed to contact the marks on the skin, and the assistant should tighten the set screws, thereby locking the bite fork, locator, and face-bow in place. Finally, loosen the axis locators. If the system is stable, their tips will not move. The patient may then open his or her mouth, and the entire assembly may be removed.

Although some articulators permit the transfer of intercondylar distance measurements, most have a preset distance. Attach the locator rods to the axes of the articulator, fasten their set screws, and place the maxillary cast in the wax indentations on the bite fork. At this stage, evaluate the position of the cast. The occlusal plane should be slightly higher in the posterior area. The cast should be supported with a block and attached to the upper member of the articulator with a mounting ring, using model plaster. After setting, use the interocclusal bite record to relate the mandibular to the maxillary cast. It is affixed with plaster to the lower or fixed member of the articulator.

All of the occlusal relationship records should be derived from the articulator. Final prosthesis balancing is accomplished as well, following these articulator-related techniques.

Study the mounted casts in respect to interocclusal distances, existing occlusal relationships, and arch forms (Fig. 4-5). If less than 7 mm of distance is found between the potential host site and the opposing natural or prosthetic occlusal surfaces (Fig. 4-6), an implant may not be used unless additional space can be created by the following:

1. Grinding the opposing occlusion
2. If edentulous, thinning the overlying gingiva and/or bone of the opposing jaw (see Chapters 6, 7, 8)
3. Reducing the alveolar height of the operative site by flattening the thin ridge (see Chapter 6, 8) (while being sure that adequate bone height remains to allow sufficient dimension to permit seating of the planned implants)

In cases of edentulous posterior mandibular quadrants, there is often extrusion of the maxillary molars or premolars directly opposing the area. In the absence of significant periodontal disease, it is the alveolar ridge that actually is thrust downward, carrying the teeth with it. In such instances, an en-

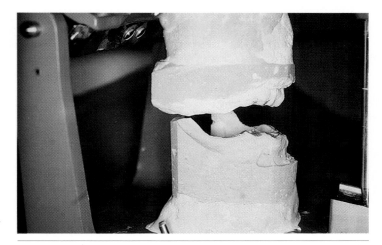

Fig. 4-5 An integral step in the diagnostic regimen is the establishment of mounted casts.

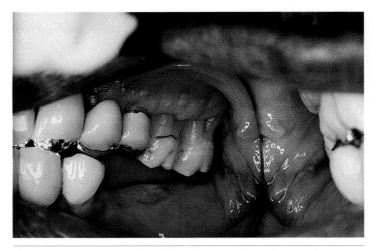

Fig. 4-6 One cause of insufficient intermaxillary distance (7 mm or less) is supereruption of the opposing dentition. This may be solved by extraction, endodontic therapy, occlusal equilibration, an increase in the vertical dimension, or subapical en bloc resection (see Fig. 4-7).

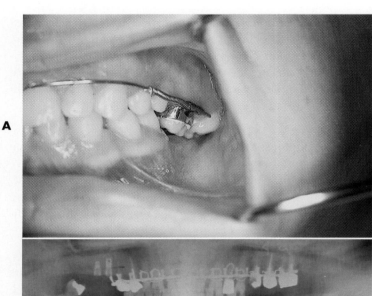

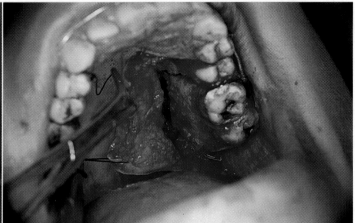

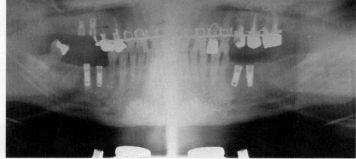

Fig. 4-7   A, The extended posterior maxillary segment prevents implants or prosthetics from being performed in the opposing mandible. **B,** A segmental osteotomy permits the intrusion of the posterior segment, which includes alveolus and teeth. After healing, a mandibular prosthesis is made possible. **C,** A postoperative radiograph shows implants placed and the maxillary quadrant successfully intruded.

bloc segmental osteotomy can be performed that will intrude the problematic area and thereby increase the intermaxillary space (Fig. 4-7).

If the articulation indicates crossbite or ridge procumbency, it is necessary to determine that the angulation of the implants will permit the final prosthesis to be in functional position. However, implants at greater than 35-degree angulations from the long axis of the ridge present significant aesthetic and functional problems. If an angle greater than this is created, forces will be exerted that may be detrimental to the longevity of implant host sites. Therefore some excellent ridges may be considered questionable if angulation places implants in compromised positions. Custom-casting using wax patterns for cementable abutments is permissible. In addition, some implant designs are available with abutments having angles of 15 degrees or even 30 degrees (i.e., Steri-Oss, Paragon). Seating these to the proper alignment, however, requires special skills (see Chapters 21 and 27).

Radiology

The next step in the diagnostic sequence is a radiologic survey. The following radiographs and their purposes are listed so that the practitioner may select the fewest possible views required to attain the optimal data:

Panoramic (Fig. 4-8): A panoramic radiograph presents an overall view of both the mandible and maxilla. Normal anatomy and existing pathologic conditions of the dentoalveolar complex and adjacent structures can be noted. The remaining natural teeth are visualized. Unpredictable

distortions of distances (25% or more) are a constant characteristic of these films.

Periapical (Fig. 4-9): A periapical radiograph gives a view of higher resolution and greater accuracy and indicates medullary and cortical bone density. Often, measurements may be made directly from these films.

Lateral cephalometric (Fig. 4-10): Lateral cephalometric radiographs are helpful for the patient with completely edentulous ridges. The cross-sectional morphology of the residual anterior ridge can be visualized along with its angles of inclination. In addition, skeletal jaw relationships may be studied. This allows an estimate of labiolingual dimension. These views may be taken with occlusal films but are best produced with a cephalometric device using high speed 8 × 10 cassettes.

Radiographic ball-bearing template: In addition to other techniques, periapical ball-bearing evaluations are of great value. Prepare a template using the second, or surgical-planning, cast. The 5-mm diameter, standardized metal marking spheres (Implant Innovations Inc.; Ace Surgical) should be counter-sunk into the cast at the crest of the ridge at each potential implant site to a depth of 1 mm using a No. 6 round bur. Sticky-wax each in place. Then, using an Omnivac machine, mold a piece of 0.02-inch gauge, clear, plastic material to the cast, which incorporates the spheres within it (Fig. 4-11). After proper trimming, the template that has been produced may be seated intraorally before periapical radiography (Fig. 4-12). If the template is nonretentive, use a small amount of denture adhesive to stabilize it. After producing long cone, periapical radiographs with the template in place, record the diameter of

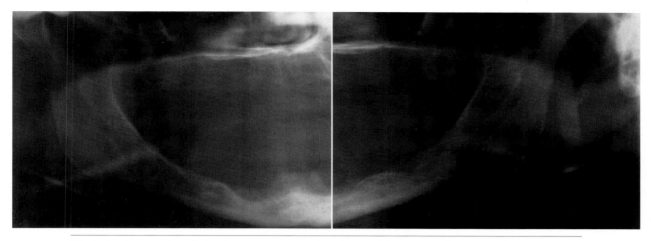

Fig. 4-8 Panoramic radiographs present a scanning view, which serves well to survey the jaws. Do not use panoramic radiographs for definitive measurements.

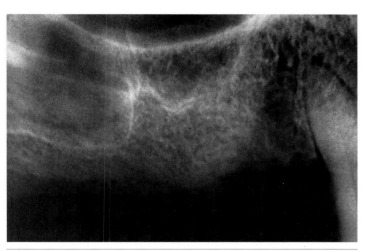

Fig. 4-9 Periapical radiographs show detail of bony architecture and offer greater accuracy of measurement. Distortion, particularly in the maxillae, still exists, but it may be minimized by using long cone techniques.

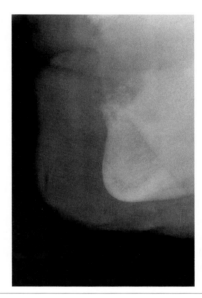

Fig. 4-10 A lateral view of the mandibular symphysis, one of the most common sites for implantation, may be taken effectively with an occlusal film. It offers some information about cortical plate angulation but is limited because only the greatest dimensions are outlined.

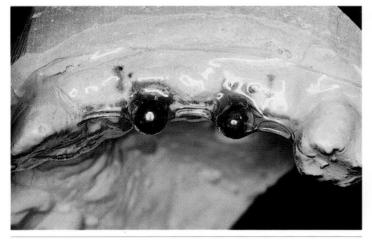

Fig. 4-11 A clear Omnivac template is processed to the preoperative study cast after placing 5-mm diameter stainless steel spheres into slightly counter-sunk holes.

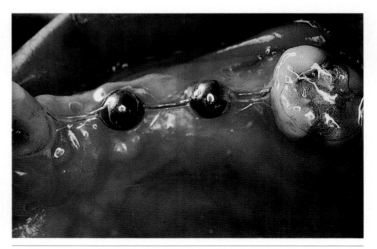

Fig. 4-12 The trimmed Omnivac template is placed into position in the patient's mouth and long cone radiographs are taken (see Fig. 4-13).

the spheres on the films (Fig. 4-13). If they are found to be 5 mm in diameter, the height and length of available bone may be measured with accuracy directly on the radiographs. If this is not the case, use the following simple algebraic equation to determine the actual bone dimensions:

$$\frac{rs}{5} = \frac{rm}{rx}$$

where rs is the x-ray sphere measurement, rm is the x-ray bone measurement, x is the actual bone measurement being sought, and 5 is the actual sphere measurement.

Retain the Omnivac guide because at the time of surgery the spheres may be removed, the template can be sterilized, and after the soft tissues are reflected, it can be used as an implant site locator. (Further elucidation of this technique is found in Chapter 9.)

An alternative method used to measure available bone is simpler but slightly less accurate. Mark the surgical-planning cast at the potential implant host sites. Then make an Omnivac template on the cast. Following this, drill a hole through the plastic template at each of the implant sites with a No. 557 bur and, using cold-cure acrylic, process a 0.045-inch orthodontic wire into each hole. Measure each wire length carefully at 5 mm. (Errors in measurement will be directly proportional to bone length distortion.) Place the template into the patient's mouth, and complete the periapical radiographic survey as in the previously described use of spheres. Since there are three known quantities, the unknown (the actual bone height) may be solved using the same formula given for the spheres. In lieu of these methods, a single, accurate technique of bone measurement and morphology may be achieved using computerized axial tomography (CT) scanning.

CT Scanning

Three-dimensional imaging enables the user to visualize any area within the parameters of the scan. CT scanning machines provide a variety of views by making 1.5-mm slices through the bone. These slices are stacked by the program's software like a deck of playing cards, and when the three-dimensional subject is completed, the company will reformat it into coronal, cross-sectional or panoramic images, which also are sliced. This program ensures that surprises are not encountered during surgery. The amount of available bone (or lack of it) may be plotted to the millimeter. The amount of bone beneath the maxillary sinus and nasal cavity may be charted for width and height. The density of bone may be observed and reported in Houndsfield numbers as well. In the mandible, the exact location of the mandibular canal in even its most tortuous course may be plotted in advance of surgery.

This information enables the clinician to plan the proper implant types, numbers, sizes, and locations. By using presurgical scanning, the possibility of being placed in the uncomfortable position of telling a patient that he or she is an unsuitable candidate for implants midway through a surgery is minimized.

The patient should be sent to a radiologist who, preferably, has a GE 9800 or GE 8800 CT unit. The radiologist must possess software that can create three-dimensional reconstruction of the maxilla and mandible such as the Columbia Scientific (3D Dental) program.

The scanner produces a series of images made from horizontal slices (Fig. 4-14). Each exposure is 1.5 mm wide, and when the series of cuts is completed within the prescribed perimeters, they are stacked by the computer. The program uses this reconstituted three-dimensional structure to supply images made in the cross-sectional (Figs. 4-15, 4-16), pano-

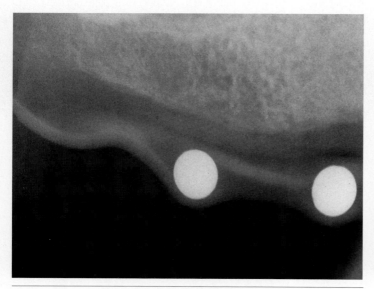

Fig. 4-13 To verify accuracy, the diameter of the spheres on the x-ray film must be compared with their actual 5-mm sizes.

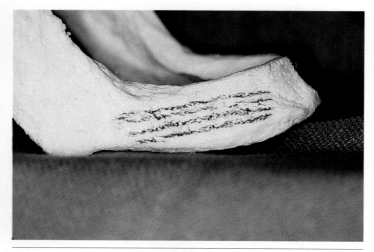

Fig. 4-14 With the patient lying on the gurney, the computed tomography (CT) scanner makes horizontal radiographic cuts of 1.5-mm width. Each image is overlapped by 0.25 mm to permit accurate continuity and the presentation of 1-mm wide views.

ramic (Figs. 4-17, 4-18), and occlusal modes (Figs. 4-19, 4-20). These images may be interpreted, area by area, so that the arch in which the implants have been planned can be plotted to the millimeter in width and depth. In addition, exact locations of all vital structures are readily identified by using the images, which the process presents in 1-mm sections.

If there are no such software programs available, radiologists may take a conventional scan of the patient on almost any CT scanner, and the resulting magnetic tape can then be sent to the Columbia Scientific Corporation. The company has the capability to translate such magnetic tapes into images containing the requisite three-dimensional information.

Currently, software and hardware (Dentascan) systems are available that allow the dentist to reformat axial images directly in the office and superimpose appropriately sized implants on them (Fig. 4-21).

Before referring the patient to the radiologist, intraoral splints designed to immobilize the lower jaw must be made if this is the area to be scanned. This is not an absolute requirement for the maxilla, however. Fabricate the splints with the following objectives in mind: immobilization, disocclusion, and orientation. Fabricate the fixation devices with the jaws in the resting position to allow the patient to keep the mandible comfortably immobilized for up to a 30-minute period. Immobilization is necessary, since any movement causes blurring or distortion of the images.

If there are teeth in the maxilla and mandible, the splints should disocclude them so that there is a space created on the images. There should be no metal allowed to remain in the teeth or incorporated into the splint of the jaw being scanned, since metal (titanium excepted) creates scatter and other masking artifacts on the images.

Establish the proper plane of occlusion in the splints and place nonmetallic radiopaque markers (gutta percha) parallel to and at the plane of occlusion. These markers tell the radiologist how to orient the patient's head for the study. They also ensure that the angle at which the cross sections are reformatted through the scanned arch is at 90 degrees to the occlusal plane. The accuracy of measurements taken from the scan is dependent on the orientation of the preliminary, or scout film. Therefore, accurate placement of the opaque occlusal plane markers is essential. The x-ray technician must position the patient's head so that the scout or first film demonstrates its orientation lines parallel to the marker (see Fig. 4-36).

Methods of Splint Fabrication

Each tooth represented in the template should have a 10-mm vertical gutta percha marker processed into it. These are transferred to the occlusal, panoramic, and transaxial images. When the template is placed into the patient's mouth, each gutta percha marker can be traced to the images so that anatomic localization is coordinated. This is of particular value during surgery, when planned host site dimensions can be pinpointed by making direct reference from them to the appropriately labeled cross-sectional views.

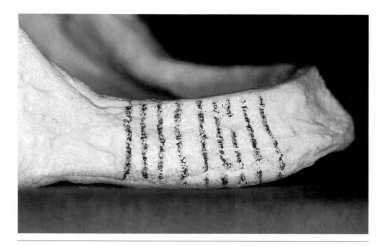

Fig. 4-15 The vertical lines indicate the cross-sectional planes or "cuts" that the CT software makes available.

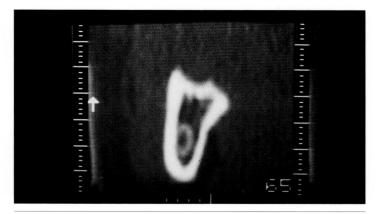

Fig. 4-16 A typical cross-sectional view of the mandible produced by CT scan dental software. Vital structures (mandibular canal, cortical plates, inferior border) may be reviewed clearly. With some systems (life-sized imaging), measurements may be made directly from the film.

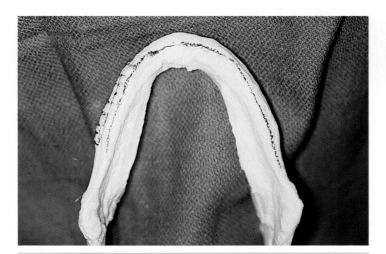

Fig. 4-17 Another valuable image produced by scanning is the panoramic. Usually five slices are made available from buccal to lingual. This mandibular model shows the middle level of the five slices marked by pencil (see Fig. 4-18).

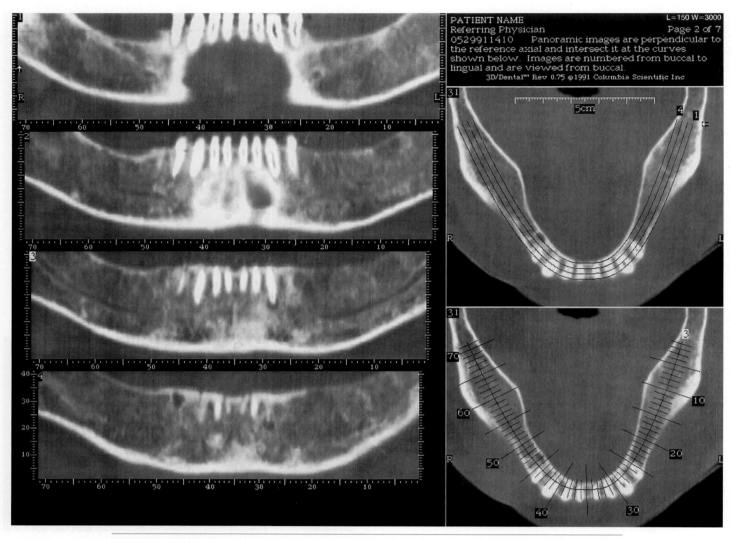

Fig. 4-18   Panoramic images at four buccolingual levels (view 31) on the right top are demonstrated in the panoramic reproductions (1-4) on the left. The lucent area in view 1 does not represent a lytic lesion. Line 1 in view 31 *(upper right)* (the most labial cut) shows that the scan passed through an area just anterior to the symphysis.

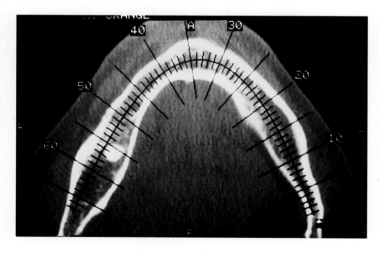

Fig. 4-19   This image represents an occlusal view made in the mid-mandible. The numbered cross-hatching indicates the cross-sectional images, each 1 mm wide, as may be noted in Figs. 4-16 and 4-37.

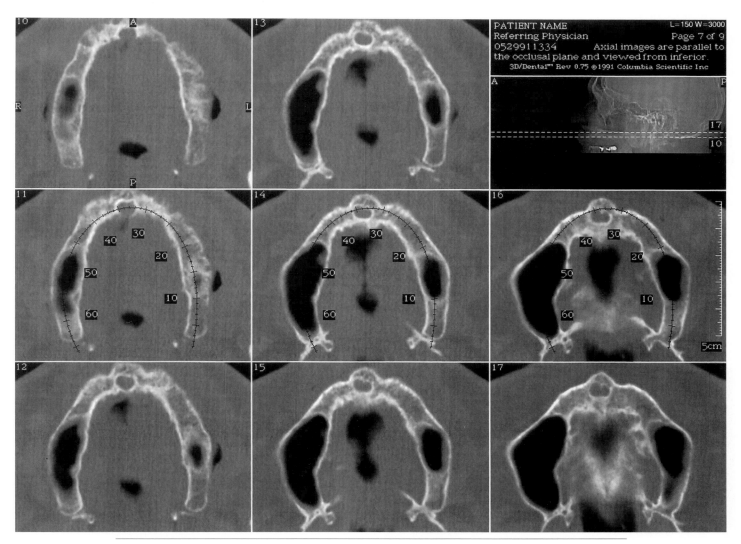

Fig. 4-20 Transaxial (occlusal) views are used for maxillae as well as mandibles. These eight images, numbers 10 through 17, offer dramatic representations of this geometrically complex structure at evenly spaced intervals (1.5 mm apart). The image at the upper right marked *A* is called a scout film and presents the inferior-to-superior perimeters of the images 10 through 17.

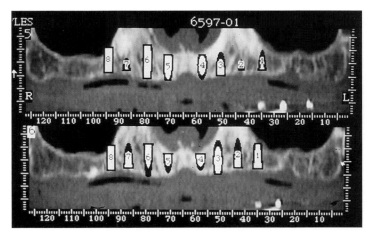

Fig. 4-21 The Dentascan program permits the computerized superimposition of implants of specific dimensions directly on the images. They may be placed on the cross-sectional as well as the panoramic views (see also Fig. 4-48).

Edentulous Arch

Make an alginate impression of the arch to be scanned and pour a diagnostic cast.

Fabricate acrylic base plates with wax rims.

Adjust the rims to the patient's correct vertical dimension, centric relationship, lip length and prominence; set the teeth for final functional satisfaction and esthetic appearance.

Try in the final wax dentures, and confirm esthetics (Fig. 4-22).

Record the patient's centric relationship position at the resting vertical dimension, and mount the trial dentures on an articulator.

Complete the dentures and replicate them in clear self-curing acrylic using a Lang denture duplicator flask (Fig. 4-23). After preliminary polymerization, it is fully cured in a pressure pot for 30 to 45 minutes (Fig. 4-24).

Seat the replicated clear acrylic trial dentures on the original cast, and fill the space between them (freeway space, by mounting casts at the resting vertical dimension position)

with additional self-curing acrylic resin, creating an inter-arch index. If the opposing arch contains teeth, then the duplicated trial denture may be luted to an opposing acrylic replica of the arch at the patient's resting vertical dimension.

Cut a 1-mm deep, 1-mm wide, and 10-mm long groove in the labial acrylic facings of each of the teeth on the appliance with a No. 6 round bur. These grooves are refined and cut perpendicularly to the established occlusal plane with a diamond point (Fig. 4-25).

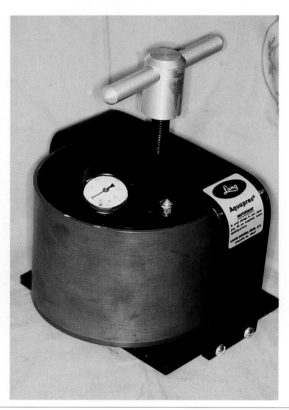

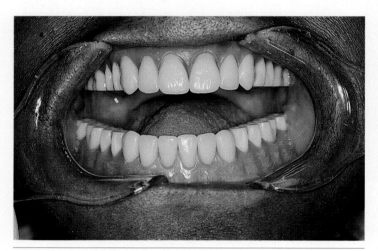

Fig. 4-22 For the completely edentulous patient, place trial dentures with the teeth set in wax to check for esthetics and function and to locate the appropriate positions of significant teeth. These relate to potential implant sites on the scan.

Fig. 4-24 Fill the pressure pot with hot water to a point of overfilling and then close it tightly, thereby permitting the acrylic to cure fully and in bubble-free condition.

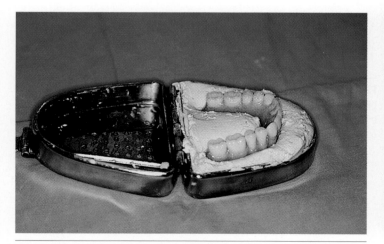

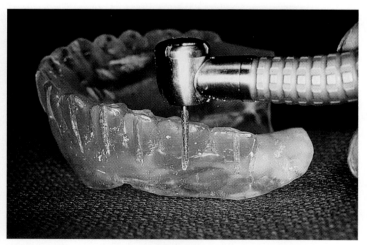

Fig. 4-23 Place the waxed trial denture into a Lang duplicating flask with alginate impression material. Complete replication in clear self-curing acrylic by closing the flask.

Fig. 4-25 Prepare the clear acrylic template for placement of 10-mm-long radiographic markers in each of the 14 teeth of the surgical template. Make each at right angles to the occlusal plane marker and fill them with a radiopaque medium.

Pack the grooves with well-condensed gutta percha or a mixture of amalgam particles and acrylic. In order to create evenly reproducible radiopaque markers, the use of a heated gutta percha gun offers greater ease and more reliable placement of the material. Alterations to the use of gutta percha that facilitate reliable marker placement include the use of composite restorative material (which, when used alone, does not present a particularly sharp image) or (for a well-defined image) a mixture of amalgam powder (¼) and acrylic powder (¾), which can be painted easily into the grooves using monomer (Nealon's technique) (Fig. 4-26).

Air holes for breathing and a suction hole for the attachment of an aspirator are required if the occlusion is extremely close or the patient produces a great deal of saliva.

Try in the appliance to the mouth to ensure that the patient can wear it comfortably during the scan.

Partially Edentulous Arch

Make alginate impressions of the mandible and maxilla and mount diagnostic stone casts (Fig. 4-27).

Replicate the models, and fabricate a diagnostic setup of the planned final restored case (Fig. 4-28).

Replicate the wax setup by making an impression of it and pouring it in stone (Fig. 4-29).

Make an Omnivac replica using 0.02-inch clear material of the stone model (Fig. 4-30).

Trim the Omnivac material so that it covers the height of contour of all teeth and extends down to the alveolar ridge in the areas where the teeth have been waxed (Fig. 4-31).

Remove the Omnivac shell from the stone model. Fill the areas in the shell where the teeth had been set with a doughy mix of clear, self-curing acrylic. Reseat the Omnivac shell back onto the original stone cast (with the edentulous areas) and cure it in a pressure pot (Fig. 4-32).

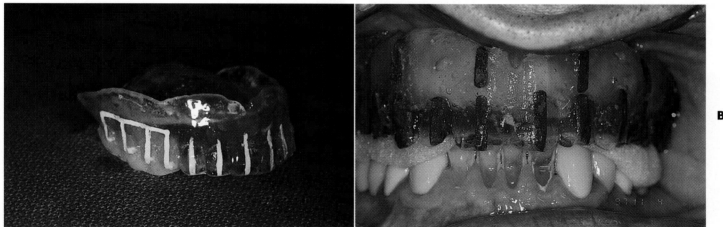

Fig. 4-26 **A,** Affix gutta percha markers into the grooves of the radiographic or surgical template. Predictable density is ensured by using the Obtura device. **B,** Amalgam powder and acrylic powder (with a 1:3 ratio applied with monomer and a paintbrush) is simple to insert into the grooves and creates a highly diagnostic image.

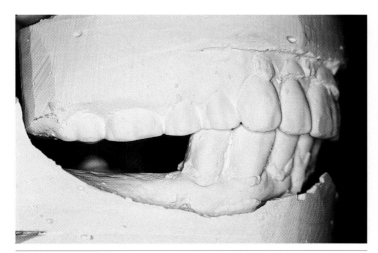

Fig. 4-27 For the partially edentulous patient, mount preoperative study casts on the articulator.

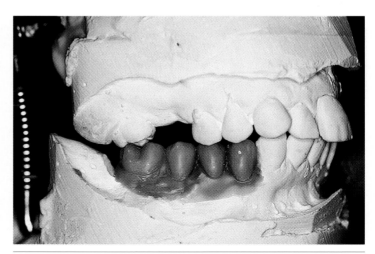

Fig. 4-28 Wax denture teeth into the planned implant host site.

After completion of curing, trim the excess acrylic.

Cut grooves (1 mm wide, 1 mm deep, and 10 mm long) through the labial surfaces of all of the natural tooth sites with a No. 6 round bur so that these grooves run perpendicular to the newly established plane of occlusion.

Fill all grooves and holes with well-condensed gutta percha (Fig. 4-33).

Try in this appliance into the patient's mouth.

Roughen the occlusal surfaces of the Omnivac appliance, and lubricate the patient's opposing dentition.

Place a doughy mix of self-curing acrylic on the occlusal surfaces of the appliance.

The patient is made to close into a centric relationship but is stopped at the resting vertical dimension (Fig. 4-34). The

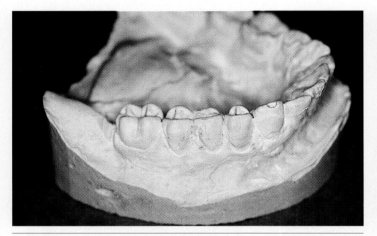

Fig. 4-29   Replicate the cast with its newly placed denture teeth in stone.

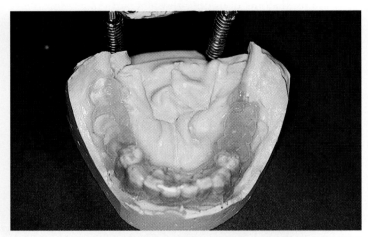

Fig. 4-32   Fill the hollow Omnivac template with clear acrylic and cure it in a pressure pot.

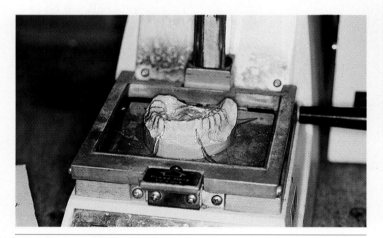

Fig. 4-30   Prepare an 0.02-inch Omnivac template over the stone cast.

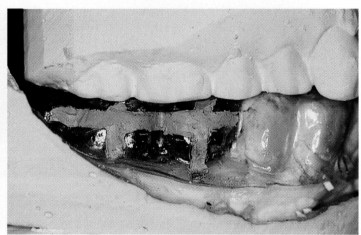

Fig. 4-33   Place diagnostic grooves in strategic positions in the cured template, fill with gutta percha points that are compacted, and smooth with chloroform.

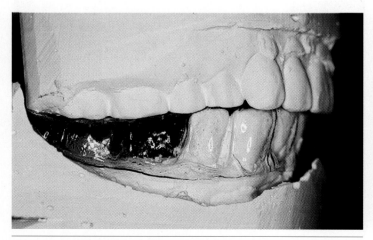

Fig. 4-31   Place the Omnivac template on the original cast after the teeth are removed.

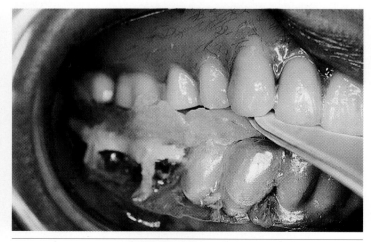

Fig. 4-34   Place the completed appliance for the partially edentulous patient into position, and add acrylic wafers to disocclude the mandible. Use several tongue blades to open the bite.

patient opens and closes his or her mouth to this position while the acrylic hardens. Complete the curing in the pressure pot (Fig. 4-35).

Insert the appliance to assess patient comfort.

Purpose of the Template

Facilitate immobilization of the patient's jaws by allowing the patient to remain comfortably in the rest position.

Radiopaque lines representing the patient's occlusal plane can be seen on the scout film. The CT scan technologist must orient the patient's head so that these lines appear parallel to the two dotted, preset orientation and perimetric lines seen on this film (Fig. 4-36).

These lines made in the long axes of the teeth represent the angulation of the proposed restorations as they relate to the angulation of the available bone at each proposed implant site (Figs. 4-37, 4-38) and localize each tooth location, thereby relating surgical sites to cross-sectional views.

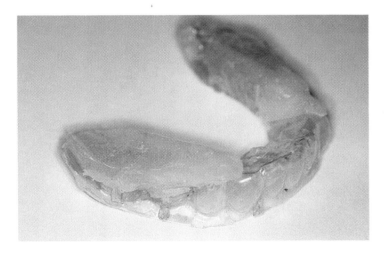

Fig. 4-35 Give the completed positioning device to the patient to be worn during the scanning procedure.

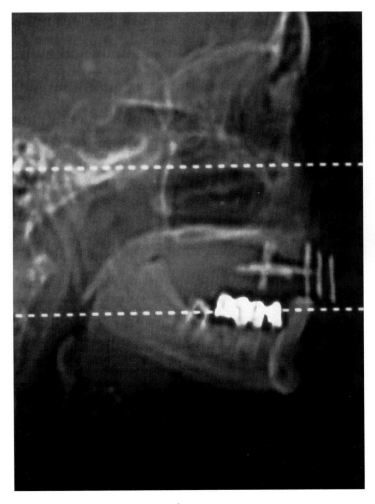

Fig. 4-36 The first film taken by the CT scanner, the scout view, must show the radiopaque horizontal occlusal line parallel to the dotted perimeters.

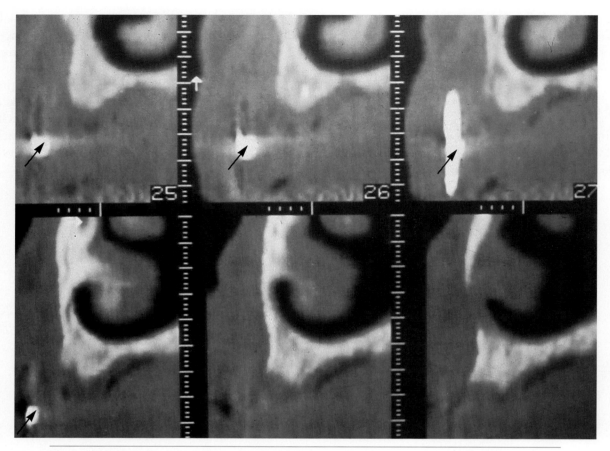

Fig. 4-37 The cross-sectional views that show the radiopaque markers *(arrows)* identify anatomic locations and axial inclinations of proposed implants. These make implant placement more precise as to site and angulation when at subsequent surgical visits, the template is used as a surgical guide.

Fig. 4-38 The surgical guide is prepared simply by removing a lingually placed trough of acrylic, which permits the ridge to be exposed but allows the labial surfaces of the teeth to remain intact so that they serve as indicators for implant placement and angulation.

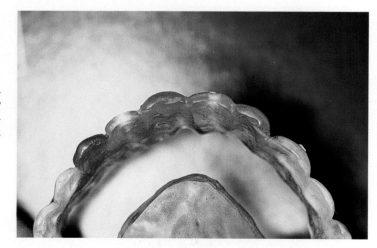

Alternate Technique

First, place the patient's denture in the replicating flask, and add alginate to both halves. After its removal, fill the dentate portion of the alginate with a mixture of 25% Hypaque (a standard contrast material used in radiology) and 75% tooth-colored polymer-monomer mixture. Complete the remaining (tissue-borne) portion of the denture with regular self-curing acrylic (Fig. 4-39). After setting, remove the denture replica from the flask; trim, polish, and give it to the patient to be worn during the scanning procedure. The result presents the radiopaque dentition clearly outlined, tooth by tooth, in its relationship to the underlying bone structures (Fig. 4-40).

The clinician may use this at the presurgical and surgical stages for localization of sites, for verification of measurements, and as a surgical template coordinating it with the cross-sectional and panoramic views (Fig. 4-41).
Now the patient is ready for the scan.

Give the following instructions to the radiologist:

Scan limits for the mandible (perimeters): the lowest cut should begin just below the inferior border of the mandible (if the scan just starts at the inferior border, valuable information will be lost). The superior limit should be above the occlusal plane of the teeth, which is marked by a radiopaque line processed into the splint.
Scan limits for the maxillae: the superior border of the scan should be placed just above the infraorbital foramina, and the inferior border should be located just below the occlusal plane of the maxillary dentition, also marked by a gutta percha line in the splint.
Make 1.5-mm-thick slices at 1-mm intervals. (This allows 0.25-mm overlapping of each cut and ensures greater accuracy.)
Make the images life-sized.
Use the splint that has been made for the patient.
Start with a scout film, the orientation lines of which should be parallel to the patient's plane of occlusion, which will be marked by a radiopaque line.

Notes

Metals cause blurring of the image, so information will be lost or distorted by artifact (Fig. 4-42). Therefore, if metals are left in the patient's mouth, the resulting films may not be diagnostic or even readable. Because these imaging programs are multiplanar, only those slices that actually contain metal restorations will contain artifacts. However, for the most accurate and diagnostic films, remove all metal restorations in the arch that is to be scanned and replace them with composite, acrylic, or other nonmetallic materials. Pure titanium does not cause severe artifacts and affects the CT minimally, if at all. Titanium alloy causes some artifact, but the films produced are usually quite readable.

It is suggested that the referring practitioner be present for scans taken of the first few patients to ensure that all instructions are followed. The radiologist and his or her techni-

cian may take a CT scan that is believed to comply with the requirements of the software program, but if the instructions are not followed carefully, the resulting films may be of little diagnostic value.

For patients who are claustrophobic, an anesthesiologist or the referring practitioner must be present (along with appro-

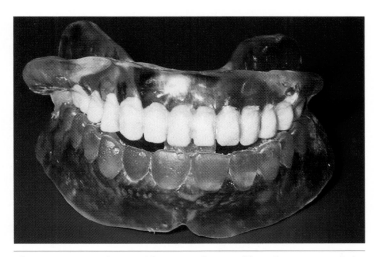

Fig. 4-39 To make a guidance appliance with radiopaque teeth for the CT scan, Hypaque, available from a surgical supply company, is mixed with self-curing acrylic in a 25% to 75% ratio for the tooth portions of the denture replica.

(Courtesy Dr. Milos Boskovic.)

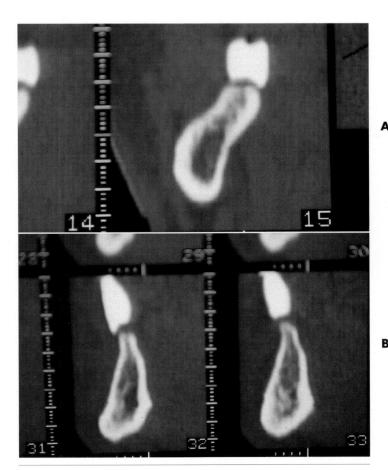

Fig. 4-40 The resulting images clearly show the position of each denture tooth as it relates to the underlying bone structure. This clarity is a result of the addition of Hypaque to each tooth indentation.

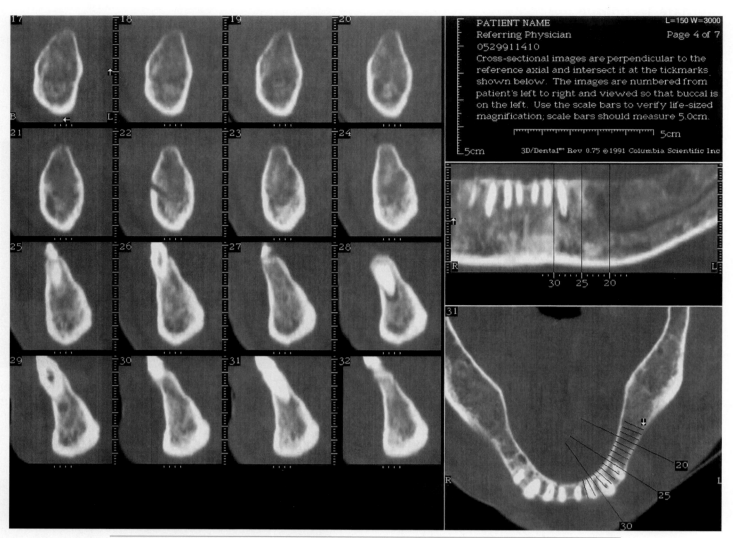

Fig. 4-41   The (mandibular) transaxial occlusal view *(lower right)* has cuts 17 through 32 of the total of more than 60 shown on the original image. Each of these lines refers to a single cross sectional image shown in the numbered boxes on the left. Box 22 demonstrates the mental foramen; box 25 demonstrates the most distal tooth, and box 19 shows the location and size of the mandibular canal. An additional dimension that may be used for substantiation is the panographic view *(upper right),* which is marked with the same cross-sectional numbers.

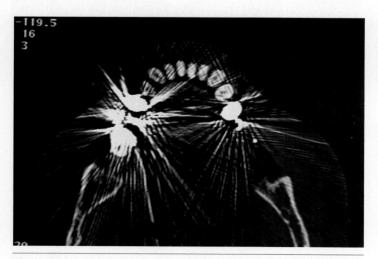

Fig. 4-42   Scatter or artifact is caused by the presence of nontitanium metals in the teeth of the jaw that is being scanned. This phenomenon renders the image useless.

priate resuscitative equipment) to administer intravenous (IV) sedation (i.e., diazepam 5 to 10 mg, midazolam 1 to 3 mg), as required. Such medication is of benefit as well for patients with neuromuscular disorders such as cerebral palsy, Parkinson's disease, or chorea.

Interpretation

The following specific instructions are for scans taken with the Columbia Scientific software.

The scout film is a lateral, two-dimensional view of the head. Two parallel dotted lines may be seen that show the superior and the inferior limits (perimeters) of the scan. These dotted lines should be parallel to the plane of occlusion set by the horizontal gutta percha–filled grooves and not to the inferior border of the mandible or the alveolar crest of the maxilla. The prescriber should be present for the first several cases because before the scanning, this view can be seen on the mon-

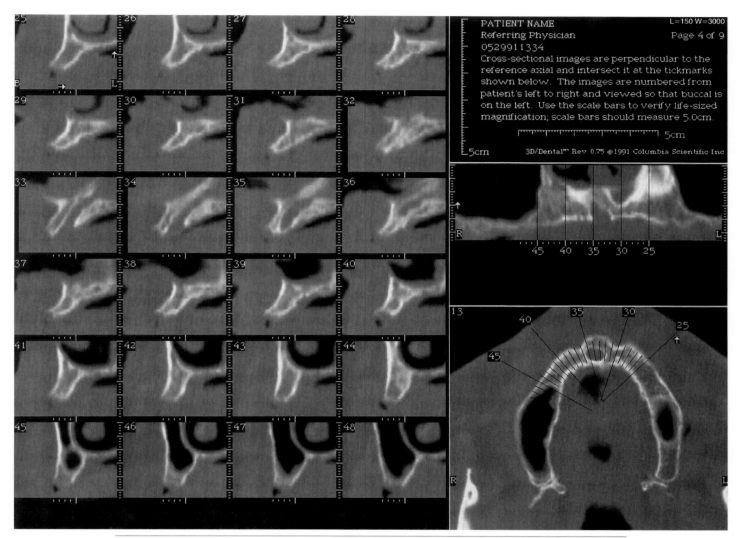

Fig. 4-43 These views of the maxillae show slices 25 to 48. Included in the cross-sectional boxes are the incisive foramen and canal (33), the anterior nasal spine and floor (35), the anterior extent of the antrum (45), and the alveolar ridge and sinus floor relationship (48). Correlations may be seen in the occlusal *(lower right)* and panoramic views *(upper right)*.

itor and corrections of head position suggested before total radiation is initiated (see Fig. 4-36).

The next view is a single horizontal (occlusal) slice through the mandible or maxilla. In this view a section through the entire arch may be seen. There are lines numbered approximately from 1 to 60 crossing from buccal to lingual. There are more or fewer lines, depending on the size of the jaw (see Fig. 4-19). These lines can be used to cross reference a series of separate cross-sectional views, each in its own small box (Figs. 4-41, 4-43).

The several horizontal (or occlusal) views are supplied with up to five orientation lines, which follow the jaw's contours proceeding from buccal to lingual (right upper). These black lines show the planes through which the five panoramic views were taken (Fig. 4-44).

Underneath each of the panoramic views are vertical lines that appear to be a scale. Each of these lines indicates the location of a cross section as numbered. These represent the

same lines as are seen in the occlusal view to the lower right, and serve as references to the numbered cross-sectional views (Fig. 4-41), as well as to the markings below the panoramic view (Fig. 4-44). The most important images for diagnostic use in planning the placement of endosteal implants are the cross-sectional views. Each is numbered for ease of cross-referencing. The number is at the bottom right corner of each image. To serve as further elucidation, there is also a segmental cross-referenced occlusal image on the side of each group of boxes to show which section of mandible or maxilla the several cross sections reproduced to its left represent.

In evaluating scans that contain the radiopaque dental markers, additional benefits accrue to the diagnostician.

Since the length of each marker is known (10 mm), dimensional accuracy can be checked by measuring them on the images (Fig. 4-45).

The occlusal views delineate the location of each marker (and therefore each tooth location) as identified by the 14 dots

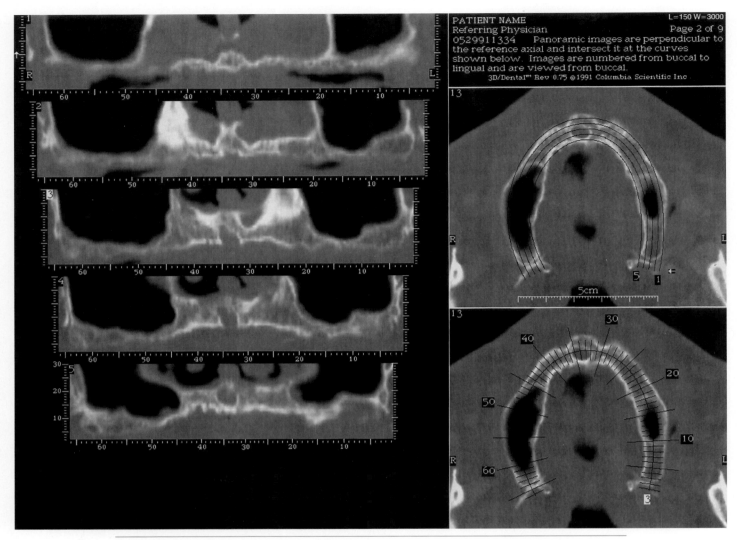

Fig. 4-44 This maxillary transaxial (occlusal) view, right at top, shows the five levels of cuts, from buccal to palatal, represented by the five panoramic images on the left. The crosscuts (1 through 67) on the transaxial image at the bottom right refer to cross-sectional boxes 25 through 48 shown in Fig. 4-43, as well as to the numbered vertical lines below the panoramic images.

and by the lines delineating the cross-sectional boxes (Fig. 4-46). These markers can then be seen in the appropriately numbered cross-sectional boxes (Fig. 4-45).

After the flaps have been reflected at stage I surgery, place the sterilized template into position. Its flange not only retracts the labiobuccal mucoperiosteal flaps, the location of each marker can be directly transferred to the underlying bone (Fig. 4-47). The density, anatomy, and dimensions of each specific clinical-surgical site can be related, at the time of surgery, to the associated cross-section (Fig. 4-45).

For purposes of extrapolating accurate measurements, there is a pointing arrow that shows where to start counting (see Fig. 4-41). In these images, there are vertical and horizontal scales in the upper right corner. Measure both scales. Each should measure 5 cm. This will confirm that the images are life-sized and may be measured in actual millimeters. If the scales do not measure 5 cm, they do not represent life-sized imaging. In such instances, the distance of interest should be measured on the image *(MD)*; then the 5-cm vertical scale

(MSC) should be measured. Place these values (in millimeters) into the following formula:

$$\frac{AD}{MD} = \frac{50\ mm}{MSC}$$

where *AD* is the actual distance; and 50 mm is the actual scale size. The equation is then solved for AD. This reveals the actual distance, compensating for distortion.

Calipers also may be used to measure the distance in question. Open them to 5 cm, and by transferring the caliper points to the 5-cm scale (provided in Fig. 4-41), count the lines between the caliper tips as if they were millimeters, thus presenting actual distances. Not all views are life-sized, however. Actual measurements may be taken only from the "master" (see Fig. 4-43). Other views can be used for cross-referencing only.

Three-dimensional images at several different angles are also shown (Fig. 4-48). These images show how the maxilla or mandible would appear if stripped of all soft tissues. They are

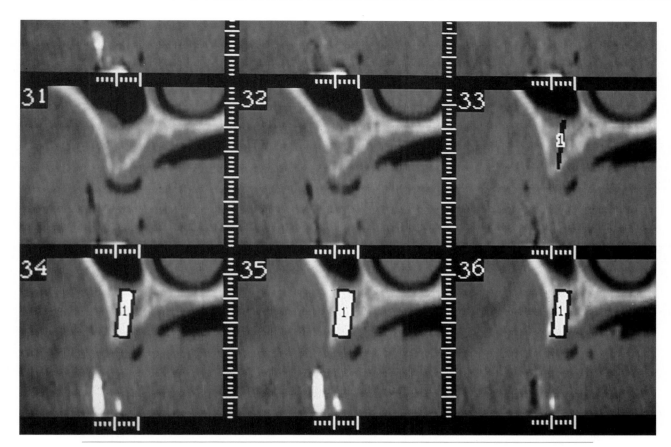

Fig. 4-45   These cross-sectional views (e.g., box 35) serve as the final arbiters in judging operative sites and the locations of vital structures. They are identified by the presence of the markers and can be localized clinically using the surgical template over the exposed bone, thereby coordinating the entire system.

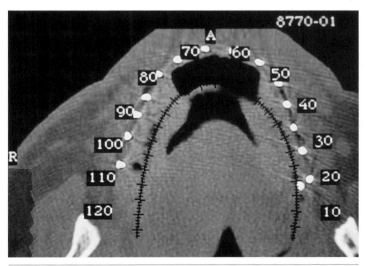

Fig. 4-46   This occlusal image clearly marks the location of each of the 14 teeth as indicated by the vertical radiopaque markings placed in the radiographic template (see well-defined dots). When this device (when used as a surgical template) is placed over the exposed bone, localization of any specific anatomic site can be made and related directly to the cross-sectional views on the Dentascan, which will be seen to demonstrate the images of the same radiopaque markers.

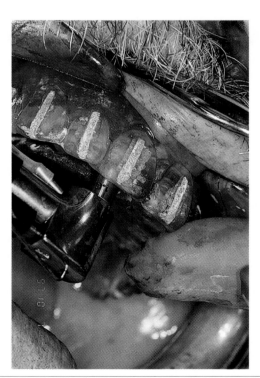

Fig. 4-47   After localizing the appropriate occlusal view by counting dots, position the surgical template over the exposed bone, and identify the site clinically.

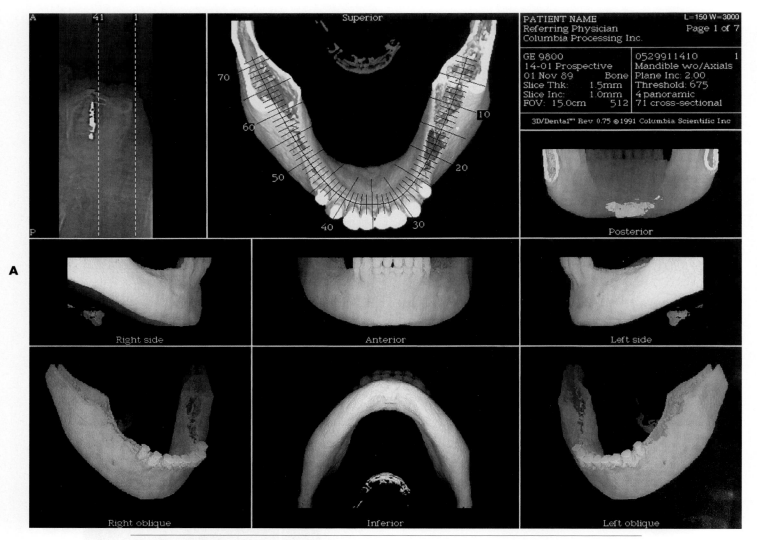

Fig. 4-48 A, The software program reconstructs the scanner slices into three-dimensional views. Not only do the images represent the bony surfaces, but also, as can be seen in the bottom row center (Fig. 4-48, *B*), a midstructural perspective through the maxillary sinuses and nose is presented with clarity. These pictures, although not of value in making measurements, point out irregularities, imperfections, and other internal and external surface characteristics.

useful only to give the surgeon a perspective on the operative areas. They may not be used for measurements. The software developed by the Columbia Scientific Corporation enables the visualization of actual implant dimensions and locations directly on the CT scans in all three dimensions. By adding the values of three-dimensional imaging to the implantologist's armamentarium, great ease and accuracy enhances his or her technical skills.

At this point, the visual, digital, bone sounding, interocclusal, radiographic, and photographic examinations have been completed, and thus the most comprehensive evaluation of the potential host sites has been acquired short of performing exploratory surgery. The available information includes ridge height, width, and anteroposterior length; location of nasal floor, antra, foramina, and canals; existing interocclusal distances; periodontal status of remaining teeth; and amounts of healthy attached gingiva. Armed with this vast body of data and the prosthetic treatment plan, the surgeon may now se-

lect the best implant modality with which to restore the patient's dentition. (The implant selection charts found in Tables 4-1, 4-2, and 4-3 offer invaluable help to the clinician in matters of implant selection.)

CAVEAT

As radiologists become more comfortable with Dentascan, they offer increasing levels of assistance by selecting implants of specific dimensions and superimposing them at sites selected by them. Although this may be of ancillary assistance, the final decision as to numbers of implants, their sizes, angulations, and locations must be left solely to the volition of the implantologist. Figs. 4-49 and 4-50, from an actual clinical case, present examples of the radiologist's suggestions and the actual sites of implantation. Not only were some of the sites inappropriately chosen, but several satisfactory sites were overlooked. Essentially, images offer great benefit to the sur-

Text continued on p. 53

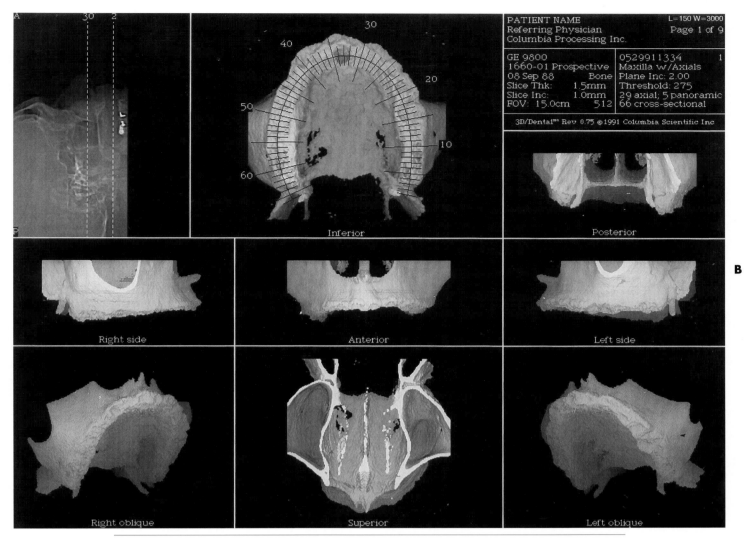

Fig. 4-48 cont'd   B, Maxillary reformatting is of significant value before soft tissue reflection, as well as for verification of CAD-CAM model accuracy.

Table 4-1   Implant Selection Chart Based on Available Bone and Bone Density

	WIDTH (A)	RIDGES DEPTH (B)	LENGTH (C)	IMPLANT TYPE RECOMMENDED
Available	0-3 mm	0-6 mm	0-7 mm	Subperiosteal D
bone	3-5 mm	>8 mm	>10 mm	Blade D
	>5 mm	>8 mm	6-25 mm	1 root form E
		>10 mm	16-23 mm	2 root forms
			24-31 mm	3 root forms
			>31 mm	1 root form for each additional 7 mm of ridge length F

NOTES:

A: If narrow crestal bone can be flattened to create a sufficiently wide plateau to permit placement of a root form implant, available depth must be reassessed (see below).

B: A measurement is made and recorded between ridge crest and one of the following four anatomic structures:
 1. Mandibular canal
 2. Antral floor
 3. Nasal floor
 4. Inferior border of mandible (symphysis area) (CT imaging helps)

C: Root form implants have diameters that vary from 3.25 to 6.3 m. and 7 to 20 mm in length. (Most often, 1 mm of additional bone depth will be required.) Table on root form selection describes each system according to available implant types.

D: If findings do not meet the bone requirements for root forms, see Chapters 11, 12, 13, 14, 15, 17, 18 (describing subperiosteal, blade, transosteal, crete mince, threaded dowels, and intramuscosal insert techniques).

E: Spacing between root form implants should equal the diameter of one implant.

F: The maximum number of implants need not be placed. Information to assist in choosing the appropriate number of implants will be found in subsequent chapters.

G: In less dense bone, the implantologist should use the largest number of implants that available space will permit, even if their diameters are of the smallest categories. Rough (TPS, HA) coatings will help as well, by presenting maximal interfacial areas.

Table 4-2   Root Form Selection Chart

Name	Material	Character and Mode	Stages	Surface	Primary Retention	Length (mm)	Diameter (mm)	Recommended RPM	Internal Cooling	Abutments	Restorative Options
3i Implant Innovations:											
Micro Miniplant Implant	Titanium CP	Threaded Screw	2	Machined and Machined/acid etched TPS	Threading	8.5, 10, 11.5 13, 15, 18	3.25	<1500	Yes	Prefabricated Threaded, UCLA, EP (Conical)	Fixed Bridges Overdentures Fixed detacha bridges
		Cylinder			Surface Texture	8.5, 10, 13, 15 8.5, 10, 11.5,	3.3				
Miniplant Implant		Threaded Screw		Machined	Threading	13, 15, 18 8.5, 10, 11.5, 13, 15	3.25				
		Cylinder		Machined/ acid etched TPS	Surface Texture	8.5, 10, 13, 15 8.5, 10, 11.5 13, 15, 18, 20	3.3				
Standard Implant		Threaded Screw		Machined	Threading	7, 8.5, 10, 13, 15, 18	3.75, 4				
		Cylinder		Machined/ Acid etched TPS	Surface Texture	7, 8.5, 10, 11.5 13, 15, 18	4				
Wide Diameter Implant		Threaded Screw		Machined	Threading	7, 8.5, 10, 13	5, 6				
		Cylinder		Machined/ acid etched TPS	Surface Texture						
Ace Surgical Supply Co.	Titanium Alloy	Threaded Screw	2	Machined	Threading	8, 10, 13, 15	3.75	<1500	Yes	Prefabricated Threaded	Fixed Bridges Overdentures Fixed detacha bridges
		Cylinder		TPS	Surface Texture		4.0				
Astra	Titanium CP	Threaded Screw	2	Machined roughened	Threading	8, 9, 11, 13, 15, 17, 19 11, 13, 15, 17	3.5, 4.0 4.5	1500	Yes	Prefabricated Threaded	Fixed Bridges Overdentures Fixed detacha bridges
Bicon	Titanium CP HA Coated TPS Coated	Threaded Screw	2	Machined	Threading	8, 11, 14	3.5, 4.0, 5.0	50	No	Locking Taper	Fixed Bridges Overdentures Fixed detacha bridges
BioHorizons Division A D1 Unit	Titanium Alloy	Threaded Screw	2	Machined RBM	Threading	9, 10	4, 5	1500	No	Prefabricated Threaded	Fixed Bridges Overdentures Fixed detacha bridges

Product	Material	Shape		Surface		Length	Diameter		Single Tooth	Abutment	Applications
D2 Unit	Titanium Alloy			Machined RBM		10, 11	4, 5				
D3 Unit	Titanium Alloy TPS			Machined		11, 12	4, 5				
D4 Unit	Titanium Alloy HA Ti alloy			Machined		12, 13	4, 5				
Division B	RBM TPS Titanium Alloy HA			Machined		12 13 9, 10	3.5 3.5 4, 5				
Division C-H	Titanium Alloy HA										
Dental Implant Systems Inc. Titanium CP		Threaded Tapering Cylinder	2	Machined and micron bead blasted	Threading	11 (not for 4.5), 13, 15	3.5, 4.0, 4.5	<1500	Yes	Prefabricated Cementable	Fixed Bridges Overdentures Fixed detacha bridges
B.A.S.I.C. Duo-Dent Titanium HA and TPS		Press fit	2	Roughened	Surface Texture	8, 10, 12, 14, 16, 18	3.25, 4	<1000	Yes	Prefabricated Threaded	Fixed Bridges Overdentures Fixed detacha bridges
Friatec Frialit-2 Titanium		Stepped Cylinder Stepped Screw Threaded Screw	2	Frios TPS	Stepped surface texture	11, 13, 15 8, 10, 13, 15	3.8 4.5, 5.5	<1500	Yes	Prefabricated Threaded	Fixed Bridges Overdentures Fixed detacha bridges
IMCOR Titanium CP		Threaded Screw	2	Machined	Threading	8.5, 10, 11.5, 13, 15, 18 8, 10, 12	3.75, 4.0 5.0	<1500	Yes	N/A	Fixed Bridges Overdentures Fixed detacha bridges
IMTEC Corporation Titanium CP		Threaded Screw Cylinder	2	Machined HA Machined TPS TPS&HA	Threading Surface Texture	8, 10, 13, 15, 20 5, 8, 11, 13 8, 10, 13, 15	3.75 5.25 3.3, 3.4, 4, 4.75	<1500	Yes	Prefabricated Threaded	Fixed Bridges Overdentures Fixed detacha bridges
Innova Titanium Alloy		Press fit	2	beaded porous	Surface Texture	7, 9, 12	3.5, 4.1, 5	700	Yes	Prefabricated Threaded	Fixed Bridges Overdentures Fixed detacha bridges

Continued

Table 4-2   Root Form Selection Chart—cont'd

NAME	MATERIAL	CHARACTER AND MODE	STAGES	SURFACE	PRIMARY RETENTION	LENGTH (MM)	DIAMETER (MM)	RECOMMENDED RPM	INTERNAL COOLING	ABUTMENTS	RESTORATIVE OPTIONS
LifeCore Restore:	Titanium CP	Threaded Screw	2	Machined	Threading	8, 10, 11.5, 13, 15, 18, 20	3.3, 3.75, 4, 5, 5.5, 6	<1500	Yes	Prefabricated Threaded	Fixed Bridges Overdentures Fixed detacha bridges
	Titanium RBM	Threaded Screw 3mm smooth neck		Machined Resorbable blast Media	Threading	8, 10, 11.5, 13, 15	3.3, 3.75, 4, 5.6				
	Titanium TPS	Threaded Screw		Machined Titanium Plasma spray	Threading	8, 10, 11, 11.5, 13, 15, 18, 20	3.3, 2.75, 4, 5				
		Cylinder			Surface Texture	8, 10, 13, 15, 18	3.4, 4, 5				
	Titanium Alloy	Cylinder		HA		8, 10, 13, 15, 18	3.4, 4				
Sustain:	Titanium Alloy	Threaded Screw		HA	Threading	8, 10, 11.5, 13, 15, 18, 20	3.3, 3.75, 4, 5				
	Titanium Alloy	Cylinder & Cylinder without machined collar		HA	Surface Texture	8, 10, 13, 15, 18	3.4, 4.2, 5				
		Cylinder		HA Internal Bevel			3.3, 4.0, 4.7				
Nobel-Biocare (Brånemark)	Titanium CP	a. threaded screw, bone tapping b. Conical	2	Machined	Threading	7, 10, 13, 15, 18, 20	3.75	2000 Bone tap, 15-20	No	Prefabricated Threaded	Fixed Bridges Overdentures Fixed detacha bridges
	Titanium CP	threaded screw self tapping	2	Machined	Threading	7, 10, 13, 15, 18	4.0		No	Prefabricated Threaded	Fixed Bridges Overdentures Fixed detacha bridges
Osteomed	Titanium CP	Cylinder	2	TPS	Surface Texture	8, 10, 13, 15	3.3	<1500	Yes	Prefabricated Threaded	Fixed Bridges Overdentures Fixed detacha bridges
Hextrac		Threaded Screw		HA over TPS							
				Machined and Machined HA Machined	Threading	8, 10, 13, 16, 20 / 8, 11, 13	3.75 / 5.2				

System	Product	Material	Shape	Stage	Surface	Feature	Lengths	Diameters			Type	Applications
Paragon (Internal Hex)	Screw-vent	Titanium Alloy	Threaded Screw	1	HA TPS Acid etched	Threading	8, 10, 13, 16	3.3, 3.7, 4.7	<1500	Yes	Prefabricated Threaded	Fixed Bridges Overdentures Fixed detacha bridges
				2	HA TPS							
	External Hex Swede-Vent (there is an external hex design available)			1	Acid Etched HA TPS		8, 10, 13, 15 18	4				
				2								
Park Dental Research	Star-Vent (star★lock system, and external hex system. Only star★lock has single stage and two stage fixtures)	Titanium CP	Threaded Screw		Machined	Threading Self tapping	8, 11, 14, 17 8, 11, 14, 17	3.3 3.8 4.5 5.0	<1000	Yes	Prefabricated Threaded Cementable	Fixed Bridges Overdentures Fixed-detacha bridges
		Titanium Plasma Spray		1		Threading	8, 11, 14, 17	3.3 3.8 4.5 5.0				
				2		Threading						
				1		Press fit	8, 11, 14, 17	3.3 4.0				
		HA Coated				Threading	8, 11, 14, 17	3.3 4.0				
				2		Threading	8, 11, 14, 17	3.3 3.8 4.5 5.0				
						Press fit	8, 11, 14, 17	3.3 4.0				
Sargon Dental Implants		Titanium Alloy	Apically expandable quintapodal screw	1	Machined	Expanded apical portion	13	3.8 expandable	Hand Placement	n/a	Prefabricated Threaded	Fixed Bridges Overdentures
Steri-Oss	Non-Hexed	Titanium Alloy	Cylinder	2	HA	Surface Texture	8, 10, 12, 14, 16, 18	3.25, 3.8	<2000	Yes	Prefabricated Threaded	Fixed Bridges Overdentures Fixed-detacha bridges
			Threaded Screw		TPS	Threading						
			Threaded Screw		Machined and HA							
	Hexed (external)	Titanium CP	Threaded Screw		Machined HA TPS	Threading		.25, 3.8, 4.5, 5, 6 (only up to 14mm)				
			Cylinder		HA and TPS	Surface Texture	8, 10, 12, 14, 16, 18	3.25, 3.8, 5				
	Replace		Threaded			Threading						

Continued

Table 4-2 Root Form Selection Chart—cont'd

NAME	MATERIAL	CHARACTER AND MODE	STAGES	SURFACE	PRIMARY RETENTION	LENGTH (MM)	DIAMETER (MM)	RECOMMENDED RPM	INTERNAL COOLING	ABUTMENTS	RESTORATIVE OPTIONS
Steri-Oss, cont'd	Titanium Alloy	Screw Solid Screw		Machined, HA, and TPS	Threading	10, 13, 16	4.3, 5, 6				
Straumann ITI Dental Implant System:	CP Titanium Titanium Plasma spray	Solid Screw	All single stage	Machined				<800	No	Prefabricated threaded, Morse taper connection Octasystem	Fixed bridges Overdentures Fixed-detacha bridges
Standard Implants		Hollow cylinder (straight and 15° angled)			Implant design	8, 10, 12	3.5				
		Solid Screw Hollow screw			Threading	8, 10, 12, 14, 16	4.1				
Reduced Diameter Implants		Solid screw				8, 10, 12, 14,16	3.3				
Wide Diameter		Solid screw				8, 10	4.8				
Narrow Neck		Solid screw		Shoulder width 3.5		8, 10, 12, 14	3.3				
Esthetic Plus		Hollow cylinder (straight and 15° angled)			Implant design	9, 11, 13	3.5				
		Solid screw									
Sulzer Calcitek	Titanium Alloy	Threaded Screw	2	Machined HA TPS Microtexture	Threading	9, 11, 13	3.3, 4.1	<1500	Yes	Prefabricated Threaded	Fixed Bridges Overdentures Fixed detacha bridges
Spline Implant		Cylinder		HA TPS	Threading	8, 10, 13, 15, 18	3.75, 5 (no 18mm)				
		Cylinder			Surface Texture		3.25, 4, 5 (no 18mm)				
Integral Implant		Cylinder		HA		8, 10, 13, 15	3.25, 4				Not for single units
Omniloc		Cylinder		HA							For single and multiple units on top
ThreadLoc		Threaded Screw		HA TPS	Threading	8, 10, 13, 15, 18	3.75				
Vancouver Implant Resources	Titanium CP	Cylinder	2	HA TPS	Surface Texture	8, 10, 13, 15	3, 3.25, 4	<1500	Yes	Prefabricated Threaded	Fixed Bridges Overdentures Fixed detacha bridges

For specific information, illustrations, and directions for insertion, refer to Chapters 10 and 11.

Table 4-3   Blade Selection Chart

NAME	MATERIAL	STAGES	SURFACE	MODIFIABLE	No. HEADS
Park Startanius	Titanium CP*	2	Fine texture	Yes	1 or 2
Park PD	Titanium CP	1	Stippled	Yes	1, 2, or 3
Miter Titanodont	Ti, Va, Al	2	Smooth	Yes	1 or 2
Ultimatics	Titanium CP	1 & 2	Textured	Yes	1, 2, or 3
Omni B-Series	Titanium CP	2	Sand-blasted	Custom designed	1
Oratronics	Titanium CP	1 & 2	Tissue-textured finish	Yes	1 and 2
Calcitek Bioblade	Titanium CP	2	Hydroxyapatite-(HA) coating	No	1 and 2
Core-Vent Sub-Vent	Titanium CP	2	Acid etched smooth	Yes	1
Stryker	Ti, Va, Al	2	Plasma sprayed or HA coating	Yes No	1 and 2
Denar	Ti, Va, Al	2	Machined smooth	Yes	1
Impladent	Titanium CP	1	Smooth, optional HA coating	No, 3-dimensional blade	1 and 2

*CP: commercially pure

geon. Nothing can compare with direct clinical views and intraoperative measurements and judgments (Figs. 4-49, 4-50).

Notes

A measurement is made and recorded between the ridge crest and one of the following four anatomic structures:

1. Mandibular canal
2. Antral floor
3. Nasal floor
4. Inferior border of mandible (symphysis area) (CT imaging helps)

If narrow crestal bone can be flattened to create a sufficiently wide plateau to permit placement of root form implants, depth will have been sacrificed and must be reassessed.

Root form implants have diameters that vary from 3.25 to 6.3 mm and from 7 to 20 mm in length. (Most often, 1 mm of additional bone depth is required.) Table 4-2 on root form selection describes each system according to available implant types and dimensions (Fig. 4-51).

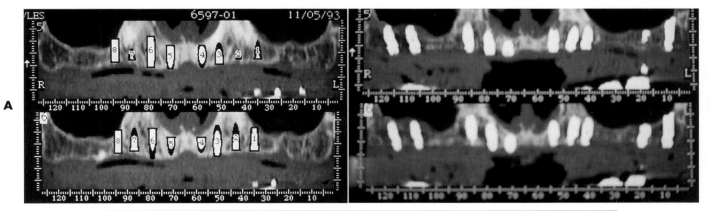

Fig. 4-49 These two panoramic images produced by Dentascan were made 6 months apart. The first view indicates the sites and locations of eight implants recommended by the radiologist. After a review of the unadorned preoperative cross sections and corroborated intraoperatively, only four of the recommended sites were selected for actual implantations, and none of the suggested sizes was chosen. Six additional sites, not recommended by the radiologist, were used.

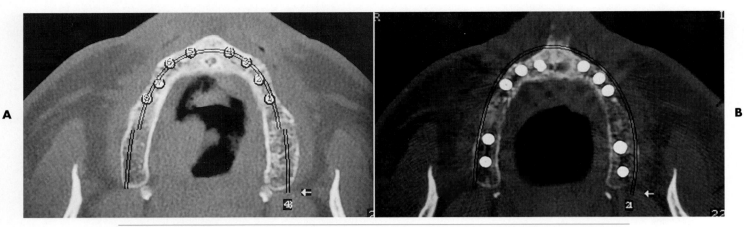

Fig. 4-50 These occlusal images reinforce the selection of 10 sites **(A)** rather than 8 **(B)** and give a more satisfactory distribution of implant locations. The averages of dimension (width and length of implants divided by the number of implants) was 40% greater clinically than those suggested. Fig. 4-50, *A* is the Dentascan with suggested host site. Fig 4-50, *B* is the image made after the actual had been placed.

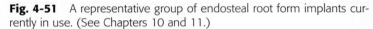

Fig. 4-51 A representative group of endosteal root form implants currently in use. (See Chapters 10 and 11.)

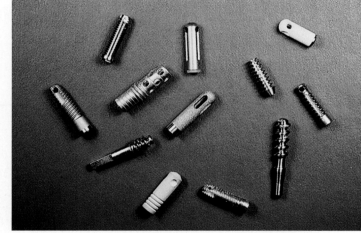

If findings do not meet the bone requirements for root forms, see Chapters 11, 12, 13, 14, 15, 17, and 18 (describing subperiosteal, blade, transosteal, Crête Mince, threaded dowels, and intramucosal insert techniques).

Spacing between root form implants should equal the diameter of one implant.

The maximum number of implants need not be placed. Information to assist in choosing the appropriate number of implants is found in subsequent chapters on prosthetic designs.

In less dense bone, the implantologist should use the largest number of implants that available space permits, even if their diameters are of the smallest categories. Rough (TPS, HA) coatings help as well, by presenting maximal interfacial areas.

Photography

A significant part of the preoperative workup must include intraoral and facial photography. The facial views should include lateral and full face with a plain beige or light blue background. Do not place the lighting so that a shadow of the patient's face and head is cast on the background.

Intraoral photography is best taken using glare-proof, plastic lip retractors and including a variety of views to demonstrate each area of importance. Front surface mirrors, warmed to prevent fogging, are of benefit in recording palatal anatomy.

Intraoperative photography is of value as a teaching aid as well as to document various phases of treatment for medicolegal reasons. For these purposes, dull-coated retractors offer the best photographic opportunities because the strobe light of the photographic unit does not disturb the image with a blinding glare. Beaver tail and other retractors can be coated with matte finished Teflon inexpensively.

There are many well-known photographic units, but the simplest to use with a high level of successful pictures is the Yashica Dental Eye Two.

Surgical Anatomy

A knowledge of anatomy is essential to the implant surgeon. Whether the plan is to insert an endosteal or subperiosteal implant, certain critical landmarks and boundaries must be kept constantly in mind. This section lists and describes those foramina canals, and their contents, natural cavities, and other potential anatomic pitfalls that can be responsible for complications and failures (Figs. 4-52 through 4-56). To prepare for a problem that might present itself during surgery despite careful presurgical planning, consult Chapter 9.

1. Foramina
   a. Infraorbital (IN)
   b. Greater palatine (G)
   c. Lesser palatine (L)
   d. Incisive (IF)
   e. Mandibular (M)
   f. Mental (ME)
   g. Cervical colli (CC)
2. Canals
   a. Mandibular (MC)
   b. Mental (MT)
   c. Palatine (PC)
   d. Incisive (IC)
3. Fossae
   a. Canine (CF)
   b. Incisive (IS)
   c. Submandibular (SF)
   d. Sublingual (SL)
4. Cavities
   a. Nasal (NC)
   b. Antral (AC)
5. Nerves and neurovascular bundles
   a. Mandibular (MN)
   b. Greater palatine (GN)
   c. Mental (ML)
   d. Infraorbital (IR)
   e. Incisive (IV)
   f. Lingual (LN)
   g. Long buccal (LB)

The anatomic structures described and illustrated demonstrate the most commonly found landmarks in the average adult patient. Of course, many variations exist, and the surgeon should be prepared for surprises, such as extra foramina (i.e., mental, lingual mandibular for cervical colli), double neurovascular bundles, deeper-than-average fossae, and plunging nasal or maxillary sinus cavities.

In addition, certain landmarks are of importance when performing the surgery described in subsequent chapters. These landmarks are as follows:

Anterior nasal spine (AS)
Zygomatic buttress (ZB)
Hamulus (H)
Lateral pterygoid plate (LP)

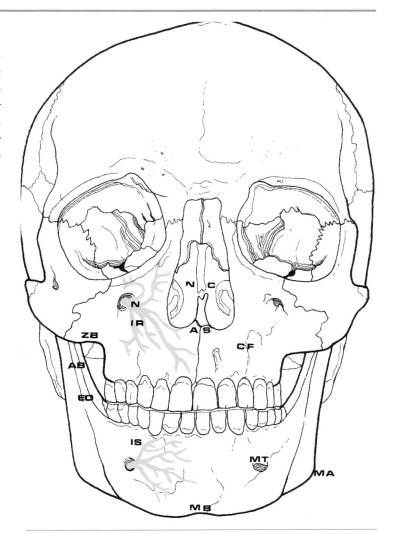

Fig. 4-52 Frontal view of the skull. *IN*, Infraorbital foramen; *NC*, nasal cavities; *ZB*, zygomatic buttress; *IR*, infraorbital neurovascular bundle; *AS*, anterior nasal spine; *CF*, canine fossa; *AB*, anterior border, mandibular ramus; *EO*, external oblique ridge, mandible; *MT*, mental foramen or canal; *MA*, angle of mandible; *MB*, mental protuberance.

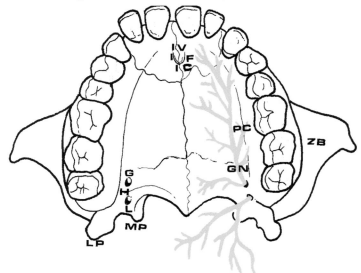

Fig. 4-53 Inferior view of maxillary and palatial bones. *IV*, Incisive neurovascular bundle; *IF*, incisive foramen; *IC*, incisive canal; *PC*, palatine canal; *G*, greater (anterior) palatine foramen; *GN*, greater palatine neurovascular bundle; *ZB*, zygomatic buttress; *H*, hamulus; *L*, lesser (posterior) palatine foramen; *MP*, medial pterygoid plate; *LP*, lateral pterygoid plate.

Medial pterygoid plate (MP)
Mental protuberance (MB)
Mylohyoid ridge (MH)
External oblique ridge (EO)
Mandibular angle (MA)
Sigmoid notch (SN)
Anterior border of ramus (AB)

Careful attention to the guidance offered on p. 27 of this chapter, Diagnostic Methods, coupled with a thorough knowledge of anatomy, places the clinician in the best position to perform the surgery with the fewest number of unexpected complications.

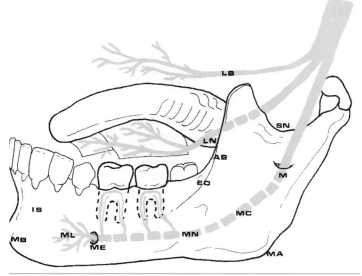

Fig. 4-55   Lateral view of mandible. *LB,* Long buccal nerve (actually crosses into buccal vestibule anterior to AB); *LN,* lingual nerve; *SN,* sigmoid notch; *AB,* anterior border, mandibular ramus; *M,* mandibular foramen; *EO,* external oblique ridge mandible; *IS,* incisive fossa; *MB,* mental protuberance; *ML,* mental neurovascular bundle; *ME,* mental foramen; *MN,* mandibular neurovascular bundle; *MC,* mandibular canal; *MA,* mandibular angle.

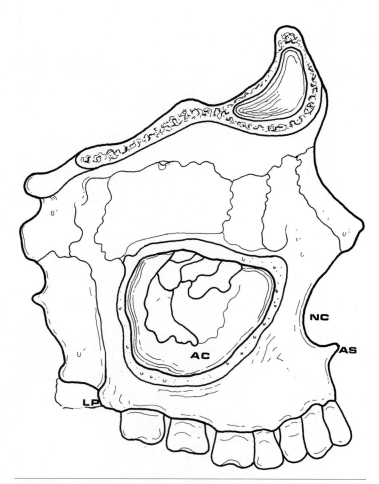

Fig. 4-54   Sagittal view of facial skeleton. *LP,* Lateral pterygoid plate; *AC,* antral cavity; *NC,* nasal cavity; *AS,* anterior nasal spine.

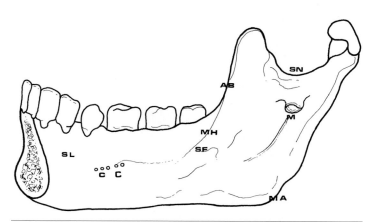

Fig. 4-56   Medial view of mandible. *SN,* Sigmoid notch; *AB,* anterior border, mandibular ramus; *M,* mandibular foramen; *MH,* mylohyoid ridge, mandible; *SF,* submandibular fossa; *SL,* sublingual fossa; *CC,* foramina for cervical colli branches; *MA,* mandibular angle.

Staging

After the implant patient who has satisfied the prescribed criteria has been selected, the diagnostic methods have been performed, and a decision made as to which implant system should be used based on this thorough workup, prepare an organized sequence of the steps of treatment. This path should be placed into the following phases:

Phase I
 Introduction
 Relief of pain
 Elimination of acute pathologic conditions, acute infections
 Extraction of hopeless teeth
 Stabilization of occlusion

 Correction and construction of provisional restorations (fixed acrylic bridges with moderate crown preparations or transitional removable dentures), which establish proper vertical dimension, arch form, occlusal plane, function, and aesthetics

Phase II
 Preparation
 Conservative periodontal therapy
 Initial endodontic therapy
 Preimplant surgery (ridge reduction, ridge augmentation, sinus lift) (see Chapter 6) unless it is to include implant placement

 Fabrication of surgical templates
Phase III
 Surgical I
 Periodontal surgery (in nonimplant areas) (see Chapter 6)
Phase IV
 Surgical II

Implant surgery (which should include requisite periodontal surgery in these sites and adjacent regions) (see Chapters 9, 10, and 11)

Phase V
 Healing
Completion of all periodontal therapy and continuation of maintenance procedures
Completion of all endodontic therapy, further crown preparations
Phase VI
 Abutment finalization
 Uncovering of implants (if using two-stage systems, see Chapter 6)
 Final healing of permucosal areas (use of healing caps and/or abutments, see Chapter 21)
 Reevaluation and mandated extraction of any remaining natural teeth with guarded prognoses
 Final preparation of teeth
Phase VII
 Prosthodontic (see Chapters 20 and 21)
 Impressions
 Abutment completion
 Placement of prostheses, selection of cementing media if any
 Occlusal equilibration (see Chapter 26)
 Occlusal splint fabrication if indicated
Phase VIII
 Maintenance
Final maintenance and hygiene visits and home care instruction (see Chapter 29).

Suggested Readings

Anderson IC et al: A review of the intraosseous course of the nerves of the mandible, *J Oral Implantol* 17:394-403, 1991.

Bolender CL: Indications and contraindications for different types of implant therapy, *J Dent Ed* 52:757-759, 1988.

Clemente CD: A*antomy: A regional atlas of the human body.* Baltimore, 1981, Urban and Schwarzenberg.

Desjardins RP: Tissue-integrated prostheses for endentulous patients with normal and abnormal jaw relationships, *J Prosthet Dent* 59:180-187, 1988.

Eckerdal O, Kvint S: Presurgical planning for osseointegrated implants in the maxilla, *Int J Oral Maxillofac Surg* 5:722-726, 1986.

Fagan MJ et al: *Implant prosthodontics, Year Book Medical Publishers,* Chicago, 1990.

Hickey JC et al: *Boucher's prosthetic treatment for edentulous patients,* St. Louis, 1982, Mosby.

Jensen O: Site classification for the osseointegrated implant, *J Prosthet Dent* 61:228-234, 1889.

Schulte JK, Peterson TA: Occlusal and prosthetic considerations, *Calif Dent J* 64-72, 1987.

Shimura M et al: Presurgical evaluation for dental implants using a reformatting program of computed tomography: maxilla/mandible shape pattern analysis (MSPA), *J Oral Maxillofac Implants* 5:175-181, 1990.

Shulman LB: Surgical considerations in implant dentistry, *J Dent Ed* 52:712-720, 1988.

Stella JP, Tharanon W: A precise radiographic method to determine the location of the inferior alveolar canal in the posterior edentulous mandible: Implications for dental implants. Part I: Technique. Part II: Clinical application, *J Oral Maxillofac Implants* 5:15-30, 1990.

Wilson EJ: Ridge mapping for determination of alveolar ridge width, *J Oral Maxillofac Implants* 4:41-43, 1989.

5

Prosthetic Options That Influence Implant Selections

*B*efore the implant type, number, and location, selection of a final prosthesis design is mandatory. The principles outlined here should be read and understood to clarify these decisions. In subsequent chapters, greater detail describes the fabrication of each implant-supported modality.

The patient presents with either a completely or a partially edentulous arch. Either condition may be restored with removable, fixed-detachable (removed only by the dentist), or cemented prostheses, which are placed directly into or onto the implant or implants or onto a bar that has been attached to them. Implant-borne prostheses often consist of two separate parts: mesostructure bars and superstructures (Figs. 5-1, 5-2). *Superstructures* are defined as the final or tooth-bearing portion of implant prostheses, and they may be single crowns, complete overdentures, or any of the variety of prostheses that fall in between, such as fixed bridges, fixed-detachable bridges, or combinations. In cases of overdentures, they are sometimes attached to coping bar splints. These splints are called *mesostructures* and can be affixed to implants or implant and tooth combinations. When planning final restorations, determine whether the prosthesis is being designed to replace teeth, teeth and soft tissue, or teeth, soft tissue, and bone. The more soft tissue and bone to be replaced, the greater the height that is required of the restoration. Depending on how much hard and soft tissue need to be replaced, planning is necessary to include more implant support in direct relationship to prosthesis size and height. Restorations supported solely by implants always require a greater number of them than the implant and soft tissue–supported prosthesis. Implant therapy allows for employment of the prosthodontic options described later.

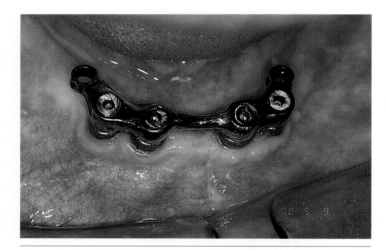

Fig. 5-1 A fixed-detachable bar using root form implants for anchorage is designed to support and retain an overdenture.

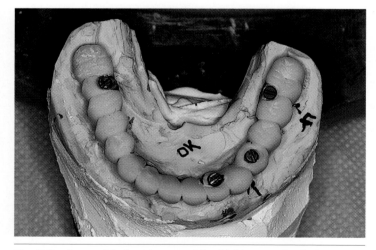

Fig. 5-2 A porcelain-fused-to-metal fixed bridge prosthesis that serves as a fixed-detachable superstructure. The natural teeth in this case are protected by cemented gold copings.

Superstructures

Overdentures

Overdentures can be classified as either soft tissue–borne and implant– or tooth-borne or purely implant-borne. Soft tissue/implant-borne overdentures are supported by the implants and the soft tissues and retained by the implants. In order for this to be practical in the parasymphyseal area, the retainers (implants or teeth) must be in a position that allows the construction of a straight bar (Fig. 5-3). This permits several internal clips to rotate around the bar and allow the posterior overdenture saddles to be soft tissue–borne so that they may take some of the stress from the implants or teeth. If the bar is placed in the anterior region and because of implant location, must be curved to conform to the shape of the arch, the overdenture will not rotate on the bar, and the posterior saddles may act as levers tending to loosen the retaining screws, cement, abutments, or the implants themselves (Fig. 5-4).

Whenever possible, splinting of implants with bars and copings rather then using them individually is the preferable approach from an engineering point of view. Depending on the location, number of implants placed, their length, the percentage of surface area surrounded by bone (osseointegration), and type of retention devices selected (clips, O-rings, Zest, Ceka, ERA), various mesostructure bar shapes and configurations are available. Bar-borne overdentures are both supported and retained by their bars (Figs. 5-5, 5-6), which, in

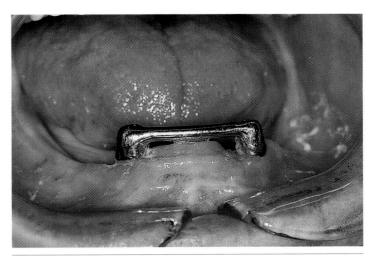

Fig. 5-3 Two root form implants support this coping bar splint. In order for the superstructure-overdenture to distribute stress to the posterior ridges, the bar must be straight to allow Hader clip retainers to rotate during masticatory function.

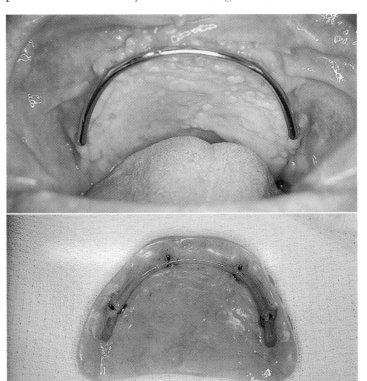

A

B

Fig. 5-5 **A,** This maxillary pterygohamular subperiosteal implant is designed with a Brookdale bar, which offers total implant-borne support of the superstructure. **B,** A denture superstructure, which is designed to be bar-retained with internal clips.

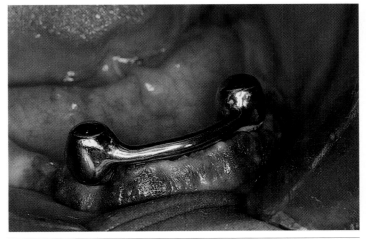

Fig. 5-4 In instances of splinting implants that require a curved bar, to allow for tongue space, the superstructure attachment must be made to permit rotation (i.e., "sloppy fit") (see Fig. 5-15).

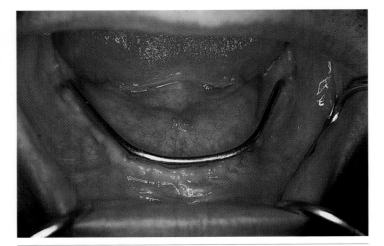

Fig. 5-6 Mandibular subperiosteal implant with a Brookdale bar designed to offer full infrastructural support.

turn, should be supported by four or more root form implants of 10 mm length or greater, by transosteals, or by subperiosteal implants.

Fixed Bridges

Fixed bridges may be supported completely by implants, or they may be used in conjunction with natural tooth abutments (Figs. 5-7, 5-8,). In both instances, construction is begun after transepithelial abutment (TEA) placement (by spline, frictional fit, or threading) and completed using the prosthetic techniques with which the clinician is most comfortable. Various attachments or interlocks between the implants and the natural abutments may be chosen (such as DE Hinges, Dalbo, Crismani, Mini Rest, Tube and Screw). These provide stress-breaking features that may be important, since the sup-

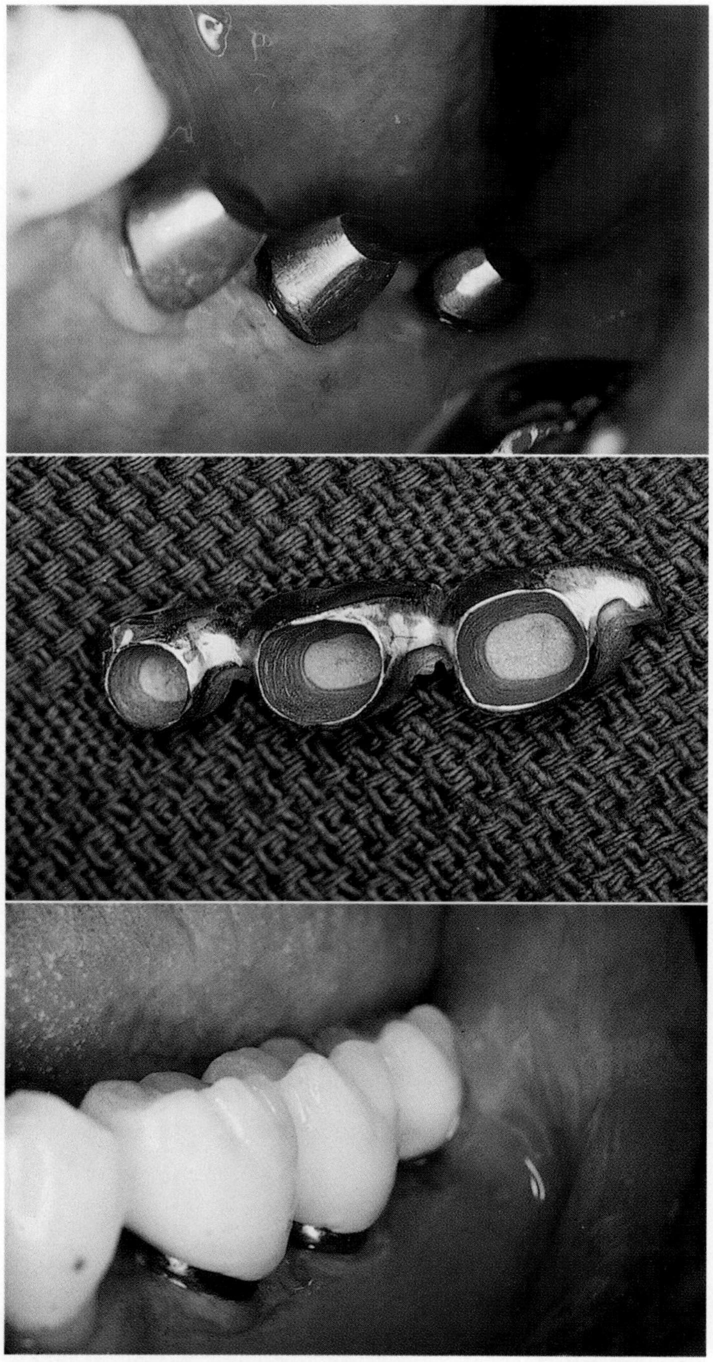

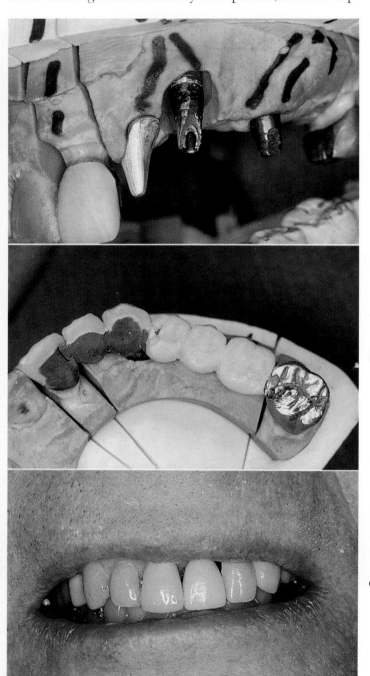

Fig. 5-7 **A,** Completely implant-supported fixed prostheses often are used when osseointegration has been established. These three abutments are prepared to receive a cement-retained bridge. **B,** These three castings were splinted to allow force distribution. **C,** The porcelain-baked-to-noble-metal fixed prosthesis is cemented into position over the three implant abutments.

Fig. 5-8 **A,** Cemented implant abutments may be coupled with those of natural teeth by the use of precision attachments or other interlock devices. Transfer of the relationship of all abutments is made to a working cast. **B,** The components of the fixed prosthesis are fabricated with interlocks placed at strategic sites. These will allow for the varying support mechanisms of natural and implant abutments. **C,** When implants are managed with interlocks, esthetic and physiologic restorations are created.

port mechanisms differ so dramatically between implants and natural teeth.

Fixed-Detachable Bridges

The fixed-detachable bridge is a prosthesis that may be removed by the dentist but not by the patient. The method of fixation is by screws that attach the bridge to the implants, to their abutments, or to an interposed mesostructure bar. These prostheses are most often completely implant borne (Fig. 5-9). However, natural tooth abutments may be incorporated into implant bridges by the use of semiprecision attachments

or internally threaded telescopic copings (Fig. 5-10). The techniques used in producing fixed-detachable bridges are by far the most complicated to perform, and the opportunities for error are high. Before selecting this method, review Chapters 22, 23, and 24. The benefits of being able to remove these bridges must be equated with the difficulties in fabrication, the costs, the potential for postinsertion complications, and the restoring dentist's willingness to manage them.

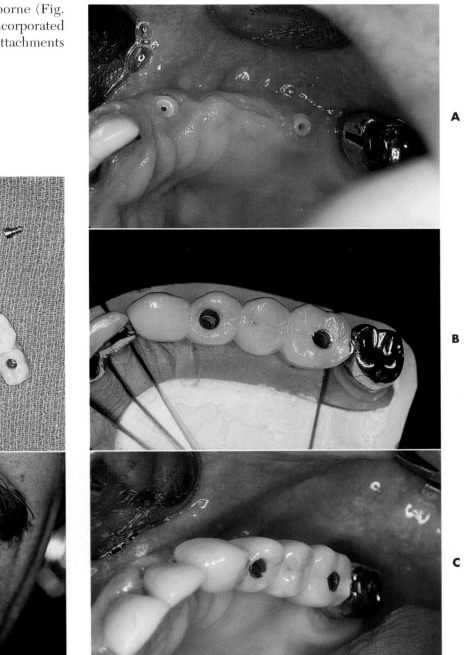

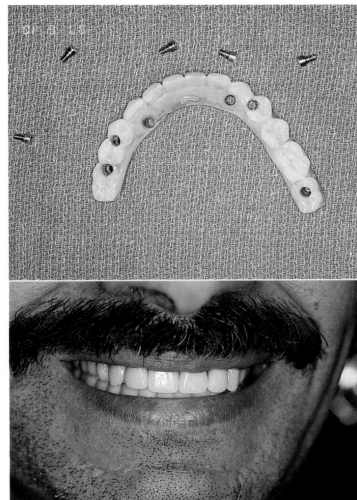

Fig. 5-9 A, A completely implant-supported fixed prosthesis requires a minimum of five to six implant abutments, but additional evenly distributed support is of benefit. Cantilevering of 10 to 15 mm bilaterally may be allowed. This maxillary prosthesis satisfies these requirements. **B,** Fixed-detachable prostheses may be completed with composite materials (Isocet) or porcelain. Hygiene is facilitated by both abutment and pontic design and the ease of removability.

Fig. 5-10 A, Two osseointegrated root form implants have been placed adjacent to a molar casting with a mesial female attachment. **B,** The completed ceramo-metal, fixed-detachable prosthesis contains a male attachment for coupling the molar and is fastened with implant-retained screws. **C,** Prostheses that are designed in this manner offer the benefits of fixed appliances with the advantage of retrievability.

Single Crowns

Single tooth prostheses may be fabricated in one of two ways. An implant-borne crown should be made that does not involve rigid dependence on any of the adjacent teeth (Fig. 5-11). It must merely abut to a single implant. Such implants must possess antirotational features (i.e., hex, spline, cold weld) (see Chapter 3). If there is a question of adequate support, an implant-borne crown may be connected with a semiprecision attachment to one or even several adjacent crowns (Fig. 5-12). Fixed rigid attachment is to be discouraged, however, unless the natural abutments are protected with telescopic copings. When such placement is performed, the practitioner must become aware of the phenomenon of natural tooth root intrusion, particularly when temporary cements have been used.

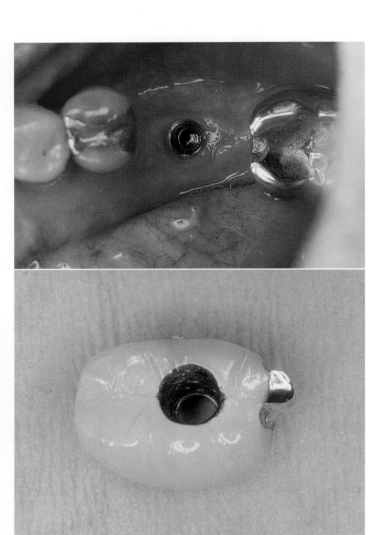

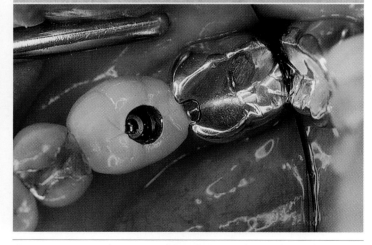

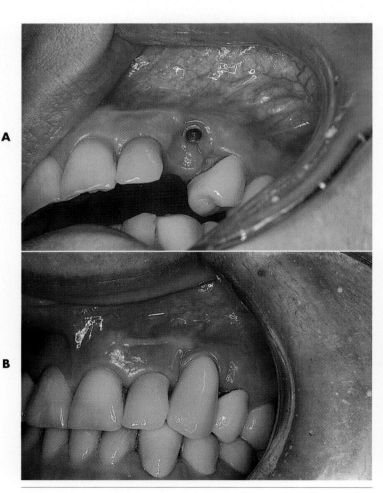

Fig. 5-11   A, Single tooth restorations may be placed on freestanding implants. The only requirement is an antirotational component, such as a hexagonal design. **B,** The completed casting is retrievable because it is screw retained.

Fig. 5-12   A, Another acceptable solution to the single tooth implant-borne replacement is to create an interlock in an adjacent natural tooth. **B,** Such an arrangement offers additional support, particularly for a longer-than-usual span, and prevents rotation as well. **C,** The completed prosthesis is functional, distributes stress intelligently, and offers an esthetic solution to the problem of a single missing molar. Generally, it is recommended that molars be replaced with two implants. (Refer to Chapter 22.)

Mesostructure Bars

The mesostructure bar acts as a connector between the implant complex (infrastructure) and the superstructure. Not all reconstructions employ such bars (Figs. 5-13, 5-14). For example, if one or several implants have been inserted and the transepithelial abutments have been attached, crowns and pontics may be made in the classic manner. In fact, all of the systems described in Chapters 10 and 11 can employ the commonly used fixed bridge superstructure design, which, when their locations allow, may be made directly on their abutments without mesostructure devices. Multiple blade reconstructions, however, because they do not osseointegrate, often employ coping bar and overdenture prostheses. Mesostructures may be designed in many forms: continuous bars or noncontinous bilateral bars, with a broad variety of shapes to permit the use of internal clips, O-rings, or withdrawable pins (i.e., Lew attachments).

Continuous Bars

Continuous bars come in different shapes. They can be round, ovoid, rectangular, or square. The amount of implant support, the location in the arch of that support, and the type of retentive devices that are chosen determines bar shape. If a desired shape is not readily available, a custom-casting is required. Superstructures may (1) simply rest on the bar ("sloppy fit," which requires occasional acrylic relining) (Fig. 5-15); (2) be attached to the bar or locked under it by the use of a variety of unique attachments, either custom made or manufactured (Fig. 5-16); (3) be secured by supplementary attachments incorporated into or onto the bar (such as O-rings, ERAs, or Zest attachments (Fig. 5-17); or (4) be used in conjunction with a fixed-detachable or cementable superstructure that was made because faulty implant angulation made fabrication of a fixed superstructure impossible to complete. In such situations, the

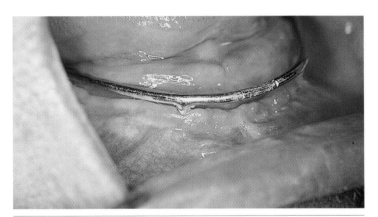

Fig. 5-13 This mesostructure bar is an integral part of a mandibular subperiosteal implant and serves as a retentive device for a denture superstructure. Such bars distribute forces more evenly than individual abutments.

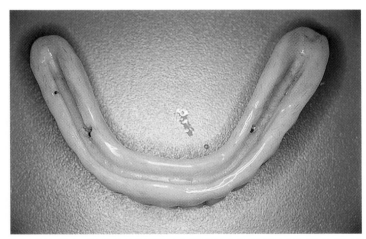

Fig. 5-15 This overdenture, designed to fit over a Brookdale bar, gains additional retention by occasional relining directly in the mouth. Such relationships are termed *sloppy fit.*

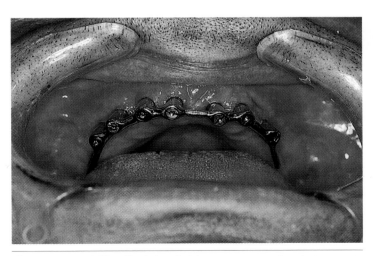

Fig. 5-14 A maxillary fixed-detachable mesostructure bar that serves to retain an overdenture is attached to root form implants by screws.

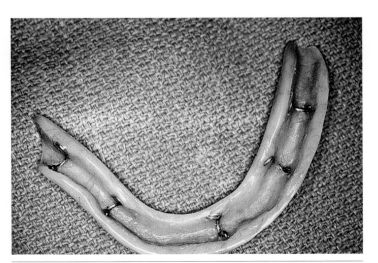

Fig. 5-16 More precise bar relationships are achieved with the use of well distributed, custom-made, high-tension steel clips (designed by Anthony Rosalia).

double-bar technique may be employed. To do this, a mesostructure bar of the optimal shape and diameter should be cast and then screwed or cemented to the malaligned implant abutments or directly into the implants themselves. This first bar must have at least three (depending on its length) internally threaded housings soldered to it and protruding at prosthetically usable angles. A second structure bar of metal or acrylic designed to hold the teeth and to be screwed into the newly fabricated first or mesostructure bar is made. Properly positioned denture teeth are processed to the second bar. (Chapter 28 offers exact details on the construction of such a double-bar prosthesis.)

Noncontinuous Bars

Noncontinuous bars fall into several categories. A mandibular subperiosteal implant with a continuous bar may have caused pain to the patient on opening the mouth. In such instances, cut the anterior (or transsymphyseal) component, thus creating bilateral bars. Some clinicians prefer this design from the outset (Fig. 5-18).

Often, because of anatomic limitations, cost, or preference, implants are placed in the canine areas, and only an anterior

bar is needed. This may be curved or straight, depending on implant location, plans of superstructure retention, and the needs for stress-breaking. Such bars are usually round in cross-section (Fig. 5-19).

In a similar manner, unilaterally placed implants, either original or residual (i.e., after other implants have been lost), may be restored with a single bar for purposes of splinting, as well as to offer a retentive source for an overdenture. These partial bar structures may use any of the attachment devices with which the clinician is most comfortable.

Methods of Bar Fixation

In almost all instances of subperiosteal implant construction, as well as in all cases of ramus frames, the bar is part of the implant casting (Fig. 5-20). In cases of the complete subperiosteal implant, the options of bar design, diameter, and location are available so that the attachments may be selected on a preinsertion basis. When a bar is prescribed for endosteal implants, it may be attached in the classic fixed-detachable manner (as described in Chapter 25) or by simple cementation. Details on bars and overdentures are found in Chapter 26.

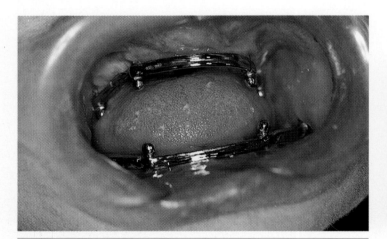

Fig 5-17   These bars have, as components of their design, round attachments designed for O-ring retention.

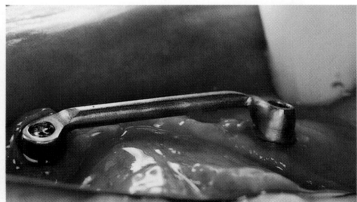

Fig. 5-19   Hader bars perform most favorably when they are straight. To make this possible, place a small offset extension on the right casting. This mesostructure complex, which is attached to two osseointegrated implants, is a single-piece casting.

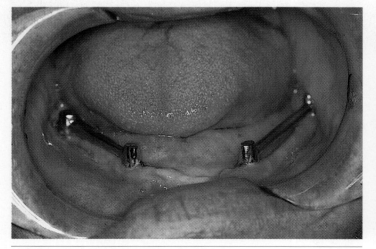

Fig. 5-18   Bilateral Brookdale bars may be used for overdenture retention in instances in which mandibular flexion is considered a factor or for other design philosophies.

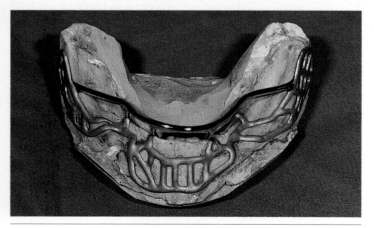

Fig. 5-20   Although bars may be attached separately to subperiosteal implants, the usual method of construction is by casting them as a single entity with the infrastructure framework, as shown in this mandibular design.

Types of Superstructure Attachments

When multiple implants have been inserted and connected with coping bar splints, several methods of overdenture retention are available. These are magnets, custom clips, Hader clips of plastic or gold, Dolder clips, Ceka attachments, Zest, Zag, anchors, Octalinks, O-rings, ERA attachments, pin locks, and Lew attachments (Figs. 5-21 through 5-25).

Make an accurate elastomeric impression of the abutments (which varries slightly from system to system), and from these, the implant prosthetic laboratory incorporates the selected attachments onto a cast bar. Table 5-1 lists the benefits and shortcomings of each of the more popular systems.

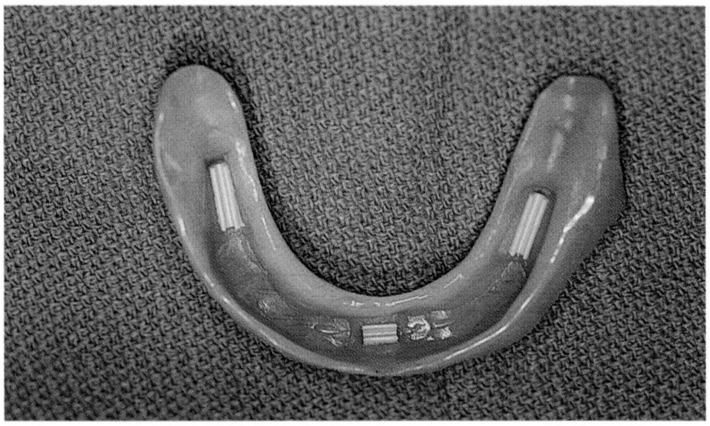

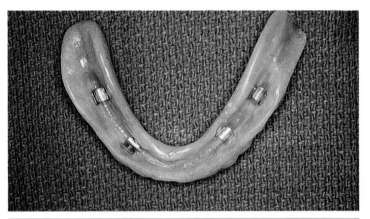

Fig. 5-21 Attachment mechanics are supplied by plastic Hader clips in this overdenture. They are easily replaceable when retention is lost.

Fig. 5-22 Gold Hader clips are more durable than plastic but more demanding to replace.

Table 5-1   Attachments

ATTACHMENT	ADVANTAGE	SHORTCOMINGS
Magnets	Easy to use Easy to repair No stress relief	Questionable retention Poor lateral stability Corrosive Loosen or unthread Expensive
Ceka, Octa-link	Easy to use Easy to repair Good retention Stress-breaking	Expensive Requires frequent maintenance Loosen or unthread
ERA	Adjustable retention Easy to replace Modest in cost	Need frequent replacement
Zest, O-rings	Inexpensive Good retention Stress-breaking Easy to use (O-rings)	Abutments must be parallel Less rigid than metal to metal Wear more quickly than metal
Hader, Dolder	Stress-breaking Easy to maintain Easy to repair and replace	Expensive
Pinlock, Lew	Easy to maintain Easy to use	Expensive

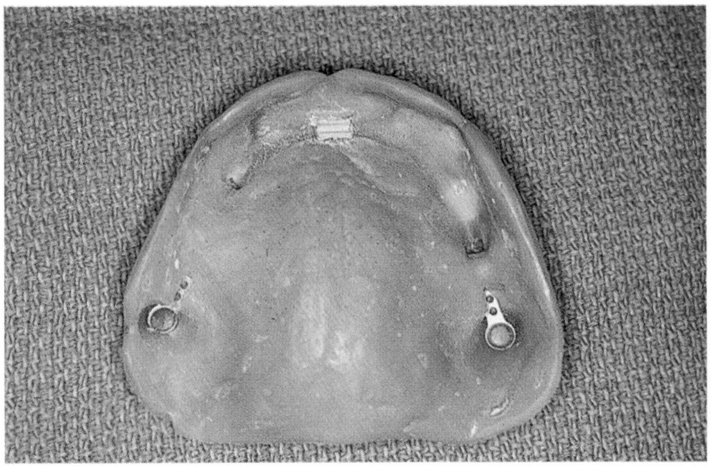

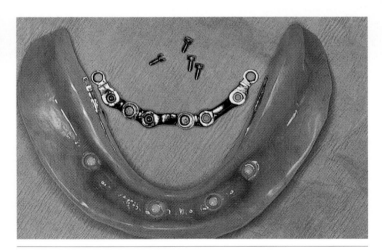

Fig. 5-23 Combinations of attachment devices, such as these anterior clip and bilateral posterior Rotherman attachments, may be used. These are of particular value when limited intermaxillary space mandates the use of short castings.

Fig. 5-24 The ERA offers male attachment placement in the overdenture and female in the mesostructure bar. The value of these devices is that the doctor may use four levels of retention by employing different males, each of which is color coded.

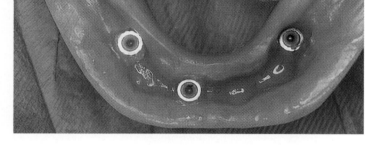

A

B

Fig. 5-25 A, Ball castings, when made part of a mesostructure bar, offer excellent sources of retention for easily renewable O-rings. **B,** The rings are snapped into special receptacles that are processed into the tissue-borne surface of the overdenture.

Transepithelial Abutments

The independent transepithelial abutment (TEA) is available for one- and two-stage (submergible) endosteal implant systems, both blade and root form (Fig. 5-26). The TEA (sometimes called *permucosal abutments*), attaches by threading directly into the implant, often passes through the soft tissues into the oral cavity and acts as an abutment for attachment of either a mesostructure bar or an anatomic superstructure (Fig. 5-27). One-stage root forms, one-stage blades, and transosteal and subperiosteal implants are fabricated with their permucosal TEAs attached. Depending on the type of submergible implant system being restored, attach the TEA to the implant in one of the following ways:

1. By screw, with or without antirotational internal or external hex, or spline
2. By press or frictional fit using the cold-weld, Morse-taper design

The portion of the TEA that is within the oral cavity can take many shapes:

1. Conventional crown preparation—straight
2. Conventional crown preparation—angled (usually at 15 to 25 degrees, but available at 30 degrees)

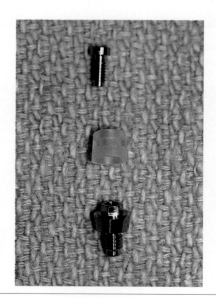

Fig. 5-26 Transepithelial abutments offer the most significant mode of attaching mesostructure bars or superstructures to integrated implants. Selection of abutments is predicated on the design of planned restorations. The middle component (pictured) represents the waxing sleeve of the superstructure that will be attached after casting to the TEA.

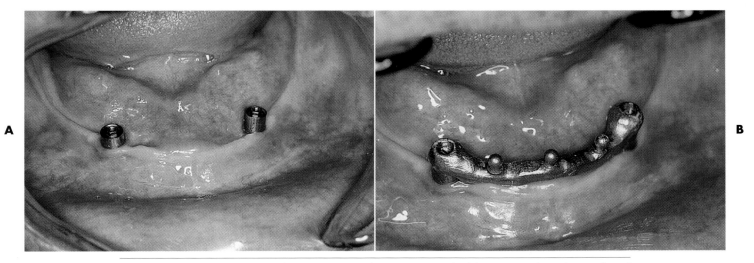

Fig. 5-27 A, The transepithelial component or abutment is attached by a screw (see Fig. 5-26) and supplies the practitioner with a variety of retention options. **B,** This mesostructure bar, one of the most frequently selected prosthetic solutions, may include any of a wide selection of attachment modalities such as these balls designed for O-rings. It is fixed to its implants by screw retention.

3. Shouldered platform
4. Shouldered platform with female attachment receptacle (e.g., Zest)
5. Shouldered platform with male attachment (e.g., O-ring)
6. Three-piece, including collars and fixation screws (e.g., Paragon)

Transepithelial abutments for each implant type are supplied by its manufacturer. However, there are some TEA systems that can be custom-cast. In addition, several companies have made a variety of abutments available that are usable with and without adaptive fittings. Individual laboratories, using manufactured patterns, may cast attachments for a wide variety of implants in any number of postures.

Since there is an overwhelming number of attachments and abutment designs available, it is recommended that practitioners become adept at using a few of the more favorite and more versatile types.

Suggested Readings

Adell R: A 15-year study of osseointegrated implants in the treatment of the edentulous jaw, *Int J Oral Surg* 6:387, 1981.

Balshi TJ: Osseointegration for the periodontally compromised patient, *Int J Prosthodont* 1:51-58, 1988.Fagan MJ et al: *Implant Prosthodontics,* Chicago, 1990, Year Book Medical Publishers.

Desjardins RP: Tissue integrated prostheses for edentulous patients with normal and abnormal jaw relationships, *J Prosthet Dent* 59:180-187, 1988.

Fagan MJ et al: *Implant Prosthodontics,* Chicago, 1990, Year Book Medical Publishers.

Finger IM, Guerra LR: Prosthetic considerations in reconstructive implantology, *Dent Clin North Am* 30:69-83, 1986.

Henderson et al: *McCracken's removable partial prosthodontics,* ed 7, St. Louis, 1985, Mosby.

Hickey JC, Zarb GA. *Boucher's prosthodontic treatment for edentulous patients,* ed 9, St. Louis, 1985, Mosby.

Misch CE: Prosthetic options in implant dentistry, *Int J Oral Implant* 17-21, 1991.

Schillingburg et al: *Fundamentals of fixed prosthodontics,* ed 2, Chicago, 1981, Quintessence.

Smith D: A review of endosseous implants for partially edentulous patients, *Int J Prosthodont* 12-19, 1990.

Sullivan DY: Prosthetic considerations for the utilization of osseointegrated fixtures in the partially edentulous arch, *J Oral Maxillofac Implants* 39-45, 1986.

6
Preparations for Implant Surgery

Armamentarium and the Operatory

M ost of the chapters in this book begin with warnings or caveats. Because this is an instructional chapter, the only warning offered is that the reader, even if he or she does not plan to perform implant surgery, should gain an understanding of the basic principles of surgery before undertaking the planning or placement of implants. Although implant surgery is less demanding and less complex than many other kinds of oral surgery presented in this chapter, the operative paths may be filled with complications. These operative paths require knowledge of management before beginning the practical endeavors in implantology. Before starting surgery, check and replenish instruments and disposable supplies as necessary. Although some of the items listed in the armamentarium may seem to be arcane or may appear unlikely to be required, their presence prepares the surgeon for virtually any unexpected occurrence (Fig. 6-1). Read this chapter at a time of leisure so that its contents can be learned completely. The reader should be able to assess the level of his or her skills before the occurrence of an incident that might require significant corrective activity.

ARMAMENTARIUM

Acrylic, self-curing
Bone files
Burs: 700 L, 701 L, 2 L, 4 L, 6 L friction grip
Curettes: surgical and periodontal
Electrical surgical unit
Explorer/millimeter probe
Forceps
    Adson (toothed and nontoothed) pickup forceps
    Gerald (toothed and nontoothed) pickup forceps
    Kelly and tonsil (curved) hemostatic forceps
    Rongeur side- and end-cutting forceps
    Wire-twisting forceps, heavy duty
Gelfoam, surgical bone wax, Avitene
Handpieces, high- and low-speed, straight and angled, Impactair
Hemostats, mosquito, Kelly
Hypodermic needles, 18 gauge disposable, 1½ inch
Local anesthetic syringes, needles, and solutions
Mallet, nylon-covered
Mirror (front surface)
3½-inch 18-gauge spinal needle with stylet for the zygoma
1½-inch needle for the mandible
Needle holders

Nerve hooks
Osteotomes: curved and straight
Periosteal elevators
Pliers
    College pliers, with plastic tips
    Titanium-tipped cone-socket pliers (2)
Polyethylene (intravenous) tubing
Prep tray for sterilizing the operative site
Retractors: sweetheart (tongue), baby Parker, blunt (Mathieu) rakes, large blunt rake, Army/Navy, beaver tail (Henahan), McBurney vein, Leahy
Sable paint brush (0-0)
Scalpel blades No. 10, 11, 12, 15
Scalpel handles (2), Bard-Parker No. 3 handles
Scissors: Metzenbaum, sharp tissue, and suture
Sponges: 2 × 2, 4 × 4
Suction tips (Yankauer and Frazier), plastic
Sutures: 3-0 black silk, 4-0 dyed Vicryl, 3-0 plain gut, 4-0 chromic gut on tapered and cutting needles
Towel clamps
Wire, monofilament No. 2 stainless steel in 12- to 18-inch lengths
Wire cutters, shears, and nippers

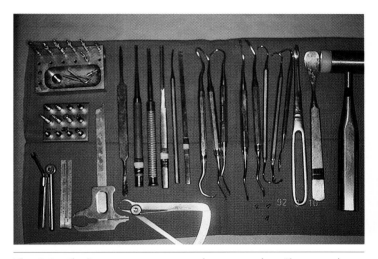

Fig. 6-1 The instrument tray serves the surgeon best if mounted on a Mayo stand, which can slide beneath the chair so that delivery can be made over the patient's chest. In addition to standard operating instruments, fiberoptic retractors, bone filters on the suction apparatus, electrosurgical equipment, and a selection of fine-toothed forceps can make the surgeon's efforts more comfortable.

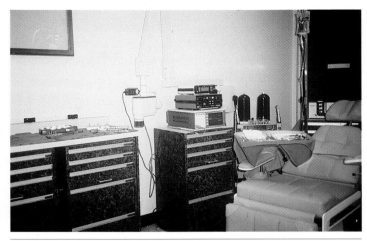

Fig. 6-2 The operatory, when possible, should be dedicated to implantology. Chair controls should be by foot, and light handles should be sterilizable. Ventilation must be excellent, and duplicate rotary instrumentation should be available. Ample countertop and storage space is mandatory, and a plentiful supply of electrical outlets and quick-release fittings for gas, air, water, vacuum suction, oxygen, and nitrous oxide provide convenience. Monitoring and resuscitation equipment, ceiling-mounted intravenous hooks, and anesthesia armboards and accouterments are helpful.

The Operatory

The office operatory is where the bulk of implant surgery procedures are performed. Attempt to incorporate the requisite equipment to perform all planned procedures so that the highest levels of convenience are afforded to the surgeon and his or her staff, and maximal comfort is available for the patient. A commodious, complete operatory helps make the treatment of patients more enjoyable. Suggestions follow in regard to some basic concepts when designing an implant operatory (Fig. 6-2).

First, make sure there is adequate space for the surgeon and two additional staff members; an operating chair; cabinetry; and sedation, monitoring, and resuscitative equipment. The chair should have foot controls to raise, lower, and recline it so that during surgery hands are not required to change its position. High- and low-power suction facilities need to be available, as well as an armboard, if sedation is planned. Positive-pressure oxygen and nitrous oxide are necessary adjuncts, and nitrogen or compressed air is required for many drilling systems. High- and low-speed handpieces as well as high-torque, low-speed implant drilling equipment are mandatory. Adequate lighting for surgery as well as appropriate side lighting for supportive procedures (i.e., mixing) should be an integral part of implant center design. A well-placed viewbox that can be seen easily during surgery must be present. An x-ray unit should be present so that intraoperative films may be taken without the necessity of moving the patient. A bracket table or Mayo stand large enough for all needed instruments must be a part of the facility. Adequate countertop and shelving area is essential to accommodate all requisite implant equipment (e.g., console, motors, handpieces, irrigation bottles), monitoring devices (e.g., Dinamap, electrocardiograph, pulse oximeter). Standby implant surgery instruments must be located conveniently and within clear visual range. An emergency tray or crash cart should be available. Other features of value are foot controls for the sink, a plentiful supply of electrical outlets above the counter (i.e., electrical strips), storage space to stock implants and prosthetic parts, a fiberoptic headlight, and adequate ventilation. All items that make for efficient, smooth, and safe treatment should be included in the plans for satisfactory implant operatory.

Surgical Delivery Systems

Ted Waller

Perhaps the most misunderstood (and most necessary) of all implant armamentaria are the surgical delivery systems. Many terms such as *consoles, motors, drills, contra-angles,* and *handpieces* are commonly misinterpreted as synonyms for delivery systems. In actuality these terms are integral parts of what make up an entire surgical delivery system. The more knowledge acquired about these components, the less time and money are spent at the time of purchase and the better chance that the acquired equipment satisfies the needs of the purchaser.

No single component is greater than the whole, and better understanding can make the difference between ease and efficacy or breakdown and failure during surgery. Despite the best maintenance, any component or system can fail. It is therefore advisable for every office to have a backup unit.

Basically, these systems are placed into one of two classes depending on the power supply. Compressed air or nitrogen gas is the energy source that most dentists use to drive their regular high- and low-speed handpieces. On the other hand, the vast majority of root form implant surgical delivery systems are powered by electricity.

Electrical Delivery Systems

Until 1985, most root form and blade implant surgery was performed using air- or nitrogen-driven surgical systems. The universal renewal of interest in the root form implant systems reintroduced the electrical surgical modalities.

Root form implant surgery called for high torque at low speeds. This created a major dilemma in regard to air- or nitrogen-powered systems. To receive more power or torque, air- or nitrogen-powered handpieces required commensurately more speed, but experimentation with electrical systems introduced higher torque at lower speeds.

Four basic components make up an electrical surgical system: console, motor, handpiece, and burs or drill bits. An in-depth examination of each component and its relationship to the others helps one to understand the entire system. It is important not only to understand the intricacies of both electrical and air- or nitrogen-powered units but also to comprehend the surgical demands made by the various implant systems as well. Some require higher speeds and less torque, and others require lower speeds and greater torque.

Console

All of the electrical circuitry, controls for speed, irrigant, handpiece selection, readout in revolutions per minute (rpm), and power are located on the console. Even the foot-controlled rheostat plugs into and is powered by the console (Fig. 6-3).

Consoles gain their power directly from any standard 110-V electrical wall outlet. They are produced as solid-state electronic devices that are explosion and spark-proof and are lightweight (between 7 and 11 lb). If implant surgery is planned in a hospital operating room, a special shockproof attachment required for the console and verification of its electrical safety must be produced for the institutional

biomedical engineers. Either the manufacturer or the hospital's engineering department is equipped to offer these services.

Electric Motors

The motor housing cord plugs into the front of the console and uses its voltage supply much the same way a cassette or CD player uses a stereo amplifier (Fig. 6-4). The tiny motors inside the housing are commonly referred to as *micromotors,* and they are designed to run at different speeds. The most commonly used motors for root form implants turn at 20,000, 30,000, and 40,000 rpm. Some motors from the same manufacturer and even the same lot can run from 2000 to 3000 rpm faster or slower than others. For simplicity, these motors may be grouped into any of the three rpm ratings. It is critical for surgeons to know their motor rating for two reasons. The first reason is that generally a 20,000-rpm motor has more torque (power) for bone tapping at lower speeds and even at equal speeds than a 30,000- or 40,000-rpm–rated motor. The second reason is that since all motors lose some speed while drilling in bone, a 20,000-rpm motor may not be capable of delivering the requisite speed to maintain the power that a high-rated motor may have. An example to illustrate this second point will clarify it.

Implant company "A" recommends no less than 1200 rpm to perform a certain procedure. Different handpieces are available that can reduce 20,000-, 30,000-, or 40,000-rpm motors down to 1200 rpm. In dense bone, electric motors often lose as much as 50 to 300 rpm per 1200 rpm (25%) while cutting. Actual top speed using a 20,000-rpm motor with a reduction handpiece might drop to as low as 900 rpm at full power, which might result in burnishing the bone. If the same handpiece is used with a 30,000-rpm–rated motor, however,

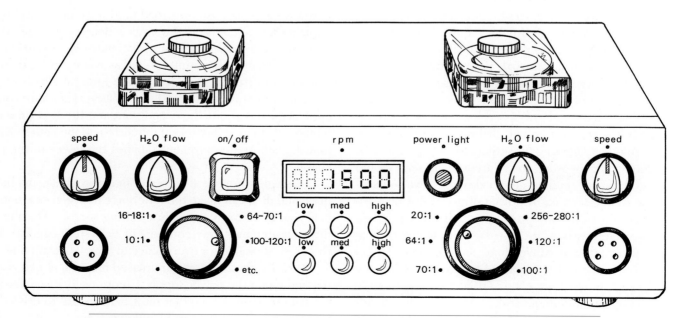

Fig. 6-3 The console, an electrical housing for low-speed, high-torque drilling equipment, should show speed in an LED readout, have adjustments to control it, have the capability to pump irrigant to the drills, be able to signal reverse direction, and when available, possess the capacity for two motors.

the speed could be increased another 600 rpm (to as much as 1500 rpm), which would compensate for the loss caused by the dense bone. As a simple rule of thumb, when speeds of over 1000 rpm are needed, a 30,000- to 40,000-rpm–rated motor should be selected. If most of a doctor's procedures demand less than 1000 rpm and many ultraslow procedures are expected (i.e., below 300 rpm), a 20,000- and 40,000-rpm motor cuts adequately at speeds well under 300 rpm, but as may be seen in the following section, the practitioner should own many more speed-reduction handpieces.

The significance of the light-emitting diode (LED) speed readout found on electrical consoles requires elucidation. If a motor is rated at 20,000 rpm and a 10:1 reduction angle is chosen, press the 10:1 selector button on the console.

The readout then shows a velocity of 2000 rpm. It is important to understand that the selector switch neither increases nor decreases actual speed. It simply calculates the change mathematically on the LED display. The only way to actually increase or decrease speed on any electrical or air- or nitrogen-powered system is by changing the posture of a hand or foot rheostat.

Most purchasers who select an electrical delivery system probably will buy the console and motor together. One manufacturer's motor may not couple with the console of another. To ensure greater accuracy in readings, use one brand of all components.

There is a choice to make between a single- or a double-motor system. A single system can accommodate one motor. A dual arrangement permits the attachment of two independent motors to a single console. The main differences between the two systems are price and versatility. With a double-motor console, the surgeon may set the motor and the handpiece for different speeds independently of each other. Motor 1, for example, can be programmed to cut at a maximum of 1200 rpm for development of the osteotomy, and motor 2 can be set to cut at 15 rpm for bone tapping. Since they cannot work simultaneously, such features as LED readout, irrigant pumps, and rheostats work only with the motor in use. If budget permits and more than one speed range is required for the performance of certain implant surgical procedures, a double-motor

system is recommended. In addition, double units eliminate the wasted time spent changing handpieces and water spray cannulas. Since most system failures occur in the motor and not the console, an additional benefit of a dual drive is the assurance of a backup device if one motor fails.

Troubleshooting

If, while using the motor, one of the following symptoms occurs, positive action must be taken.

1. The actual "feel" of loss of speed with vibration of the handpiece head. (This can cause gear stripping and handpiece failure.)
2. The bur wobbles or chatters during cutting. (This causes friction to the handpiece and can burn and injure the bone.)
3. The actual "sound" of the motor changes or it begins to growl or buzz. (This may indicate a dropping of speed and power as a result of an internal problem in the gear housing.)
4. The motor and handpiece begin to feel warm and get progressively hotter over time. (This may represent a worn gear assembly.)

In such instances, use the rheostat to increase motor speed. This may help to reduce the difficulties. To avoid such problems, make smaller increases in drill diameters (see Chapter 9); use new, sharp burs and drills at appropriate velocities, and change them often (see section in this chapter on burs and drills); and stay within proper handpiece power zones (see section on handpieces and Tables 6-1 and 6-2).

Sterility of electric motors is an issue involving cost and versatility. The majority of available autoclavable motors are three times more expensive than motors that cannot be so treated. Autoclavable motors usually are rated at no more than 20,000 rpm and run hotter than nonautoclavable motors, since they have no vents for cooling.

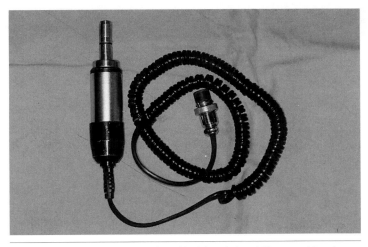

Fig. 6-4 Electric motors are hand-held and should be capable of a variety of speeds and torques. Backup equipment is recommended in case of motor failure during the procedure.

Table 6-1	**20,000 rpm Electric and 90 psi 20 k Air or Nitrogen Motors**	
CONTRA-ANGLE REDUCTION	**APPROXIMATE SPEED RANGE (RPM)**	**APPROXIMATE POWER RANGE (RPM)**
1. 10:1	200 - 2000	1700 - 2000
2. 16:1	78 - 1250	950 - 1250
3. 17:1	70 - 1175	875 - 1175
4. 18:1	60 - 1110	850 - 1100
5. 20:1	50 - 1000	800 - 1000
6. 64:1	25 *- 312	50 - 312
7. 70:1	20 *- 285	50 - 285
8. 100:1	18 *- 200	40 - 200
9. 120:1	15 *- 166	25 - 166
10. 256:1	10 *- 78	15 - 78
11. 280:1	8 *- 70	15 - 78

*Minimum speeds at which bur will cut without stalling.

Nonautoclavable motors, however, can be used with sterile transparent drapes (i.e., Steridrapes, which are supplied with adhesive). These wraps are inexpensive and disposable and fit any standard electric motor (Fig. 6-5). They cover the connections at the console and permit the use of the controls through them.

Handpieces

The term *handpiece* is one of the most misused words in dentistry. Simply defined, a handpiece is any apparatus attached to an electric or air- or nitrogen-powered motor that accepts a bur. There are two types of handpieces: contra-angle and

straight (Fig. 6-6). With these two types, the ability to increase or maintain a motor's speed with reliability is ensured.

Handpieces that reduce a motor's top speed are referred to as *reduction handpieces.* These are rated by the ratio of speed decrease of which they are capable. For example, a 16:1 reduction handpiece reduces a motor's top speed by 16 times. As speed is decreased, torque is increased by the same ratio.

Conversely, when using reduction handpieces, it should be noted that they have more power at higher speeds than at lower speeds. This phenomenon is called the *handpiece power zone.* With a 16:1 reduction on a 20,000-rpm motor, power is greater at 1250 rpm than at 500 rpm. Table 6-1 shows that a 16:1 reduction handpiece has near maximum power between speed ranges of 950 and 1250 rpm. Below 950 rpm, both speed and power are lost rapidly. If the same 16:1 reduction handpiece is placed on a 30,000-rpm motor, the top speed increases to 1875 rpm, and the power zone is found at the 1200-rpm level. It is critical for the surgeon to know the motor's top-rated speed and the handpiece power zone.

Universally, green stripes on a handpiece denote reduction capabilities. If a handpiece is not marked, mark the reduction ratio on its surface with a bur.

Instruments that increase a motor's highest velocity are referred to as *speed-increasing handpieces* and universally are marked with a red stripe. As speed is increased by a certain ratio, power is decreased by the same ratio. Because of this, speed increases are contraindicated for root form surgery. They should be used primarily for placing blade implants.

Be aware that both speed-increasing and speed-reduction handpieces demand high maintenance and are up to three times more expensive than ordinary handpieces. Generally, the higher the reduction ratio, the higher the cost.

Handpieces that do not increase or reduce speed are commonly known as *1:1 handpieces.* They are universally marked with blue stripes.

Table 6-2 30,000 rpm Electric and 90 psi 20 k Air or Nitrogen Motors

CONTRA-ANGLE REDUCTION	APPROXIMATE SPEED RANGE (RPM)	APROXIMATE POWER RANGE (RPM)
1. 10:1	300 - 3000	2500 - 3000
2. 16:1	115 - 1875	1200 - 1875
3. 17:1	100 - 1765	1150 - 1765
4. 18:1	90 - 1660	1100 - 1660
5. 20:1	75 - 1500	850 - 1500
6. 64:1	50 *- 468	60 - 468
7. 70:1	40 *- 428	50 - 428
8. 100:1	25 *- 300	40 - 300
9. 120:1	20 *- 250	25 - 250
10. 256:1	10 *- 119	20 - 119
11. 280:1	10 *- 107	15 - 107

*Minimum speeds at which bur will cut without stalling.

Table 6-3 Handpiece Selection

	DIFFERENT CONSOLE JACKS FOR DIFFERENT SPEEDS	DIFFERENT MOTORS FOR DIFFERENT SPEEDS	DIFFERENT CONTRA ANGLES FOR DIFFERENT SPEEDS	TAPPING CAPABILITY	REVERSE CAPABILITY	AUDIBLE SOUND ALARM	AUTO-CLAVABLE MOTOR	INTERNAL IRRIGATION	SINGLE UNIT (1 MOTOR)	DOUBLE UNIT (2 MOTORS)	ELECTRIC
Aseptico	–	–	*	*	*	*	*	*	*	*	*
Bicon	*	*	*	*	*	–	–	–	*	*	*
Duo-Dent	–	–	*	*	*	*	–	*	*	*	*
Dynasurg	–	–	*	*	*	*	–	*	*	*	*
Medidenta	–	*	*	*	*	–	air only	*	electric only	air only	*
NobelBio	–	–	*	*	*	*	–	*	*	–	*
Osada	–	–	*	*	*	*	*	*	*	–	*
Osteomed	–	–	*	*	*	*	–	*	*	*	*
Physiotron	–	–	*	*	*	*	*	*	–	*	*
Steri-Oss	–	–	–	*	*	*	*	*	*	*	*
Stryker	–	*	*	*	*	–	*	*	*	–	*
Sulzer	–	–	*	*	*	*	–	*	*	*	*
W&H	–	–	–	*	*	*	*	*	*	–	*

*: YES; –: NO

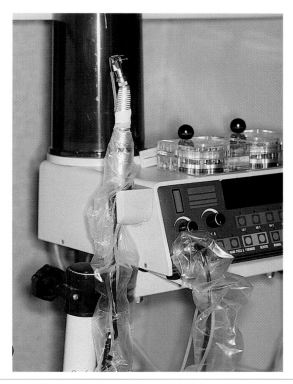

Fig. 6-5 A disposable plastic sleeve, which is inexpensive and simple to place, permits motor and cord use without the necessity of autoclaving them.

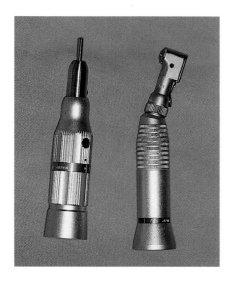

Fig. 6-6 Both straight and contra-angle handpieces are necessary for the surgeon.

Power Ranges of Handpieces

Every handpiece has more power at higher speeds than at lower speeds. It is important to know the speed at which the torque of each system is highest. The vast majority of problems occur during root form surgical procedures because changes in drill diameter are not made at sufficiently small increments and because dull drills are not changed with sufficient frequency. If the following six simple rules are understood and the power ranges found in Tables 6-1 and 6-2 are observed, the chances for problem-free surgery are greatly enhanced.

1. Allow for a one-third drop of top speed.
2. Increase speed if handpiece vibration begins.
3. Increase speed if bur wobble (chatter) occurs.
4. Allow several seconds for the bur to get up to speed before cutting in bone.
5. Never apply pressure to the handpiece head during cutting procedures. It is a natural reaction to do so if a handpiece begins to stall or drop in speed. This causes gears to strip, and thermal injury to the bur and bone results.
6. Hold the handpiece with a "featherlike" touch and let the motor, handpiece, and drill do the cutting. The surgeon's fingers should simply guide the handpiece.

Table 6-3 provides a list of currently available systems with some of their specifications. If a desired cutting speed is 200 rpm, handpieces 1 to 8 theoretically offer 200 rpm. In reality, angles 1 to 5 stall at that speed. Looking at the "approximate power range" column, angles 6, 7, and 8 have a capacity of 200 rpm with acceptable power. Since it is necessary to allow for a one-third drop in speed, only angles 6 and 7 would allow a one-third increase in speed at the high end of the speed range (285 to 312 rpm).

If the desired speed is 1500 rpm, handpieces 1 to 5 should cut at that speed. From a practical point of view, only handpieces 2 to 5 have adequate power at 1500 rpm. Allowing for a one-third drop of maximum speed (so that speed may be increased if needed), only angles 2, 3, and 4 are good choices.

Commensurate values can be extrapolated similarly for 40,000-rpm–rated motors.

Burs and Drills

All burs and drills for either blade or root form implant surgery have an absolute minimum speed at which they cut.

GAS OR AIR	VARIABLE SPEED	FOOT CONTROL	VARIABLE IRRIGATION PUMP FLOW	OUTPUT DISPLAY (RPM)
—	*	*	*	*
air only	*	*	—	*
—	*	*	*	*
—	*	*	*	*
*	*	air only	*	—
—	*	*	—	—
—	*	*	*	*
—	*	*	*	—
—	*	*	*	*
—	*	*	*	*
—	*	*	*	—
—	*	*	*	*
—	*	*	*	*

Keeping in mind that electric motors lose up to one third of their maximum speeds and air or nitrogen motors even more, it is not suggested that burs be rotated at their minimum cutting speeds. Speed ranges for the most common types of blade and root form burs and drills are discussed next.

BLADE IMPLANTS   The majority of burs used for blade implants are friction-grip, fissure burs that perform best between 30,000 and 100,000 rpm. These burs are used with external irrigant only. They always should be new, and the motion should be a light, brushing one.

Some clinicians start their blade osteotomies with wheels or disks (Paragon); others use oscillating mini saws. Mini saws are technique sensitive, but they do establish a more precise outline in the cortical bone. Completion of these osteotomies must be made with a high-speed bur.

ROOT FORM IMPLANTS   Most pilot burs and twist drills (Fig. 6-7) are available with cannulas for internal irrigation, but they are often run with external coolant as well and cut best at speeds between 300 and 1200 rpm. Those without provision for internal coolant are used with an external source only.

The next three categories of burs are the most critical in regard to speed. It was thought in the past that the slower the speed, the more protected the bone. Unfortunately, little was known about motor torque, handpiece power, and efficient cutting speeds. If a bur cuts too slowly, it may splinter bone, create chatter, and contribute to handpiece failure.

Drill progression according to size is also a factor in efficient cutting. A rule of thumb: the larger the drill size, the more speed required for it to cut. It should become a practice never to increase diameters by more than 0.5 mm with each change. Slight speed increases in such instances are warranted as well.

The drills that are known as the *intermediate stage* and *finishing stage* are designed as *saddle*, *bispade*, and *trispade* shapes. Most are internally irrigated but should also be supplied with external saline sprays.

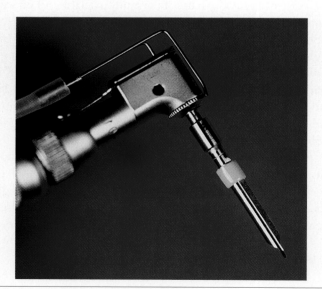

Fig. 6-7 A reduction gear angled handpiece with a Brasseler fluted bone drill mounted. This system uses both internal and external irrigation. The drill has a sterile length marker (yellow Disposaboot) attached to its shank.

Air- or Nitrogen-Powered Systems

Systems of 90 pounds per square inch (psi) using 20 and 30 k air- or nitrogen-powered motors are the selections of choice. All motors are fully autoclavable. Air- or nitrogen-powered systems, however, do not offer accurate speed readouts. The surgeon should know the desired speed range, allow for between one-third and one-half speed loss, select a proper handpiece power zone (Tables 6-1, 6-2), and run the handpiece at full speed. In other words, if 1200 rpm are required and a 30-k motor is being used, the best handpiece would be capable of 16:1, 17:1, or 18:1 ratios. If a 16:1 is selected, the top speed is 1875 rpm. At full speed, allowing for a one-third decrease in velocity, the safe range would still be maintained. Air- or nitrogen-powered motors have fewer moving parts and probably serve longer than the electrical types before requiring service.

Important Aspects of Selecting a Delivery System

1. For safety's sake, purchase either a double-motor system or two single-motor systems.
2. If more than one implant type is to be used and there is a need for different procedures (i.e., bone tapping, counter-sinking, threading, cutting, seating of implants) and different speed ranges, a double-motor system that offers variable torque control with a handpiece speed-ratio selection on the console is best. This permits the reading of actual speeds rather than the need for the surgeon to make mental conversions.
3. If handpiece changes are made to that of a new manufacturer, the console motor company should be able to recalibrate speed readouts on the console that can conform to the newly acquired handpiece speed ratios.
4. Variable flow and good pressure from the water pump should be available.
5. All water tubing should be made of silicone.
6. If two different sizes of tubing are used, the connections should be watertight and at a reasonable distance from the console so that if water leaks occur, they will not cause the pump motors to rust.
7. Choose a foot-controlled rheostat. Reverse and forward directions that can be made from the foot pedal are important features. When in reverse mode, an audible signal is a significant requirement.
8. A colleague who is near each implant office with similar devices is important so that arrangements can be made to exchange equipment when necessary.
9. Two motors and two handpieces should be available so that if one fails, the surgical procedure can be completed. Handpieces break down more often than all the other components combined.
10. If saline is used as an irrigant (which is highly recommended), flush handpieces and silicone tubing with water after completion of every case.
11. Equipment is mechanical and, as with all machinery, regular maintenance is essential. Staff members must be taught maintenance procedures as directed by manufacturers.

Surgical Principles of Value to the Implantologist

Preoperative Regimen

Routine care should include bringing a well-rested patient into surgery. Therefore, an oral sedative given the night before, such as lorazepam (Ativan) 2 mg, flurazepam (Dalmane) 30 mg, or pentobarbital (Nembutal) 100 mg, will offer a relaxed and receptive patient. If local anesthetic agents are to be used, a good breakfast is beneficial. (Patients will not be very hungry after surgery.) Procedures scheduled in the morning are best for the surgeon and the patient.

For the sensitive patient, 600 mg of ibuprofen (Motrin) 30 minutes before surgery elevates the pain threshold. If patients are to have sedation of any kind, including nitrous oxide or general anesthesia, instruct them not to eat or drink for 12 hours immediately before surgery.

Regarding antibiotics for prophylactic and therapeutic use, the American Heart Association (AHA) continues to review and revise its recommendations on prophylaxis for subacute bacte-rial endocarditis. At present (1999), for patients considered to be at "normal risk" (patients with the most usual congenital heart malformations, rheumatic and other acquired valvular dysfunctions, hypertrophic myopathies, and mitral valve prolapse with valvular regurgitation), the AHA recommends 2 g of amoxicillin orally 1 hour before surgery and nothing postoperatively. For those who report allergies to penicillin, 600 mg of clindamycin 1 hour before surgery is recommended. For patients unable to take oral medications and not allergic to penicillin, administer 2 g of ampicillin intramuscularly or intravenously 30 minutes before the procedure. For patients unable to take oral medications and allergic to penicillin, administer clindamycin 600 mg intravenously 30 minutes before the procedure (see Appendix M).

Phlebotomy skills are not difficult to acquire, and every implantologist should seek the benefits of such a technique. Patients with prosthetic valves and surgically constructed shunts require antibiotic prophylaxes. In addition, anticoagulant therapy is an integral part of their regimens. These factors can contribute a sufficient number of complications intraoperatively and postoperatively so that implants must be considered only for the most demanding cases. In instances when implants are selected for patients on anticoagulant therapy, assess patients as either moderate risk, that is, hypertension (HTN), transient ischemic attacks and with an international normalized ratio or prothrombin time (INR) of IB or high risk, that is, prosthetic (but not porcine) heart valves in which discontinuation of anticoagulants for 3 days is dangerous. The moderate-risk patient should be admitted to the hospital, where the warfarin (Coumadin) is discontinued for 3 days with monitoring of the patient until a point at which surgery can be performed without risk of excessive bleeding. At this time, perform surgery. Primary closure and use of bovine thrombin and Avitene should provide adequate hemostasis. Monitor the surgical site for 12 hours postoperatively. After 12 hours if a stable surgical site with stable clot formation is present, administer a bolus of 5000 U of heparin IV followed by 1000 U IV per hour until partial thromboplastin time (PTT) reaches 60. After 3 days of heparin, warfarin (Coumadin) can be started with a 24-hour overlap of the two medications until INR or prothrombin time (PT) levels reach presurgical therapeutic levels.

Severe-risk patients are to be admitted to the hospital and immediately discontinue warfarin (Coumadin). These patients should start receiving heparin 5000 U with IV bolus followed by 1000 U IV per hour and should wear antiembolism stockings. When the PTT reaches 60 and INR is at 2.0, discontinue the heparin. One hour from this time, commence surgery if the immediate preoperative PTT levels remain at an acceptable level. Postoperative management is identical to the moderate risk patient with emphasis on bed rest until presurgical therapeutic coagulation values are achieved.

On the other hand, antibiotic prophylaxis for the healthy patient with a good state of oral hygiene is unnecessary and may actually cause harm by creating bacterial resistance or drug sensitivities. If it is believed that antibiotic therapy is important, one dose preoperatively and a second (and final) dose after the completion of surgery may be given.

Methods of Anesthesia

When performing implant surgery, most practitioners feel comfortable with the use of local anesthetics. (Refer to Chapter 4 for guidance regarding nerve blocking.) Mepivacaine (Carbocaine) without vasoconstrictor is a poor choice because it lacks depth and longevity. Experience shows that trying to renew or supplement anesthesia during the course of a procedure is difficult to achieve. If a patient is not a good enough risk to be given lidocaine with 1:100,000 epinephrine, he or she should not be considered a suitable candidate for elective implant surgery in the ambulatory setting. For an average-sized adult, the limit, for at least the first 90 minutes, is eight anesthetic cartridges. Therefore, adminsiter each one with effectiveness and care.

When planning the placement of anterior mandibular (parasymphyseal) implants, infiltration into the vestibule is satisfactory, although the lingual side of the ridge must be anesthetized as well. Avoid the mental foramen block. It may result in a higher-than-expected number of long-lasting dysesthesias. Sound anesthesia can be achieved by an injection in the general area of the neurovascular bundle, but avoid the foramen itself. In the posterior mandible it is preferable to use infiltration anesthesia rather than nerve blocks. Soft tissue and bone anesthesia can be achieved with satisfactory depth, but the lower lip will not become anesthetized. As a result, if rotary instruments approach the mandibular canal, the patient is able to offer a warning: the lip will begin to tingle, or a sensation of heat may be expressed. Therefore, by infiltrating, a significant safety factor can be built into the procedure.

Nerve blocks are required for both mandibular and maxillary subperiosteal procedures, particularly for the first or impression-making stage. The surgeon should become comfortable with the Gow-Gates technique, which requires that the surgeon aim high for the medial surface of the condylar neck. When doing this, the possibility of entering the internal maxillary artery exists, so be cautious and be sure to aspirate. If failure greets repeated mandibular blocks, it is important to remember the benefits of infiltrating the lower lingual gingivae in the premolar area with the hope of blocking branches of the cervical colli nerves.

The infraorbital block is facilitated by knowing the location of the foramen. Most often, it is found below the medial quarter of the infraorbital rim rather than at the midway point. The neurovascular bundle can be approached only if the needle enters the upper labial mucosa at a point midway between the vestibule and the vermilion border. Palpate the foramen through the skin with the index finger while the lip is retracted using the thumb and middle finger of the same hand. The direction of the syringe should be upward and inward toward the area of the foramen through the soft tissues and the anesthetic discharged only when the presence of the needle is felt against bone beneath the palpating forefinger. Entering the gingiva as if to give a canine tooth infiltration prevents the advancement of the needle to the infraorbital nerve because of the deep concavity of the canine fossa.

The maxillary (second division) block is important in implant surgery. It is given by entering the anterior (greater) palatine foramen, which may be found by piercing the mucosa in the middle of the operative side of the hard palate at the mesial level of the first molar. Inject a few drops followed by a pause to permit the tissues to become anesthetized, and then advance the needle tip is stepped about until it falls into the foramen. Propel the needle in an upward and forward direction. Use a 27-gauge, 1½-inch needle if the block is to be effective, since it has to pass through the canal to its full length. Make injections very slowly because the space is restricted and rapid discharge of the solution will cause the patient severe pain. Use at least two anesthetic tubes. As a general rule, but particularly with this block, never inject as the needle is being advanced. It is extremely painful, tears the tissues, and negates the value of a sharply pointed needle. If the second division block is correctly given, symptoms of numbness of the ipsilateral upper lip, nasal ala, facial tissues, and lower eyelid result. Avoid intravascular injections. In the adult population, a fully patent canal can be encountered approximately 65% of the time. If full needle-length entry cannot be achieved, the injection should still be given, and at the least, anesthesia of the hard palate, ridge, and buccoalveolar gingivae up to the second premolar is achieved.

Also of importance are the incisive and posterior superior alveolar blocks that give greater operating time and more profound anesthesia than can be obtained from using simple infiltrations.

Sutures and Suturing

Suture Materials

Table 6-4 presents the available types of suture material, their characteristics, and possible uses. Complicated implant clo-sures, for example, require a synthetic resorbable suture such as Vicryl or Polysorb (polylactic acid/polyglycolic acid or Bio-Syn) because such a suture permits the use of long, continuous, and complicated closures and eliminates the necessity of removing all parts of the suture material.

Sutures made of silk, nylon, Dexon (polyglycolic acid), Vicryl, plain gut, and chromic gut, all sizes from 1-0 to 6-0, or even finer, are available. Some are made in braided form (silk Dexon, Vicryl) and others come in monofilament form (nylon, Biosyn and gut). The braided types are easier to use because of the softness, compliance, ease of tying, and stability of knots. On the other hand, they serve as wicks (particularly silk) that may cause retrograde infection, which the monofilaments discourage.

Silk and nylon are nonresorbable. Some patients may be sensitive or allergic to it because it is a foreign protein. The other products are resorbable. Vicryl and Polysorb are synthetic polymers and resorb very slowly (from 30 to 45 days). Most dentists are accustomed to using silk. It must be remembered, however, that all of its remnants have to be removed. When a complicated closure such as that over a subperiosteal implant is performed using a continuous mattress suture with much pericervical wrapping, it may be extremely difficult to remove all remnants of the suture material. In these cases, therefore, Vicryl or Polysorb is recommended. They are available in dyed purple form, and once the surgeon becomes comfortable with them, the convenience and ease of management (despite their relative expense) make their use worthwhile. Deeper layers (i.e., periosteum, muscle, subcuticular tissues) may be closed with 3-0 plain gut (which resorbs in about 5 days), chromic (which resorbs in about 30 days), or one of the synthetic polymers (30 to 45 days). Nylon usually is reserved for skin.

Suture Needles

Needles may be tapered (round in cross section) or cutting (either outside or inside) or be straight (for skin closure) or curved irregularly or regularly in ⅜, ½, and ⅝ circles of varying sizes. The preferable needle for use in intraoral surgery, including implant closure, is a ⅜ circle, inside cutting needle mounted atraumatically to the suture material (an eyeless needle swaged to the suture material). Cutting needles are preferable for use in intraoral closures, particularly for keratinized tissues, because too much resistance is presented for easy passage when the use of tapered needles is attempted. However, 5-0 silk or Vicryl on tapered needles is indicated for closure of fine, thin, fixed gingiva such as the type found in the anterior portion of the mouth overlying the alveolar ridge (e.g., for apicoectomies). When a cutting needle is used, pass it evenly and smoothly, one flap at a time, pushing it in the direction of its own arc. In this manner, the cutting edge assists in needle passage and does not excessively incise the tissues through which it is being passed.

Grasp the needle holder the way scissors are held, through the loops. Many surgeons hold needle holders in a palm-thumb grasp, which gives good tactile control. However, when

Table 6-4 Suture Types

NAME	MATERIAL/ CHARACTERIZATION	RESORB-ABLE	TIME TO RESORB	PURPOSES/SIZE	VALUES	PROBLEMS
Silk	Braided, black, natural	No	–	Mucosal closure-3.0, tongue and flap retraction-2.0	Slides and knots easily, knot doesn't slip	Acts as a wick, needs to be removed, not very strong
Plain gut	Monofilament, clear, animal	Yes	5-7 days	Subcuticular & mucosal closure 3.0	Resorbs quickly, good for noncritical wounds	May create sensitivity, doesn't hold knots well, unreliable for critical wounds, bothers the tonge intraorally, weak
Chromic gut	Monofilament, gut, beige, natural	Yes	28 days	Deep muscle closure 3.0, 4.0	Resorbs slowly, dependable	May create sensitivity, not applicable for intraoral use, holds knots poorly, weak
Nylon	Monofilament, blue/ black, synthetic	No	–	Skin closure	Strong, discourages wicking	Holds knots poorly, has plastic memory, requires removal
Tevdek	Braided, green, Teflon coated dacron, synthetic	No	–	Skin closure	Strong, knots well	Acts as wick to some extent, requires removal
Dexon	Braided, white or dyed, polyglycolic acid, synthetic	Yes	28-45 days	Deep suturing, mucosal closure	Strong, holds knots well, after removal residual deep components may be left behind & will resorb eventually	Causes some wicking, requires removal when used intraorally because 28 days is too long, when wet neither slides nor knots as well as silk
Vicryl	Braided, white or dyed violet, polylactic acid, synthetic	Yes	28 days	Deep suturing, muscosal closure		

the needle is passed halfway through the flap, open the needle holder so that the needle can be released. In order to do this, wriggle the fingers backward, seeking the instrument's scissors holes or loops, which must be engaged to allow the jaws to snap open. These potentially traumatic machinations often cause the grasped needle to tear the tissues. Some surgeons acquire the skill of releasing the needle holder using the heels of their hands. If this technique cannot be mastered, keep the fingers in the scissors holes during all the steps. By so doing, the surgeon is able to pass sutures and open and close beaks without disturbing the posture of the needle. An alternative is to use a "loopless" needle holder, such as a Crile or Mathieu, which opens easily when the handles are squeezed together.

Another technique that should not only hasten closures, but make them more accurate, is to acquire the custom of using a toothed pickup forceps (Adson or Gerald) to hold, position, and stabilize the flaps. This is not an easy technique to master, although few, if any, surgeons who operate in other fields spear the tissues without supporting them. An assistant is needed to retract so that the surgeon's other hand can remain free to stabilize the tissues to be sutured. Once the technique is mastered, however, it becomes an effective method to close wounds quickly and accurately. A good way to practice is on a towel or bedspread.

Surgical assistants must be reminded that they are not to suction after the first suture throw (two clockwise turns). Allow the first half of the knot to lie flat and untouched until the second (counterclockwise) throw is completed, which locks and

fastens it. Suctioning or wiping disturbs and loosens the knot, therreby slowing progress.

Methods of Closure

There are several methods of closure (Fig. 6-8) that offer advantages when employed for different types of incisions and at varying locations.

Interrupted Sutures

Interrupted sutures are the classic type used by most practitioners for simple closures (Fig. 6-8, A). A good alternative to assist in performing firm, accurate knots is to make the first throw singly clockwise (rather than twice as is generally taught). Tighten the turn and lay it flat. Follow with a second clockwise throw, thereby creating a granny knot. In most cases (particularly with new silk and nylon), it may still be drawn tight because the granny permits some beneficial slipping and tightening. The knot at this stage remains stable and firm while the final counterclockwise turn locks the knot (Fig. 6-9). As braided suture becomes moistened, the granny technique may become more difficult to affect.

The problem with interrupted sutures in general is that they bring very thin mucosal edges together, which have the potential of not healing primarily. In addition, interrupted sutures present areas of intermittent ischemia, which may offer a further impediment to healing, collect food and debris, and serve as general sources of annoyance to the tongue and lips.

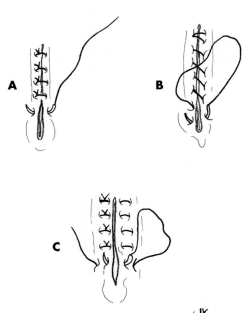

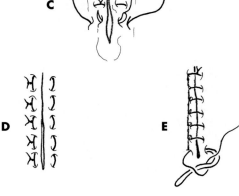

Fig. 6-8 **A,** Interrupted sutures. **B,** Continuous sutures. **C,** Vertical mattress sutures. Stabilize the flaps and pass the needle through each of the flaps 1 mm from the incision. Then reverse the needle and pass it in the opposite direction 4 mm from the wound margins. The exit and entry points are both on the buccal flap. They are tied in a surgical knot. **D,** Interrupted horizontal mattress sutures. **E,** Continuous box-lock sutures. This technique is valuable for closure of crestal incisions. Entry is made from buccal to lingual each time as for a continuous suture. Before tightening each pass, however, lift the loop from the tissue, turn it once clockwise, and pass the needle through it. When tightened, a locked-box configuration will result.

Horizontal Mattress Sutures

The continuous horizontal mattress suture avoids the problems previously cited, apposes 1- to 2-mm-wide zones of bleeding periosteum, and presents the greatest opportunities for primary healing (Fig. 6-8, *D*). With a little practice, skills in using this technique can be acquired. Stringing a series of single horizontal mattress sutures together makes the continuous horizontal mattress.

To perform this maneuver, the mouse tooth pickup forceps grasps the distal end of the buccal flap, and the needle pierces it (Fig. 6-10, *A, B*). Perform the same procedure through the inside (or periosteal surface) of the distolingual flap. Reverse the needle and pass it from the mucosal surface of the lingual flap 2 to 3 mm mesially and then from the periosteum of the mucosal surface of the buccal flap in parallel posture, moving anteriorly.

At this juncture, four penetrations have been made, thus creating a ∪ of suture material (Fig. 6-10, *C*). It starts from the buccal and ends at the buccal and therefore the needle and the trailing end both protrude through the buccal flap 3 mm apart. This constitutes an interrupted horizontal mattress suture. Tie these ends using a standard surgical knot described previously. Cut the trailing, or free, end, leaving a 3-mm tail. Turn the needle on itself to face the mucosal surface of the buccal flap 3 mm mesially. Use the mouse tooth forceps again for tissue stabilization and pass the suture through this flap and then through the lingual flap, as had been

performed on the previous pass. Continue the pattern at 3-mm intervals, lingual through buccal followed by buccal through lingual (Fig. 6-10, *D*).

Continue the closure to the anterior end of the incision, and at this point and plan for the final knot at the last buccal-to-lingual pass. Do this by leaving a small loop (L-p) protruding from the buccal side, which the assistant holds taut to prevent the entire system from loosening (Fig. 6-10, *F*). Then guide the needle through both flaps from lingual to buccal (M) and tie the knot using the protruding loop as one end and the needle end as the other. Then cut both ends and leave three tails at the final suture (Fig. 6-10, *G*).

If after each pass the system is tightened by pulling on suture material, the flaps give the appearance of the welt of a mattress edge (Fig. 6-10, *H*). If the coaptation of the flaps does not appear satisfactory, place appropriate supplementary horizontal mattress sutures to achieve a more reliable closure.

When an implant with a protruding cervix is reached (as in subperiosteal and nonsubmergible implant forms), make one pass distal to the abutment with the suture being carried around its mesial surface and made to exit on the lingual, distal to the cervix. Initiate the returning lingual-to-buccal pass mesial to the cervix, with the suture passing distal to it exiting on the mesial side of the buccal flap. This makes a "figure 8" configuration and gathers the tissues around the cervix in the form of a purse string. The continuous closure may then be completed (Fig. 6-10, *E*).

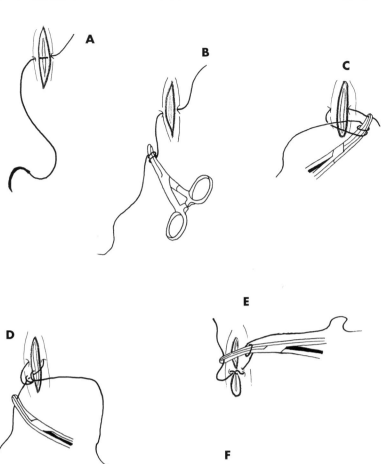

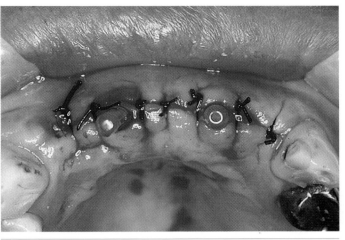

Fig. 6-9 Simple interrupted suture. **A,** Pass the needle through both flaps. **B,** Wrap the needle end of the suture twice around the needle holder in a clockwise direction. **C,** Then, open the beaks and grasp the free end. **D,** Pull the free end through the double loop and fasten it snugly alongside the incision. **E,** Now, wind the needle end counterclockwise one revolution around the needle holder, and grasp the free end with the beaks. **F,** Pull the free end through the loop and, when tightened, it creates a stable square knot. The knot should not be allowed to rest directly on the incision, but should lie alongside it. The cut ends must be left sufficiently long to permit easy access for removal. **G,** Clinical view of closure with interrupted sutures.

Vertical Mattress Sutures

Vertical mattress sutures have few uses intraorally but are of great benefit for skin suturing when the possibility for primary closure needs to be enhanced, such as in the case of a transosteal or staple implant (Fig. 6-8, C). This is a technique that can be used in the form of interrupted sutures only.

Pass the needle (a straight needle makes this technique easier) from one flap to the other, with the entry and exit both made 1 mm from the incision. Next, elevate the two flaps by lifting the entering and exiting suture ends, leaving extra suture material protruding at the needle end. With the wound margins lifted, pass the straight needle back from the second flap to the first in the same vertical plane but 4 mm more removed. As the knot is tied, the two flaps evert, creating the first component of the requisite mattress welt. As additional vertical mattress sutures are placed, the eversion occurs from one end of the incision to the other. Time and physiology offer reliable healing with subsequent flattening of the welt.

Continuous Box-Lock Sutures

The box-lock technique offers a type of nonmattress continuous closure that is more reliable than a simple continuous or a series of interrupted sutures. It may be used after alveoloplasties, multiple extractions, or other procedures that result in linear gingival defects (Fig. 6-8, E).

The procedure is initiated with a simple interrupted suture, which should be tied with a surgical knot. Lift the labial flap with the pickup forceps and pass the needle through it and then through the lingual flap but not pulled tight. Instead, leave a loop. Make one twist in the loop, and pass the needle through it. Then pull the suture tight. A locked box occurs. Repeat these steps, and when papillae are present (as after extractions), they may be interdigitated so that the underlying bone becomes covered. Continue these locked boxes until the entire closure has been completed. Do not draw the final box loop tight because it is used as one end for tying the final knot with the other or protruding needle end (Fig. 6-11).

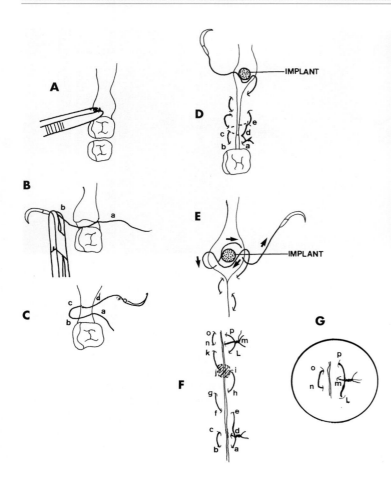

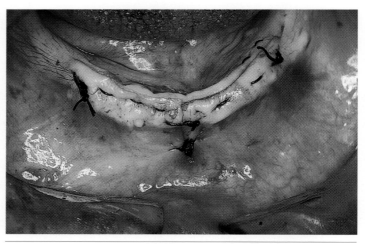

Fig. 6-10 Continuous horizontal mattress suture. **A,** Use the mouse tooth forceps to stabilize the flaps. **B,** Pass the needle through the buccal and lingual flaps (*a* to *b*) at the beginning of the incision. **C,** Then reverse the needle and pass it from lingual to buccal (*c* to *d*). **D,** Tie a knot between ends *a* and *d,* cut the loose end, and pass the needle from buccal to lingual at point *e.* Continue the pattern from lingual to buccal and buccal to lingual until the mesial surface, of the one-stage implant is encountered. Enter the buccal flap at a point distal to the abutment, wrap it to its mesial surface, and exit distal to the cervix through the lingual flap. **E,** Bring the needle mesially (see arrow on lingual) and pierce the lingual flap mesial to the abutment. The arrows indicate that the suture then passes distal to the cervix and exits mesially through the buccal flap, and on this fourth pass, when the suture is tightened, the tissue will be gathered, purse string fashion around the cervix. **F,** Continue the suture pattern through points *k, l, n, o,* and *p* and suture at point *m.* **G,** Make the final closure by taking end n and tying it to loop *pl,* creating knot *m.* **H,** Clinical view of continuous horizontal mattress suture. Rapid and reliable healing is a characteristic of this kind of closure.

Fig. 6-11 Continuous box-lock suture. This technique is valuable for closure of crestal incisions. Entry is made from buccal to lingual surfaces each time, as for a continuous suture. Before tightening each pass, however, lift the loop from the tissue and turn it once clockwise and pass the needle through it. When tightened, a locked-box configuration will result (See Fig. 6-8, *E*).

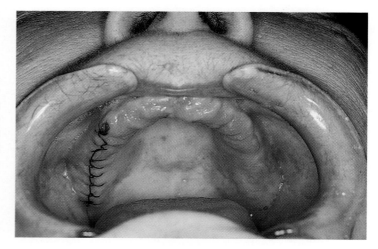

Periodontal Sling Sutures

Begin the continuous sling (periodontal closure) technique by entering a facial papilla at the distal end of the wound and then pass the needle through the lingual papilla. Return the needle to the facial side by passing it over the two papillae through the greater embrasure and tie a square knot tied. Cut the short end and pass the needle over the papillae through the same greater embrasure to the lingual side. Now bring the needle mesially around the lingual cervix of tooth no. 1 and pass it above the mesial lingual papilla and through the buccal papilla. Next, return the needle over the same buccal papilla back through the embrasure and pass it through the lingual papilla.

Tighten the system and return the needle over both papillae. Next, wrap the suture mesially over the buccal papilla of tooth no. 2. The next papilla should not be pierced but passed over through the embrasure so that the lingual papilla can be pierced. Next enter the buccal papilla in this fashion, and draw the flaps tightly into the dental interspaces, directly (rather than obliquely) and without distortion. Make three passes between each tooth: the first to catch the buccal papilla, the second to pierce the lingual, and the third to simply return over them to the buccal. With each successive pass, reverse the pattern; the effect is the same.

Complete the suturing in the same manner as for all continuous closures by leaving a loop to be used for one end of the knot and the needle end for the other.

As an alternative to the technique described, periodontal sling suturing may engage only the buccal papillae proceeding in the distal direction and the lingual papillae in returning (Fig. 6-12, A-G). Make the final knot at the anterior facial papilla, tying the protruding needle end to the original suture end (Fig. 6-12, H, I).

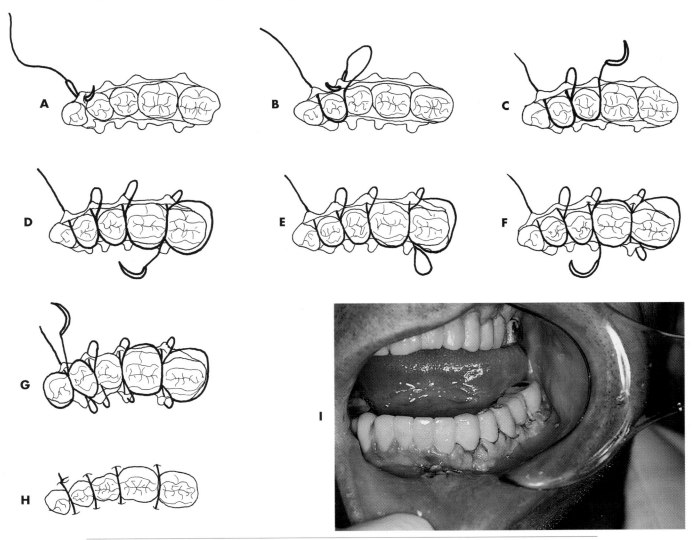

Fig. 6-12 Periodontal sling suturing. **A,** Entry is made through the first buccal papilla. **B,** Pass the needle to the lingual through the greater embrasure, wrap it around the lingual cervix of the first tooth, and then pass it through the second buccal papilla. **C,** Return the needle over this second papilla through the second embrasure, again to the lingual flap, and wrap it around the second tooth. **D,** In this fashion the buccal flap is brought firmly to place. At the distal portion of the last tooth, after passing the suture through the buccal papilla, it passes to the lingual and enters this papilla. **E and F,** In similar fashion, all of the papillae of the lingual flap are engaged. **G,** Make the final pass around a tooth anterior to the incision so that the suture will come directly from lingual to buccal at the mesial surface of the first tooth. Before tying the two ends, tighten the system by tugging gently at each loop. **H,** Tie the knot at the mesiobuccal papilla of the first tooth. **I,** Clinical view of a properly executed periodontal sling suture.

Ligating a Splint, Stent, or Prosthesis

Circumosseous Ligation

Circumosseous ligatures are of value for securing prostheses to the jaws after preprosthetic procedures such as ridge augmentation, the insertion of intramucosal insert prostheses, and in the fixation of stents after vestibuloplasties and other oral plastic operations. In order to achieve a snug fit of ligature wire against bone, most techniques require that the skin be incised directly down to the bone (mandible or zygoma) or, at the least, that the ligature be forced through the soft tissues by using a sawing motion. This procedure is time consuming, fraught with the dangers of injuring a nerve or blood vessel, causes a skin scar, and requires the sterile precautions of a hospital operating room. The methods described in the following paragraphs are suitable for ligating a splint either to the mandible or to the maxilla by using the zygomatic arch or alveolar processes and are quick, safe, and avoid the need for incisions. The armamentarium is minimal and readily available in any office or clinic.

Use a new needle for each ligature. Hug the bone to avoid garroting soft tissues. Avoid the regions of the mental nerve and facial vessels, and retract Wharton's duct and the lingual nerve medially so that they are not injured.

Circummandibular Ligation Procedure

Palpate the inferior border of the mandible. Avoid the regions of the anterior facial artery and vein and the mental foramen.

Prepare the skin with a chlorhexidine or hexachlorophene soap followed by saline; then dry it and paint liberally with povidone-iodine. Insert a 1½ inch 18-gauge needle in an upward vertical direction until it contacts the inferior border of the mandible. Then, use a sweetheart retractor to compress the tongue and sublingual tissues medially. Slide the needle being manipulated by the other hand off the inferior border medially and direct it toward the mucosa. The tip should hug the cortex.

Once the needle has perforated the floor (Fig. 6-13, A), thread a piece of No. 2 stainless steel monofilament ligature wire through its lumen. Grasp the end of the wire as it emerges through the needle's tip with a Kelly hemostat (Fig. 6-13, B). Hold the hemostat with one hand while the other hand withdraws the needle so that it hugs the bone during its retraction. Do not withdraw the needle withdrawn any farther than the inferior border. At this point, swing it around to the lateral side of the inferior border and push it upward toward the buccal vestibule, again using a retractor to stretch the tissues laterally (Fig. 6-13, C). As the needle is pushed upward, a double thickness of vertically ascending wire is carried with it: one thickness within the needle, the other alongside it. If the wire that protrudes from the submandibular skin is pulled taut, it will bend sharply over the lumen of the needle and folds back parallel to the needle shaft, thus allowing the point to be the advancing structure. This makes pushing it easier and less traumatic. The wire from the intraoral (hemostat) end

must be fed as the needle is advanced. Since extra wire is needed for this purpose, a sufficient length of it should have been passed into the mouth at the initial threading through the lumen.

After the needle has perforated the mucobuccal fold (Fig. 6-13, C), grasp the double-thickness wire protruding from the needle tip with a second Kelly hemostat. Hold the wire while the needle is withdrawn directly downward through the skin at its original and only point of entry. Now pull the portion of wire still protruding through the skin up into the mouth through the fold by using a thin instrument in the protruding loop (Fig. 6-13, D)

An end of the wire extends from both buccal and lingual vestibules. Twist these ends over the prosthesis; cut and tuck them in and cover them with a bit of self-curing acrylic (Fig. 6-13, E). There may be reason to cut a receptacle for the wire and its twisted end before covering it. As many circummandibular ligatures as needed may be placed for prosthesis stabilization (Fig. 6-13, F), but three such anchors usually suffice.

Circumzygomatic Ligation Procedure

Circumzygomatic wiring is initiated by palpating the superior surface of the zygomatic arch. After the skin is prepared with a chlorhexidine gluconate and povidone-iodine scrub, insert a 3½-inch, 18-gauge spinal needle with stylet until it contacts the superior bony surface of the arch. Next, direct the needle medially to the arch, and with the forefinger of the opposite hand, place it into the mucobuccal fold as far superoposteriorly as possible, aiming the needle toward the finger. Compress the tissues laterally, and the needle should be made to hug the maxilla so that it is not pushed through the mandibular sigmoid notch (Fig. 6-14, A). This assisted by having the patient partially close his jaw.

When the needle has perforated the maxillary mucobuccal fold, pass a length of No. 2 wire through its lumen, pulled down at least 30 cm and grasped with a Kelly forceps (Fig. 6-14, B). Then withdraw the needle along its path of insertion only as far as the superior surface of the zygomatic arch while the intraoral wire end is stabilized. Pass the needle tip and its wire wrapped around and over the zygomatic arch and force it downward around its lateral side while the wire is being fed from its intraoral source. Again, direct the needle toward the same spot: an intraorally placed finger (Fig. 6-14, C). Make an effort to have the wire emerge from or near the first point of perforation. Grasp the doubled end of the wire from the needle tip with a second hemostat and hold it in place while the needle is withdrawn (Fig. 6-14, D). Finally, pull the double-looped end into the mouth. Make the ligation through a hole in the denture flange or around a buccally placed lug, intermaxillary hook arch bar, or mucosal insert on the prosthesis flange (Fig. 6-14, E, F). To ligate a full splint or denture, repeat the procedure on the contralateral side, and pass a third

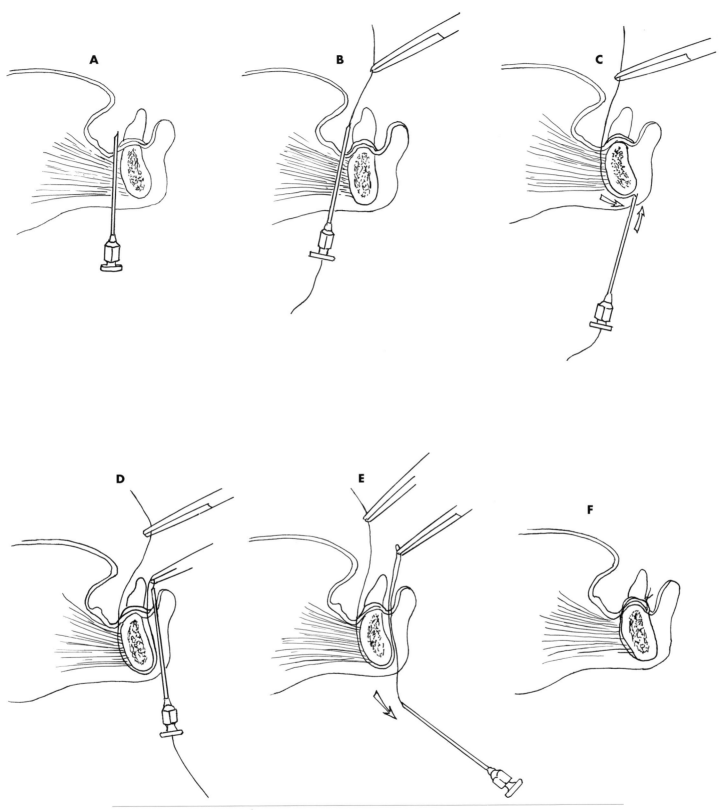

Fig. 6-13   Circummandibular ligation. **A,** Dentures, stents, splints, and other prostheses often must be fastened to the mandible. This may be accomplished without incision by using a disposable 18-gauge needle and No. 2 stainless steel ligature wire. It may be done with local anesthesia. Pass the needle through the submandibular skin, and permit it to exit through the lingual vestibule. **B,** Pass the wire through the lumen and grasp it intraorally with a hemostatic forceps. Withdraw the needle but only to the level of the inferior mandibular border. At this point redirect it around the border and push with the wire in its lumen through the buccal vestibule, hugging the bone. Avoid the mental bundle. **C,** Grasp the protruding wire loop from the needle end and hold it with a hemostat while the needle is withdrawn. **D,** Pull this looped end up through the floor of the mouth. **E,** Twist the buccal and lingual ends to lock the prosthesis into place. **F,** Repeat the procedure contralaterally.

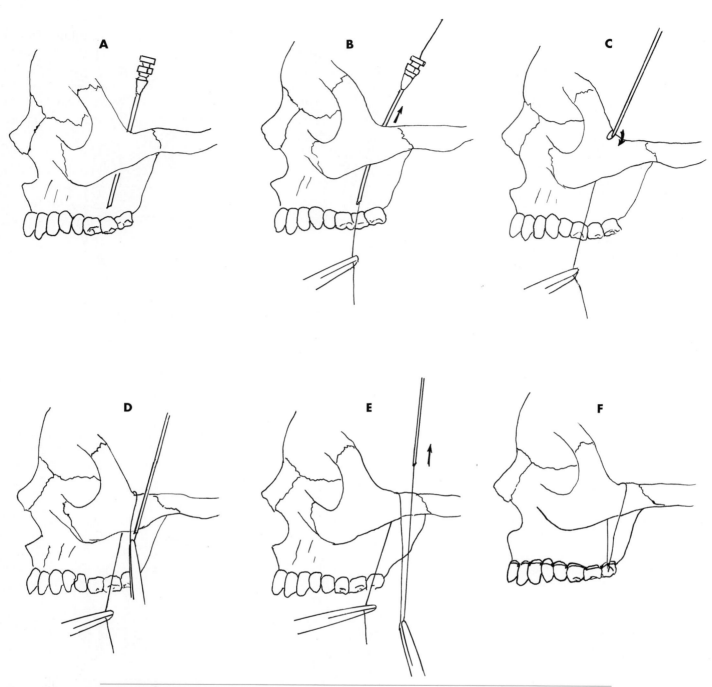

Fig. 6-14   A, Passing ligatures around the zygomatic arch to stabilize maxillary prostheses may be done using local anesthesia. Spinal needles, 18 gauge, 3½ inch long, are required. Make the first entry through the skin above the arch. **B,** The needle point should contact the superior surface and then be directed medially to enter the buccal vestibule in the tuberosity area. **C,** Use your forefinger of your other hand to retract the buccal tissues and to serve as a directional guide. **D,** Once the needle pierces the mucosa, grasp and stabilize the wire exiting from its lumen with a hemostat, withdraw the needle, and pass it subcutaneously over the arch on to its lateral side and use it to carry the wire back to the same vestibular site. Use a second hemostat to grasp the protruding double end of the ligature, and withdraw the needle. Draw the free end of the wire down into the mouth. **E** and **F,** Then twist the two ends around an intermaxillary hook processed into the prosthesis flange.

wire over or through the anterior nasal spine. Do this by making an incision, reflecting the tissues, exposing the spine, and threading the wire over it or into a drill hole made through it. One flange hole on either side of the frenular notch serves for anterior splint retention. These ligatures, too, should be covered with self-curing acrylic.

Transalveolar Ligation Procedure

A simpler method of ligating a prosthesis or splint to the maxilla for the time period during which root form implants are

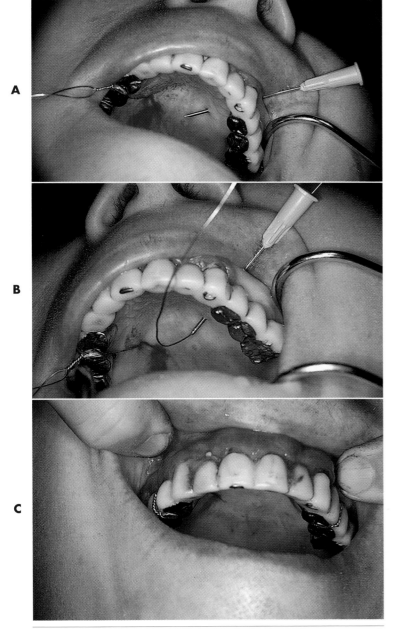

Fig. 6-15 Transalveolar ligation. **A,** A disposable 18-gauge hypodermic needle is passed through the buccal mucosa and is tapped with a surgical mallet until it emerges through the palatal mucosa. **B,** Pass a No. 2 stainless wire through its lumen and grasp it at the protruding end. **C,** Withdraw the needle and twist the wire tightly over the prosthesis. Occasionally a drill or motor-driven Kirschner wire will be required to make a pilot hole in cases of bone resistant to needle-tapping.

becoming integrated or for other purposes requiring stabilization of a stent or splint is by transalveolar ligation. This may be done in most (but not all) cases simply by selecting a site in the buccal mucosa above the apical level of the teeth or implants and placing a disposable, 18-gauge hypodermic needle through the soft tissues and against bone. Aim the needle in a direction that permits it to emerge through the opposing palatal tissues when tapped with a surgical mallet (Fig. 6-15, *A*). After the needle has emerged from the palatal side, pass a 20-cm length of No. 2 SS wire (Fig. 6-15, *B*) through its lumen, grasp the protruding end, and withdraw the needle.

Twist the two ends tightly over a prosthesis (Fig. 6-15, *C*), denture, or splint; this ligature (alone or in multiples) serves as an anchor for periods of up to 6 months. Antibiotic therapy may be required if incipient symptoms of retrograde infection are noted.

When a patient is missing most or all of the teeth in the maxillae and cannot or will not wear a removable prosthesis during the period of osseointegration, a temporary fixed prosthesis may be fabricated and fixed to the maxillae using transalveolar ligatures, sometimes with the addition of a distal end one-piece implant (i.e., ITI) or a two-stage implant with abutment attached. These can be included or removed at the time of implant exposure when healing collars or abutments are placed. They can be put into service immediately as abutments for transitional fixed or fixed-detachable prostheses if they have osseointegrated (Fig. 6-16).

Ligature Removal

Before removing intraoral portions of ligatures, they must be disinfected, cleaned, and made aseptic with povidone-iodine. Then push the mucosa should be pushed apically, exposing a portion of the buried wire. Snip it at this point and, with a needle holder, pull it out from the other end. Removal is rapid, painless, and clean if performed in this fashion. Local anesthesia is not required. If the intraoral portions of the wire are not sterilized, contaminants will inoculate the soft tissues as the wire is withdrawn, and serious infection may result.

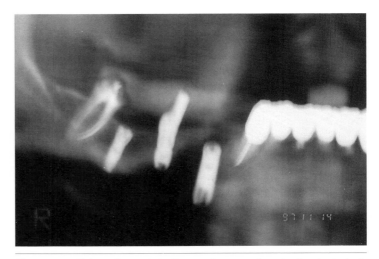

Fig. 6-16 This radiograph indicates the use of a pier implant abutment, with immediate placement of its TEA to support an all-acrylic interim prosthesis. (See Chapter 20.)

Preprosthetic Surgery

There are a number of procedures, mostly preparatory in nature, with which every implant surgeon should become comfortable. Removal and reduction of nonneoplastic structures (such as ridge undercuts, tori, and tuberosities) and recontouring of soft tissue aberrations or malformations (such as high frenular or muscle attachments, absence of fixed gingivae, and epulides fissurata) should be completed before implant placement. The following paragraphs serve as a surgical guide that the implantologist may use throughout the preimplantation period.

Tori Removal

Tori may be found in the palatal midline as well as attached to the mandible, lingual to the premolars. They may appear to be sessile but are always pedunculated and are found in single or multiple configurations. They are covered by normal-appearing epithelium except for the presence of an occasional superficial traumatic ulcer. Removal requires flawless incision, flap and osteotomy planning, and careful hard and soft tissue management.

Palatal Tori

Make the incision directly over the middle of the bony growth extending from the soft palate anteriorly almost to the incisive papilla (Fig. 6-17, A). Use a sharp periosteal elevator, since the tissues are resistant to reflection, particularly at the base of the tori (which are undercut). Start the reflection at the anterior end and continue posteriorly until the superficial portion of the torus is uncovered. The reflection then proceeds down to the hyperostotic base. If the tissues do not come away without the threat of tearing, substitute a No. 12 blade for the elevator and carefully detach the mucosa using the blade point in gentle stroking maneuvers. Use the No. 12 blade with great care to avoid the stigma of perforation complete the exposure by uncovering the base fully around the periphery. Establish a zone of normal hard palate, 5 mm in all directions, (Fig. 6-17, B). When the torus is fully visible, use a No. 1 L round bur in the high-speed Impactair or a Hall drill with copious irrigation to make perforations at the base of the torus 2 to 3 mm apart completely around it. Direct the bur through the cortex and parallel to the palatal vault.

A 701 L fissure bur is used to cut the torus into quarters from its top directly down to the levels of the expected palatal contour. Throat packs or curtains must be used to protect the patient from aspiration of bone fragments.

Fig. 6-17 A, To remove a palatal torus, two elliptical incisions are required. They should be made quite close to each other, over the bony protuberance. **B,** Each flap is reflected laterally beyond the torus. Tori are pedunculated, which makes the reflection a difficult one. Care must be exercised not to tear the tissue. **C,** After making No. 2 bur holes at the base, resection of the torus is facilitated by using a mallet and osteotome. The bed is smoothed with a Vulcanite bur and a primary closure made with interrupted sutures.

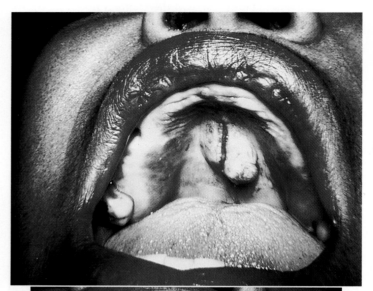

A

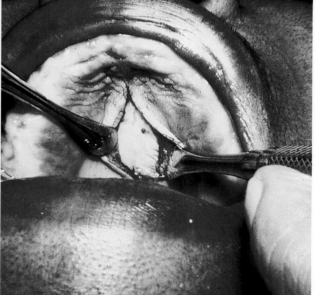

B

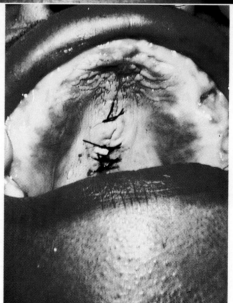

C

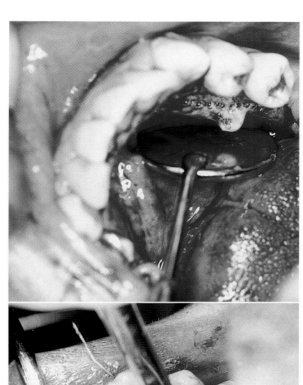

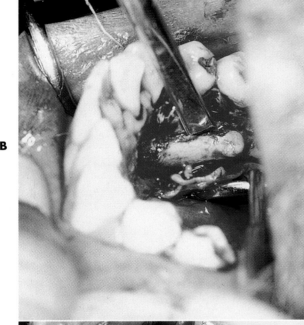

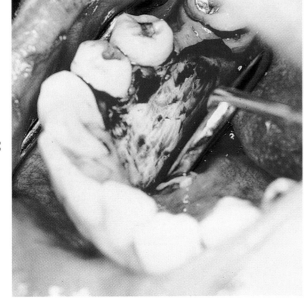

Place a curved osteotome of appropriate width at the points of perforation in the base of the torus with its curvature following the contour of the palatal vault. Firm tapping with a mallet causes the torus to cleave from its base, in most cases, at the correct level. When this step is completed at several locations, insert the osteotome into one groove of the cruciform osteotomy and turn it. The four quarters fall away, one by one. Complete the contouring and smoothing of the base bone by using a large, round, water-cooled vulcanite bur.

Perforation of the bony palate is a rare but dangerous complication. If this does occur, the careful handling of the soft tissues during their reflection is a valuable asset because a primary closure over the defect using a continuous horizontal mattress suture of 4-0 dyed Vicryl is mandated to contribute to the prevention of an oronasal fistula (Fig. 6-17, *C*).

Mandibular Tori

Management of mandibular tori is not dissimilar from that of the palatal torus. Make the incision at the lingual marginal gingiva from molar to midline. The curvature of the arch permits the reflection to be completed inferiorly without the benefit of inferiorly vertical relieving incisions (Fig. 6-18, *A*). Again, since mandibular tori are pedunculated, detaching the gingiva at their bases takes great care. Once the entire bony mass is fully exposed, use a No. 1 L round bur to perforate the tori bases at 2- and 3-mm intervals parallel with the lingual cortex. Simple tapping with a sharp curved osteotome placed in the perforations allows them to cleave from the mandible, usually in a satisfactory plane (Fig. 6-18, *B*, *C*). Use bone files or egg-shaped vulcanite burs to smooth the bone, and make an anatomic closure with a periodontal sling suture. (See the section, Sutures and Suturing, in this chapter.)

Tuberosity Reduction

Tuberosities that are in need of reduction should present few problems. To begin, make a determination, with panoramic or periapical x-rays and by probing, whether these enlargements are bony or fibrous (Fig. 6-19, *A*). If they consist of soft tissue, make a crest-of-the-ridge incision over the tuberosity directly to bone (Fig. 6-19, *B*). Start at the distal end and advance it anteriorly to the first premolar area. Make reflections buccally and palatally (Fig. 6-19, *C*, *D*) and with the flaps being supported with a toothed Gerald forceps; fillet (thin) each one (thinned) by removing 50% or more of its internal layers from the periosteum outward. Taper the cuts so that as the scalpel advances buccally and palatally away from the incisions to the bases of the flaps, the layers to be removed are thinned to a fine

Fig. 6-18 **A,** Mandibular tori, often multiple, are exposed most easily by making incisions in the gingival crevices above them. **B,** After these hyperostoses are exposed, make small bur holes tracing their bases. Then, apply a curved osteotome at the bur perforations. **C,** These tori cleave predictably in most instances. On their removal, the bone may be further smoothed with a bur or bone file, and a closure made using the periodontal sling technique.

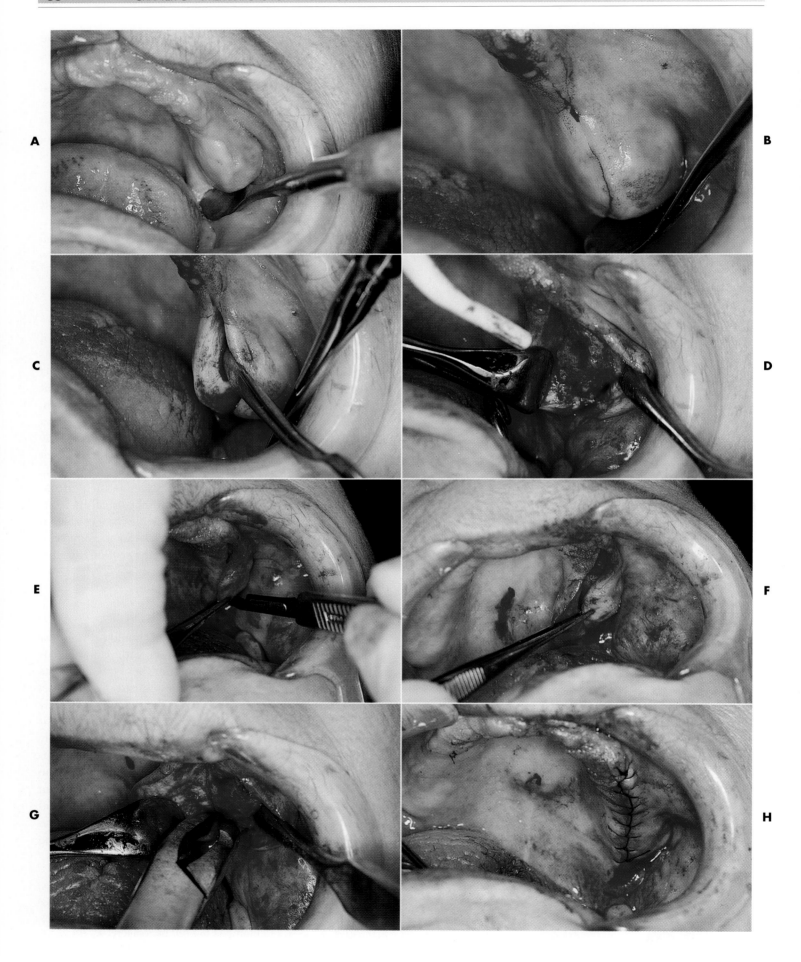

Fig. 6-19 **A,** Large tuberosities may be osseous, connective tissue, or a combination of both. **B,** The initial incision should start from behind the tuberosity at the pterygomandibular raphe attachment and come forward over the crest of the ridge to the premolar area. **C,** Periosteal elevators serve to reflect the flaps. **D,** Make the exposure to the base of the tuberosity. **E,** Hypertrophic soft tissues are reduced in thickness by stabilizing them and filleting with a No. 15 blade. Thin each flap in this manner. **F,** After thinning, draw together the flaps and tailor them to fit snugly against each other to permit a primary closure. **G,** Trim excessive bone with rongeurs and bone files. **H,** Tissues are brought together, and suturing may be done using a continuous box-lock closure.

edge (Fig. 6-19, *E*). When the newly reduced flaps are brought together, there is an excess of tissue, and the flaps will have to be trimmed so that their margins meet comfortably in the midline without redundancy at the suture line (Fig. 6-19, *F*).

If the tuberosity is bony, make the same incisions and reflections but the ridge requires trimming with a side-cutting rongeur forceps or a saline-cooled, slow-turning large ovoid surgical bur (Fig. 6-19, *G*). Follow this with the use of a bone file, and tailor to fit the excess soft tissues at the wound margins. This may be completed successfully by suturing with a continuous box-lock mattress closure (Fig. 6-19, *H*).

Alveoplasty

Alveoplasty is a technique with which all surgical practitioners must become competent. Knife-edged ridges may require planing, undercut reduction, or the removal of sharp, spinous processes before making implant osteotomies. Make incisions at the ridge crests and perform reflections of soft tissues with care to preserve the sanctity of the mucoperiosteal flaps (Fig. 6-20, *A*). With rosette and flame-shaped burs (always saline-cooled), rongeurs, and bone files (Fig. 6-20, *B, C*), the reduction, contouring, and smoothing of the bone can be performed with precision. Running a piece of gauze over the bone can test results. It should pass easily over the ridge without the shredding or pulling of any of its threads (Fig. 6-20, *D*). When the alveolus passes this test, perform closure with either a box-lock or continuous horizontal mattress suture (Fig. 6-20, *E*). (See the section on suturing in this chapter.)

Correction of High or Hypertrophic Muscle Attachments

There are some simple soft tissue manipulations that should be mastered. Frenula and other high muscle attachments often require elimination (Fig. 6-21, *A*). In cases of the high buccinator attachment in the mandibular region, avoid the mental nerve. After infiltration anesthesia, make incisions through the soft tissues and down to bone on either side of the frenulum or muscle attachment, starting at its apex and widening elliptically until the vestibule is reached. These incisions are facilitated if the assistant pulls the cheek or lip taut. When cutting through fixed gingivae, the knife must stay against

bone. As the scalpel passes into mucosa, control the depth of the incisions to the muscle level. The widest point between the two incisions should be at the depth of the vestibule. Then curve the incisions toward one another through the labial mucosa, on either side of the muscle attachment until they touch at the point where the frenulum or muscle attachment ends, thereby creating an ellipse. Use a thin, sharp periosteal elevator to lift the alveolar end of the frenulum from the bone. Grasp the liberated segment with an Allison forceps, and as it is pulled gently forward (Fig. 6-21, B, *C*), snip it neatly from the orbicularis oris or buccinator muscle with the tips of a baby Metzenbaum scissors.

Lift each soft tissue flap with the toothed Adson or Gerald forceps and undermine them laterally for about 5 mm, until the flaps may be drawn together easily and closed with interrupted, dyed, or continuous horizontal Vicryl sutures (Fig. 6-21, *D*). Obviously, it will not be possible to draw the tissues overlying the alveolar bone together, since they are fixed, but this portion of the wound should be sutured across despite the lack of primary closure. If more than 1.5 mm of bone is exposed, place Coe-Pak or the periodontal dressing of choice beneath the sutures. This protects the bone while secondary intention healing takes place (Fig. 6-21, *E*).

Epulides Fissuratum and Other Hyperplasias

Such excessive growths are best trimmed and contoured using a 5-mm-diameter electrosurgical loop set on "cutting" current (Fig. 6-22, *A*). Move the loop smoothly and rapidly, thus encouraging bleeding and minimizing necrosis of the tissues. If metal restorations or implants are adjacent to the operative field, be careful not to touch them. If proximity is a problem, insulate the metal with a square of rubber dam. Alternatively, a scalpel blade may be used (Fig. 6-22, *B*).

After completing the resection, use the patient's own denture as a stent and line it with a noneugenol containing periodontal dressing such as Coe-Pak (Fig. 6-22, *C*). The stent may be ligated to the jaw, as described in the section on ligating in this chapter, or sutured with 2-0 nylon through submandibular buttons placed against the submandibular skin (Fig. 6-22, *D*). (See Chapter 7.) After removal of the stent, acceptable postoperative healing with good fixed tissue control should be expected (Fig. 6-22, *E*).

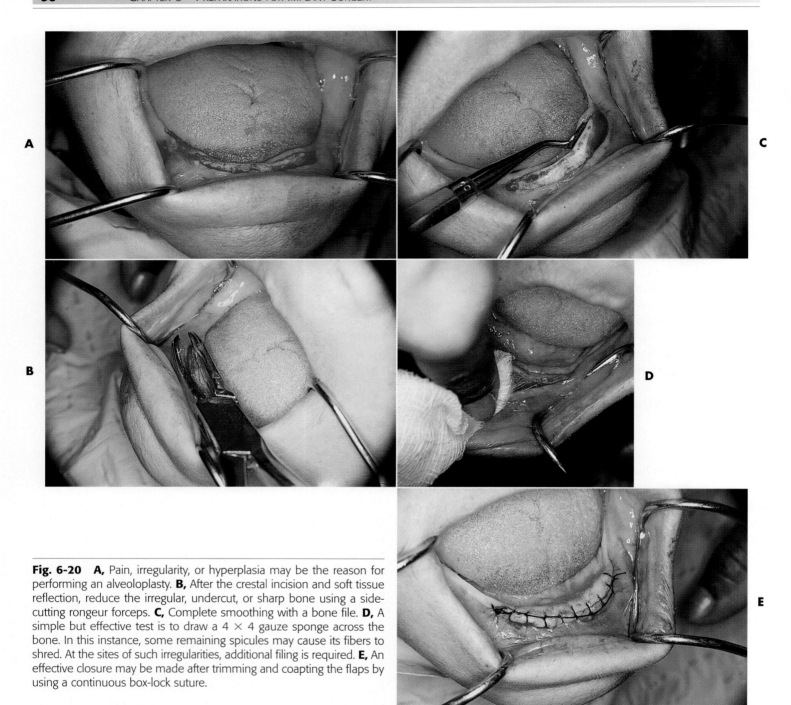

Fig. 6-20 **A,** Pain, irregularity, or hyperplasia may be the reason for performing an alveoloplasty. **B,** After the crestal incision and soft tissue reflection, reduce the irregular, undercut, or sharp bone using a side-cutting rongeur forceps. **C,** Complete smoothing with a bone file. **D,** A simple but effective test is to draw a 4 × 4 gauze sponge across the bone. In this instance, some remaining spicules may cause its fibers to shred. At the sites of such irregularities, additional filing is required. **E,** An effective closure may be made after trimming and coapting the flaps by using a continuous box-lock suture.

A   B   C

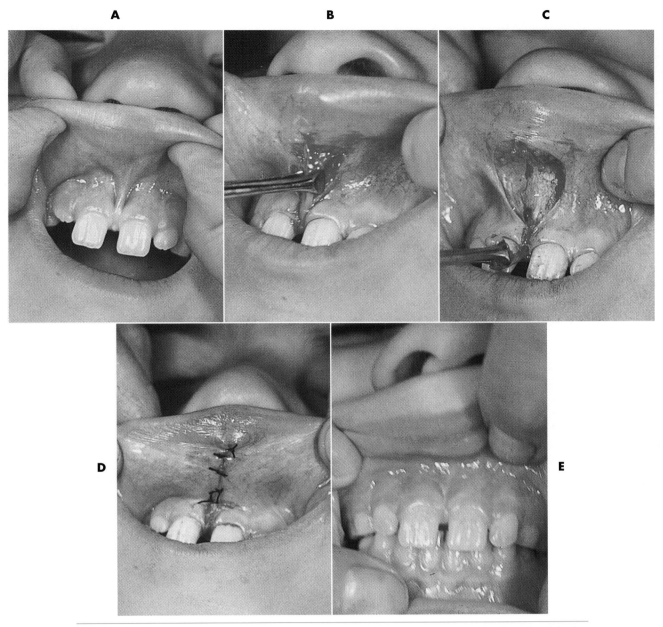

D   E

Fig. 6-21   A, High muscle attachments, like this labial frenulum, may cause postimplantation irritation and tissue loss. Remove before definitive surgery. **B,** Grasp the frenulum after anesthesia, using an Allison forceps. **C,** Incisions on either side create an elliptical defect. The soft tissue will not come away, however, unless a periosteal elevator is used to detach those portions that emanate from the fixed gingival zones. **D,** A simple vertical closure completes the procedure. **E,** If the frenulectomy has been performed aggressively, its deleterious effects often correct themselves. In this case the diastema partially closed without benefit of orthodontic therapy.

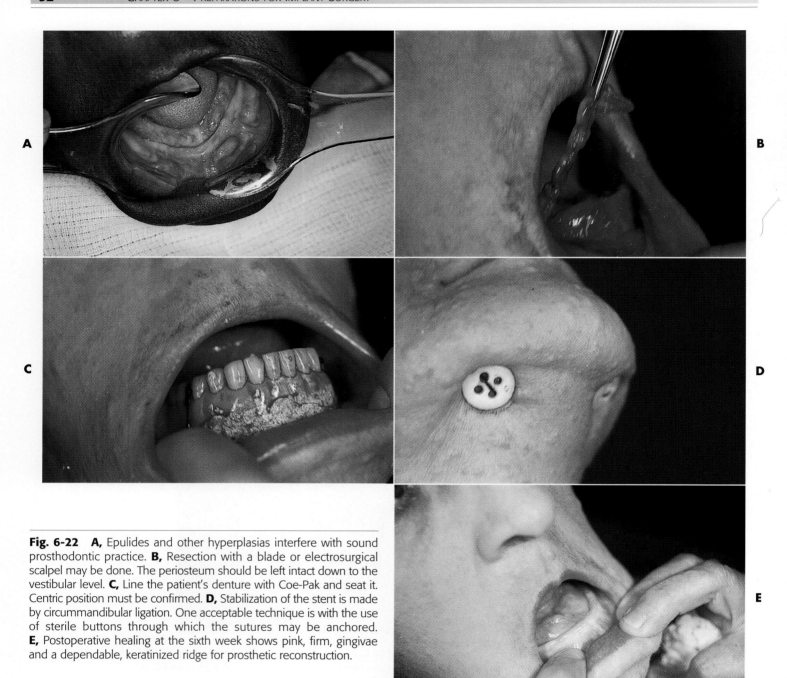

Fig. 6-22   A, Epulides and other hyperplasias interfere with sound prosthodontic practice. **B,** Resection with a blade or electrosurgical scalpel may be done. The periosteum should be left intact down to the vestibular level. **C,** Line the patient's denture with Coe-Pak and seat it. Centric position must be confirmed. **D,** Stabilization of the stent is made by circummandibular ligation. One acceptable technique is with the use of sterile buttons through which the sutures may be anchored. **E,** Postoperative healing at the sixth week shows pink, firm, gingivae and a dependable, keratinized ridge for prosthetic reconstruction.

Suggested Readings

Babbush CA: *Dental implants: principles and practice,* Philadelphia, 1991, WB Saunders.

Babbush CA: *Surgical atlas of dental implant techniques,* Philadelphia, 1980, WB Saunders.

Bahat O: Surgical-planning for optimal aesthetic and functional results of osseointegrated implants in the partially edentulous mouth, *J Calif Dent Assoc* 20(5):31-46, 1992.

Bahat O: Treatment planning and placement of implants in the posterior maxillae: report of 732 consecutive Nobelpharma implants, *Int J Oral Maxillofac Implants* 2:151-161, 1993.

Becket W, Becket B: Flap designs for minimization of recession adjacent to maxillary anterior implant sites: a clinical study, *Int J Oral Maxillofac Implants* 11:46-54 1996.

Bedrossian E, Gongloff RK: Considerations in placement of implants through existing split-thickness skin graft vestibuloplasty: a case report, *J Oral Maxillofac Implants* 5:401-404, 1990.

Brisman D: The effect of speed, pressure, and time on bone temperature during the drilling of implant sites, *Int J Oral Maxillofac Implants* 11:35-37, 1996.

Cranin AN: *Oral implantology,* Springfield, Ill., 1970, Charles C Thomas.

Eriksson RA, Albrektsson T: Temperature threshold levels for heat-induced bone tissue injury, *J Prosthet Dent* 50:101, 1983.

Fonseca R, Davis WH: *Reconstructive preprosthetic oral and maxillofacial surgery,* Philadelphia, 1986, WB Saunders.

Hallman W et al: A comparative study of the effects of metallic, non-metallic, and sonic instrumentation on titanium abutment surfaces, *Int J Oral Maxillofac Implants* 11:96-100, 1996.

Hjorting-Hansen E, Adawy A, Hillerup S: Mandibular vestibulolingual sulcoplasty with free skin graft. A five year clinical follow-up study, *J Oral Surg* 41:173-176, 1983.

Jensen S et al: Tissue reaction and material characteristics of four bone substitutes, *Int J Oral Maxillofac Implants* 11:55-67, 1996.

Koole R, Bosker H, Noorman van der Dussen F: Secondary autogenous bone grafting in cleft patients comparing mandibular (ectomesenchymal) and crista iliaca (mesenchymal) grafts, *Cranio Maxillofac Surg* 17(suppl J):28, 1989.

Kruger GO: *Textbook of oral and maxillofacial surgery,* ed 6, St. Louis, 1984, Mosby.

Linkow LI: Bone transplants using the symphysis, the iliac crest, and synthetic bone materials, *J Oral Implant* 11:211-247, 1983.

MacMillan HW: Structural characteristics of the alveolar process, *Int J Orthodont Oral Surg* 12:722-730, 1926.

Marx RE: Principles of hard- and soft-tissue reconstruction of the jaws, *Abstract ML* 315, American Association of Oral and Maxillofacial Surgeons, New Orleans, 1990.

Misch C: Density of bone: effect on treatment plan, surgical approach, healing, and progressive bone healing, *Int J Oral Implant* 6:23-31, 1990.

Misch C, Crawford E: Predictable mandibular nerve location a clinical zone of safety, *Int J Oral Implant* 7:37-40, 1990.

Quayle AA: Atraumatic removal of teeth and root fragments in dental implantology, *J Oral Maxillofac Implants* 5:293-296, 1990.

Venturelli A: A modified surgical protocol for placing implants in the maxillary tuberosity: clinical results at 36 months after loading with fixed partial dentures, *Int J Oral Maxillofac Implants* 11(6):743-749, 1996.

7

Soft Tissue Management and Grafting

ARMAMENTARIUM

Bougies: whalebone-olive tipped
Buttons: sterile
Forceps: Adson and Gerald (toothed and nontoothed)
Forceps: hemostatic-mosquito
Needle holders
Retractors: Blunt Mathieu, beaver tails, Sweetheart
Scalpel blades: BP 15, 12
Scalpel handles: BP No. 3
Scissors: Baby Metzenbaum
Scissors: Goldman-Fox
Sutures: Biosyn 3-0, 4-0 on C13, C14 on F1, F2 cutting needles
Sutures: Polysorb or Vicryl 3-0, 4-0 on C13, C14 cutting needles 5-0
  6-0 on CV 23 tapered needles
P10 cutting needles

CAVEATS

When there is a paucity of mucosa, a variety of soft tissue grafting
  strategies may be undertaken. In planning pedicle grafts, rigidly
  observe certain guidelines:

a. The pedicle cannot be more than two and a half times longer
   than it is wide.
b. The flap must be well vascularized.
c. Suturing must be tension free.

Impeccable tissue handling offers assurance that the highest levels
  of functional and cosmetic success result.
Perform creation of pedicles with care. Do not make mucosa too
  thin, or devascularization may result. If excessive connective tissue
  is permitted to remain, the graft may be bulky, unsuitable, and esthetically displeasing.
Employ the sharpest instruments, the finest sutures that will serve
  satisfactorily, and the gentlest use of tissue forceps.
Regional block anesthesia is preferable to infiltration because the tissues requiring plastic surgery respond best if they are not bloated
  with anesthetic solution (which causes distortion) and ischemia
  from the vasoconstrictor.
Careful dissection for undermining demands attention to the surface
  of the mucosa as the scissors are dissecting beneath the flap. In
  this fashion, perforation can be avoided.

Soft tissues are required to cover bone, transport vascular channels, enclose implant host sites, and bring
functional and esthetic contour to critical anatomic areas. Defatted or split-thickness skin and mucosa derived from
the patient serve best as free grafts. These grafts may be taken
by dermatome from the lateral thigh, from skin found behind
the ear and overlying the mastoid process, and from the palate.
Mucosa to be used as pedicle grafts is derived primarily from
the superior and inferior vestibular areas. To a lesser extent,
mucosa to be used for purposes of closing oroantral fistulae is
derived from the palate. Gingival faults may be repaired reliably with palatal split-thickness, connective tissue, free-grafts
covered by gingivomucosal pedicles.

The plastic surgical manipulation of oral tissues plays an
integral role in implant-borne oral habilitation and should become an essential skill of all implant surgeons.

Incisions

Making incisions properly offers rapid and consistent primary wound healing by causing fewer postoperative sequelae such as edema, pain, and bleeding and creating a surgical environment that protects the sanctity of the implants that have been placed.

Counsel surgical assistants that suctioning, particularly when it is powerful, has the potential of doing harm. It can tear tissues, injure small blood vessels, encourage the continuation of bleeding, and as the tip sweeps back and forth, disturb the alignment of flaps. In addition, suctioning aspirates the organisms floating in the aerosol above the wound directly into it, inviting infection. Use suction only for purposes of permitting the surgeon to see the operative field and to evacuate the pharynx. If no need exists for these two uses, keep the suction tip away from the operative site and counsel the surgical assistant to use sponges first. Observe the following rules:

1. Use only sharp scalpels. Change blades frequently.
2. For dentoalveolar surgery, make incisions at the crest of the ridge. No. 15 BP blades are the preferred design. Each edentulous ridge has a linea alba centered directly on its superior surface. This represents an avascular scar that resulted from the trauma of extractions and the pressure from denture saddles. Recent research indicates that there is no blood flow from buccal to lingual sides of each ridge as a result of the lack of capillary anastomoses across this whitish line (Fig. 7-1). Unique, innovative, or unconventional incisions such as the S type or the labial vestibular visor present risks of retarded healing, implant dehiscence and ischemia or necrosis of that portion of the flap that is to be found between the incision site and the linea alba.

3. Press the scalpel firmly to the bone to avoid retracing incisions. If the incision is not made cleanly, periosteal reflection is resistant, the danger of tearing tissue is significant, and postoperative pain and swelling increase. Make incisions once and make them correctly. Multiple slices of the periosteum decrease vascularity and retard healing. If the ridge is sharp or knife-edged, be careful to prevent the blade from slipping off to the side.
4. Extend incisions adequately: anteriorly by at least one tooth and posteriorly over the tuberosity or through and beyond the retromolar pad. This may eliminate a need for vertical or releasing incisions that can cause pain and swelling and may retard healing as well. When required to gain further exposure of an operative site, releasing incisions should be oblique with broader bases and must always include full papillae. Hemisectioned papillae are difficult to suture and present poor prospects for predictable healing.
5. A No. 12 BP blade is important. Because of its curvature, this blade permits the extension of incisions through the gingival crevice of the most distal tooth present and makes surgical separations accurately and cleanly in all the crevices (Fig. 7-2).
6. Before making the first incision, plan the procedure on a study cast. Small or inadequate incisions may be a major reason for surgical failure. Make larger rather than smaller incisions; they heal just as rapidly. Improved access to the operative site contributes to more precise surgery. In addition, retraction is gentler, causing the tissues to respond more kindly to the trauma caused by surgery.

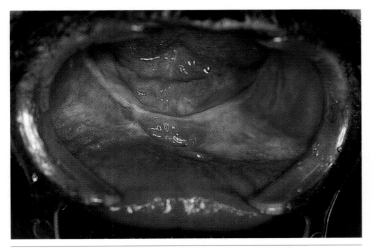

Fig. 7-1   Linea alba, a fine white crestal line found on edentulous ridges, is avascular and does not permit cross-ridge capillary anastomoses. After novel incisions (e.g., S-shaped or visor types), the site may break down or heal slowly and cause bone loss around implant cervices.

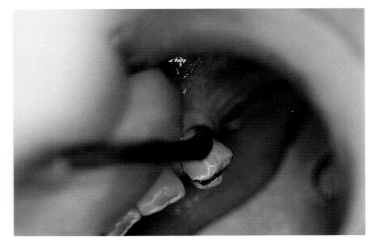

Fig. 7-2   The use of No. 12 scalpel blades enables the surgeon to make sharp incisions in inaccessible places.

Flap Design, Elevation, and Retraction

Careful, thorough, and complete flap design and elevation, without tearing or injuring the periosteum, is necessary for a smooth operative and postoperative course. This demands that new or freshly sharpened periosteal elevators be available (Fig. 7-3). Do not rip or tear the fibers. Instead, sharply incise them at the cortical bone level. To do this, a keen-edged elevator is required. Before each operation, the auxiliary staff should be sure that the elevators are as flawless and as sharp as new ones.

Flaps that have releasing incisions should have bases that are wider than their alveolar margins, essentially trapezoidal (Fig. 7-4). If tooth areas are to be included in the surgical exposure, the gingival papillae should never be split but should instead be included totally in the flap. Elevation of such gingival tissues must be made gently with a fine-pointed elevator only after thorough incision.

In areas that have experienced previous surgery or trauma, where evident scarring is present, or in other cases where the investing tissues have been found to be resistant to easy and

complete reflection, the procedure can be expedited by using a technique that performs this challenging task with ease and consistency. It involves the use of a small-toothed pickup forceps (Adson or Gerald) and a scalpel armed with a new No. 12 BP blade (Fig. 7-5). Use the forceps to lift an edge of the flap so that the tip of the blade may gently stroke the scarred adherent fibers in the fashion of a periosteal elevator. Proceed, a bit at a time, carefully elevating the flap until a zone is reached at which conventional periosteal separation is permitted. Do not attempt this technique for the first time on a patient. Practice on a cow mandible (which can be obtained from a butcher) until a high level of confidence is achieved in regard to full-thickness reflection without perforating the mucoperiosteum, which is a serious, but not always irrevocable, incident. If the blade tip is kept against the bone and the strokes are made in a short and gentle fashion, the technique can be mastered readily. If the overlying mucosa is perforated, keep the laceration to a minimal length and continue the reflection and subsequent surgery completion. After suturing and closure, close the iatrogenic laceration with 6-0 Vicryl or Polysorb continuous horizontal mattress sutures using a fine tapered (SH) needle. (Refer to the Sutures and Suturing section of Chapter 6.)

In two areas, the palatal and the mandibular facial, be very careful in the reflection of mucosal flaps so that the greater palatine and mental neurovascular bundles are protected. Such efforts are abetted if a 2 × 2 gauze sponge is inserted beneath the flap. By pushing the sponge with a peri-osteal elevator, the surgeon can enlarge the separation with safety and accuracy (Fig. 7-6). In this fashion, as a foramen is approached, it comes into view in a trauma-free fashion, sparing injury to its neurovascular bundle.

Once the flaps are reflected, manage them gently. Keep them well hydrated with saline-moistened sponges. The man-

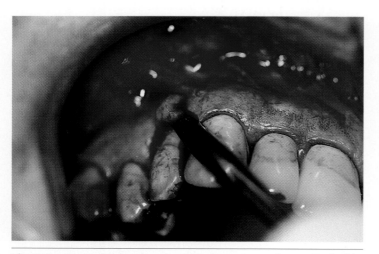

Fig. 7-3 Periosteal elevators should incise, not tear, tissues. To do this, keep them sharp.

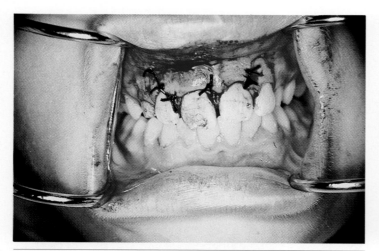

Fig. 7-4 Flaps heal fastest when their bases are wide. Wide bases ensure the greatest amount of vascularity.

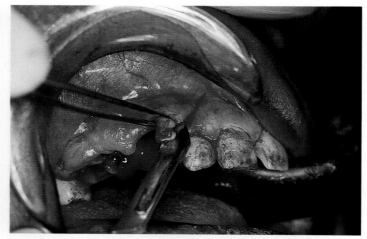

Fig. 7-5 Adherent or scarred tissue is often resistant to elevation. This procedure is facilitated by grasping an end of the mucoperiosteum with an Adson or Gerald forceps and stroking beneath the flap gently with a No. 12 scalpel blade. This will permit the lifting of the flap atraumatically and without effort.

ner in which they are kept retracted also plays a role in subsequent healing. Retractors should be smooth surfaced; these include Henahans, Seldins, beaver tails, or blunt-toothed rakes (Mathieus) (Fig. 7-7). The staff should make sure that they are not nicked or scratched. All the rakes in the armamentarium should have blunt, not sharp, tips.

A suitable and convenient alternative to manual reflection is autoretraction by using sutures. Buccal flaps may be sutured to the buccal mucosa. Palatal flaps may be sutured into a midline bundle, which keeps these tissues out of the operative field. Unilateral palatal flaps may be sutured to the teeth on the contralateral side, which keeps the surgical site well exposed without the need for refractors. Bilateral mandibular lingual flaps may be sutured to each other across the dorsum of the tongue,

not only serving as an excellent retraction source but also as a competent tongue depressor (Fig. 7-8). Unilateral mandibular flaps may be kept retracted by suturing them across the dorsum of the tongue to teeth on the unoperated side.

In planning and designing flaps, do not split papillae, frenula, and muscle attachments but include them totally within the flap design. When palatal flaps are planned, make all incisions in the gingival crevices or at the ridge crest and never across the palatal mucoperiosteum. In this fashion only full-thickness, total palatal mucosa is reflected (Fig. 7-9). If palatal tissues are segmented, as a worst case scenario, the risk of cutting the palatine artery exists; at best, such incisions retard healing and cause considerable pain. In order to elevate a full palatal flap, it is permissible in the area of the incisive neurovascular

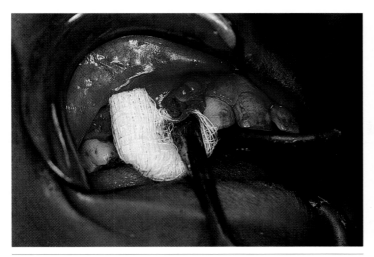

Fig. 7-6 A method to elevate flaps in mucosal areas with minimal trauma is to tease them away from the bone by pushing a 2 × 2 sponge ahead of the periosteal elevator. When the neurovascular bundle is reached, it will be clearly visible and remain uninjured because of the gentleness of the sponge (see Figs. 7-8, 7-9).

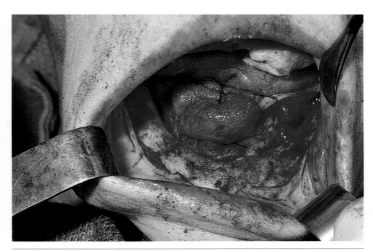

Fig. 7-8 Sutures serve as excellent retractors. In surgery of the mandible that involves both sides, the two lingual flaps may be tied together across the dorsum of the tongue in a shoelace configuration. This not only keeps the lingual flaps out of the field, but it also stabilizes the sublingual adnexae and immobilizes the tongue. In unilateral procedures, the contralateral teeth may be used as anchorage for the retracting sutures.

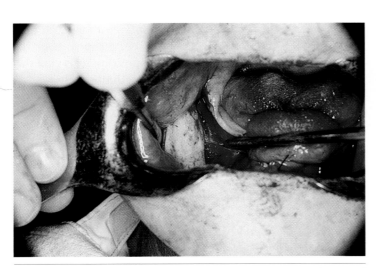

Fig. 7-7 Polished edges on retractors prevent tissue injury. The use of blunt rake, smooth Henahan, beaver tails, and Seldins is to be encouraged. Retractors cause the least damage when you permit them to rest against bone.

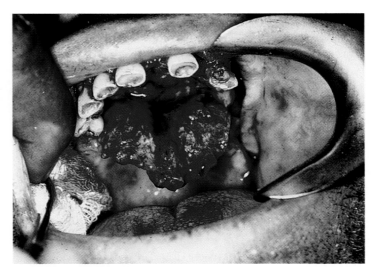

Fig. 7-9 Operations performed on the palate should be made with crevicular incisions only. The resulting full-thickness, complete palatal reflections remain well vascularized and offer the greatest possibilities for primary healing.

bundle to cut this structure while doing the reflection. Surprisingly, little or no bleeding results and no noticeable dysesthesia or retardation of healing is noted postoperatively.

Filleting or thinning of soft tissue flaps should be performed with great care. After incision and reflection, lift the flap to be thinned with an Adson (short) or Gerald (long) forceps and excise the deep layers at a depth that permits the required thickness of mucosa to remain (Fig. 7-10). Exercise care when dissecting in a plane parallel to the mucosa so that it does not become perforated or overly thinned. By using the technique of filleting, the implantologist is able to thin and streamline many tissues, such as those covering the ridges or tuberosities. In addition, use sheets of such salvaged uninjured connective tissue as substitutes for synthetic membranes, either with a poncho design or over synthetic grafting materials placed to cover a cortical plate perforation. (See Chapter 8, sections on Periodontal Defect Correction and The Use of Guided Tissue Regeneration Membranes.)

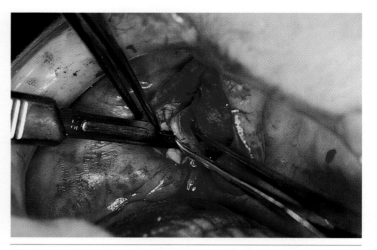

Fig. 7-10 Flaps often require thinning. To do this, stabilize them with a toothed forceps so that a sharp scalpel blade can be used to fillet the deeper layers. Although the tissue reduction is being performed beneath the flap, the surgeon's eyes should be focused on the mucosal surface so that flap perforation will be avoided.

Soft Tissue Grafting, Vestibuloplasty, and Pedicle Grafting

Sometimes there is not an adequate amount of tissue available to create a primary closure, that is, to bring the margins of the wound together firmly so that the underlying bone and implants are covered. One cannot be assured of primary healing or osseointegration if the flaps are sutured under tension. This is particularly important when using guided tissue regenerative membranes (GTRMs). Flaps may not be pulled, stretched, caused to blanch, or allowed to become ischemic. Unfortunately, it is not always possible to create a quiescent, tension-free closure. The major key to surgical success is the mastering of a technique called *undermining* and in so doing, creating an easy closure (Fig. 7-11). This is a simple technique, although many practitioners may be unfamiliar with the method or its inestimable value.

Undermining involves picking up a buccal or labial flap (it cannot be done on the palatal or lingual sides) with a toothed Adson or Gerald forceps. As the surgeon looks beneath the elevated flap, it is noted that muscle fibers (buccinator or orbicularis oris) are attached to it. Although these fibers are stretchable and compliant, they do have the memory of isometricity. If they are pulled or drawn excessively in order to permit a closure of flaps across a wound, the muscle fibers immediately begin to retract the tissues to their original positions, thus causing a wound dehiscence.

To prevent this, carefully use baby Metzenbaum scissors (which are curved and blunted) to snip the muscle fibers from the overlying flaps. This permits the flaps to cover the bony operative site without tension (Fig. 7-12, A-C). The surgeon must be wary when undermining in the vicinity of the mental nerve, and, when operating in the maxillary first molar area, Stensen's duct may present a potential hazard. If doubts exist about the location of the duct, dry the tiny carunculum that indicates its presence in the midbuccal mucosa, and milk the

gland with one hand and retract and pull forward the cheek to straighten the premasseteric kink with the other hand. While a drop of saliva is secreted, pass a fine olive-tipped bougie or lacrimal probe into the orifice. After the duct is entered, have the assistant stabilize it while a 3-0 black silk circumferential suture is passed through the tissues and tied around the probe to anchor it in place. Subsequent undermining is simple because the presence of the probe provides information as to exactly where the duct is lying in relationship to the dissection (Fig. 7-12, D).

Early undermining efforts may cause mucosal perforation, although such defects may be repaired. To prevent such accidents, do not look at what you are cutting from the undersurface of the flap but rather view the dissection and the snipping of the shears from the intact mucosal surface above. After the flap has been mobilized so that it may be drawn over the wound with ease, suture it into its new position. It is vital that implant surgeons become comfortable with this technique.

Split-thickness grafting offers additional benefits (Fig. 7-13, A). To avoid loss of vestibular depth, which is caused by producing a tension-free undermined pedicle flap, separate the newly liberated tissue, mucosa from periosteum (Figs. 7-13, B, C). The deeper layer is used to cover the implants and ridge while the superficial layer may be employed to maintain the vestibular depth by closing it short of the crest and tacking it to the periosteum with several 5-0 Vicryl or Polysorb sutures (Fig. 7-13, D). The denuded crestal periosteum, closed with a periodontal dressing, is covered within 5 days by new secondary-intention epithelium (Fig. 7-13, E, F). Within 3 weeks, a stable zone of fixed gingiva becomes established (Fig. 7-13, G).

Pedicle (attached base) grafting is also of value. The three rules governing management must be followed for successful results. Using these rules, you can intelligently make flap de-

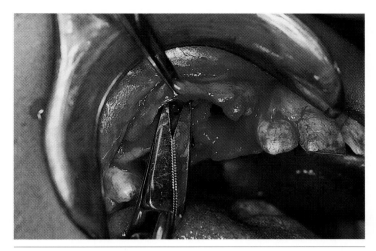

Fig. 7-11 When there is not adequate tissue available to cover the bone, it may be made attainable by undermining mucosa from the buccinator or orbicularis oris muscles. This is done by lifting its edge and detaching it from its muscular bed using baby Metzenbaum or other curved scissors. The surgeon's eyes should remain on the mucosal surface despite the fact that the dissection is being carried out beneath it. On drawing the newly made flap across the denuded bone, it will not demonstrate tension nor will it show signs of blanching.

signs. Make them more generous in dimension than you deem adequate. When possible, elevate them from the donor site with neurovascular bundle included. This permits primary coverage of fistulous sites, antral communications, dehiscent implants, or ridge augmentation devices (Fig. 7-14, *A*).

When such grafts are sutured to the adjacent host site mucosa, be sure that a well-vascularized, bleeding, muscular bed is present to receive it. When creating pedicles, leave behind an exposed donor site of either bone or muscle. Dress these donor sites with iodoform or Xeroform gauze or a periodontal pack using splints, stents, or sutures to hold them in place. Design and create palatal, labial, and buccal mucosal pedicles by dissecting the mucosa from its bony or muscular bed by elevating or undermining. Flaps generated from buccal and labial areas should be mobilized and brought over the area to be covered only after a bleeding host site has been created to receive them on the lingual or palatal surfaces over healthy bone. In similar fashion, palatal flaps with neurovascular bundles may be developed, elevated, and rotated 90 degrees across the ridge, where they can be sutured into newly made, bleeding, buccal pockets (Fig. 7-14, *B, C*). To do this, make a

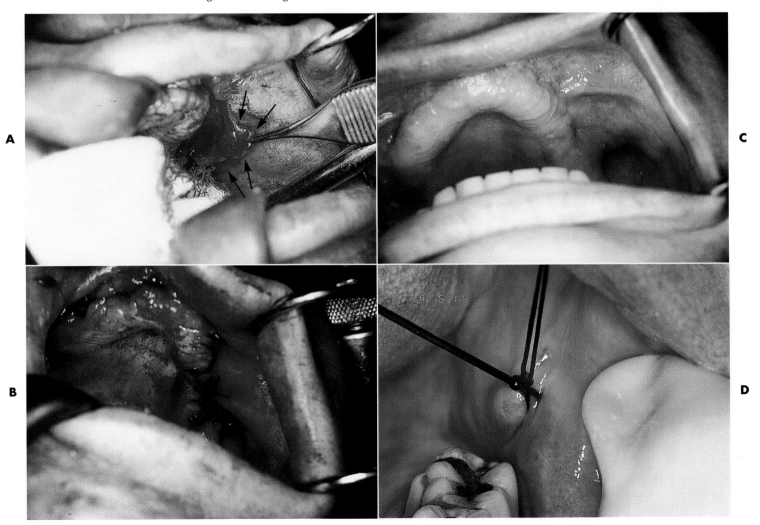

Fig. 7-12 **A,** The buccal mucosa is a generous donor site for creating pedicle grafts. During undermining, hold the flap *(arrows)* with a toothed forceps (Adson), while the Metzenbaum scissors is used to detach it from the musculature. **B,** A tension-free closure is mandatory if primary healing is to take place. **C,** Two weeks postoperatively, good tissue tone and color indicate a successful graft. **D,** If Stensen's duct is close, it is best avoided by suturing a whale bone bougie or lacrymal probe into it.

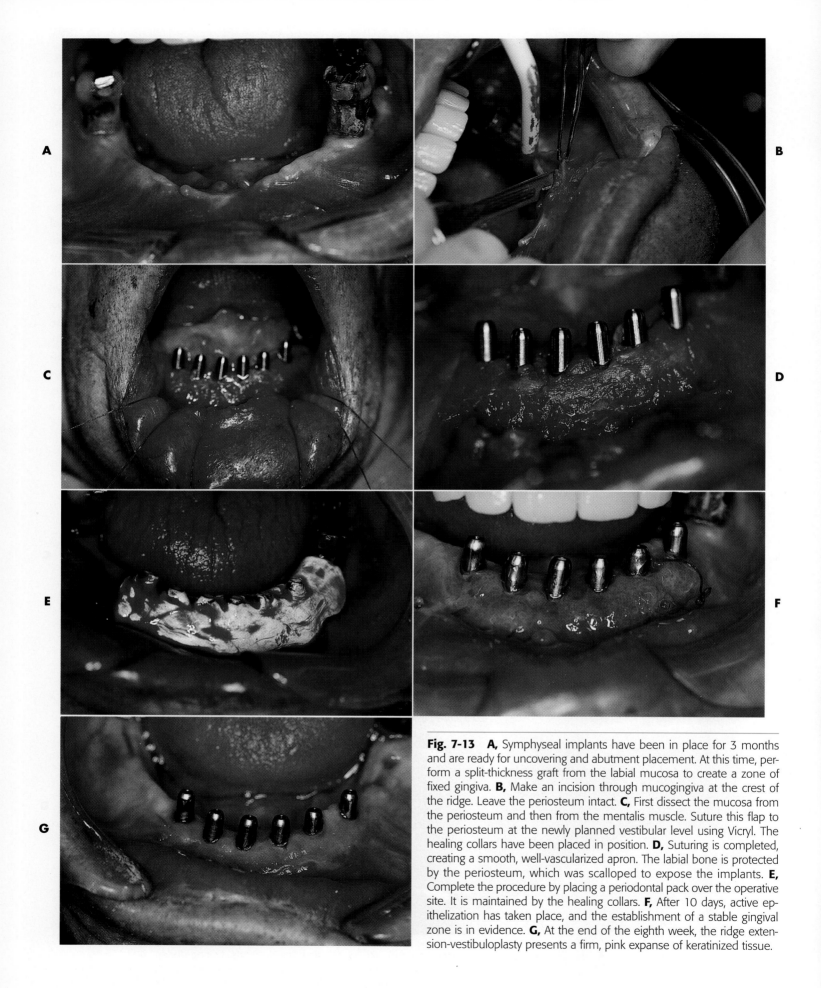

Fig. 7-13 **A,** Symphyseal implants have been in place for 3 months and are ready for uncovering and abutment placement. At this time, perform a split-thickness graft from the labial mucosa to create a zone of fixed gingiva. **B,** Make an incision through mucogingiva at the crest of the ridge. Leave the periosteum intact. **C,** First dissect the mucosa from the periosteum and then from the mentalis muscle. Suture this flap to the periosteum at the newly planned vestibular level using Vicryl. The healing collars have been placed in position. **D,** Suturing is completed, creating a smooth, well-vascularized apron. The labial bone is protected by the periosteum, which was scalloped to expose the implants. **E,** Complete the procedure by placing a periodontal pack over the operative site. It is maintained by the healing collars. **F,** After 10 days, active epithelization has taken place, and the establishment of a stable gingival zone is in evidence. **G,** At the end of the eighth week, the ridge extension-vestibuloplasty presents a firm, pink expanse of keratinized tissue.

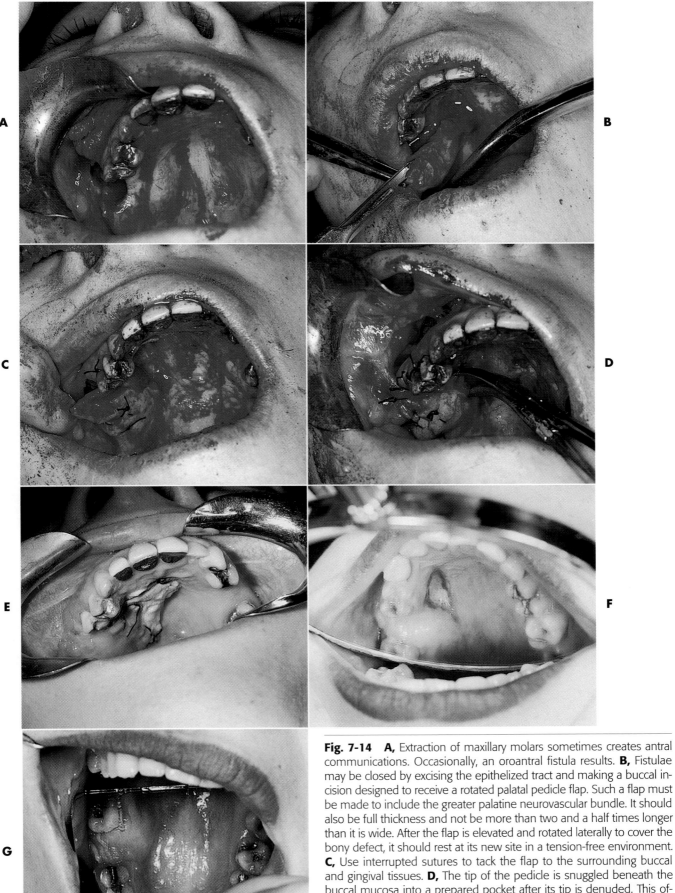

Fig. 7-14 A, Extraction of maxillary molars sometimes creates antral communications. Occasionally, an oroantral fistula results. **B,** Fistulae may be closed by excising the epithelized tract and making a buccal incision designed to receive a rotated palatal pedicle flap. Such a flap must be made to include the greater palatine neurovascular bundle. It should also be full thickness and not be more than two and a half times longer than it is wide. After the flap is elevated and rotated laterally to cover the bony defect, it should rest at its new site in a tension-free environment. **C,** Use interrupted sutures to tack the flap to the surrounding buccal and gingival tissues. **D,** The tip of the pedicle is snuggled beneath the buccal mucosa into a prepared pocket after its tip is denuded. This offers double assurance of primary healing. **E,** Permit the donor site to heal by secondary intention. During this period, it is protected with iodoform packing stabilized by crisscross silk sutures. **F,** The well-vascularized flap indicates good healing at the fourth week. The palate has yet to epithelize. **G,** By the eighth week the palate has filled in fully with keratinized tissue, the rugae have recurred, and the pedicle's rugae are present and will remain so for the remainder of the patient's life.

horizontal incision in the buccal margin of the wound, separating mucosa from muscle. Dissection should extend 1 cm into the buccinator muscle. Denude the transported palatal flap of epithelium from its tip for a distance of 1 cm, using a scalpel blade or a sterile abrasive heatless wheel. Then slip this tip into the buccal pocket and tack it in place with several deep 4-0 Vicryl sutures. The double layer created in this manner offers additional assurance of a primary closure (Fig. 7-14, D).

After healing, cover the primary defect by the transported mucosa, and fill in the donor (palatal) site, which had been protected by pack, with secondary-intention epithelium (Figs. 7-14, E, F). In most cases the patient's vestibule has been sacrificed. A subsequent vestibuloplasty may be required (Fig. 7-14, G).

A more predictable procedure is the vestibuloplasty made with a pedicle graft (Fig. 7-15, A). Three sides of the graft must be outlined on the labial mucosa with a No. 15 BP blade. Its two sides should extend from the vestibule to a length equal to the height of the planned zone of fixed gingiva. Connect the lateral incision across the mucosa parallel to the vermilion border, leaving an intact base at the vestibule (Fig. 7-15, B). Lift and undermine the flap as described in earlier paragraphs of this chapter. Follow the three cardinal rules for pedicle flap design listed previously. When the mucosa is dissected from the orbicularis oris muscle to its full extent, lift it with two Adson forceps, and reveal the periosteum against the anterior mandible (Fig. 7-15, C). Push the attached muscle fibers apically with a periosteal elevator to the depth of the an-

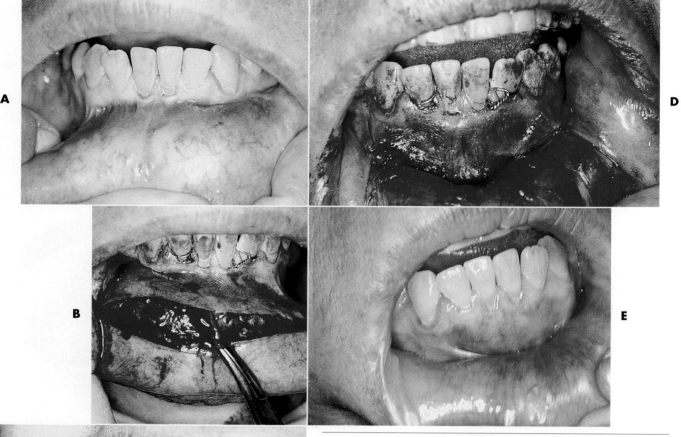

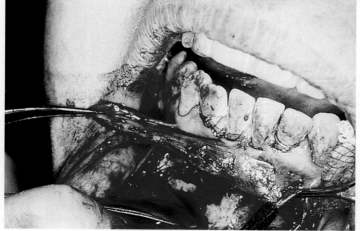

Fig. 7-15 **A,** A common site that requires vestibuloplasty is the anterior mandible. When the labial muscle fibers are attached close to or at the gingival margins, recession, bleeding, and soreness may lead to alveolar atrophy. **B,** An effective solution is the creation of a lip-based pedicle flap. This is done in the reverse manner of the procedure described in Fig. 7-13; the base in this technique is at the gingival side. The incisions that extend onto the labial mucosa should create a generous zone of fixed tissue. **C,** After the flap is outlined, a toothed forceps grasps one corner, and, with dissecting scissors, it is lifted from its muscle bed. Carry the elevation toward the mandible, but leave the periosteum unscathed. Push the attached musculature at the base of the flap inferiorly to a level at which the zone of fixed gingiva is planned. **D,** Turn the flap downward and tack it into position by using an SH tapered needle with 5-0 Vicryl sutures, which suture it firmly against the periosteum. Place brass ligatures around the teeth to serve as armatures for pack maintenance. **E,** Postoperatively, the well-keratinized zone of fixed gingiva has created a stable periodontal environment.

ticipated correction that is equal to the length of the flap. The periosteum must be permitted to remain in place, and press the elevated pedicle flat against it, thereby extending it apically and expressing entrapped blood and air. Tack it to the periosteum at its corners with 5-0 dyed Polysorb using a tapered needle. Use additional sutures, as needed, to keep it securely in place.

If teeth are present, place brass ligature wires between them, leaving extended twisted loops to act as retentive devices for a protective Coe-Pak dressing (Fig. 7-15, *D*). The pack serves as a stabilizer and also keeps the opposing labial donor site more comfortable while it is healing by secondary intention (Fig. 7-15, *E*). As an alternative, simplify this operation by using an appropriately sized piece of Alloderm.

Free Grafting Mucosa and Connective Tissue

Free grafting has its place in implant surgery, particularly during the preparatory phases when areas of implantation need to be altered so that zones of fixed gingiva can be created (Fig. 7-16, *A*). Such conditions may be acquired with vestibuloplasty, which is done either with free dermal or mucosal grafting.

Mucosal Grafting

When a free graft is planned, do not take it until the host site has been prepared. This keeps donor tissues most viable. First, make a vestibular incision at the base of the fixed gingiva, if any exists. If none is available, make the incision at the gingival margins of the teeth. Push the mucosa apically to the

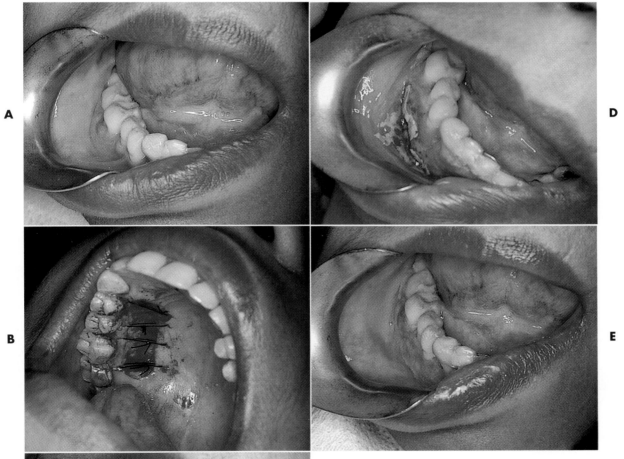

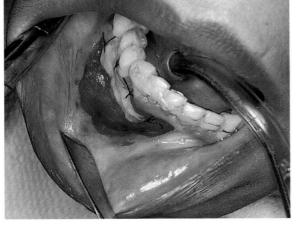

Fig. 7-16   A, The mandibular premolar area demonstrates a lack of fixed gingiva, causing chronic soreness and irritation. **B,** The palate as a donor site offers opportunities to harvest large quantities of keratinized mucosa. After the tissue is removed in split-thickness fashion, dress the wound with xeroform gauze Vicryl membrane, which is stabilized with shoelace sutures. Healing will take place by secondary intention. **C,** Prepare the host site by depressing the mucosa overlying the periosteum and then applying the graft to the exposed, bleeding surface. Peripheral sutures of a fine diameter (5-0 Vicryl) are used to stabilize it. **D,** Ten days postoperatively, remove the sutures. The area is inflamed, but its color indicates viability. **E,** By the fourth week, healing has progressed to a point at which one can be assured of a successful graft with a wide zone of pink fixed gingiva.

planned depth of the zone of fixed gingiva, but leave the periosteum intact against the bone, thus creating a split-thickness flap. Place a small saline-soaked sponge into the wound and take a free split-thickness graft from the palate using No. 15 and No. 12 BP blades (Fig. 7-16, *B*). The lateral portion of the palatal vault is the best donor site. It is important to perform the dissection superficially, taking only mucosa and avoiding injury to the greater palatine artery. The size of the graft should be 2 mm larger in each dimension than the host site requires, and the corners should be rounded.

Place the graft over the exposed host site periosteum immediately after harvesting and press it in place with a saline-moistened surgical sponge. Then use 5-0 dyed, Vicryl, interrupted sutures (with a tapered, not a cutting, needle) to tack it

down in strategic locations on all four sides. Complete the closure with interrupted sutures 2 mm apart. The graft at this point is blanched (Fig. 7-16, *C*). Dress and protect the palate and graft areas with previously prepared acrylic stents, each lined with periodontal pack.

Within 1 week after pack removal, evidence of graft success is forthcoming on inspection. It appears pink and well attached to host tissues (Fig. 7-16, *D, E*). By using Alloderm, similar success may be achieved without the necessity of harvesting. A full description of its use may be found in the last paragraphs of this chapter.

Free grafting is effective for creating vestibules in edentulous jaws as well. Perform this procedure before the placement of implants (Fig. 7-17).

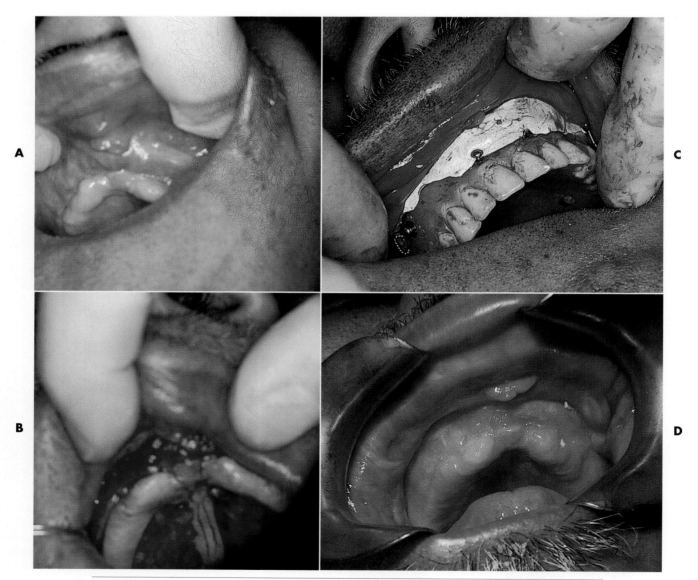

Fig. 7-17 **A,** Edentulous maxillae that are being considered as candidates for implants should demonstrate zones of fixed gingivae before implant placement. **B,** Make incisions in the labial mucosa down to, but not including, the periosteum. The mucosa is elevated superiorly, leaving well-vascularized host sites against the labial surface of the bone. This step is followed by the split-thickness dissection of the palatal mucosa, which will serve as the graft material. Each palatal half is taken to serve as the ipsilateral graft. Only the avascular palatal midline is left intact. **C,** Trim, place, and tack each graft into position with fine sutures, and ligate a preoperatively, prepared stent lined with Coe-Pak to the zygomatic arches. **D,** Four weeks postoperatively, after stent removal, the grafts have been accepted, and a significant zone of fixed gingiva presents itself. The patient may now undergo implant placement via crestal incisions.

Alloderm

Allogenic Mucosal Grafting

Alloderm, described later, is a homologous material. In 1994, this acellular dermal matris was introduced. It is processed from human skin and is reported to have an intact basement membrane, retained collagen, and absence of epidermal and fibroblast cells. It is treated so that it is immunologically inert, and it is packaged in a dehydrated state.

Use of Alloderm requires rehydration with two saline baths, each for 5 minutes. Unlike other membranes previously described, this allogeneic material is not used as a GTRM but rather as a substitute for gingiva or mucosa. It has a smooth side, to be placed against the underlying bone or connective tissue, and a roughened side, which should be externally faced. In addition, to avoid the significant error of placing the improper side down, an orientation slit is found in each specimen. This slit must be horizontal on the surgeon's upper left or lower right corners. Use of such a surface graft is suggested when inadequate soft tissue is available to create a primary closure and undermining is not an acceptable alternative; when the potential overlying flap has been torn, damaged, or devascularized; or when the ridge has been enlarged significantly by spreading, splitting, or grafting. Instead of taking palatal tissue, which is time consuming and painful, this graft material serves as a satisfactory substitute.

After rehydration, it becomes soft, compliant, and amazingly strong. If the graft is not large enough (the largest size commercially available is 2 × 4 cm), two or more pieces may be sutured or micro-stapled together (Fig. 7-18).

The finally sized graft, after cutting, tucking, and contouring, should be large enough to extend peripherally to healthy cortex and is stabilized by membrane tacks or sutured with Polysorb, Vicryl, or Biosyn to the adjacent periosteum. In order to retain its morphology, place a periopak (Coe-Pak) stent over it for a period of 7 to 10 days. If the graft remains undisturbed, it becomes vascularized within 1 week.

Protection of the site becomes less important after 3 weeks, when the originally pallid Alloderm becomes pinker, and, under the best of conditions, becomes keratinized at the end of 6 weeks. Simple precautions should be recommended: no tooth brushing, a pureed or liquid diet, and gentle management postoperatively for 3 weeks (Fig. 7-19).

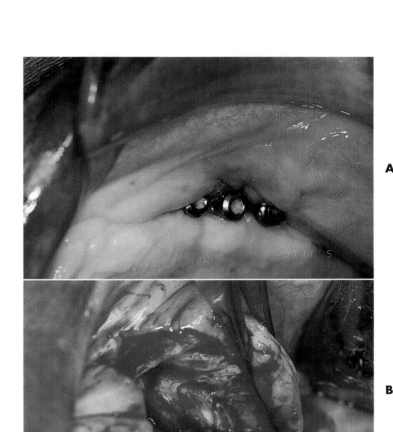

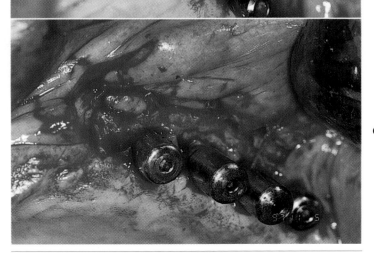

A

B

C

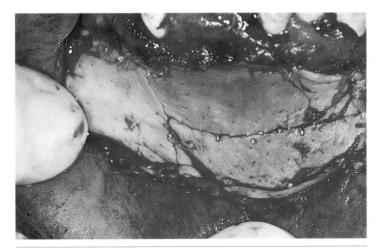

Fig. 7-18 Pieces of Alloderm can be patched together using mini staples to satisfy the requirements of a large or irregular host site.

Fig. 7-19 **A,** An overgrowth of buccal tissue occurred adjacent to these three root form implants. **B,** After an incision is made at the crest of the ridge, elevate the buccal flap, permitting the periosteum to remain in place. **C,** Thin the flap by filleting, and suture its lower edge to the periosteum at the planned new height.

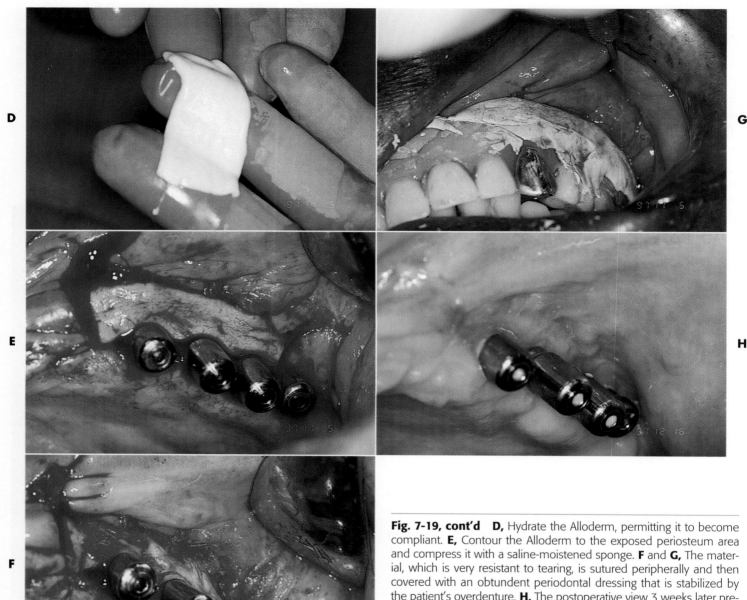

Fig. 7-19, cont'd D, Hydrate the Alloderm, permitting it to become compliant. **E,** Contour the Alloderm to the exposed periosteum area and compress it with a saline-moistened sponge. **F** and **G,** The material, which is very resistant to tearing, is sutured peripherally and then covered with an obtundent periodontal dressing that is stabilized by the patient's overdenture. **H,** The postoperative view 3 weeks later presents a satisfactory zone of fixed gingiva.

Connective Tissue Grafting

Autogenous connective tissue serves as an excellent substitute in grafting. It provides the overlying epithelium with a vascular bed and some requisite bulk. It accepts sutures well and is resistant to tearing. It is particularly valuable in reconstructing cervical dental and implant areas denuded because of gingival atrophy (Fig. 7-20, *A*).

In such cases, isolate the gingival margin with two parallel vertical incisions that include the papillae. After the reflection and development of this pedical flap by undermining, curette and condition the exposed root or implant with citric acid, and bring up the flap to the level of the C-E junction or cervix to verify its capability to cover the area without tension (Fig. 7-20, *B-D*). Retrieve a connective tissue specimen of the appropriate size to cover the exposed root surface from the palate by means of a crevicular incision, reflection of the full thickness flaps, removal of the connective tissue by filleting and primary closure by periodontal sling suture (Fig. 7-20, *E*).

Place the free graft over the root defect, tailored to fit the

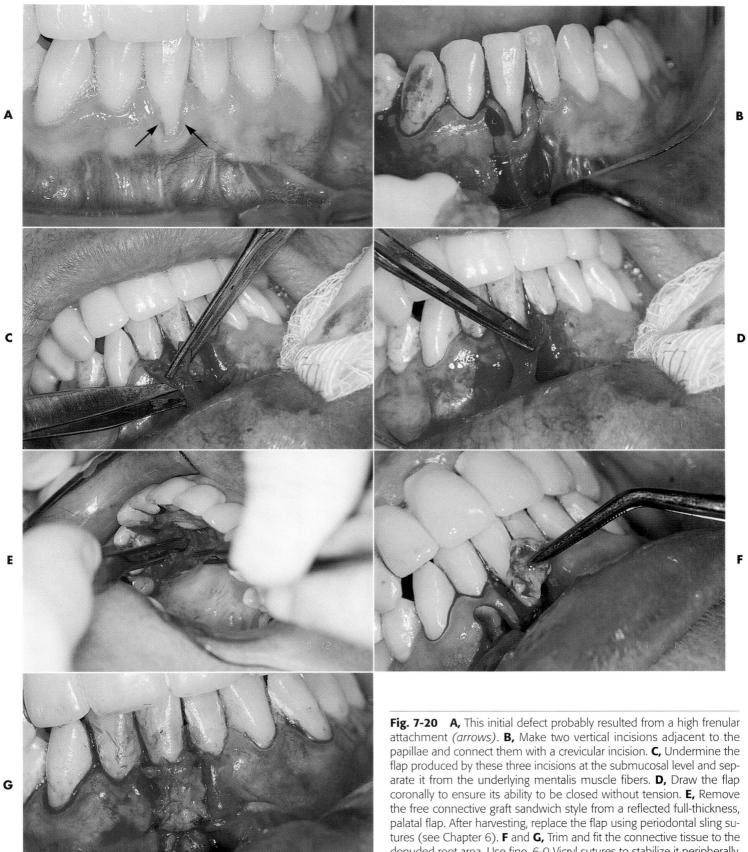

Fig. 7-20   A, This initial defect probably resulted from a high frenular attachment *(arrows).* **B,** Make two vertical incisions adjacent to the papillae and connect them with a crevicular incision. **C,** Undermine the flap produced by these three incisions at the submucosal level and separate it from the underlying mentalis muscle fibers. **D,** Draw the flap coronally to ensure its ability to be closed without tension. **E,** Remove the free connective graft sandwich style from a reflected full-thickness, palatal flap. After harvesting, replace the flap using periodontal sling sutures (see Chapter 6). **F** and **G,** Trim and fit the connective tissue to the denuded root area. Use fine, 6-0 Vicryl sutures to stabilize it peripherally.

H

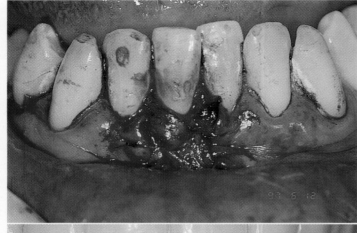

I

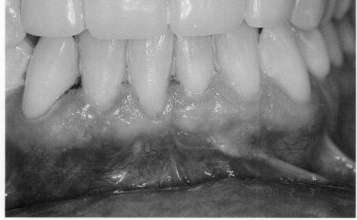

Fig. 7-20, cont'd   H, Bring the mucosal pedicle to its final position of repair and suture it with 6-0 Vicryl. **I,** A 6-month postoperative view of the site reveals a satisfactory result.

available area, and suture it peripherally with 5-0 Vicryl (Fig. 7-20, *F, G*).

Then, bring the gingival pedicle coronally to cover the connective tissue and suture it peripherally and to the lingual papillae interproximally (Fig. 7-20, *H*).

The result 6 months later indicates a high level of home care and the appearance of a keratinized repair (Fig. 7-20, *I*). On the fourth postoperative day, section the gingival pedicle free at the vestibular level to convert it to a free graft, thereby freeing it from muscular tension.

Suggested Readings

Babbush CA: *Surgical atlas of dental implant techniques,* Philadelphia, 1980, WB Saunders.

Bahat O: Osseointegrated implants for the maxillary tuberosity: report on 45 consecutive patients, *Int J Oral Maxillofac Implants* 7:459-467, 1992.

Bahat O: Surgical planning for optimal aesthetic and functional results of osseointegrated implants in the partially edentulous mouth, *J Calif Dent Assoc* 20(5):31-46, 1992.

Bedrossian E, Gongloff RK: Considerations in placement of implants through existing split-thickness skin graft vestibuloplasty: A case report, *J Oral Maxillofac Implants* 5:401-404, 1990.

Cranin AN: *Oral implantology,* Springfield, Ill, 1970, Charles C. Thomas.

Fonseca R, Davis WH: *Reconstructive preprosthetic oral and maxillofacial surgery,* Philadelphia, 1986, WB Saunders.

Hjorting-Hansen E, Adawy A, Hillerup S: Mandibular vestibulolingual sulcoplasty with free skin graft. A five year clinical follow-up study, *J Oral Surg* 41:173-176, 1983.

Kruger GO: *Textbook of oral and maxillofacial surgery,* ed 6, St. Louis, 1984, Mosby.

Quayle AA: Atraumatic removal of teeth and root fragments in dental implantology, *J Oral Maxillofac Implant* 5:293-296, 1990.

8

Hard Tissue Surgery and Bone Grafting

Antibiotics (tetracycline, gentamicin)
Antral membrane elevators (Tatum)
Atwood, 347 diamond drill
Autopolymerizing resin
Autostaple skin closures
Bone marrow gouges
Bone wax
Bard-Parker, No. 3 handles; No. 11, 12, and 15 blades
Bone files
Bougies whalebone, olive-tipped, or lacrimal probes
Burs: 699 L, 700 L, 701 L, 2 L, 4 L, 6 L friction-grip
Curettes, antrum
Curettes, surgical and periodontal
Electrosurgical unit
Forceps: curved mosquito and baby right angle, Kelly, and tonsil forceps
Forceps, rongeur and Kerrison
Forceps: (Adson and Gerald) toothed and nontoothed pickup
Graft material, particulate (20 and 40 mesh) and block forms, solid and porous
(hydroxyapatite) HA, (tricalcium phosphate) TCP, (demineralized freeze-dried bone DFDB, Bioglasses, hard tissue replacement (HTR), xenografts (Bio-Oss, Osteograft N),
Irradiated bone, bioreactive glass, collagen sheets, plugs, and microfibrillar form
Guided tissue regeneration membranes (GTRM), Gore-Tex (4 and 6), Vicryl mesh, other resorbable polymers, Lambone, Resolute, TefGen, Biomend, Regenetex, GBR-2000, and other PTFE products
Handpieces: high- and low-speed, straight and angled
Handpiece: Impactair high-speed
Hemostats: mosquito, Kelly, tonsil, Carmalt
Implant osteotomies (Steri-Oss) (Brookdale augmented set)
Implant osteotomies (Summers 3i)

Ligature wire: No. 2, No. 3 stainless steel
Local anesthetic syringes, needles, and solutions
Mallet (plastic covered)
Mandibular mortise form (Ti mesh), titanium, contouring pliers
Membrane tack or fixation set (IMZ/Steri-Oss), Imtec, Straumann, 3i Osseofix
Mortar and pestle
Needle holder
Needles: 18 gauge disposable, 11/2-inch hypodermic
Nerve hooks
Nylon-tipped amalgam carrier
Orangewood or cottonwood sticks
Osseous coagulum trap suction tip
Osteotomes: curved and straight, spatula, regular
Penrose drain, 1/4, 1/2, 1 inch
Periosteal elevators, double-ended
Retractors: baby Parker, blunt Mathieu (rake), beaver tail (Henahan), sweetheart (tongue)
Rongeur forceps (side-cutting and end-cutting)
Sable paint brushes (0 and 0-0)
Scissors: Metzenbaum, sharp, and suture scissors
Sheers: wire-cutting
Staples, for skin closure
Sterile cotton-tipped applicators
Sterile dappen dishes
Sterile saline
Sutures: 3-0 black silk, 4-0 dyed polyglactic acid (Vicryl, Polysorb), Biosyn, 3-0 plain gut on tapered and cutting needles
Syringes (for delivery of particulate graft material)
Titanium miniplate set with taps, screws, and screwdrivers
Tourniquet
Towel clamps
Wire, monofilament, No. 2, No. 3, stainless steel
Wire cutters

CAVEATS

Implant graft materials directly against bone. Remove all interposed connective tissue or integration will fail.

Follow the guidelines for preimplantation tunneling to facilitate ridge augmentation with great care, or permanent injury to the mandibular or mental nerves may result. Do not undertake it if the canal is dehiscent. Overaggressive tunneling pierces the vestibular attachment and permits ectopic migration of graft material particles.

Do not use grafting materials if infection exists near or within the proposed operative site.

Periodontal and other defects must have at least two remaining bony walls before grafting.

Do not expect more of the grafting materials than they have the potential to offer. Most of these materials conduct bone (i.e., they facilitate bone growth in areas where bone would ordinarily regenerate). Their presence merely makes osseous repair more efficient, better contoured, more rapid, and stronger. The only osteogenic material is autogenous bone. It is recommended for the repair of all but three walled defects for which mixtures of osteoconductive (HA, TCP) and osteoinductive (DFDB) materials may be used. For lesions requiring more substantive grafting assistance, add autogenous bone or use it alone.

General Guidelines

Bone Management

The best protection for bone is the maintenance of an uninjured periosteal envelope. The dangers of overheating bone should also be of concern. Temperature elevations beyond 47° C for as short a time as 30 seconds may cause serious, unalterable injury. The staff must be sure that burs, twist and spade drills, trephines, and bone taps are sharp and replaced with frequency (i.e., depending on bone hardness, after every sixth to tenth implant). After every use, make a notch on the shank so that an accurate count of the number of uses is available. Always keep replacement drills at hand. When possible (because not all systems have this feature available), use internal as well as external irrigation, and clean hollowed drills immediately after each use to ensure their future patency (Fig. 8-1). It is not always necessary to use the drilling systems supplied by the implant manufacturers. There are generic consoles, motors, handpieces, and drills that offer irrigation systems (thus keeping endosteal sites cool), which assist in the performance of all the final steps involved in the making of osteotomies (see Chapters 9 and 10 for specifics). The use of drills with 0.5-mm diameter increments injures the bone minimally and permits the use of drills for a greater number of times.

When doing alveoloplasties, osteoplasties, sinus floor elevations, or bone-tapping procedures, maintain a steady, copious source of irrigation to the bone and on all cutting instruments. If attention must be diverted from the operative site, keep the site dressed with saline-soaked sponges at all times to prevent dehydration.

Use electrosurgical units for implant surgery only when the greatest care is being exercised. Vascularity must be encouraged to ensure the best prognosis for healing. If an electrode tip should touch any part of an implant, the current is conducted throughout the entire implant body (although at dissipated intensity), creating the possibility of widespread injury to the bone.

Preserve bone grindings when possible by placing a filter in the suction system (Fig. 8-2). The recovered osseous coagulum can be used (mixed with a synthetic particulate grafting material if necessary) for bone repair, after implant placement, or in the floor of the maxillary sinus after an elevation procedure.

Understanding and use of synthetic bone grafting materials (Table 8-1) should become a part of every implantologist's

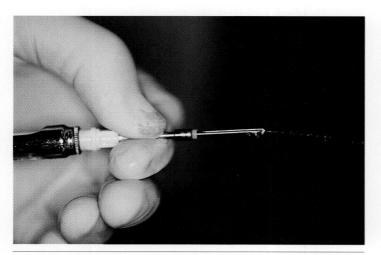

Fig. 8-1 An anesthetic syringe with a 27 gauge, 1½-inch needle fits comfortably into the hollow drill lumens. On forcing a tube of solution through it, bone fragments and debris will be expressed.

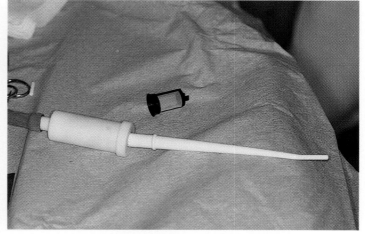

Fig. 8-2 This filter, which is attached to the suction tubing, is available from Ace Surgical. It collects bone grindings produced during osteotomies. The retrieval material, osseous coagulum, may be used for grafting purposes.

Table 8-1 Categories of Grafting Materials

	VALUES	SHORTCOMINGS

AUTOGRAFTS

This type of bone is "self-donated" by the patient
Source:

	VALUES	SHORTCOMINGS
Iliac crest	Patient's own bone / Osteogenic / Availability	Second site morbidity / Requires general anesthesia / Prolonged postoperative recovery
Ascending ramus or symphysis of mandible	Patient's own bone / Osteogenic / Availability	Second site morbidity / Prolonged postoperative recovery
Torus	Patient's own bone / Osteoconductive	Host site availability / Second site morbidity / Cortical bone only
Rib or tibial plateau	Patient's own bone / Osteogenic / Availability	Second site morbidity / Requires general anesthesia / Prolonged postoperative recovery
Calvarium	Patient's own bone / Osteogenic / Availability	Second site morbidity / Requires general anesthesia / Prolonged postoperative recovery

HOMOGRAFTS/ALLOGRAFTS

This type of bone is donated from a human source other than the patient
Source: bone banks
Types available:

	VALUES	SHORTCOMINGS
Demineralized freeze-dried bone* (DFDB)	Availability / Osteoinductive/conductive / Biologic acceptability / Replaced by patient's own bone	Cost / Patient may not accept
Freeze-dried bone matrix	Availability / Osteoconductive / Biologic acceptability / Replaced by patient's own bone	Cost / Patient may not accept
Irradiated bone	Availability / Osteoconductive / Biologic acceptability / Replaced by patient's own bone	Cost / Increased concerns about disease transmission due to decreased processing
Fresh frozen bone	Availability / Osteoconductive / Replaced by patient's own bone	Cost / Significant risk of disease transmission and graft-host reaction
Human bone ash (Osteomin)	Availability (Pacific Coast Tissue Bank) / Osteoconductive (human HA) / Resorbable / No risk or disease transmission	Cost / An HA based on human bone

XENOGRAFTS

Mineralized bone matrix from a species other than man:
Source: Bovine
Types:

	VALUES	SHORTCOMINGS
Bio-Oss, Osteograf N	Availability / Osteoconductive / Patient acceptance / Biologic acceptability	Cost / Similar to HA

*Available in various forms: cortical or cancellous powder, cortical chips, monocortical or bicortical blocks, as a gel in combination with glycerol (Grafton/Osteotech) or thin cortical sheets to be used as a membrane (lambone/Pacific coast Tissue Bank).

Continued

Table 8-1 Categories of Grafting Materials—cont'd

	VALUES	SHORTCOMINGS
ALLOPLASTS		
These are synthetic bone materials		
Source: a variety of manufactures		
Types:		
Nonresorbable		
Polymer : (HTR)	Availability	Cost
	Osteoconductive	Nonresorbable
	Hydrophillic	
	Patient acceptance	
	Biologic acceptability	
	Nonresorbable	
Ceramic: HA (i.e. Calcitite, Osteograf D, Interpore)	Availability	Cost
	Osteoconductive	Nonresorbable
	Patient acceptance	(HA component)
	Biologic acceptability	
	Nonresorbable	
Ceramic HA (35%) in a resorbable medium	Availability	Cost
CaSO$_4$ (65%) (Hapset)	Osteoconductive	Nonresorbable
	Patient acceptance	
	Nonresorbable (HA component)	
Resorbable	Availability	Cost
Ceramic (TCP)	Osteoconductive	Absorbability
(i.e. Augmen, Synthograf)	Patient acceptance	Questionable
	Biologic acceptability	Predictability
Ceramic (HA)	Availability	Cost
i.e. Osteogen, Osteograf LD, Osteograf N	Osteoconductive	Absorbability
	Patient acceptance	
	Biologic acceptability	
Bioactive Glass—	Availability	Cost
(i.e. Biogran, Perioglas)	Osteoconductive	Absorbability
	Biologic acceptability	
	Patient acceptable	
Bone Banks		
For bone banks see Appendix for members of the		
American Association of Tissue Banks.		

area of competence. It offers a constant source of benefit and may be needed at unexpected times.

Grafting for purposes of repair, augmentation, osteosynthesis, or morphologic maintenance may be performed either with autogenous or allogeneic bone, with xenografts, or with synthetic (particulate or porous solid, block forms) of both resorbable and nonresorbable osteoconductive biomaterials. The names and other significant characteristics of these grafting materials are found in Table 8-2. The techniques for use are essentially the same for all of them except that some have different handling characteristics. Indications for the use of some of the synthetic bone materials (i.e., tricalcium phosphate [TCP] and other resorbable substances) differ. The clinician may be able to change both the quantity and the quality of a patient's bone by using bone-replacement materials. An essential aspect in the application of grafting materials is the use of membranes (GTRMs) both resorbable and nonresorbable. Although there is a small but stalwart contingent of practitioners who remain loyal to the traditional nonresorbable designs, these designs of-

fer no advantages over their resorbable counterparts and require a second operation for purposes of removal.

The first section of this chapter is reserved for the more basic procedures of bone grafting such as ridge maintenance, ridge augmentation, and the general application of membranes and techniques for their fixation. The background provided serves as a guide for the second section, which is dedicated to the description of bone alteration and grafting techniques designed for the ridge with dimensional deficiencies, which prevent routine implant procedures. The methods of selecting donor sites and obtaining grafts are included as well.

Basic Grafting Procedures

Periodontal Defect Correction

Only teeth that are or can be made clinically firm should be included in the treatment plan. If mobile, they must be bonded

Table 8-2 Membranes (GTRM)

NAME	MATERIAL	RESORBABLE OR NONRESORBABLE	MANUFACTURER	VALUES	SHORTCOMINGS
Gortex	Expanded Polytetra fluoroethylene (e PTFE)	Nonresorbable	W.L. Gore & Associates	Proven track record Established good standard Available with titanium reinforcement variations	Nonresorbable requires removal surgery Exposure results in inflammation possible reduced results
Tef Gen-FD	Non-expanded PTFE	Nonresorbable	Lifecore Biomedical	Some clinical studies suggest primary closure not 100% necessary Nonporous surface inhibits bacterial colonization	Nonporous structure may result in increased exposure Nonresorbable
Regenetex TXT-200/ GBR-200	Non-expanded PFTE	Nonresorbable	Osteogenics Biomedical	Some clinical studies suggest primary closure not 100% necessary Nonporous surface inhibits bacterial colonization	Nonporous structure may result in increased exposure Nonresorbable
Bio-Mend	Bovine Type I Collagen	Resorbable	Sulzer Calcitek	Resorbable	Difficult to manipulate once wet
Bio Gide	Porcine Type I & III Collagen	Resorbable	Osteohealth	Resorbable Approved by FDA for use around implants	Short track record
Vicryl Mesh	Polyglactin 910 (9:1 ratio of polylactic acid and polyglycolic acid)	Resorbable	Ethicon	Resorbable Easy to position and place	Easily collapsible into defect
Resolute Resolute XT	Polyglycolide and Polylactide polymers	Resorbable	W.L. Gore & Associates	Resorbable Retains form once shaped	Stiff, difficult to bend and adapt
Guidor	Polylactic Acid & Citric Acid ester	Resorbable	J.O. Butler	Resorbable Malleable	Product discontinued as of Oct. 97
Atrisorb	Poly DL–Lactide in N-Methyl 2 pyrolidone	Resorbable	Block	Chairside fabrication Resorbable Mildly adherent to tooth	Short track record Learning curve Can be difficult to adapt
Lambone	Freeze dried Demineralized Allogenic laminar bone sheets	Replaced by bone	Pacific Coast Tissue Bank	Replaced by bone Available in variable thickness	Needs to be rehydrated in saline for 5-30 minutes Thicker pieces more difficult to adapt Patient may not accept
Capset	Calcium Sulphate	Resorbable	LifeCore	Resorbable Custom adapted at time of placement Does not require bone tacks or suturing	Somewhat technique-sensitive

with stainless steel wire, with acrylic intracoronal splints, or in some other fashion be provided with total immobilization. If there is a possibility of periodontal-endodontic involvement, presurgical pulp canal therapy is mandatory (Figs. 8-3, 8-4).

Plan flaps carefully with incisions at least one tooth anterior and one tooth posterior to the anticipated surgical site. Make crevicular incisions with a No. 12 blade using the inverted bevel design so that involved epithelium as well as granulomas are left in situ to facilitate their excision. Connect the crevicular incisions with those that are vertical/oblique. Flaps should be widest at their vestibular bases. Papillae should never be split, but rather, included in their entireties within the flap (Fig. 8-5).

Make reflections with great care so that flaps are not torn. A sharp, fine periosteal elevator or sharpened No. 7 wax spatula is beneficial. It is not necessary to expose the alveolar bone any more than 1 to 2 mm apically beyond the periodontal defect. Serious postoperative sequelae (pain, swelling) occur when reflections extend apically beyond the attached gingival level. Of course, depending on anatomic factors and pocket depth, it may be necessary to reflect beyond the vestibular attachments.

When facial and lingual flaps have been reflected, use impeccable care to curette and plane all exposed root surfaces. Do not blunt, ramp, or alter the bone in any manner. The higher the residual walls, the better the prognosis for osseous

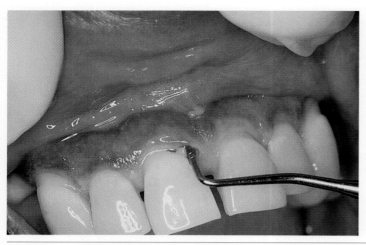

Fig. 8-3 A thorough examination, including periodontal probing, is essential before surgical intervention.

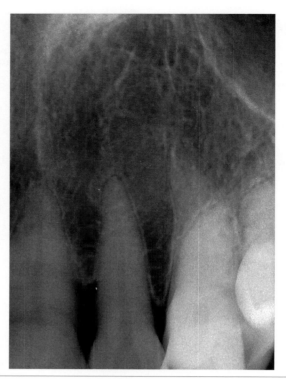

Fig. 8-4 Perform a radiographic survey to further assess the prognosis of the involved teeth.

repair using grafting materials. Cortical perforations made with a No. ½ round bur offer additional sites for retention.

Hemostasis must be achieved to ensure particle stabilization, but slight bleeding is important, since blood is necessary for particulate incorporation and the encouragement of osseous repair. Active bleeding, on the other hand, often washes the new graft material away. Periodontal particulate grafting material should be of a fine grain size (40 mesh or 250- to 350-μm diameter). When mixed with the patient's blood and permitted to remain in the dappen dish for 15 minutes before use, the material takes on a texture that allows easy handling. It clumps quite naturally and remains reliably in position. Of course, improper condensing, poor suturing, brisk bleeding, or incorrect operative design (i.e., defects without walls) may be responsible for a less-than-perfect result.

When the operative site is absolutely free of granulomas, plaque, and calculus, the grafting material can be placed within the defect. It may be delivered with a nylon-tipped amalgam carrier. The old-fashioned all-plastic, back-end plunger type, kept sterile and reserved only for grafting use, is preferable.

After the graft material has been placed into the furcation or against one of several (at least two) remaining bony walls and tamped with a moistened cotton applicator, use firm

pressure until fibrin becomes incorporated into and stabilizes the particles (Fig. 8-6). Suturing should follow, using 4-0 violet-dyed polyglactic acid or glycomer on a cutting needle as is described in the section, Sutures and Suturing, in Chapter 6. Watertight closures serving to replace each papilla accurately are mandatory so that particle fixation is ensured (Figs. 8-7, 8-8).

When a bony periimplant defect exists adjacent to an edentulous area, perform classical wedging. After a full-thickness flap has been reflected, treat the pocket and opposing implant surface as described in the section concerning failing implants in Chapter 28. Following this, a spatula osteotome placed at the crest of the ridge and 3 to 4 mm from the lesion is tapped gently with a mallet to a depth equal to that of the pocket. Direct it inferoobliquely toward the failing implant. When the osteotome reaches the depth of the defect, use it as a lever to mobilize this newly created triangle of bone. Push the wedge against the denuded implant surface and maintain it in this position by pressing some nonresorbable 40 mesh HA particles into the donor site from which the triangular graft has come. A simple closure completes the procedure.

Do not attempt pocket measurements for at least 3 months and, even after that, attempt them only with great care (Fig. 8-9).

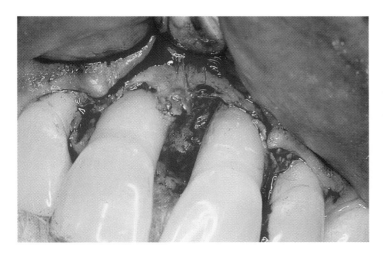

Fig. 8-5 A full-thickness periodontal flap is planned in such a manner that at least one tooth anterior and posterior to the defect are included. The base of the flap must be wider in order to establish an adequate vascular supply. A sharp, fine periosteal elevator will allow careful flap management without tissue perforation.

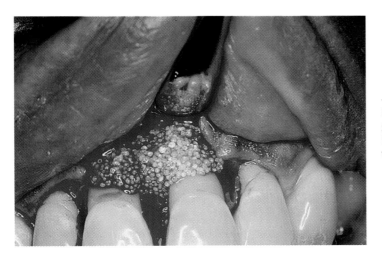

Fig. 8-6 Before placement of the graft material, thoroughly debride all granulomatous tissue. Place this material in such a manner as to restore ideal anatomic contours. Proper condensation must be carried out to prevent particulate loss and soft tissue ingrowth.

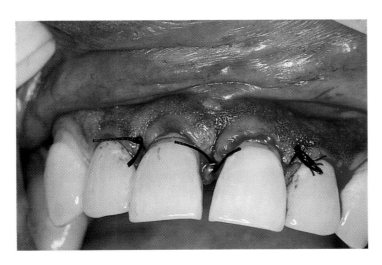

Fig. 8-7 Primary closure is imperative for successful grafting results. A variety of suturing techniques may be needed to achieve this outcome.

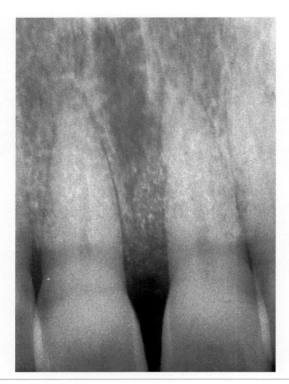

Fig. 8-8 Take immediate postoperative periapical radiographs using a standardized technique so that future assessments for comparison can be made.

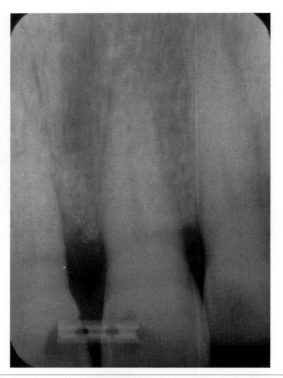

Fig. 8-10 Replicate the radiographic examination at semiannual recall visits. Note changes in bone morphology and use them in conjunction with other diagnostic tools to evaluate long-term prognoses.

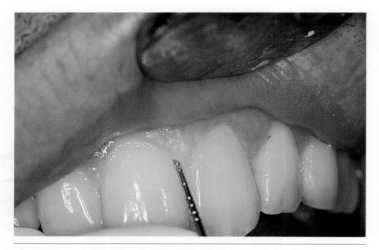

Fig. 8-9 Periodontal probing can be made 3 months postoperatively. Carry out these measurements gently so that the newly formed attachment will not be compromised.

If expectations are realistic and home and office care regimens satisfy the stringent requirements presented by most periodontal strategies, the results may be quite salutary (Fig. 8-10). The grafting of periimplant and other defects mentioned in this and other chapters is made simpler and more successful if GTRMs are used (see Table 8-2).

The Use of Guided Tissue Regeneration Membranes: Resorbable and Nonresorbable

The use of membranes to cover osseous repairs does not offer automatic assurance of improved prognosis. In fact, employing them might be responsible for delayed healing, suture line breakdown, and compromise of the operative site.

There is a wide variety of membranes. Before selecting one, however, decide whether such a choice would be beneficial.

Essentially, membranes are used if there is questionable primary soft tissue closure, a void in the osseous operative site, a mucosal pedicle is required, the graft material is physically unstable, or additional bone height or width is required. Conversely, if the operated area presents no irregularities and a closure can be accomplished without tension, avoid the use of membranes.

The use of GTRMs may be applied with or without bone-grafting materials for perforations of the cortical plates, saucerization phenomena (Figs. 8-11 through 8-18), thin ridges, exposed implant cervical areas, other intraosseous defects, voids remaining after implants have been placed into immediate extraction sites, or ridge maintenance after extractions with the use of accompanying synthetic grafting materials.

Some membranes require rehydration, and others have a crystalline or granular composition; some are grossly porous, while others are microporous or nonporous.

The resorbable membranes generally are polymers that hydrolyze over time (usually about 40 days). A homologous resorbable membrane that serves more than just a barrier function is laminar bone, which is retrieved from human specimens and treated with demineralization and sterilization techniques.

The nonresorbable groups are synthesized. They most often consist of PTFE or nonporous or microporous material. They may require either primary soft tissue coverage (i.e.,

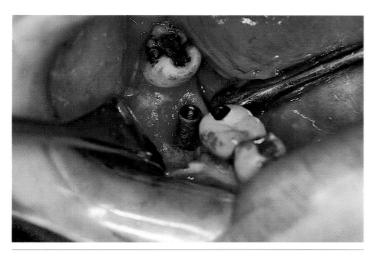

Fig. 8-11 The use GTRMs is a valuable adjunct to the correction of bony defects associated with implants caused by saucerization phenomena. Before placement of the GTRM, thoroughly curette the defect of all soft tissue.

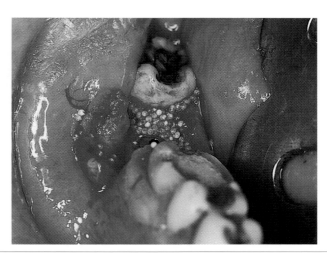

Fig. 8-12 Before membrane placement, condense a selected bone-grafting material firmly into the defect.

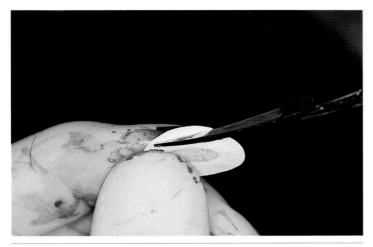

Fig. 8-13 Tailor the membrane precisely to fully cover the osseous void and overlap the peripheral cortex by 3 mm.

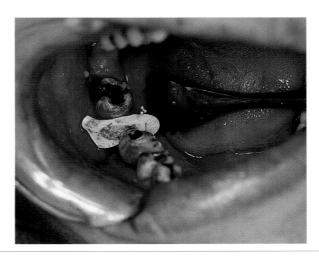

Fig. 8-14 Meticulously place the GTRM and fix its periapical margins below the periosteum. If possible, it is desirable to employ the surgical healing screw of the implant in order to stabilize the GTRM.

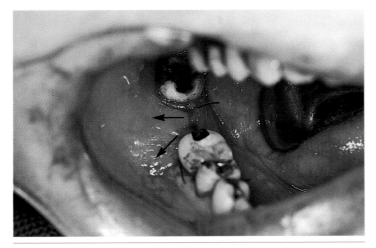

Fig. 8-15 Primary closure is mandatory for success of this procedure. Lack of total coverage of the GTRM will lead to its exposure and a less positive prognosis. In order to achieve this closure, a buccal pedicle *(arrows)* had to be undermined from its buccinator bed so that tension-free suturing would result.

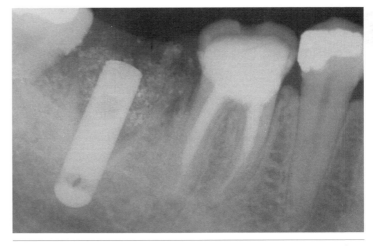

Fig. 8-16 Although the GTRM is not radiopaque, take a periapical radiograph to confirm graft position and stability.

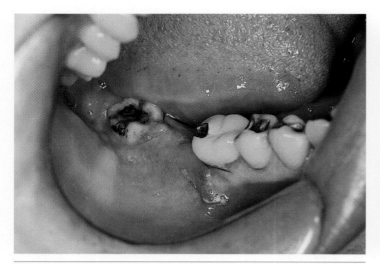

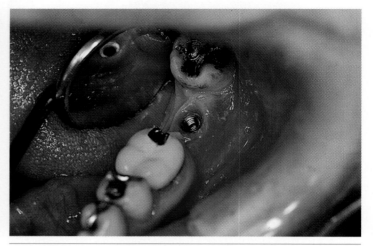

Fig. 8-17 At the 2-week postoperative visit, healing is taking place by primary intention. Observation of the area is carried out bimonthly until removal of the membrane.

Fig. 8-18 Reentry of the site is accomplished to remove the GTRM. Satisfactory soft tissue healing with good lingual and buccal zones of fixed gingivae are seen 1 month after membrane removal.

Gore-Tex) or may be used without the wound flaps coming into direct contact, thereby allowing the membrane to be exposed (i.e., TefGen or Cytoplast GBR 200). The surgeon must make the choice. The decision is influenced by familiarity with the product, ease of use, cost, compliance, and the desire to avoid a second or retrieval operation.

Membranes require reliable fixation. In most instances, undermining the surrounding mucosa and wedging the membrane periphery firmly beneath it will satisfy this. If this technique is not practicable, place membrane tacks or miniscrews at strategic sites. Ordinarily, the device (membrane, slurry, or laminar bone) should fit intimately over the operative site. Its purpose is to discourage epithelial ingrowth. Accuracy of adaptation encourages this goal. Make tucks and alterations when indicated; complete these maneuvers and ascertain the capability of primary flap closure before placing the graft material. If not performed in advance, membrane manipulations and flap undermining disturb the stability of particulate graft material. On completion of the operative procedure and graft placement, slip the precontoured membrane back into position, fasten and tuck it as needed, and complete a primary closure.

At sites that require dimensional enlargement, the guided tissue device must be "tented." This is sometimes a challenging procedure, particularly when using a soft or compliant membrane. Contour corrections are most readily completed using firmer devices such as laminar bone or Gore-Tex with titanium reinforcement. Of course, a less stiff membrane is required when supported by underlying graft material.

In order to permit the GTRM to fulfill its function, which is the promotion of bone proliferation into a defect, a space equivalent to the area that requires filling must be left beneath it. Saucerization defects and similar problems allow this space to occur quite naturally, since the lesion's peripheral bone margins maintain the membrane in a tented configuration. On the other hand, cortical plate perforations, protruding implant apices or bodies, or knife-edge ridges require grafting material to be used in block or particulate form over which membrane is to be placed.

Before using any grafting material, eliminate all residual infection, treat the implant appropriately (see Chapter 28, Failing Implants), and ensure adequate available tissue for primary closure with mattress sutures.

Incisions should be crestal, not S shaped or visor, in order to protect the vascularity of the flaps.

After the site has been exposed adequately (4 to 5 mm of normal bone on all sides of the defect), select a membrane of the closest proper size and trim it with sharp scissors to fit competently over the entire area. Avoid sharp corners and create a 3-mm overlap to cover adjacent cortex. If a natural tooth exists adjacent to the operative region, circumvent its periodontal space. Perform the tailoring of the GTRM with precision. If space beneath the membrane is required, place a selected bone-grafting material and firmly tamp it into position, followed by membrane implantation (Figs. 8-19 through 8-29). If a convex configuration is required, make one or several nips and tucks to permit the formation of an additional dimension. Fibrin should be allowed to maintain it in its new shape before closure.

Fixation of GTRMs before wound closure is essential for ultimate success in bone-generation procedures. The peripheral margins of the membrane may be wedged gently beneath the periosteum or even sutured with an absorbable material to the periosteum at strategic peripheral locations. Small fixation tacks are available from Steri-Oss, which in most maxillae, can be forced into the bone using finger pressure. These sharp, titanium tacks are made available in a set that includes an instrument that grasps them by their heads and carries them to the site at which the membrane is to be stabilized. The mandible, having a denser cortex, usually does not yield to the sharp point of the tack unless a preliminary bur hole starts the process (the bur is supplied in the kit), followed by a few light mallet taps applied to the end of the seating instrument (Figs. 8-30 through 8-35). Additional tack and screw systems are supplied by Straumann, 3i, Ace Surgical, and others.

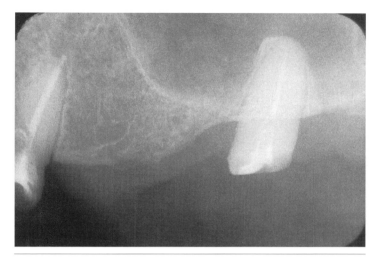

Fig. 8-19 Preoperative radiographic assessments fail to determine the buccolingual dimension of the alveolar ridge.

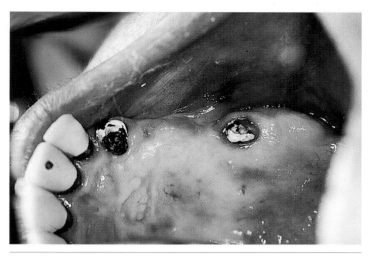

Fig. 8-20 Clinical visual examination and bone sounding sometimes fail to define the osseous topography of the area.

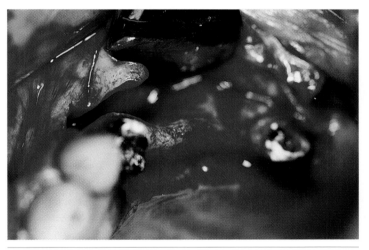

Fig. 8-21 On flap reflection, an inadequate width of bone is seen. This problem can be managed with the use of bone grafting with a GTRM.

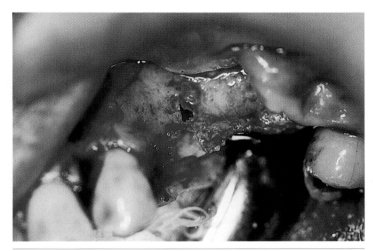

Fig. 8-22 Preparation of the uncorrected implant host site may lead to buccal plate fenestration of the bone in narrow ridges, like the one above.

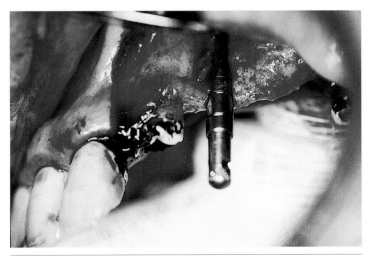

Fig. 8-23 An implant body try-in is used to determine the surface area of exposure of the planned implant. A lack of stability of the device at this juncture mandates grafting of the host site.

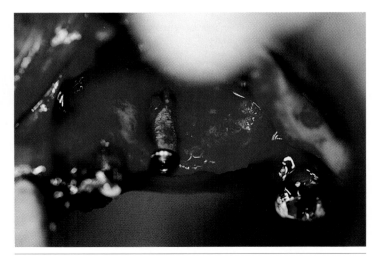

Fig. 8-24 When positive retention can be achieved, the implant is placed, and its exposed surface is given GTRM coverage, with or without graft material depending on tenting capabilities.

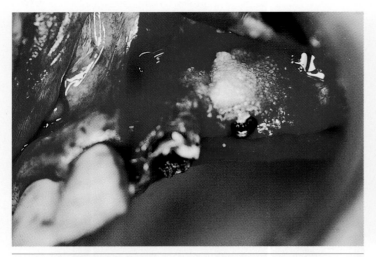

Fig. 8-25 A space for bone ingrowth is necessary between the implant surface and the membrane. If this cannot be achieved by tenting with a firm GTRM (e.g., Lambone), select a graft material to elevate the membrane away from the implant.

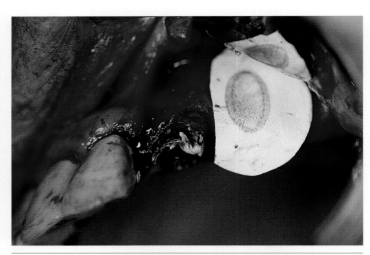

Fig. 8-26 Trim the GTRM to overlay intact peripheral bony margins.

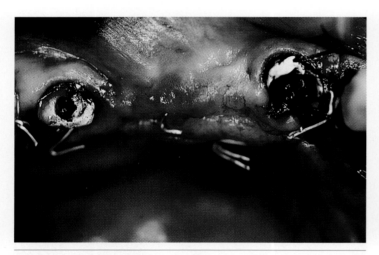

Fig. 8-27 Closure of the mucoperiosteal flap is accomplished in the usual fashion. PTFE suture material offers minimal adverse reactions.

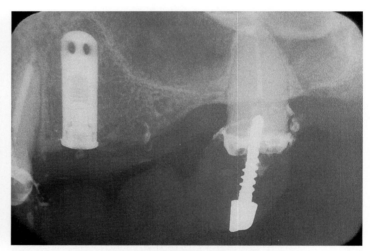

Fig. 8-28 A postoperative radiograph shows proper implant placement and good osseous support.

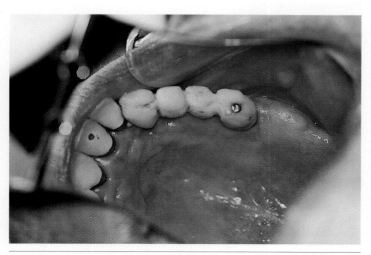

Fig. 8-29 Clinical healing has taken a place without complication 2 weeks postoperatively.

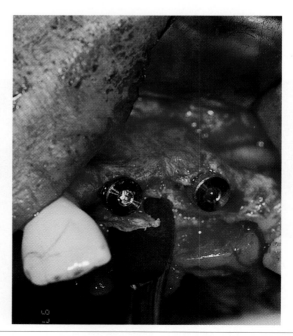

Fig. 8-30 Two Paragon implants have been placed into this osteotomized split ridge. The adjacent defects, between the implants require grafting.

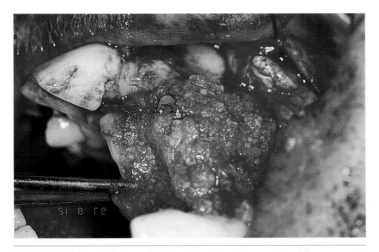

Fig. 8-31 The graft material, demineralized freeze-dried bone moistened and carried with the patient's blood, is placed in generous quantities over the entire operative site and tamped into the defects and osteotomy grooves adjacent to each implant.

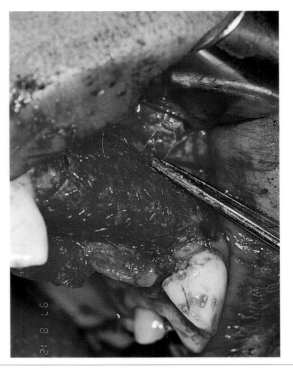

Fig. 8-32 After proper graft contouring, fit a tailored resorbable membrane like this Resolute design over the site and extend it to intact peripheral bone margins. The instrument is being used to tuck the membrane beneath the adjacent soft tissue flaps.

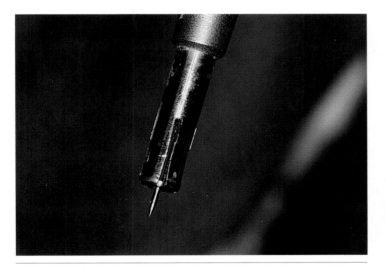

Fig. 8-33 The sharply pointed membrane fixation tack is held by its delivery instrument.

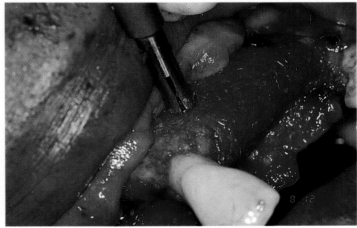

Fig. 8-34 Pressure applied by the delivery instrument through the membrane into the underlying bone forces the tack into place.

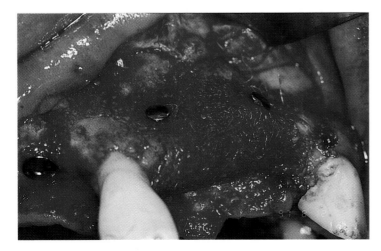

Fig. 8-35 After reliable fixation with tacks placed in strategic locations, perform suturing.

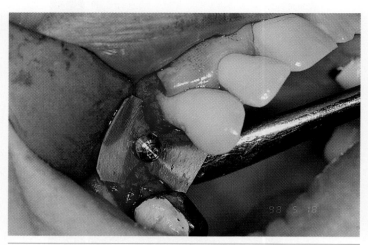

Fig. 8-36 This laminar bone (Lambone), after being hydrated in saline, is shaped to fit over the implant host site, and a hole is made at the appropriate position to accommodate the healing screw, which, when tightened, will stabilize the Lambone.

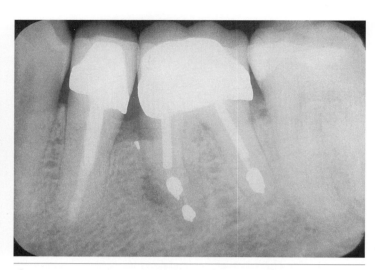

Fig. 8-38 GTRMs are of significant value when used in conjunction with the immediate placement of implants into extraction sockets. Radiographic evaluation reveals a planned extraction site.

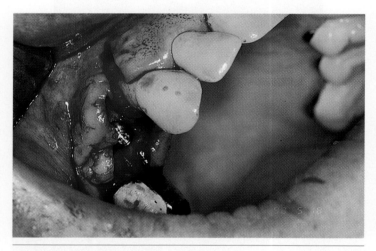

Fig. 8-37 After the membrane (laminar bone, in this case) is fastened firmly into place, suture the wound.

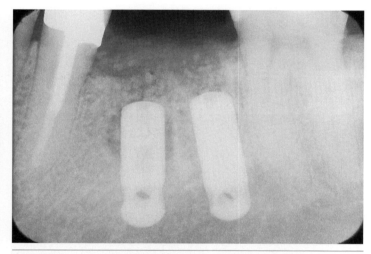

Fig. 8-39 Carry out extraction in the most atraumatic fashion possible so that the integrity of the buccal and lingual plates is preserved. Clinical judgment must ensure the absence of acute infection before any implants are inserted. Thorough debridement of all soft tissue must be accomplished. Use curettes judiciously to avoid any injury to vital anatomic structures. Then place implants, using the maximal amount of apical bone available to ensure their stability. Lay the GTRM over the implant in the classic manner, tamp grafting materials peripherally, and close the flap.

If the area to be repaired is pericervical and the ailing implant has a healing screw, cut a hole in the membrane with a diameter only large enough to permit entry of the threaded portion of the screw. After the grafting material has been placed, position the GTRM poncho fash-ion and tighten the cover screw to anchor it firmly (Figs. 8-36, 8-37).

Perform closure with polyglactic sutures and complete it using the horizontal mattress technique. Exercise care so that the membrane does not become wrinkled, is firmly fixed, and so that its rounded margins extend well beyond the defect on the cortical bone. Do not suture the overlying flaps under tension (see Undermining, Incisions, Flap Design, and Sutures and Suturing sections in Chapters 6 and 7); an absolute primary closure must be achieved (Figs. 8-38 through 8-42).

Remove sutures after 7 to 10 days, or permit them to resorb. If the selected membrane is nonresorbable, remove it at any time after 3 months. If a greater period of time is permitted, the intimate relationship of the overlying soft tissues to the membrane may make its removal troublesome and threaten the integrity of the mucosa.

If the membrane becomes exposed because of a dehiscent suture line, although the prognosis becomes less positive, encourage its continued presence by gentle Peridex irrigation and debridement. Teach the patient to practice this on a daily basis between professional visits. It is possible that bone regeneration will take place successfully despite the loss of integrity of the wound.

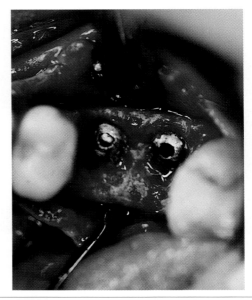

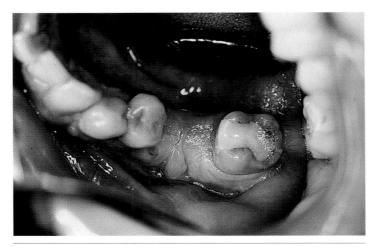

Fig. 8-40 If uneventful healing takes place, leave the membrane in position until the time of second-stage surgery or until it resorbs.

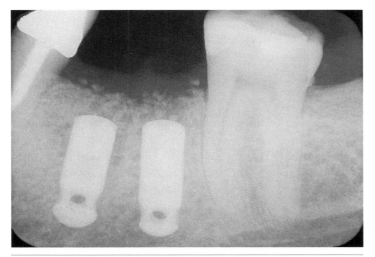

Fig. 8-41 The result of grafting appears satisfactory in a standardized radiograph. It is of importance to note that two implants should be used for the replacement of molars whenever feasible. (See Chapter 22.)

Ridge Maintenance

In most cases, maintaining alveolar ridge morphology after dental extractions is a worthy preventive measure and potentially offers patients the ridge form, height, and shape that make denture fabrication simpler and more successful and fixed prosthesis pontic construction more realistic looking, hygienic, and comfortable. In addition, if implants are planned, it may be expected that larger and more generous host sites in which to place them will result.

There are two instances when maintenance procedures may be of more immediate and tangible value to a patient. The first is after mandibular third molar extraction, and the second is after molar hemisection procedures. For the latter, endodontic therapy must be performed on the planned residual root before sectioning. In both cases, use of grafting avoids the potential hazards of significant bone loss to adjacent teeth and spares a predictable array of periodontal complications. In

Fig. 8-42 Careful removal of the nonresorbable GTRM is done by sharp dissection, using a scalpel blade and a toothed forceps. Meticulous removal of exuberant bone overlying the cover screw must be accomplished by using a sharp operative chisel or small round bur.

each situation, perform the technique of placing particulate graft material and membrane at a deficit site by completing the extraction with preservation of as much bone as possible. Sectioning molars makes this goal easier to achieve. Debride the vacated sites thoroughly, remove all granulomata and epithelia, and encourage fresh bleeding. Introduce the 20 mesh graft material (650- to 850-μm diameter) by syringe or periosteal elevator, tamp it firmly to avoid spaces, and then, after overlapped bone coverage with a membrane, complete the procedure with primary closure. If there is a paucity of tissue, interdigitation of facial and lingual papillae often solves the problem. Details of these procedures are found in the following paragraphs.

Technique

Make broad-based facial and lingual full-thickness crevicular incisions before tooth removal. They should include whole papillae and result in well-vascularized flaps of generous dimensions. Make mucoperiosteal reflection with great care down to but not beyond the vestibular level.

CAVEATS

In order to avoid packing graft material into the antrum or mandibular canal, ascertain whether an opening has been made into one of these structures. Chapter 28 presents the symptoms of antral or canal penetration. If such a finding is confirmed or, in fact, even suspected, tailor a piece of Colla Cote or Colla Plug to fit the defect and lay it or tamp it gently at its base with a saline-moistened plug of cotton. This serves as a protective dam against which the particles may be placed. Control bleeding before implantation, or the graft material will be carried away. Tamponade is a sound maneuver for achieving hemostasis and stabilizing the fibrin-particulate slurry.

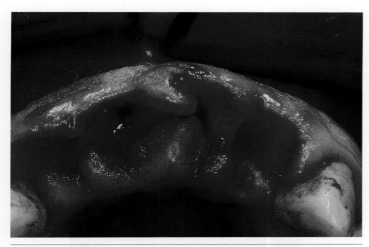

Fig. 8-43 Preservation of existing bone is accomplished through surgical extractions after full-thickness mucoperiosteal flaps are elevated.

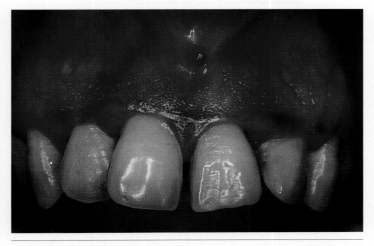

Fig. 8-44 Removal of severely periodontally involved teeth often results in osseous defects caused by bone loss in both buccolingual and occlusocervical dimensions.

Next, complete the extractions, hemisections, or impaction removals in the usual manner, being careful to preserve as much of the bony socket as possible (Figs. 8-43, 8-44).

Inspect the operative sites carefully. Eliminate all forms of follicles, cysts, and granulomas by sharp dissection using a No. 12 or No. 15 blade (described in Chapter 6, Surgical Principles) and follow it with the aggressive application of periodontal and surgical curettes.

After clean, bony beds are evident, confirm the ability of the flaps to close primarily over the entire operative site. If they do not come together anatomically, attempt to slide the facial and lingual flaps one-quarter tooth in opposite directions from one another. This often permits the papillae to interdigitate into a saw-toothed relationship. Bone is valuable and should not be removed to allow the flaps to close. The buccolingual plates are necessary for long-term ridge maintenance width and height. The graft materials alone cannot supply the area with bone, nor will the achieved level result in a dimension greater than the highest level of bone. If all else fails, the surgeon's undermining skills must be brought into use to achieve primary closure. (Chapter 7 reviews this and other soft tissue procedures). After primary coverage capabilities have

been ascertained or created, the assistant should retract the flaps so that irrigation, debridement, and hemostasis can be achieved.

Depending on the defect size, a special syringe or amalgam carrier may be used to deliver the graft materials (Fig. 8-45). If the plan is to use a particle-loaded syringe, add moisture to the material while it is still within the barrel. This may be done using a nonvasoconstrictor local anesthetic solution, sterile saline, or the patient's blood. There is reason to believe that blood derived from bone marrow offers greater possibilities of osteogenesis as compared with peripheral blood. In addition, it is easier and more convenient to aspirate blood using a 3-ml syringe (sans needle) from a bony wound than from a phlebotomy.

A simple method is to place the diluent of choice into a sterile dappen dish and add the particles of graft material. Then, using an amalgam carrier or the blade of a periosteal elevator, carry the mixture to the host site where it can be tamped firmly into the defect (Fig. 8-46).

An alternative method of wetting the particles may be satisfied by withdrawing the syringe plunger almost to the breach of the barrel and, while supporting the syringe with one hand, injecting the blood or fluid from another syringe with a fine needle that has been inserted directly into the particles (Fig. 8-47).

Allow the syringe or carrier to remain untouched for 2 to 3 minutes. Then, into each well-controlled and visualized defect, gently but firmly introduce a slurry of particles to occupy a level just to the highest point of bone. Tamp the particles with a moistened cotton applicator to condense them. Confirm that blood has impregnated the entire mass. A continuous box-lock configuration of 4-0 dyed polyglactic suture is best used for closure. Before dismissing the patient, confirm stable hemostasis (Fig. 8-48, A, B).

Take well-oriented, long-cone, standardized, reproducible radiographic views before dismissing the patient, since a baseline must be established from which subsequent comparisons of particle retention and host-site density and morphology are made.

Do not undertake prosthodontic efforts until at least 12 weeks have elapsed. If it is planned to place endosteal implants into these ridges, allow 6 months for osseous maturation (Fig. 8-49). If it is the surgeon's plan to use the grafted sites for endosteal implants, nonresorbable HA cannot be used, since it prevents precise and effective drilling for implant placement. Either a resorbable ceramic (TCP, osteogen), an allograft (DFDB), a xenograft (Bio-Oss), an alloplast (HTR), or, preferably, autogenous bone (from a nearby tuberosity) is recommended.

Ridge Augmentation

Even if a ridge has not been maintained with grafting materials at the time of extractions and is found to be resorbed, it may be augmented with a natural or synthetic biomaterial. Flat, atrophied, or knife-edged ridges may be treated with a variety of resorbable and nonbiodegradable materials, as may

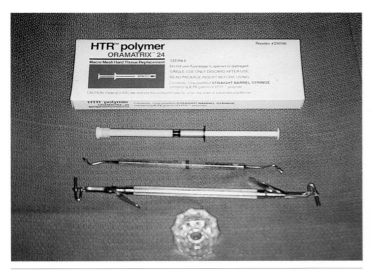

Fig. 8-45 The armamentarium needed to deliver the bone substitute material into the fresh extraction sockets consists of a sterile dappen dish, a Teflon-coated amalgam carrier, and a condenser. Alternatively, a syringe can be loaded to transfer the material to the socket.

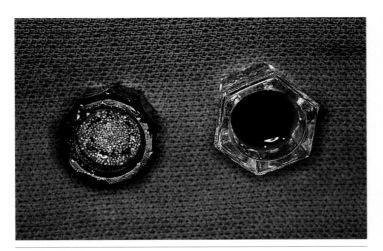

Fig. 8-46 Draw the patient's blood, preferably from an intraosseous site, and mix it with the graft material.

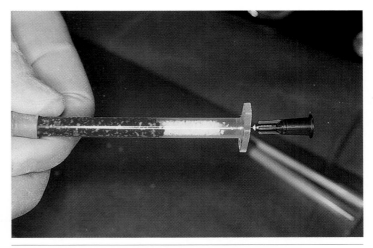

Fig. 8-47 When using a syringe, the blood can be injected into the barrel to inundate the graft material completely. The needle extending from the syringe serves as a vent.

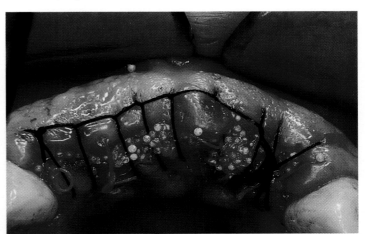

A

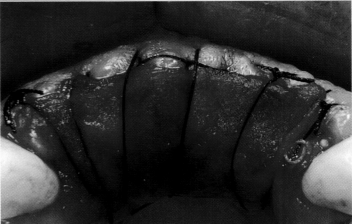

B

Fig. 8-48 **A,** Firmly condense the bone replacement material. Attempt primary closure. **B,** If primary closure cannot be achieved, suture a collagen sheet over the graft.

be noted in Table 8-1. These materials are available in two forms: particulate (syringe loaded) and porous block. They may be inserted by either "closed" (tunneling) or "open" (incision-flap-reflection) techniques. Each approach has its advocates, and each form (blocks or particles) has its proponents.

From an operative point of view, tunneling would appear to be less invasive and certainly faster. Fewer sutures and much shorter incisions are made, and a closure over or even near the implanted allograft will not be encountered. However, there are other factors that may influence the selection of this surgical approach.

If the mandibular canal appears to be dehiscent radiographically or the mental foramen is seen to be less than the width of the periosteal elevator blade from the crest of the ridge, a potential exists for creating an iatrogenic neuropathy if tunneling is used. Open procedures in such instances are safer because vital structures may be observed and thereby avoided.

Techniques

TUNNELING If a closed procedure is the chosen approach for the mandible, follow these steps:

Achieve anesthesia by infiltration, not block.

If the ridge is high but knife-edged, and the mentomandibular bundles are well below the crest and encased in canals, make a vertical incision in the labial gingiva of each canine

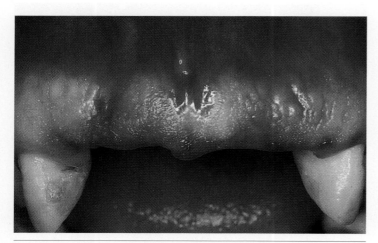

Fig. 8-49 Three-month postoperative healing demonstrates maintenance of ridge morphology.

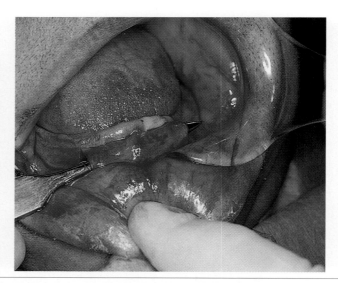

Fig. 8-51 Many ridge augmentation procedures can be completed by a technique of elevating the mucoperiosteum through several strategically placed small vertical incisions. These maneuvers are called *tunneling*. Each tunnel is created by passing the elevator beneath the periosteum in the area to be augmented.

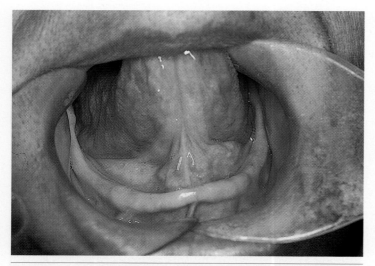

Fig. 8-50 Edentulous ridges often require augmentation. These ridges may be atrophied or as in this patient, require correction of undercuts.

area from crest to vestibule (Fig. 8-50). The incision must be of sufficient dimension to admit the wide end of the periosteal elevator and, of course, the muzzle of a delivery syringe or an augmentative block.

Insert the elevator beneath the periosteum using the palm-thumb grasp, with the palm facing upward, and slide it beneath the periosteum over the defective portion of the ridge. There must be enough room above the mental bundle to permit continuous passage of the elevator blade all the way back to the retromolar pad. After this has been completed on both sides, reenter and tunnel the right or left incision anteriorly until the elevator blade protrudes from the opposing incision. There now are one anterior and two posterior tunnels (Fig. 8-51).

Elevate each of the three tunnels using a Gerald forceps or a silk retracting suture as if the mucoperiosteum were a tent. Evaluate whether there is sufficient dimension for an adequately augmented ridge shape. If not, the tissues at the vestibular level may require detachment and, of course, a subsequent secondary vestibuloplasty will be required us-

ing free or pedicle natural or reconstituted (AlloDerm) mucosal grafting (see Chapter 7 for further instructions on these procedures).

In cases of knife-edged ridges, elevation labially and buccally must be made to allow for lateral augmentation. In instances of mental foramina in proximity to the crest of the ridge when tunneling is still the procedure of choice, two incisions, each distal to the foramen, are required. A third incision is made in the anterior midline. Tunneling can be carried out posteriorly to the retromolar pads from each lateral incision, and the anterior tunnel can be started in the midline and carried to the right and left sides up to but not including the mental areas. If this second technique is selected, the areas just over the foramina will remain unaugmented.

The question of whether to use a block or particles requires analysis. Blocks are valuable because they may be easily placed and remain unchanged in shape, whereas particles have a tendency to drift, migrate, and settle. There are several kinds of porous blocks: permanently rigid ones are available in the replaminaform (coraline) design. Rigid blocks that become compliant after implantation as a result of their dehydrated collagen matrices may be used. Blocks consisting of HA beads that are strung together with polyglycolic acid threads (Ceramed) may also be chosen. The latter consists of HA particles that are bound together with a collagen floss that becomes hydrolyzed by body fluids (or water) and, as it softens, releases the HA particles, permitting blood infiltration. Upon completion of that event, wound organization is well advanced.

Soak rigid blocks in a mixture of the patient's blood and aqueous antibiotic solution (i.e., 80 mg genta-micin in 10 ml of sterile saline) for 20 minutes before implantation. The collagen vehicle cannot be treated in this fashion because it allows the block to become soft before insertion, thus impeding its placement.

The major disadvantage of the use of rigid porous blocks is that if a dehiscence occurs and causes exposure of even the tiniest portion of its surface, the possibilities of preserving the block or any part of it are lost. No matter how aggressively one attempts to salvage a dehiscent porous block, surgical efforts will fail. Exposure mandates block removal.

Autogenous bone blocks from ribs or iliac crests or precut DFDB slivers or wedges from the Pacific Coast Bone Laboratory, on the other hand, are choices that offer greater chances for success.

Once a decision has been made regarding the material and the form in which it is to be used, perform the implantation.

If the particulate form of graft material has been chosen, elevate the tunnel opening and retain it with a suture or a toothed Gerald or Adson forceps. Insert the barrel of the syringe into the tunnel (after wetting the particles and removing the breech cap if any) to its most distal extent (Fig. 8-52). Stabilize the plunger with the opposite hand while the barrel is withdrawn. This permits the extrusion of a smooth, symmetrical, blood-soaked, cylindrically shaped slurry of particles, deposited in the center of the tunnel. Exercise care not to make the tunnel larger than the minimal size required to accommodate the syringe or to permit it to penetrate beyond the vestibular attachment. Impeccably made tunnels determine postimplantation particle stability and graft success (Figs. 8-53, 8-54).

If a block is planned, retract the lip of the tunnel. Trim the block using a rongeur forceps to a size (Fig. 8-55) that permits its admission. Blocks may not be ground or adjusted with rotary instruments because grinding clogs the surface pores. Slide the block into place by pushing gently with a cotton-tipped applicator, and maneuver its position by using the thumb and forefinger on the overlying tissues (Figs. 8-56 through 8-58).

Complete the augmentations in the two other tunnels and close the incisions with a few 4-0 polyglactic interrupted sutures (Fig. 8-59). Take a panoramic radiograph to judge the positions of the blocks.

Fixation of the particles or blocks is a valuable postimplantation adjunct. If the patient has a denture, ream its saddle aggressively and reline it with a tissue conditioner such as Coe-Comfort or Viscogel. After the denture flanges have been trimmed and polished, stabilize the denture, which retains the blocks or particles in position, by employing circummandibular or circumzygomatic ligation, the techniques of which are detailed later in this chapter.

Prescribe a pureed diet. The opposing denture should be removed whenever possible and a week of antibiotic therapy should be instituted.

Maxillary augmentations are a bit easier to complete because the tissues are thicker and there are no significant foramina or vital structures with which to cope.

Open Flap

If the choice is made not to tunnel for ridge augmentation, make an incision at the crest of the ridge in the linea alba, re-

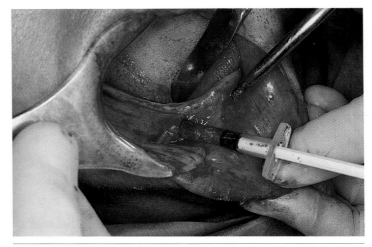

Fig. 8-52 When the enhancement is to be performed using particulate grafting material often supplied in syringes, these devices are inserted into the full depth of the tunnel and the material expressed evenly into the undercut areas or at the ridge crest.

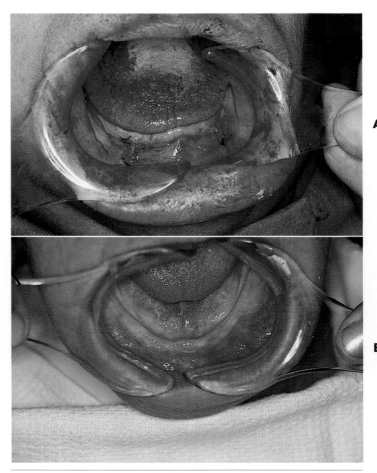

Fig. 8-53 **A,** After deposition of the graft material, each small incision is closed with several simple sutures. **B,** After healing, the ridge demonstrates an improvement in morphology.

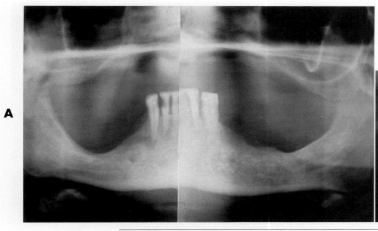
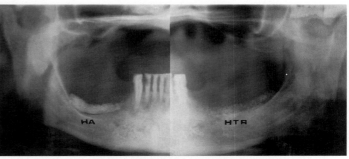

A

B

Fig. 8-54   A, The preoperative radiograph of this mandible with posterior ridge atrophy indicates a significant need for augmentation. **B,** Augment the ridges by tunneling, using two different but equally effective grafting materials. The difference in radiodensity of the two is not representative of their stability or competence.

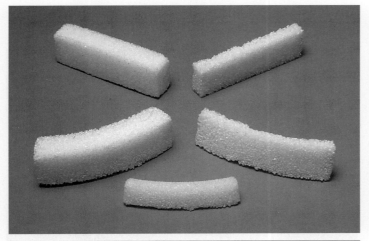

Fig. 8-55   A more reliable form of synthetic bone material for augmentation is the block. It is less likely to migrate, and portions of it will not be lost. On the negative side, if it becomes dehiscent, the entire graft will be lost.

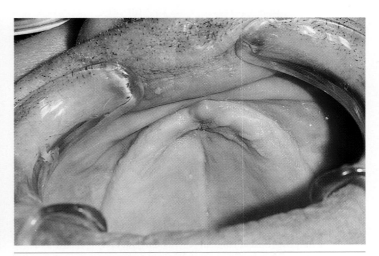

Fig. 8-56   These maxillae are severely atrophied. The palate is flat, and the tuberosities are nonexistent.

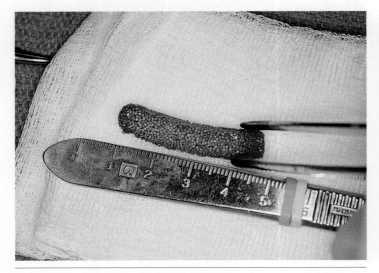

Fig. 8-57   Porous blocks are soaked in the patient's blood and a soluble antibiotic solution (gentamycin) before their insertion.

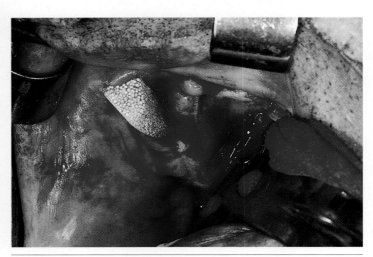

Fig. 8-58   Tunneling is the most appropriate technique for block placement. After removing the block from the solution, place it into the tunnel and gently advance it to its position of repose. Simple suturing will close the small vertical incisions.

flect the flap, and place the graft materials directly against the bone. Circumvent the mental neurovascular bundle and attempt to keep the particulate graft material in integrated form by allowing the patient's blood to clot within it before suturing. The fibrin acts as a preliminary cementing medium.

In open procedures, it is more important that the operating team be prepared to retain the grafted particles with a splint. Make this in advance to a projected ridge shape by rebuilding the ridge on a study cast with wax and then using the augmented model to fabricate a clear acrylic template. Close the flaps, and seat the clear plastic splint to ascertain that it

causes no blanching. When this criterion has been met, suture the flaps with a horizontal mattress closure (see Chapter 6). Carry out undermining when necessary to permit a tension-free flap relationship. Affix the splint with significantly shortened flanges to the mandible or maxilla with No. 2 stainless steel, monofilament, ligature wire following the instructions in this chapter. Keep it in place for at least 3 weeks.

If the plan is to augment with blocks by an open surgical procedure, incise and reflect the tissues, adopt the blocks to the residual ridge using a rongeur forceps and place them into position (Figs. 8-60 through 8-62). Follow this with suturing

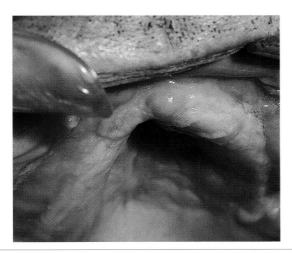

Fig. 8-59 Postoperatively, the ridge morphology is changed significantly as a result of porous block augmentation.

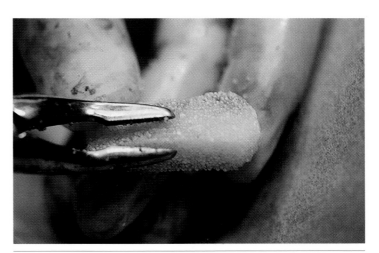

Fig. 8-61 Trim a hard tissue replacement polymeric block to fit the defect using rongeur forceps.

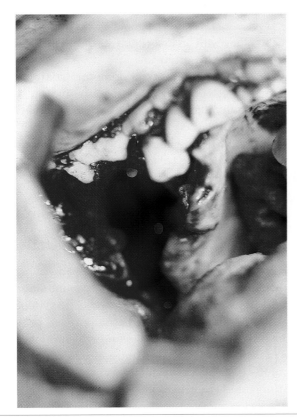

Fig. 8-60 Blocks may be used successfully for reconstruction of major jaw defects. A recurrent ameloblastoma was responsible for a hemimaxillectomy. The resultant discontinuity was significant.

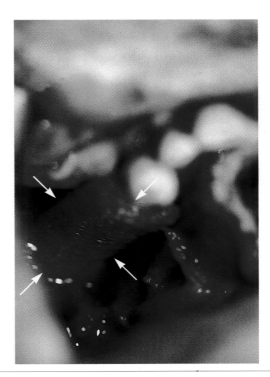

Fig. 8-62 If sized properly, the porous block (arrows) will be self-retained by wedging it between the alveolus of the canine and the anterior surface of the pterygoid plates.

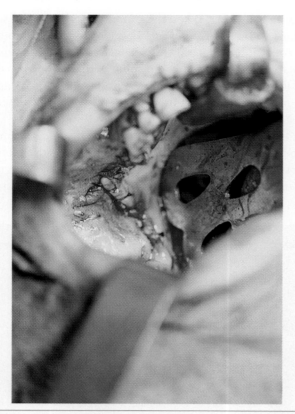

Fig. 8-63 Undermining to create a primary closure with well-vascularized pedicle grafts completes the reconstruction.

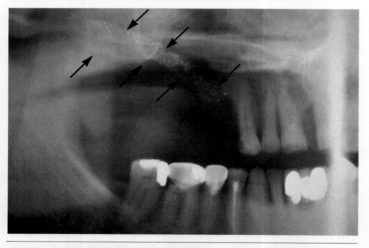

Fig. 8-64 A postoperative radiograph indicates that the block *(arrows)* has served well to recompartmentalize the antrum.

and, if necessary, ligating with a prefabricated splint following the same techniques presented in the previous paragraphs for use with particulate grafting material (Figs. 8-63, 8-64). If the choice is an HA-collagen block, do not trim it, because, as it becomes hydrated with body fluids, it adapts itself to the bone's morphology. The pressure from an overlying fixation splint will threaten to flatten an HA-collagen block, so do not use one. When splints are indicated, 3 weeks of fixation will protect the grafts and offers greater possibilities for their adhesion to the underlying bone. Place both root form and blade implants into such sites after a 6-month period of maturation but only if a graft material has been placed that presents an environment that allows the preparation of an osteotomy (e.g., DFDB, autogenous bone) (Fig. 8-65).

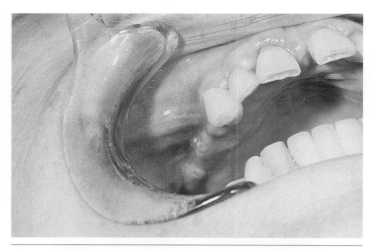

Fig. 8-65 Clinically, primary healing has taken place, incorporating the graft material as a biologic substitute. Vestibular and ridge morphology are restored.

Maxillofacial Reconstruction

Lesions and defects of the facial soft and hard tissues may be managed using bone-grafting materials.

Certain exclusion criteria must be employed, including the following:

1. Any acute or chronic infectious process at or near the intended implant site
2. Severe cardiovascular, respiratory, endocrine, renal, hepatic, or collagen disease that contraindicates elective surgery or anesthesia
3. Uncontrollable diabetes mellitus
4. Progressive, severe, or malignant blood dyscrasias
5. A malignancy with an associated short life expectancy
6. Uncontrollable hypertension
7. Any disease causing marked demineralization of bone (e.g., severe osteoporosis, hyperparathyroidism, multiple myeloma. sarcoidosis, Paget's disease, or vitamin D deficiency or intoxication)
8. Patients receiving or who recently received radiation therapy to the areas to be treated
9. Immunologically suppressed individuals
10. Hypersensitivity to all antibiotics
11. A documented history of mental incompetence or deficiency
12. Anticipated patient nonavailability for regular follow-up procedures and evaluations

Workups should include preoperative panoramic and periapical radiographs and photographs, medical and dental evaluations, photographs, and study casts. Surgical procedures should involve careful flap design, thorough curettage, proper creation of well-vascularized host sites, preparation and stabilization of the graft material, and impeccable primary closure.

Use implanted grafts in either particulate or block form as plumpers for cosmetic purposes or within bony defects to serve as scaffolds to encourage new bone growth. Employ the block forms as cosmetic prostheses for genioplasty, malar prominence matrices, and to solve problems caused by large

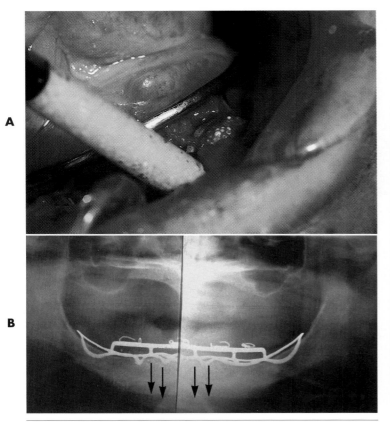

Fig. 8-66   A, A submandibular fistula resulted from a blow to the chin 11 years after the placement of a subperiosteal implant. An incision was made in the vestibule, the tract of drainage was excised, and an HA barrier was inserted by syringe. **B,** The postoperative result separated the oral from the submandibular spaces (note the HA barrier) *(arrows)* and restored health to the implant host site.

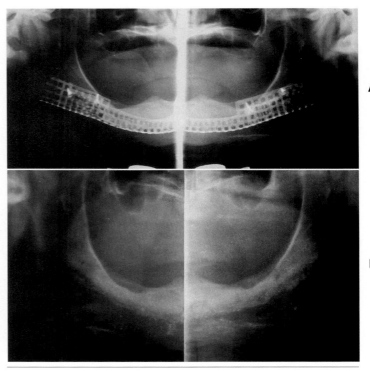

Fig. 8-67   A, For severely atrophied mandibles, autogenous bone grafts placed into titanium mortise forms can double their height and volume. The original height of the mandible can be seen through the mesh. (After the technique of Philip Boyne, DDS.) **B,** After the mesh is removed (in order to prevent stress shielding), the amount of well-mineralized augmentation is clearly visible.

fistulas and continuity defects. The procedures undertaken often require the use of a specific form of grafting material and respond most successfully when autogenous bone is used.

Particulate

1. Vestibular compartmentalization (Fig. 8-66)
2. Mandibular inferior border augmentation (Fig. 8-67)
3. Mandibular fracture defects (Fig. 8-68)
4. Large cyst reconstruction (Fig. 8-69)
5. Mandibular continuity defects (Fig. 8-70)

Block Form

1. Infraorbital rim, malar defects (Fig. 8-71)
2. Ridge augmentation, maxillary and mandibular (Figs. 8-50 through 8-54)
3. Hemimaxillectomy repair (Figs. 8-60 through 8-65)
4. Genioplasty (Fig. 8-72)
5. Mandibular continuity defects (Fig. 8-73)

Platelet-Rich Gel

Natural cementing media offer the benefits of stability when the surgeon is using large quantities of particulate graft material. This material might be pure marrow, marrow mixed with ground cortex, or combinations of synthetic, autogenous, and alloplastic shavings. Often, even when the patient's blood or fibrin is used as a vehicle, maintaining its integrity in a mass becomes difficult because of the large quantity of graft material and the complex anatomic role it is being used to serve. Recent predictable benefits of stability have been experienced with the use of platelet-rich gel.

Although the preparation of this biologic glue probably is too complicated for most practitioners to use with small grafts, large ones (i.e., major ridge replacement, inferior mandibular border augmentation, continuity defects) benefit greatly from the addition of platelet-rich gel.

At the onset of the procedure, draw blood from the patient by phlebotomy in quantities of 50 to 500 ml depending on the volume and size of the graft.

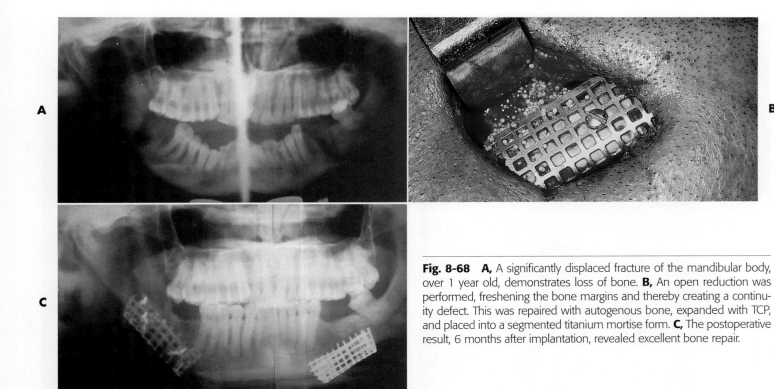

Fig. 8-68 **A,** A significantly displaced fracture of the mandibular body, over 1 year old, demonstrates loss of bone. **B,** An open reduction was performed, freshening the bone margins and thereby creating a continuity defect. This was repaired with autogenous bone, expanded with TCP, and placed into a segmented titanium mortise form. **C,** The postoperative result, 6 months after implantation, revealed excellent bone repair.

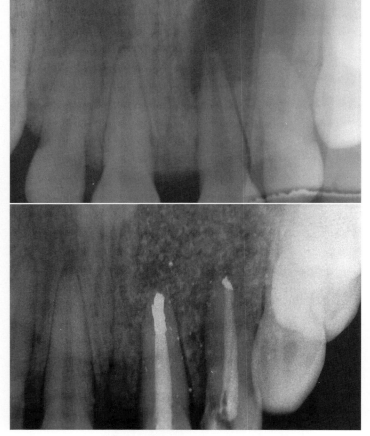

Fig. 8-69 **A, B,** Do not repair cysts with graft material because its presence prevents radiographic evidence of recurrence. However, there are instances when grafting is acceptable because both facial and palatal cortical plates have been lost. These defects will never fill in with bone, thereby leaving a permanent radiolucency if not grafted.

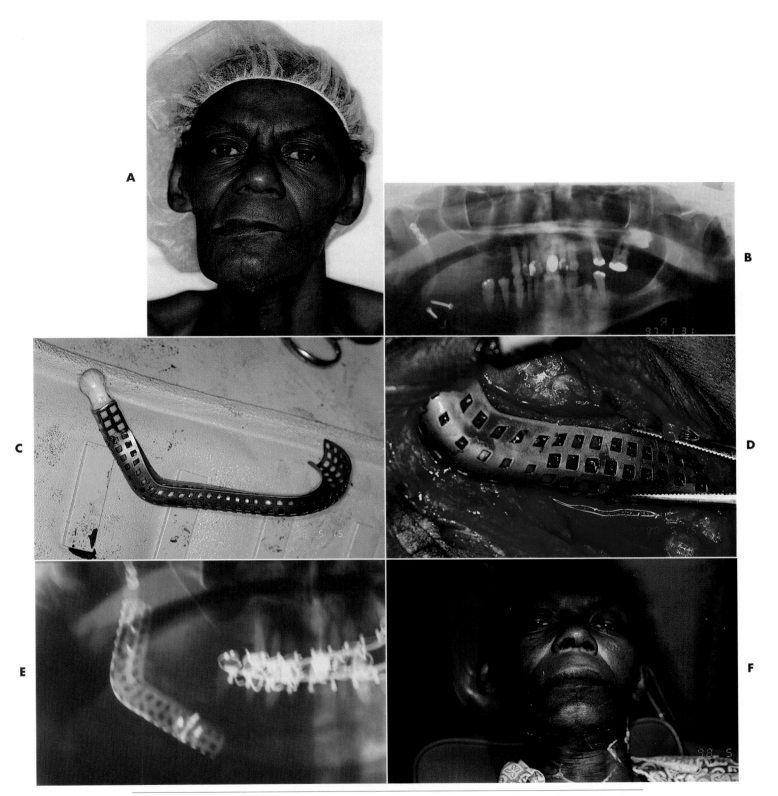

Fig. 8-70 **A** and **B,** A significant continuity defect was created after mandibular resection resulting from an intraoral squamous cell carcinoma. **C,** A titanium mortise-form prosthesis with an added acrylic condyle was fabricated to serve as an anatomic replacement. **D,** An intraoperative view of the titanium mortise-form containing particulate autogenous cortical and cancellous bone harvested from the anterior iliac crest and augmented with HA-N. **E,** A postoperative radiographic view of the mortise-form in place. **F,** Postoperative photograph demonstrates restored facial symmetry.

A   **B**   **C**

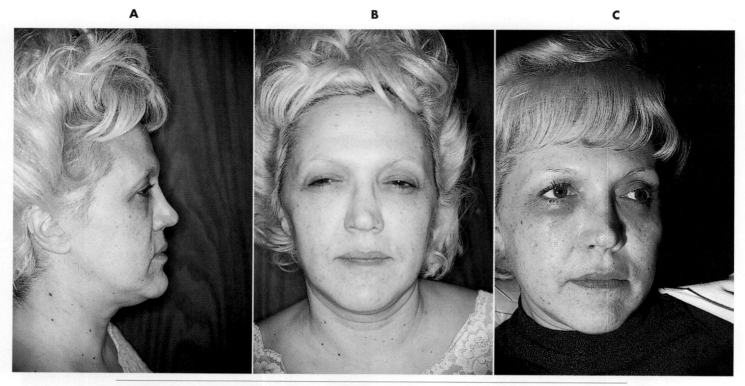

Fig. 8-71   A and **B,** Profile and frontal views of a patient with congenitally deficient malar prominences. **C,** This postsurgical view after bilateral augmentations using carved silicone blocks demonstrates a significantly enhanced malar region and an overall improvement in facial esthetics.

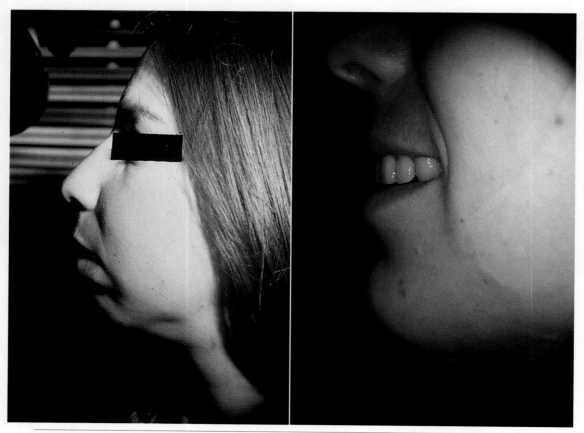

Fig. 8-72   Before and after profile views of a patient who had a deficient chin augmented with a contoured silicone block. The approach was via a submental skin incision.

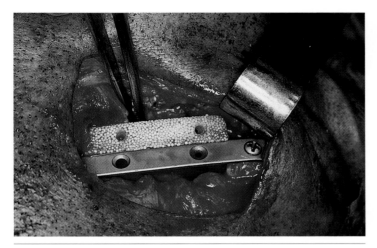

Fig. 8-73 Porous blocks, although possessing poor structural strength, can serve as plumping or scaffolding devices for maxillofacial reconstruction in conjunction with metal plates or armatures that offer the requisite rigidity. This HTR block accepts drilling and tapping to accommodate the self-tapping Vitallium screws, which attach it to the Luhr fracture plate. This has already been used for splinting these two mandibular segments.

Place the blood in a centrifuge (there are machines that do the entire procedure, but for small quantities, a manual operation is available) and spin it to separate the plasma from the cells (Fig. 8-74). The platelets are buff in color, and they are removed from the precipitated cell mass. If the total quantity of blood withdrawn was large, return the cell-free plasma to the patient via the intravenous route. Keep the platelets in a covered container until the graft material, usually in an anatomically designed titanium mortise form, is ready to be transferred to the host site. At that time, gel activity is induced by the addition of a mixture of calcium chloride and thrombin, creating a physiologic glue that is placed atop the particles just before implantation of the complex (Fig. 8-75). Manipulation, fixation with screws, and other adjustments that might otherwise disturb the sanctity of the graft are discouraged because of the stabilizing influence of the adherent, glutinous, biologic addition.

If the planned grafting procedure is a minor one to be performed in the doctor's office, platelet-rich gel can be produced from small quantities of blood using an inexpensive countertop centrifuge. In these instances, do not reinfuse the blood to the patient.

Periimplant Support and Repair

Many blade, transosteal, or root form implants that show radiographic signs of host-site deterioration may be treated as if they were periodontally involved teeth by making flaps followed by curettage and implantation. Details may be found in Chapter 27, "Diagnosis and Treatment of Complications" as well as in Section II of this chapter. Do not undertake the repair or salvage of endosteal implant host sites unless the implant is completely firm and the bony defect is of reasonable size. GTRMs offer greater assurance of repair stability (Fig. 8-76). Subperiosteal implants also may be found in failing modes. Chapter 28 describes how particulate grafting can contribute to salvage operations in this category as well (Fig. 8-77).

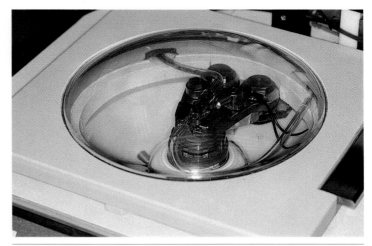

Fig. 8-74 The Electromedic centrifuge that separates the blood cells from the plasma. This is the first step in preparing platelet-rich gel.

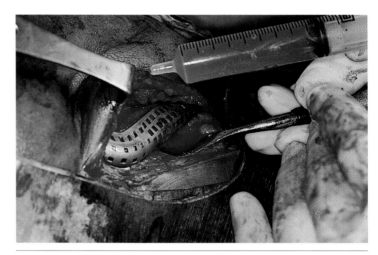

Fig. 8-75 Addition of the platelet gel to the graft before implantation, lends stability to it and simplifies management of the bone-filled titanium mortise-form.

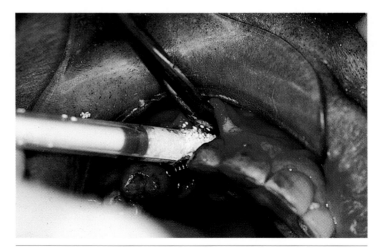

Fig. 8-76 Implants that have periodontal defects are salvageable by using grafting materials if the management of the problem is controlled carefully and the principles governing periodontal surgery are observed strictly.

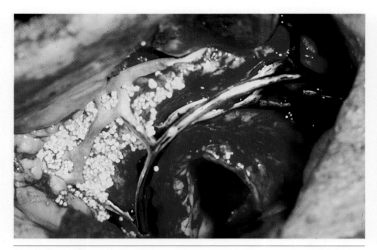

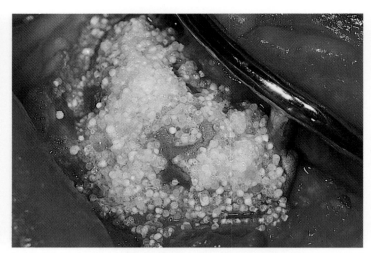

Fig. 8-77 If host bone suffers resorption, subperiosteal implants (either at the time of insertion or subsequently) respond well when particulate grafting material is used to augment osseous deficiencies. Thorough curettage and adequate soft tissue flaps for primary closure are mandatory.

Fig. 8-78 When accuracy is lacking, particularly with CAD-CAM castings, particulate graft material serves as a satisfactory grout.

Blade implants do well when, on their placement within their slotted osteotomies, particles are used to support ridge contours over and about their shoulders.

Root form implants can be inserted into extraction sites that are larger in diameter than the implant bodies or infrastructures by using grafting materials and membranes. This is described in detail in Chapter 9, "Root Form Implant Surgery: Generic."

The new bone interface, after extraction, should be developed either from 40% of additional bone apical to the alveolus, or from within it if its diameter is narrow enough to permit a freshly cut enlargement to accommodate the implant.

If there is an inadequate amount of bone in the cervical area after the implant has been placed but it is found to be stable, use particulate grafting to correct the deficiency. Place the implant below the alveolar margins, tamp the graft material meticulously around its periphery, and place a healing screw, which should be used to stabilize a GTRM so that postintegration healing is encouraged.

Primary closure requires the technique of creating pedicle flaps by undermining as described in Chapter 7.

CAD-CAM subperiosteal implants, particularly maxillary, in cases of inaccurate apposition, require particulate augmentation (Fig. 8-78). This can be reviewed in Chapters 14 and 15.

Bone Grafting for Root Form Implant Host Sites of Inadequate Dimension

The following sections are devoted to the management of potential implant host sites that are not sufficiently wide or high enough to permit the placement of implants. In addition to containing descriptions of the methods of obtaining graft materials, this section is divided into four anatomic sections: anterior and posterior maxillae and anterior and posterior mandible, as listed in the following box:

I. Mandible
  A. Anterior
    1. Width
      a. Alveoloplasty
      b. Monocortical block grafting
    2. Height
      a. Monocortical block grafting
      b. Inferior border augmentation
  B. Posterior
    1. Width
      a. Alveoloplasty
      b. Monocortical block grafting
    2. Height
      a. Mandibular nerve repositioning

II. Maxilla
  A. Anterior
    1. Width
      a. Alveoloplasty
      b. Splitting and expanding
      c. Osteotome expansion
      d. Monocortical block grafting
    2. Height
      a. Nasal floor elevation
  B. Posterior
    1. Width
      a. Alveoloplasty
      b. Splitting and expanding
    2. Height
      a. Antroplasty
      b. Antroplasty and miniplate
      c. Osteotome (Summers)

CAVEATS

The harvesting of autogenous bone (the most reliable of materials) is not without complications. Exercise care so that as little trauma as possible occurs in these second operative sites.

At the primary or host sites, make sharp, full-thickness incisions and elevate the periosteum, without tearing it.

Attention to the neurovascular bundles as well as to the foramina must be constant when the symphysis is being used as a source of bone. Stop arterial bleeding from the mandibular artery beneath the incisor apices, which may be brisk, using either bone wax or an electro-surgical tip.

When drilling holes for bone graft fixation screws, make them of a proper size to encourage firm fixation. Stripped holes can cause bone loss and often deprive the surgeon of a second strategic site for screw placement.

Use of the lag screw technique makes monocortical block placement simple by eliminating the awkward event of graft spinning. Using a lag screw achieves firm fixation by pressure from the screw head as its shaft passes unencumbered through the graft. The procedure is performed by making the hole in the graft sufficiently large so the screw threads do not engage its sides and making the hole in the host sufficiently small so that the threads lock into the underlying bone. Of course, the hole in the graft must be made small enough so that the head serves as a locking device (Fig. 8-79).

When using osteotomes, mallet taps must be controlled to prevent penetration of vital structures.

Osteotome techniques for ridge splitting and expansion cannot be used in the mandible because the bone is too dense and inelastic. In the maxilla, good judgment, experience, and tactile skills are essential tools when ridge expansion and splitting are undertaken. Danger of fracture always threatens the effort to expand the bone beyond its physiologic limit. Acquiring a sense of the elastic limits of the operative site is essential if fracture is to be avoided. Such an event, of course, mandates abandoning the procedure. Chapter 27 offers instruction on how to proceed should such an event occur.

Minimal reflection of the mucoperiosteum at the site to be grafted or expanded is of benefit because this ensures optimal vascularity. In addition, if a fragment of bone is fractured and remains attached to its overlying periosteum, there is an excellent possibility that it will heal properly after an anatomic closure.

Management of the inferior alveolar neurovascular bundle in nerve repositioning must be gentle, and the osteotomy performed to expose it must be sufficiently wide to allow its impeccable manipulation. Nonetheless, transient paresthesia should be expected.

The handling of the maxillary sinus membrane must be performed with skill to avoid tearing it. Use of Tatum instruments is of benefit in achieving this goal. If torn, repair the membrane by suturing or placing collagen sheets.

Although most surgeons use a round bur to scribe the bony lateral wall overlying the maxillary sinus, as it passes through the eggshell-thin bone, it sometimes catches and tears the membrane. By using a round diamond instead, a definitive oblong osteotomy can be completed with virtually no threat to the translucent, fragile membrane.

Although autogenous bone can be harvested from the cranium, fibula, tibial plateau, anterior or posterior iliac crests, and ribs (as well as a variety of intraoral sources), not all of these sites are described in this section. Those selected were chosen because of their excellent yields and the broad familiarity that maxillofacial surgeons have with them. Of course, there are morbid complications related to bone harvesting in all situations, which mandates that the surgeon must weigh risk as compared with benefit.

Intraoral sites such as osteomas and palatal and lingual tori should not be seriously considered for service as grafts because they are constituted of almost pure cortex, and as such, they cannot supply significant sources of osteogenic or osteoinductive activity. They may be used, however, as expanders when minced and added to marrow, which serves to increase graft quantity.

Techniques for Obtaining Autogenous Bone

Anterior Iliac Crest

The most reliable and predictable grafting material is autogenous bone marrow. The easiest and safest place from which to harvest it in adequate quantities is from the anterior iliac crest.

There are a few possible complications involved in exposing the anterior iliac crest and several vital structures to be encountered during the dissection, which should be performed in an operating room under general anesthesia. The surgeon should be aware of the femoral cutaneous nerve, which is encountered lateroinferiorly on rare occasions.

After skin preparation, apply a Steri-drape and then, after palpating the crest, make an incision through the overlying skin and fascia (Fig. 8-80, A). When, on occasion, the femoral cutaneous nerve, which should be sought, is damaged, the patient is left with a sensory deficit of the skin overlying the anterolateral thigh. Clamp and electrocoagulate bleeders, and continue the sharp dissection through fat, muscle fibers, fascia lata, and periosteum. Reflect the periosteum medially just over the full thickness of the crest and laterally down over its

undercut for a distance of 4 cm. Do this from the anterior to the posterior tubercles. Use a sharp, 2-cm-wide osteotome to bisect the crest in its long axis to its fully exposed length (Fig. 8-80, B). Connect this osteotomy with two vertical cuts, one anterior and one posterior, that are carried down through the lateral cortex just beneath the periosteal attachment. Next, use the osteotome as a lever to pry this "trapdoor" open laterally, allowing it to rotate downward on its periosteal hinge. Use bayoneted medullary gouges to lift the marrow from between the cortical plates with gentle, undulating, pushing movements (Fig. 8-80, C). Avoid perforating the cortical plates. A perforation of the medial plate could lead to a pelvic infection, so avoid pressure of the gouge against this cortex. Store the harvested marrow in a saline-filled medicine glass (Fig. 8-80, D). When the marrow cavity yields a sufficient amount of material, follow with thorough irrigation (Fig. 8-80, E). Employ tamponade or platelet gel to minimize intraosseous bleeding, and, when controlled, reset the cortical trapdoor into its anatomic position. Drill two fine holes through it and the adjacent intact

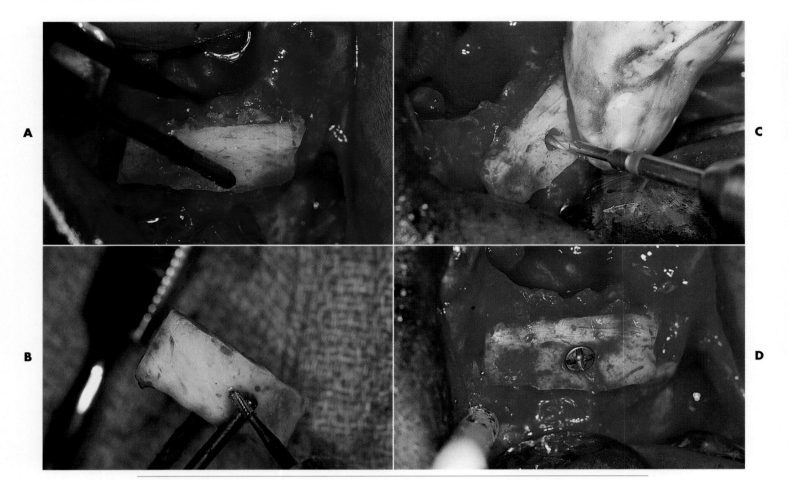

Fig. 8-79   Lag screw technique. **A,** Place the monocortical graft, marrow side down, against the potential host site. **B,** Use a 701 bur (which has a larger diameter than the planned fixation screw shaft) to make an osteotomy in the graft, which initiates the lag screw technique. **C,** Refit the graft, and mark and deepen the center of the osteotomy in the host cortex using a 700 SL bur. This serves to pre-tap the screw hole in the host bone. **D,** Place the final screw through the graft without touching its walls. Its threads, however, cut into and grasp the host bone beneath it. As the screw is tightened, its head locks the graft firmly against the host site.

crestal cortical plate, and achieve fixation with two 2-0 Biosyn sutures (Fig. 8-80, *F*). If an insufficient quantity of bone is harvested, the cortical trapdoor may be removed, particulated, and added to the harvested material. When the cortex is sacrificed, anatomic contours can be retained by grafting the donor site to the former level of the crest with particulate or block (HA) graft material (Fig. 8-80, *G*). Then irrigate and suture the soft tissues in carefully restored layers. Pay attention to the fascia lata and other structures so that an anatomic closure results. Use a 3-0 chromic suture for the subcuticular tissues, and close the skin quickly and efficiently with an Autostapler (Fig. 8-80, *H*). Place a small Hemovac, which applies constant, gentle suction to the interior of the wound for evacuation of pooled blood, under the periosteum and allow it to exit through a point 2 cm beyond the inferior end of the incision (Fig. 8-80, *I*). This is made possible by use of its sharp-tipped trocar. Withdraw the tube so that its perforations are left deep in the wound. Remove the trocar, and trim the tube to proper

Fig. 8-80   **A,** Place a Steri-drape over the prepared skin in the anterior iliac crest region using a BP No. 10 blade and make the incision through the plastic drape, the skin, and into superficial fascia. **B,** After the crest is exposed use a 2-cm-wide osteotome to make a midcortical groove from the anterior to posterior ends. Use vertical osteotomies at either end to create a trapdoor that is wedged open with the osteotome (see Fig. 8-80, *F*). Its hinge is the intact periosteum at its base. **C,** Use gouges, which are bayonet shaped, to remove the osteogenic marrow. **D,** Store the graft complex, spongiosa, synthetic particles, and when needed, particulated cortex, in the patient's marrow derived blood, with 80 mg of gentamycin added. **E,** The requisite amount of bone has been removed from between the cortical plates, and hemostasis has been achieved. **F,** Close the trapdoor of lateral cortex, described above (Fig. 8-80, *B*) after two drill holes are made in it and matching holes made in the stable medial crest. Use Biosyn sutures (2-0) to close and stabilize the door. **G,** If a greater bulk of bone was required than was available from the marrow harvesting, mince and add the cortex. In order to restore the contours, use a synthetic graft material to replace the cortex. **H,** Skin closures in areas not demanding the highest level of esthetics are completed quickly and efficiently with staples.

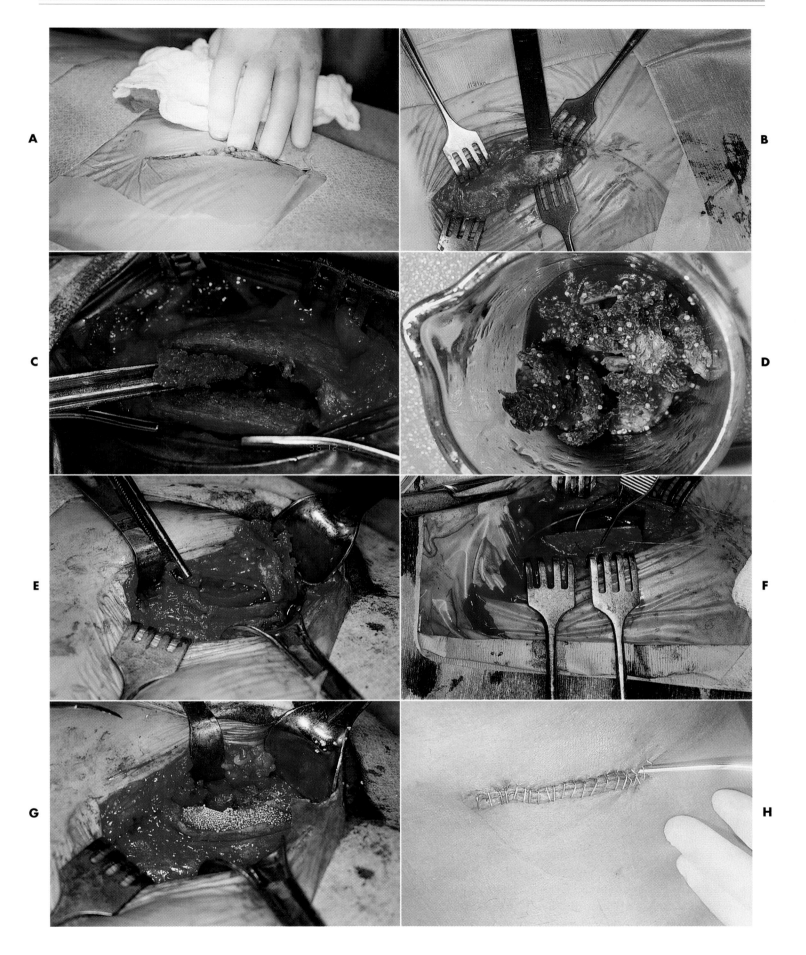

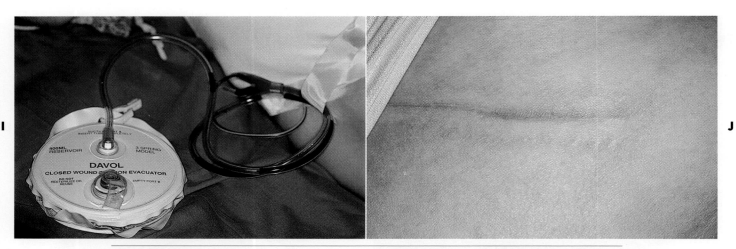

Fig. 8-80, cont'd   I, A Hemovac is manually armed to maintain gentle negative pressure in the depth of the wound and mediated via a multiple perforated polyethyhene tube. This evacuates oozed blood and discourages pooling and subsequent infection. **J,** The appearance of the operative site after staple removal.

length, suture it to the skin with 2-0 nylon, and connect it to the bellows. Then dress the wound, and arm the Hemovac by compressing its walls. Examine the container periodically and, when necessary, recompress it (about every 8 hours). Remove it in 24 to 48 hours, depending on how productive the bleeding appears to be. Ambulate the patient no later than the second day with the help of a walker or crutches, and encourage physical activity. Remove staples on the fourteenth day using the specialized extractor after carefully preparing the area with povidone-iodine (Fig. 8-80, *J*).

Rib

Wedge the patient's back with sheets to support the rib cage in an upward direction and apply a Steri-drape. Place an incision in the inframammary crease to best hide the scar (Fig. 8-81, *A*). This incision should be carried through the periosteum overlying the donor, which is either the fifth or sixth rib. Incise the periosteum sharply to bone and use an elevator to expose the rib (Fig. 8-81, *B*). Be careful not to pierce the lung or enter the thoracic cavity. Were this to occur, pneumothorax would result, requiring placement of a chest tube.

If cartilage is required, it can be harvested with the rib by incising with the scalpel 1 cm medial to the costochondral junction. If this cartilage is not needed, the rib graft may be sectioned at the costochondral junction and at a lateral posterior site that is determined by the length of bone required. If an acute curve of the rib is desired, score it deeply to allow it to be bent without fracturing (Fig. 8-81, *C, D*).

Perform bone sectioning with a rib cutter or a small oscillating saw with saline irrigation for cooling. Store the graft in saline, and perform an anatomic closure in layers with 3-0 chromic gut and Autostaples for the skin. If the periosteum is allowed to remain, a new rib ossifies. If periosteum is desired (as it might be for a mandibular continuity defect), remove the rib with its investing membrane intact. Natural rib replacement will not ensue. The patient, after such a harvesting pro-

cedure, should have a firm occlusive chest dressing placed, and the surgical team should be observant of the operative site for 2 weeks at which time the skin staples can be removed.

Tuberosity

The instructions for incision making are the same as for tuberosity reduction in Chapter 6. Before making the incision, however, if it is bone that is being sought, pay careful attention to a periapical radiograph for the presence of mineralized rather than soft tissue and the location of the antral floor.

After exposure of the underlying bone (Fig, 8-82, *A*), which is rich in marrow, use a side-cutting rongeur to remove the quantity required (Fig. 8-82, *B*), with special concern exhibited to circumvent the sinus floor (Fig. 8-82, *C*).

Closure follows the technique described for tuberosity reduction (Fig. 8-82, *D*).

Anterior Border of the Mandibular Ramus

The anterolateral border of the mandibular ramus on the same side as the sinus that is to be grafted should be palpated. Anesthetize the donor site using infiltration procedures laterally and medially. Make the incision with a No. 15 BP blade, proceeding vertically over the anterior border of the ramus from a point 1 cm below the coronoid tip downward and forward to a point level with the mandibular third molar area. By keeping the instruments directly against the anterior border, the lingual nerve is not disturbed. Reflect the flaps laterally and medially with a sharp periosteal elevator, creating adequate access to the anterior surface of the ramus (Fig. 8-83). Initiate the osteotomy with a No. 2 round bur in a straight handpiece or Impactair (a regularly designed contra-angle makes it difficult to place the bur holes). Place the holes made with this bur in a 2-cm-diameter, semilunar pattern in the lateral cortex, at the midlevel of the ramus. Connect them with the gentle strokes of a No. 700 L bur and copiously cool them

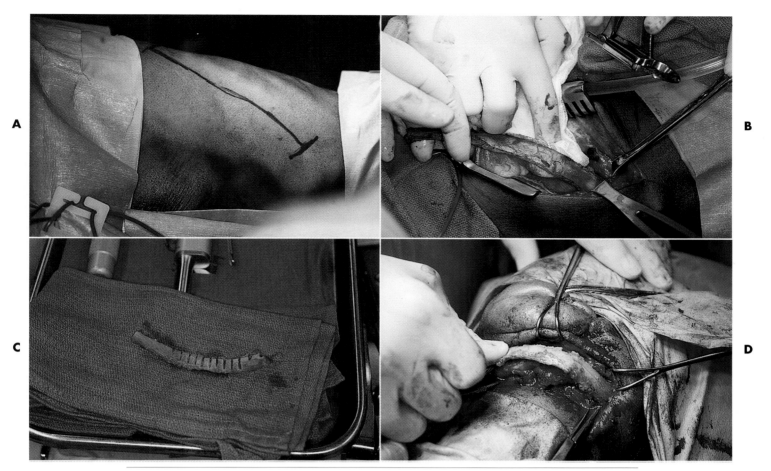

Fig. 8-81 **A,** Outline the area overlying the rib that is planned for removal with a skin marking pen. **B,** Expose the rib by sharp dissection to the full extent required for the graft. Observe care to avoid causing pneumothorax. **C** and **D,** In order to create a significant arc in a rib, deeply score the side of the lesser curvature to permit bending without fracture. Ribs should be made self-sustaining so that they will not require plates or mesh for support.

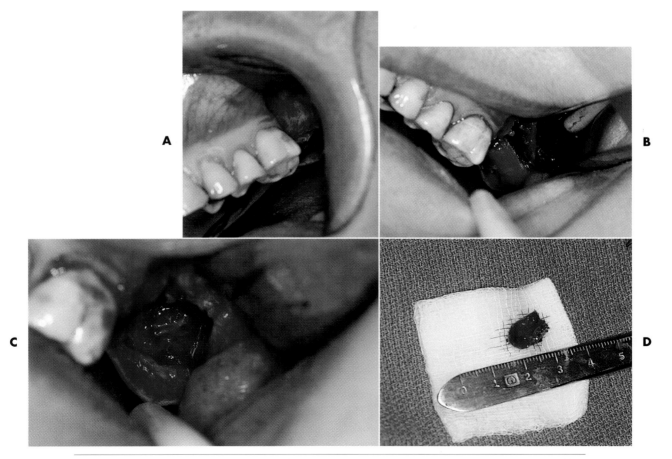

Fig. 8-82 **A,** Expose the bony tuberosity by crestal incision extending distally to the pterygomandibular raphe followed by mucoperiosteal reflection. **B,** Remove the portion of the tuberosity designed to serve as a donor using a spatula osteotome. **C,** Smooth the residual bone, and eliminate sharp corners. **D,** A generous quantity of viable marrow is made available from the tuberosity area.

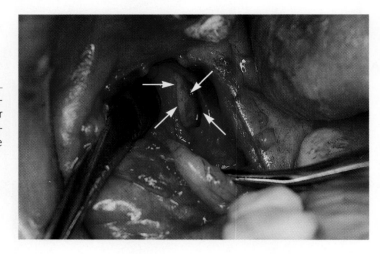

Fig. 8-83 The anterior border of the mandibular ramus is readily exposed with small risk of injuring vital structures. After the anterior border *(arrows)* has been made available, use small burs, rongeur forceps, osteotomes, and a mallet to remove a significant amount of bone. Little medullary material is included in the ramus.

with saline. Deepen the groove until a properly directed tap with a spatula osteotome produces a predictable fracture and the entire half circle of bone from lateral to medial cortices is retrieved in a single piece. Be constantly aware of the presence of the mandibular canal. The harvesting may have to be completed by using a mallet, curved osteotomes, and rongeur forceps. Finally, file smooth the donor site and suture the tissues with a 4-0 Vicryl continuous horizontal mattress closure. Grind the harvested bone into fine particles with the rongeur forceps, mixed with an expander such as TCP or DFDB in accordance with the instructions presented in previous paragraphs, and store it in sterile saline or the patient's marrow-derived blood.

Lateral Border of the Mandibular Ramus/Body

A unique disposable osteotome/collector called the *Maxillon MX-grafter* enables the surgeon to remove thin strips of lateral cortex by a planing action.

Make the exposure of the posterior lateral mandible by crestal incision, on the side at which the host site is located. After adequately denuding the external oblique ridge and the area beneath it, apply the blade and strip the bone surface in narrow lengths. Sufficient quantities can be harvested to fill tooth pockets, repair periimplant defects and serve, with allografts, as an osteogenic nidus when larger volumes are required. As the shavings are removed, compact them with blood in a posterior storage chamber of the MX-grafter handle. The instrument also serves as a direct delivery device (Fig. 8-84).

Mandibular Symphysis

MANUAL RETRIEVAL
In most cases the mandibular symphysis offers a rich source of bone marrow. Evaluate the site on a basis of the presence, location, and length of the incisors and canines, the total mass of the symphysis, and the positions of the mental foramina and canals.

If the boundaries appear to be acceptable, the harvest may take place using regional and field block anesthesia.

Augment bilateral mandibular blocks with mental and deep vestibular infiltrations, and with the assistant drawing the lower lip outwardly with thumbs and forefingers, make an incision from canine to canine through mucosa in the areolar gingiva (Fig. 8-85, *A*). Make a second, deeper incision through mentalis muscle, and, finally, using a new blade, incise the periosteum at the incisor apical level for the full length of the incision (Fig. 8-85, *B*).

Periosteal elevation is achieved from mental foramen to mental foramen and from above the apical areas of the teeth to the curvature of the inferior border (Fig. 8-85, *C*). Place Henahan, McBurney, or other retractors, electrocoagulate bleeders, and use a half round bur in the Impactair to outline the donor sites with separate dots about 4 mm apart (Fig. 8-85, *D, E*). The bur holes should pass through cortex and into medullary bone. If a maximum quantity of bone is required, the superior horizontal outline should be below the dental apices, its apposing one just above the inferior border cortex, the posterior vertical dotted lines, 6 mm anterior to the mental foramina and the anterior ones, 4 mm lateral to the midline. This leaves an 8-mm central zone that is to remain untouched. The purpose of preserving the midmandibular spine is to protect the sanctity and esthetic appearance of the chin, the mentolabial fold, and the function of the vestibule and mentalis muscle. The overlying cortex is of little value, but its underlying marrow can be harvested.

When the outline of the donor area appears to be satisfactory, connect the dots transcortically with a No. 700 L surgical bur (Fig. 8-85, *F*). Complete the osteotomies using a mallet and spatula osteotome, which can be used as a lever to elevate the cortical plates (Fig. 8-85, *G*).

On their removal, set aside the specimens in saline so that they can later be denuded of any clinging marrow and, if needed, particulated for purposes of graft quantity expansion.

Use sharp surgical curettes and small marrow gouges to harvest the exposed, highly vascular medullary bone (Fig. 8-85, *H*). Aspirate the accompanying blood by syringe and place it with the stored bone. As it clots, it makes a reliable and biocompatible transfer medium and osteogenic matrix.

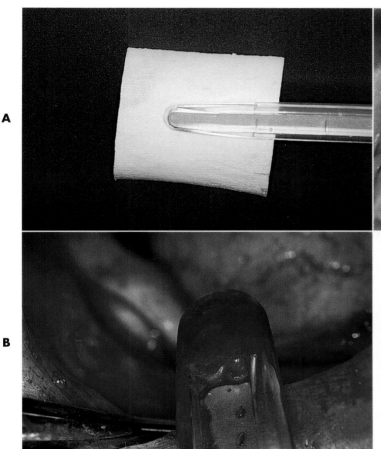

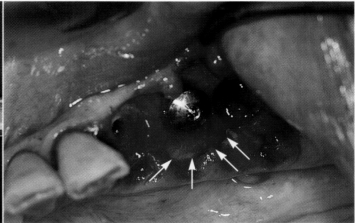

Fig. 8-84 **A,** The disposable Maxillon osteotome shaves bone with an acutely sharp steel blade. **B,** Thin strips of bone come away from even the densest mandibular cortices. **C,** The quantity of bone recovered is sufficient to fill an implanted extraction site with ease *(arrows)*.

Be careful to protect the anteriorly looping mental bundles, the mandibular inferior border, its lingual cortex, and the dental apices.

When you have obtained all of the available medullary bone, control bleeders, and tamp dense, 20 mesh HA particles firmly into the oblong defects (Fig. 8-85, *I*). Then cover them with a resorbable membrane (Fig. 8-85, *J*) and close them in two layers: periosteum and muscle first, with interrupted 4-0 Polysorb or Biosyn (Fig. 8-85, *K*), and the mucosa with the same material in a continuous, horizontal mattress configuration (Fig. 8-85, *L*). Keep the harvested cortex (which should be particulated), spongiosa, and blood in a covered, glass container. Transient postoperative paresthesia of the lips and chin may be experienced.

A firm pressure dressing across the chin assuages postoperative edema and pain, and presages a well-healed and functional vestibule (Fig. 8-85, *M*). When a smaller monocortical graft lined with medullary bone is required, retrieve it from the symphysis using the technique outlined in the previous section (Fig. 8-86). If a specifically sized specimen is required for a monocortical graft, a smaller block of bone can be harvested. Using a sterilized sheet of periapical x-ray lead foil as a template, and transferring it from the deficient site to the donor will permit this. The bur dots are used to outline the template (Fig. 8-86, *A-D*).

Mandibular Symphysis: Trephine Retrieval

As an alternative to shaping and developing square or oblong osteotomies, which is performed by hand with a high-speed handpiece, burs, osteotomes, and mallets, a far more rapid technique can be employed by the use of surgical trephines driven by latch-type contra-angles or straight handpieces. They are available from Ace Surgical in 10-, 8-, 6-mm, and smaller diameters. They cut efficiently and remove plugs of cortical marrow bone quickly and cleanly (Fig. 8-87, *A-C*). Each has depth markings on its side to avoid injuring the lingual cortex.

These bony specimens do not yield quite as much graft material as the oblong segments because the osteotomies are smaller. Greater quantities can be harvested if multiple round cuts overlapping one another are made. Following the use of the trephine, use gouges and curettes to retrieve additional marrow from beneath the cortical margins. Exercise care not to cut through the lingual plate of bone. Since the surgeon's fingers will have developed high levels of tactile sense, brief experience with the trephines is instructive in regard to this important point. After removal of the donor plugs and marrow, fill the sites with HA covered with Vicryl mesh and make a closure in two layers (Fig. 8-87, *D*).

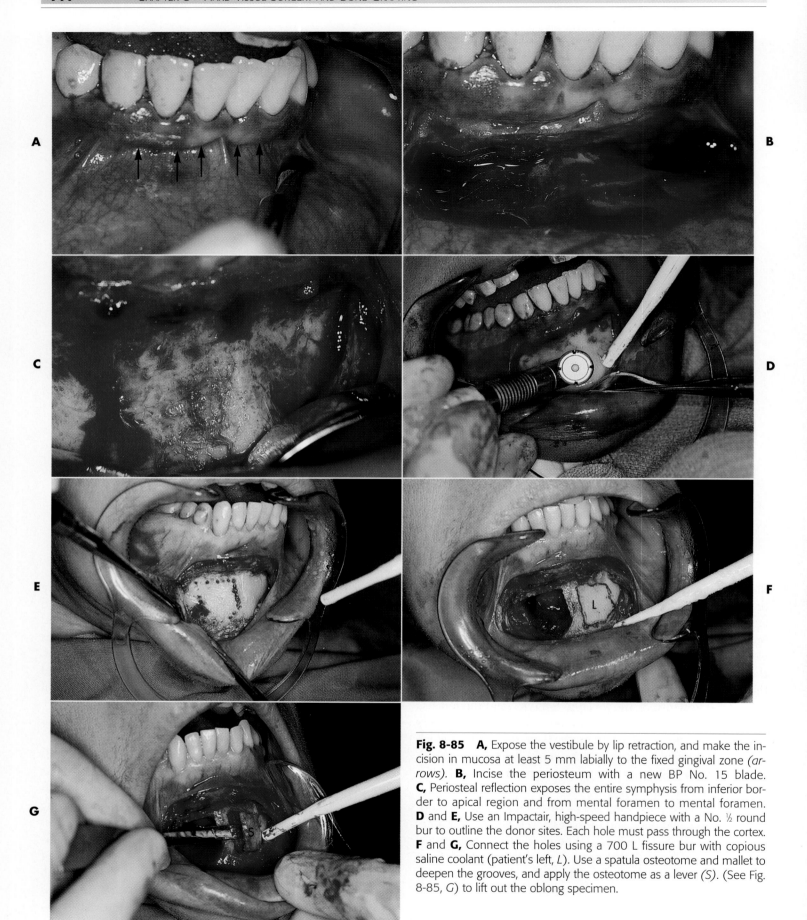

Fig. 8-85   A, Expose the vestibule by lip retraction, and make the incision in mucosa at least 5 mm labially to the fixed gingival zone *(arrows)*. **B,** Incise the periosteum with a new BP No. 15 blade. **C,** Periosteal reflection exposes the entire symphysis from inferior border to apical region and from mental foramen to mental foramen. **D** and **E,** Use an Impactair, high-speed handpiece with a No. ½ round bur to outline the donor sites. Each hole must pass through the cortex. **F** and **G,** Connect the holes using a 700 L fissure bur with copious saline coolant (patient's left, *L*). Use a spatula osteotome and mallet to deepen the grooves, and apply the osteotome as a lever *(S)*. (See Fig. 8-85, *G*) to lift out the oblong specimen.

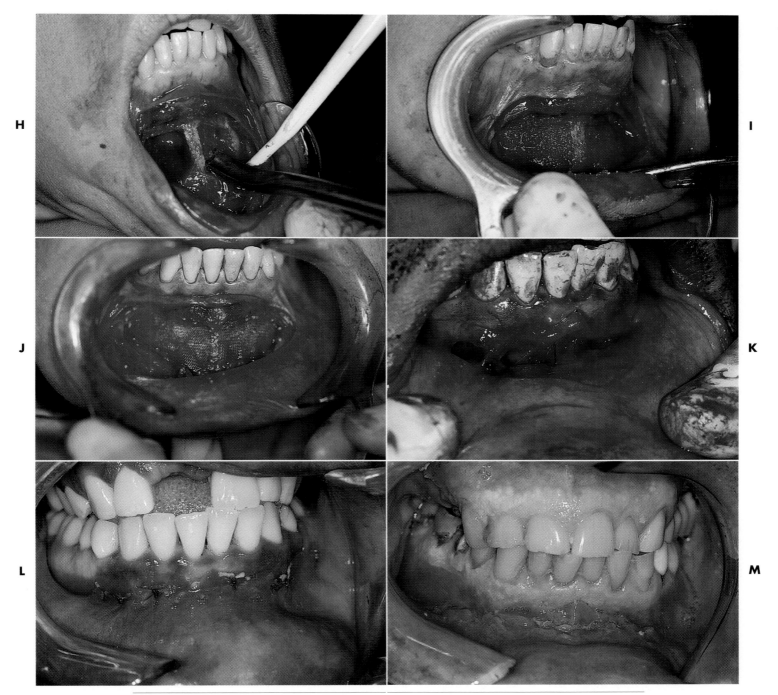

Fig. 8-85, cont'd   H, Use a narrow gouge (or a curette or both) to scoop the osteogenic spongiosa from the donor site. After the block has been removed, retrieve the marrow from beneath its former site, exercising great care not to damage dental apices or mental nerves. **I,** After completion of the harvesting procedure, tamp particulate HA into the defects. **J,** The HA particles are covered by a Vicryl mesh resorbable membrane, which remains stable as a result of the accrued fibrin. **K,** Make a deep closure of periosteum and mentalis fibers with 4-0 polyglactic acid sutures. **L,** Suture the mucosa in a horizontal mattress configuration. **M,** Healing, 6 weeks postoperatively, demonstrates good tissue tone and a compliant, unencumbered vestibule and lip.

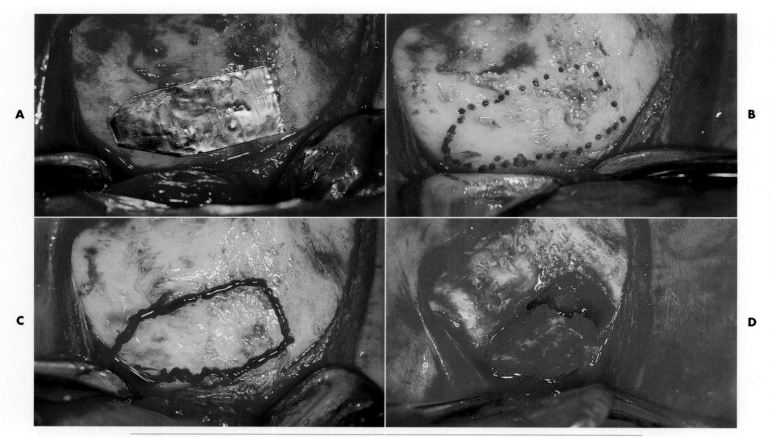

Fig. 8-86   A, Trim a sterilized, lead-sheet template (from an x-ray film) over the defect and place it in the parasymphyseal donor area. **B,** Transfer the outline to the bone with a No. ½ round, high-speed bur passed transcortically. **C,** Connect the holes into well-defined intramedullary grooves with a 700 L fissure bur. **D,** The graft can be removed easily after deepening the grooves with a spatula osteotome and then using it for leverage. Store the graft in the patient's marrow-derived blood until it can be attached with lag screws to the host.

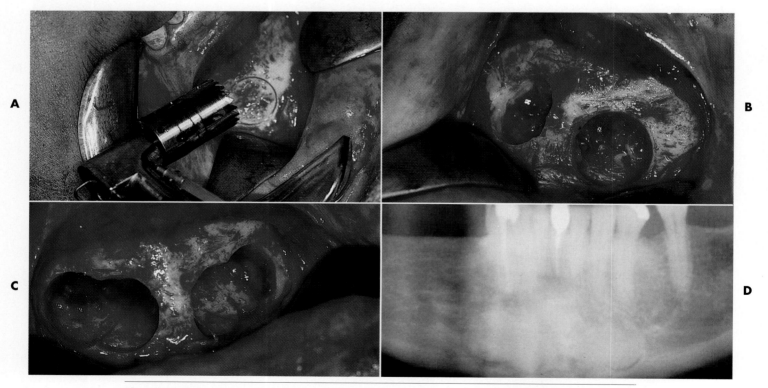

Fig. 8-87   A and **B,** Use the largest available trephrine (10-mm diameter) to make two transcortical, intramedullary osteotomies. These osteotomies do not need further refinement with burs or osteotomes. Note the depth markers on the surface of the trephine. **C,** Additional bone can be retrieved by superimposing additional circular cuts. Removal of the donor specimens is predictable; they snap out cleanly when leverage is applied. They can be employed as monocortical block grafts or may be particulated for use in antral floors or at other sites. Each round segment yields approximately 2.5 cc of particulated bone. **D,** A postoperative Panorex shows the outlines of the grafts, now filled with HA.

Grafting to Improve Ridge Dimension for the Accommodation of Implants

Anterior Mandibular Width Deficiencies

Alveoplasty

Alveoloplasty is a technique with which all surgical practitioners should become competent. Knife-edged ridges may require planing, and undercut reduction, or removal of sharp, spinous processes before making implant osteotomies. Make the incisions at the ridge crest and perform reflection of soft tissues with care to preserve the integrity of the mucoperiosteal flaps. With rosette and fissure burs (always saline cooled), rongeurs, and bone files, perform the reduction, contouring, and smoothing of the bone with precision (Fig. 8-88). By correcting the spinous or knife-edge ridge, create a plateau at the crest, which will offer a broad enough surface to permit accommodation of the planned root form implants. Of course, this alveoloplastic procedure sacrifices height, and a reassessment of available vertical dimensions must be made up on its completion. Running a piece of gauze over the bone can test results. The gauze should pass easily over the ridge without shredding or pulling of any of its threads. When the altered alveolus passes this test, place implants and make a closure with either a box-lock or continuous horizontal mattress suture. (Refer to Chapter 9 for a complete set of illustrations).

Monocortical Block Grafting

Affixing a block of bone (Fig. 8-89, *A, B*), can augment the width and height of the anterior mandibular ridge. This block may be obtained from a bank or, preferably, from an autogenous source. Since some cortex is required as well as an underlying marrow bed, the mandibular symphysis is an ideal site for harvesting the requisite specimen. Outline it by using a sterilized periapical film lead sheet as a template (Fig. 8-89, *C-E*). Instead of mincing the retrieved bone, preserve it in its solid retrieved condition, and after the alveolus is exposed and smoothed, tailor the block to satisfy the needs of the deformity (Fig. 8-89, *F*). It must be wide enough to serve as a labial

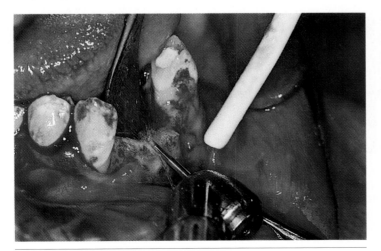

Fig. 8-88 The Impactair is used effectively with a fissure bur to broaden a ridge before implantation.

mantle from the crest to its tapered inferior level that is found to be of a sufficient width.

If the defect is so significant that it makes a graft from the symphysis inadequate, some practitioners use a rib. Ribs do have curvatures that are suitable for anterior mandibular use, and, when split longitudinally, their interior surfaces contain marrow. Gentle handling permits more acute curvature, but if they fail to yield to finger pressure, bur cuts made on the lesser curvature at right angles to the rib facilitate their compliance.

Whichever choice you make, prepare the outer surface of the host and the inner surface of the graft so that maximal contact is created. However, cortex-to-cortex and cortex-to-marrow contact are both acceptable relationships.

When this itimacy is achieved, either for a small defect or for an arch segment, fixation may be performed by lag screw placement at strategic sites.

Hold the graft in position with a Babcock clamp or have it held manually by the assistant, and use an Atwood 347, tapered diamond drill with saline coolant to drill through it and well into the host alveolus.

The titanium screw selected can be taken from any micro- or mini-fixation kit (Synthes, Osteomed, Leibinger, and others). Enlarge the hole in the overlying graft with the Atwood drill so that the screw threads do not bite, but it should not be so large that the head is not be able to lock the graft to the host site.

For small blocks, one central screw is satisfactory. For longer ones, two or three are required. After screw fixation (Fig. 8-89, *G*), fill the donor site with HA and cover it with a resorbable GTRM.

Closure of the host site is not achieved readily. Be prepared to undermine the labial mucosa in order to complete a tension-free pedicle suture line (Fig. 8-89, *H, I*). The results are usually of benefit to ridge improvement suitable for the placement of implants 6 months later (Fig. 8-89, *J*).

Anterior Mandibular Height Deficiencies

Monocortical Grafts

The technique for adding height is the same as that used for adding width to the ridge. Preparation of the graft is different, however. In conditions requiring additional vertical dimension, the block must be hollowed and made saddlelike to fit over the ridge. It is vital that residual marrow be left on the internal surface. The lag screw fixation is best performed on the labial flange of the graft at appropriate inferior locations. Taper both the labial and lingual aprons so that they merge gently against the residual ridge.

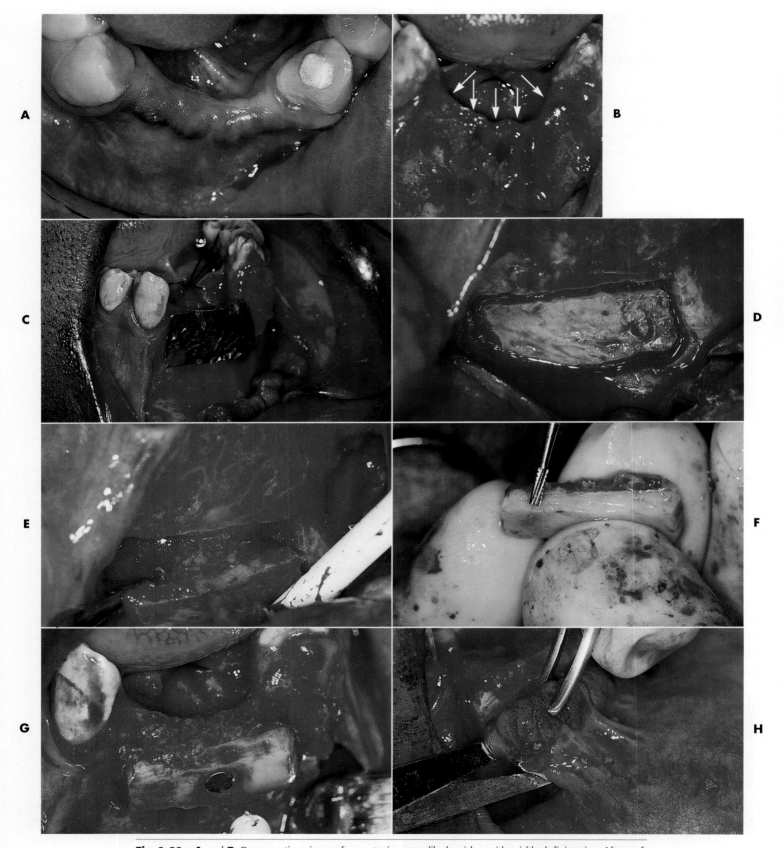

Fig. 8-89   A and **B,** Preoperative views of an anterior mandibular ridge with width deficiencies. After soft tissue reflection, a knife-edged bony ridge is noted *(arrows)*. **C,** Make the template from the lead foil found in the x-ray packet. Sterilize it by autoclaving. **D,** Use the template to outline the required mono-cortical block from the symphysis. This is completed by reflecting the tissues via the original crestal incision. **E,** Remove the donor block with a generous marrow lining by using a thin osteotome as a lever. **F,** Use rongeur forceps and cooled burs to tailor the block to the intended host site for purposes of accuracy of adaptation. **G,** After an intimate relationship is verified, complete fixation of the graft with a single lag screw. Techniques for lag screw placement are found in Fig. 8-79. **H** and **I,** Final closure will not be possible without the completion of aggressive undermining to supply a generous and tension-free pedicle flap. **J,** Six months postoperatively, a wide ridge is available for implant placement.

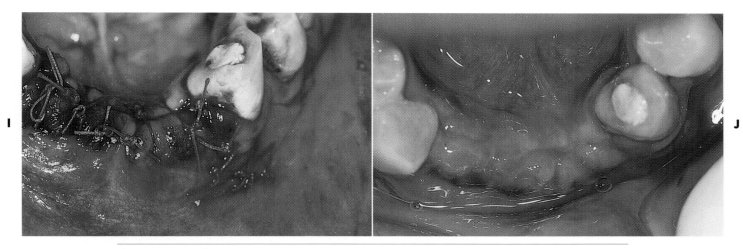

Fig. 8-89, cont'd
For legend, see opposite page.

Inferior Border Augmentation

If a patient has an extremely atrophied mandible (i.e., 1 to 6 mm thick), despite the fact that the only viable approach to its rehabilitation is the subperiosteal implant, problems may be created even with this modality, which are caused by settling. This may result in total resorption of the residual mandible with subsequent submental skin fistulization and even exposure of a peripheral strut through the skin (Fig. 8-90). A variety of techniques may be employed that can increase mandibular size before implant placement. One approach is alveolar ridge augmentation with biologic or synthetic materials.

Another therapeutic solution is the alteration of a CAD-CAM–generated model by adding up to 1 cm to its alveolar height by using wax. The model so created is reproduced in Velmix stone. The implant is designed to rest only minimally on this new area, with the peripheral struts gaining the greatest support by being extended to unaltered original cortical areas (i.e., inferior border, symphysis, genial tubercles, and rami). When the implant so produced is seated, there is a large void representing those areas that had been built up in wax. Before closing, but after seating and assessing the stability of the infrastructure, fill the voids and all struts with a synthetic mesh particulate graft material mixed with DFDB.

A third method is to increase mandibular height by augmenting its inferior border (Fig. 8-91). Patients with redundant neck tissues, collapsed lower facies, or protruding or pouting lips will not witness improvement of any of these problems while undergoing intraoral surgery, changes in ridge structure or morphology, or changes in vertical dimension. When, after inferior border augmentation has been completed, root forms or a subperiosteal mandibular implant is planned, place them into or atop the original, cortical bone. This offers the advantage of discouraging less subimplant and periimplant resorption than would be expected were the implants to be placed on or into newly grafted bone.

FIRST-STAGE PROCEDURE   In the operating room, harvest marrow from the anterior iliac crest as described earlier in this

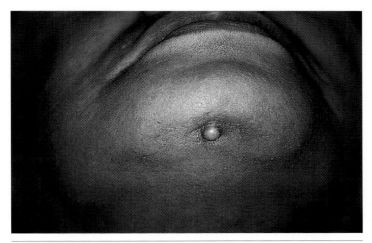

Fig. 8-90   Submandibular fistulas are seen when mandibular subperiosteal implants settle as a result of resorption.

chapter. Store it in a saline-moistened, covered glass container (Fig. 8-92, A).

Hyperextend the patient's head, place some sheets under the shoulders, and prepare and drape the face and neck. Make a curved incision 3 cm medial to the inferior border of the mandible through skin (Fig. 8-92, B). Change the blade, clamp and tie bleeders, and continue the dissection through fascia and platysma. The procedure is designed to be sufficiently medial so that injury to the rami marginalis mandibulae is unlikely. The digastric muscles appear, and they should be detached from the inferior border to expose the investing periosteal envelope.

Use a new No. 15 blade to incise the periosteum directly at the mandibular inferior border, and expose the lateral surfaces up to the mental foramina anteriorly and even higher in the rami regions. On the medial (lingual) surfaces, about 4 mm of exposure is required to accommodate the flange of a titanium mortise mesh, which demands that the aponeurosis must be elevated to that extent (Fig. 8-93). With the assistant exposing one side of the mandible only using Army/Navy retractors, insert the first end of the mortise mesh in place. Then, retract the contralateral flaps so that the other end of the mesh can be slipped into position. Note the length of the mesh at each end

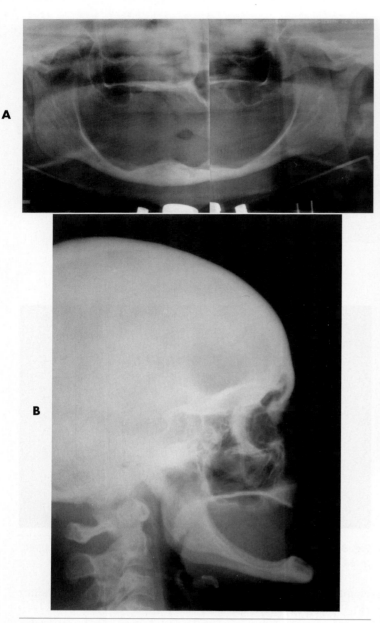

Fig. 8-91 **A,** Panorex of a severely atrophied mandible. In such instances, even a subperiosteal implant may not be indicated without augmentation. **B,** The cephalometric view offers another dimension of extreme atrophy.

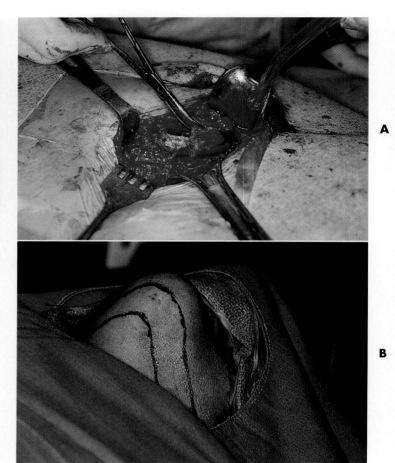

Fig. 8-92 **A,** Autogenous bone for mandibular augmentation is harvested marrow from the anterior iliac crest. **B,** Inferior border augmentation, performed in the operating room, shows a skin scribe locating the mandible and a second one indicating the location of the incision.

by palpation and inspection. Its adaptation to the inferior border and the angles is of principal importance, which mandates that it be cut and trimmed, as required, for purposes of precise accommodation. Small slits may be made so that the contouring pliers are able to create optimal conformity. Smooth all peripheral margins, and rehearse the seating of the prosthesis several times until it is carried out with predictable ease. Line the mesh with a precut, sterilized, 4-μm Millipore filter, and tamp it gently with moist cotton balls to keep it well adapted. Fill it with the harvested marrow, or marrow and particulated cortex if needed, and place it over the inferior border following the exact rehearsal protocol (Fig. 8-94). The upper layer of fenestrations of the mesh must remain uncovered by the bone graft material to allow it to overlap the mandible for screw fix-

ation. Pay careful attention to the posterior ends of the mesh. Contour them so that a clear and well-delineated angle is presented at each end.

Have the assistant surgeon maintain the loaded mesh in place with upward pressure while a single hole is tapped through a mesh fenestration into the mandible at a site near the inferior cortex designed to avoid nerve injury. Use the Atwood 473 diamond point in the Hall drill for preliminary tapping, and then employ a titanium screw (Synthes or Osteomed) with a titanium-tipped screwdriver. Three to five additional screws, strategically placed, hold the bone-filled mesh firmly and securely in place against the mandible (Fig. 8-95).

Irrigate and close the wound anatomically in layers. Suture detached digastric, mylohyoid, masseter and medial pterygoid fibers with 4-0 Polysorb or Vicryl on a tapered needle to fenestrations in the mesh, thereby anatomically reattaching them. Close skin with 5-0 or 6-0 nylon. Excise redundant skin, if any, which creates a cervical rhytidectomy, but avoid suturing under tension. Complete the operation with a skin dressing with Telfa, fluff, and 4-inch Elastoplast (Fig. 8-96).

SECOND-STAGE PROCEDURE Allow 6 months for maturation of the inferior border graft, and at that time return the patient

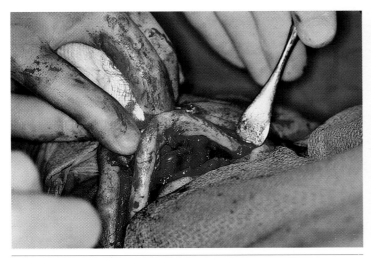

Fig. 8-93 After dissection and reflection, the inferior border of the mandible is exposed fully.

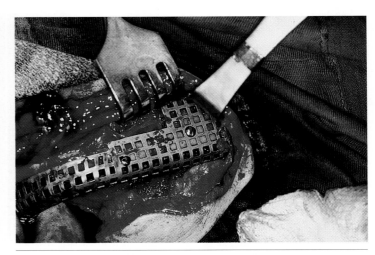

Fig. 8-95 Affix the mesh prosthesis filled with graft material to the mandible with self-tapping screws.

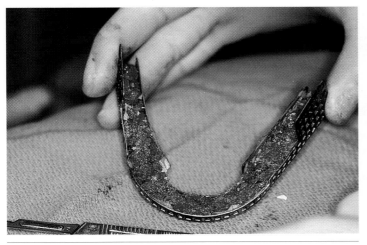

Fig. 8-94 An Osteomed titanium inferior border mortise-form mesh is lined with Millipore filter and filled with iliac crest marrow seen being harvested in Fig. 8-92, *A*.

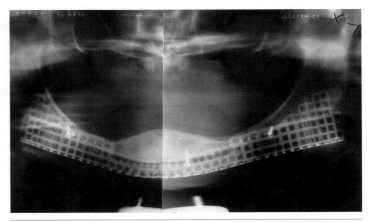

Fig. 8-96 The graft material consolidates after 3 months and becomes bonded to the inferior border, thereby augmenting it. This acts as a safeguard to implant settling.

to the operating room and remove the metal mesh. To do this, retrace or excise the old incision. After exposure of the mesh, back out the screws, cut the mesh into three or four segments using the Atwood diamond, and remove each segment separately (Fig. 8-97). Make the closure in the same manner as was done previously.

The graft material will have become smoothly incorporated onto the mandible, and both mandibular and lower facial dimensions will have increased attractively (Fig. 8-98).

Eight weeks later, a CAD-CAM or classically constructed subperiosteal implant or root forms, as desired, may be placed in accordance with descriptions found in appropriate sections of this atlas.

If patient or surgeon is reluctant to remove the mesh, which prohibits the use of a CT scan for CAD-CAM fabrication, a two-stage subperiosteal implant by direct bone impression may be fabricated and placed 6 months after the inferior border augmentation has been completed (Fig. 8-99).

As an alternative, parasymphyseal root forms may be placed into the newly grafted mandible.

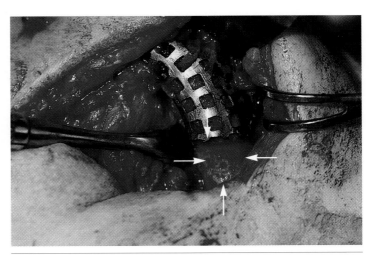

Fig. 8-97 Removal of the titanium reveals the presence of new, cortically enhanced bone within its contours *(arrows)*.

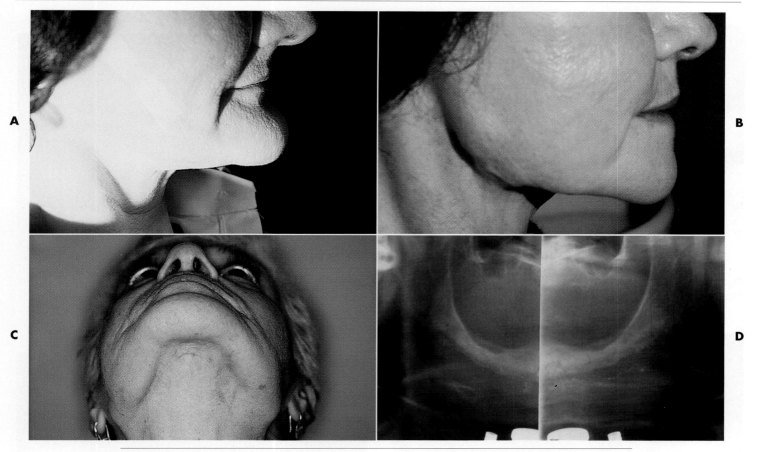

Fig. 8-98   A, Preoperative lateral view of a woman in need of mandibular augmentation. **B,** Postoperative view after augmentation. Note the increase in height of the lower face, improvement in appearance of the skin of the neck and improved mandibular posture. **C,** If the incision is placed strategically, the postoperative results will be esthetically pleasing. **D,** Panorex of mandible after removal of titanium mesh shows mineralization and consolidation of the inferior border graft.

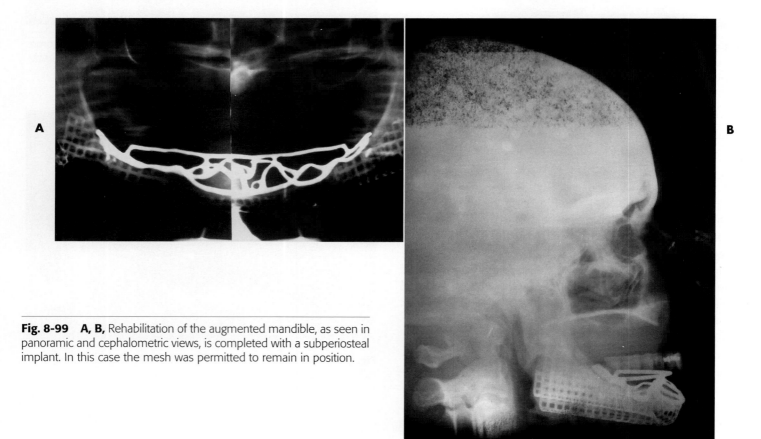

Fig. 8-99   A, B, Rehabilitation of the augmented mandible, as seen in panoramic and cephalometric views, is completed with a subperiosteal implant. In this case the mesh was permitted to remain in position.

Posterior Mandibular Width Deficiencies

Alveoloplasty

Alveoloplasty in cases of knife-edge ridges, as described earlier for the anterior mandible, may serve the required needs to prepare the posterior ridges for implant placement. However, in so doing, height will be lost, which may force the surgeon to seek a solution by grafting.

Monocortical Block Grafting

Symphyseal monocortical block onlays may be used as well in the region posterior to the mental foramina. They may be added to the buccal, lingual, or both surfaces in the form of sandwiches (Fig. 8-100). There must be sufficient alveolar bone above the mandibular canal to permit fixation screw entry without threat to the neurovascular bundle.

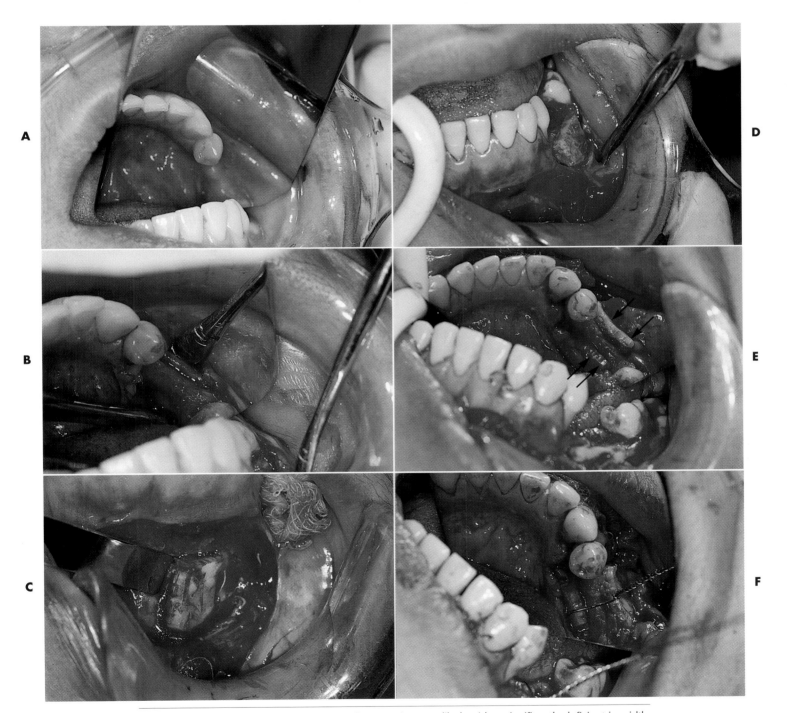

Fig. 8-100   A and **B,** Preoperative views of a posterior mandibular ridge, significantly deficient in width. **C,** Place lead foil templates for both buccal and lingual ridge surface deficiencies over the exposed parasymphyseal cortices in the classical manner, and harvest right and left monocortical blocks. **D** and **E,** Lateral and occlusal clinical views reveal the apposition of the two tailored blocks, one on the lingual surface and the other on the buccal surface of the narrow ridge *(arrows)*. **F,** Fixation of the two blocks is made by a single circummandibular steel wire ligature, the instructions for which are found in Fig. 6-13, *A-F.*

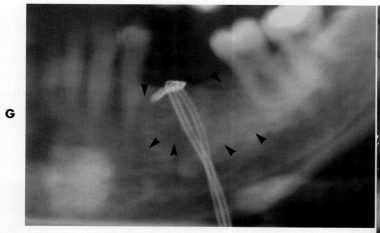

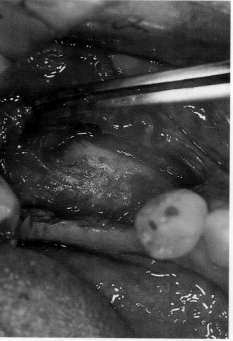

Fig. 8-100, cont'd   G, Radiograph shows circummandibular ligature stabilizing sandwich grafts *(arrows)*. **H,** Six months after grafting, the area has been re-exposed and the ligature removed. The dramatically widened ridge presents an excellent site for implantation.

Posterior Mandibular Height Deficiencies

Monocortical Block Grafting

Block grafting may be used for correction of atrophy as described for the anterior mandible. If this can be completed, significant or total loss of the vestibules is a predictable sequelum. Secondary vestibuloplasty, as described in Chapter 7, is required, either with the use of free palatal grafts, buccal split-thickness pedicles, or an alloplast (AlloDerm).

Mandibular Neuroplasty and Nerve Management

If it becomes important to find additional vertical height by placing an implant below the level of the mandibular canal, remove the neurovascular bundle from within its confines (Fig. 8-101, *A, B*). Make an incision at the crest of the ridge from the retromolar pad anteriorly to the most distal tooth in position, continue it in the crevicular gingivae to the canine, and then curve it forward toward the inferior border.

Use a sponge to elevate the mucoperiosteum to the level of the mental foramen. The emerging neurovascular bundle will be seen (Fig. 8-101, *C*). Protect it with a periosteal elevator or other small retractor. Then, using a No. 8 round bur in a high-speed Impactair handpiece, starting at a point 1 cm distal to the foramen, brush the bone away from the mandibular cortex overlying the canal with gentle light strokes. Continue the procedure posteriorly to a point at least 3 cm past the most distally planned implant site until an oblong osteotomy is outlined. Remove this cortical block using a spatula osteotome as a lever (Fig. 8-101, *D*). With careful effort and exquisite technique using sharp spoon excavators or a slowly turning round bur in

a straight handpiece, the neurovascular bundle lying within the canal becomes exposed. A Kerrison forceps enlarges the osteotomy, until the full diameter of the canal is accessible. Then with a blunt nerve hook, lift the bundle from its canal. Line the internal environment of the canal with ossicles that cling tenaciously to the bundle. Gentle teasing releases it. Retraction of the thin, fragile structure is best done using a length of ¼-inch Penrose drain, which is passed readily using a baby right-angle hemostatic forceps (Fig. 8-101, *E, F*). A "nerveless" mandible has been created, which now is available for more aggressive implantation. The implants, after the neuroplasty, may be placed the full distance to the inferior border (Fig. 8-101, *G, H*). Lay the displaced neurovascular bundle gently into position over a tailored length of Colla Cote shield that is interposed between it and the implants (Fig. 8-101, *I*). Use a second Colla Cote strip to cover the bundle, place a synthetic graft to the level of lateral cortex, and suture the flaps for an anatomic closure (Fig. 8-101, *J*).

As an alternative procedure, although more invasive and complicated, the mental and mandibular bundles may be mobilized as a single unit by eliminating the entire distal half of the foramen. This may present significant difficulties because of the complex and labyrinthine course taken by the mental branch. It does offer, however, far greater flexibility in regard to retraction of the neurovascular bundle.

Use a sponge to evaluate the mucoperiosteum to the level of the mental foramen. The emerging neurovascular bundle will be seen (Fig. 8-101, *K*). Protect it with a periosteal elevator or other small retractor, and using a No. 8 round bur in a high-speed Impactair handpiece, brush the bone away from the foramen's distal periphery with gentle light strokes, directly through the lateral mandibular cortex. Continue the procedure posteriorly to a point at least 2 cm past the most

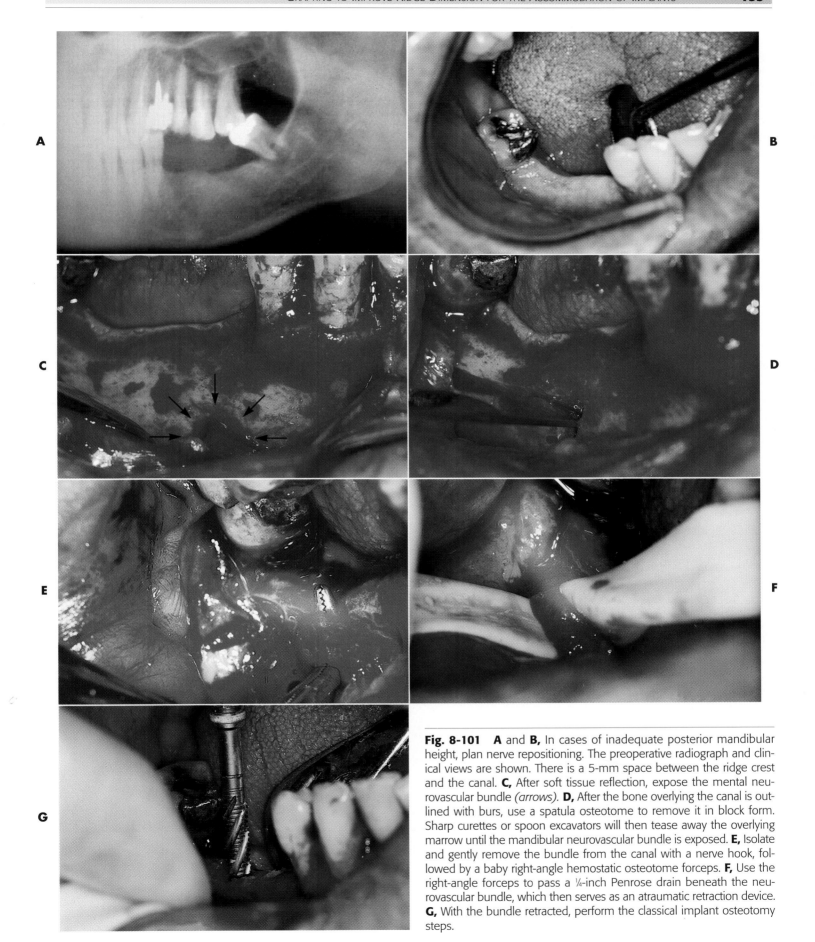

Fig. 8-101 **A** and **B,** In cases of inadequate posterior mandibular height, plan nerve repositioning. The preoperative radiograph and clinical views are shown. There is a 5-mm space between the ridge crest and the canal. **C,** After soft tissue reflection, expose the mental neurovascular bundle *(arrows)*. **D,** After the bone overlying the canal is outlined with burs, use a spatula osteotome to remove it in block form. Sharp curettes or spoon excavators will then tease away the overlying marrow until the mandibular neurovascular bundle is exposed. **E,** Isolate and gently remove the bundle from the canal with a nerve hook, followed by a baby right-angle hemostatic osteotome forceps. **F,** Use the right-angle forceps to pass a ¼-inch Penrose drain beneath the neurovascular bundle, which then serves as an atraumatic retraction device. **G,** With the bundle retracted, perform the classical implant osteotomy steps.

distally planned implant site (Fig. 8-101, *L*). With careful and patient effort, the neurovascular bundle lying within the canal becomes completely visible. Enlarge the osteotomy until the full diameter of the canal is accessible. Change the bur to a No. 6 round diamond, and, protecting the mental bundle, brush away the distal or posterior half of the foramen to an eggshell thickness. Remove the remainder with sharp spoon excavators. Now lift the combined mandibulomental bundle from its crypt using a nerve hook (Fig. 8-101, *M*).

For surgical procedures of the palate, never cut the greater palatine bundles when elevating a flap. The integrity of these nerves and particularly, the arteries must be maintained or the flap will fail. The incisive bundle, however, may be sacrificed with small risk.

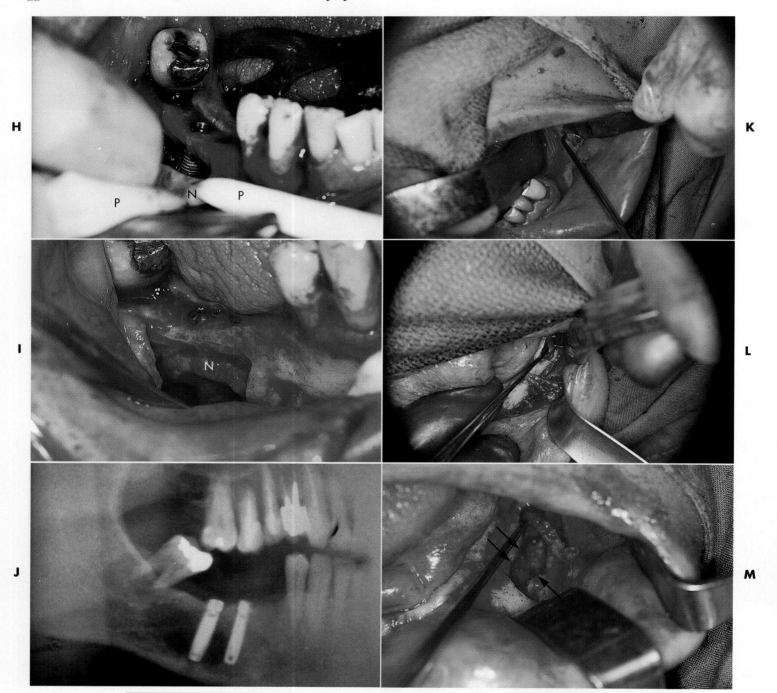

Fig. 8-101, cont'd   H, These Steri-Oss implants have been placed almost to the inferior border of the mandible, with the neurovascular bundle *(N)* being retracted with the Penrose drain *(P)*. **I,** After placing the requisite Colla Cote to cushion the implant infrastructures, gently replace the neurovascular bundle, insulate it with a moistened collagen sheet and close the wound. **J,** The postoperative radiograph shows the extent to which an altered mandible may be used. **K,** As an alternative to removing the mandibular neurovascular bundle from the canal alone, which sometimes is physically restrictive, a mentomandibular bundle continuum may be mobilized. This is done by exposing the mental foramen and using this as a guide to locate and expose the contents of the canal. **L,** Use the round bur followed by the round diamond to extend the initial osteotomy anteriorly until the posterior osseous rim of the mental foramen is picked and curetted away. **M,** On the removal of the distal half of the foramen *(arrows)* and its canal, the contiguous defects so created permit the comfortable retraction of the mentomandibular bundle, permitting wider access to the potential implant host site.

Anterior Maxillary Width Deficiencies

Monocortical Block Grafting

In addition to monocortical block grafting, which is performed using the same technique as for the mandible, the relatively elastic anterior maxillary ridge permits a number of more versatile and diverse techniques for width augmentation (Fig. 8-102).

Expansion by Longitudinal Splitting

After making a crestal incision and reflecting the mucoperiosteum with care to avoid tearing it, flatten and refine the lower edge of the ridge with a side-cutting rongeur and bone files to present a plateau sufficiently wide to allow entry of first a No. ½-round and then a No. 699 XXL high-speed bur (Fig. 8-103, *A, B*). Make perforations using this bur to the full depth of its cutting surface (Fig. 8-103, *C*). If the bur holes are well aligned and oriented in a midcortical direction, connect them into a groove. Deepen this groove to the depth of the planned implants with great care to prevent perforations of the labial or palatal plates (Fig. 8-103, *D*). This is followed by the placement of a spatula osteotome into the osteotomy. Tap it with a mallet to the planned depths in a step-wise methodical pattern, until an evenly created, full-length groove has been placed in the entire operative area. Use the osteotome as a lever, gently expanding both labial and palatal walls (Fig. 8-103, *E*). Skill and sensitivity are essential qualities in carrying out these expansion maneuvers, or a cortical fracture will occur, which may mandate withdrawal from the operative field. If the two bone plates can be expanded to the width of the proposed implants (minimally 3.25 mm) and, even better, some medullary bone remains as an internal lining, the implants may be placed with confidence. Use of the Steri-Oss or similar osteotomes at each site, pushed and rotated directly upward with gentle finger pressure, offers additional assistance in achieving the requisite dimensions.

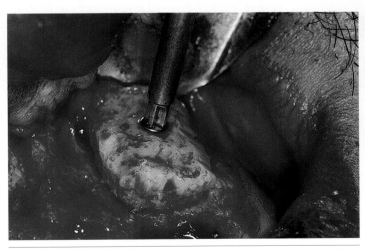

Fig. 8-102 Anterior maxillary width deficiencies can be improved using the same block grafting techniques described in previous sections (Fig. 8-89, *G*). This is an illustration of a chin-derived monocortical onlay block graft to the anterior maxilla, affixed with a single titanium lag screw.

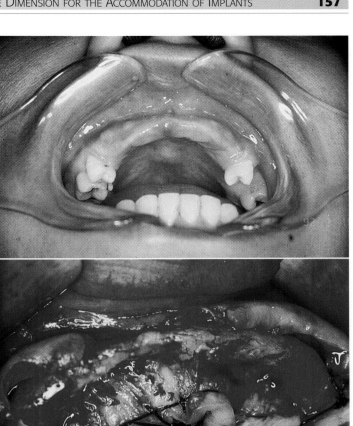
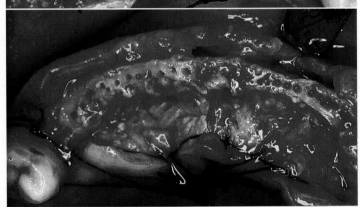
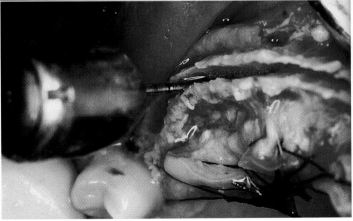

A

B

C

D

Fig. 8-103 **A,** The preoperative appearance of an extremely narrow anterior maxillary ridge is illustrated. The compliant nature of this bone permits dramatic expansion procedures. **B,** Expose the ridge after mucoperiosteal reflection. Retract the palatal tissues by bundling with a 3-0 silk suture. **C,** Place bur dots midcortically, tracing the outline of the ridge. **D,** These small perforations are connected with a 699L fissure bur into a continuous osteotomy.

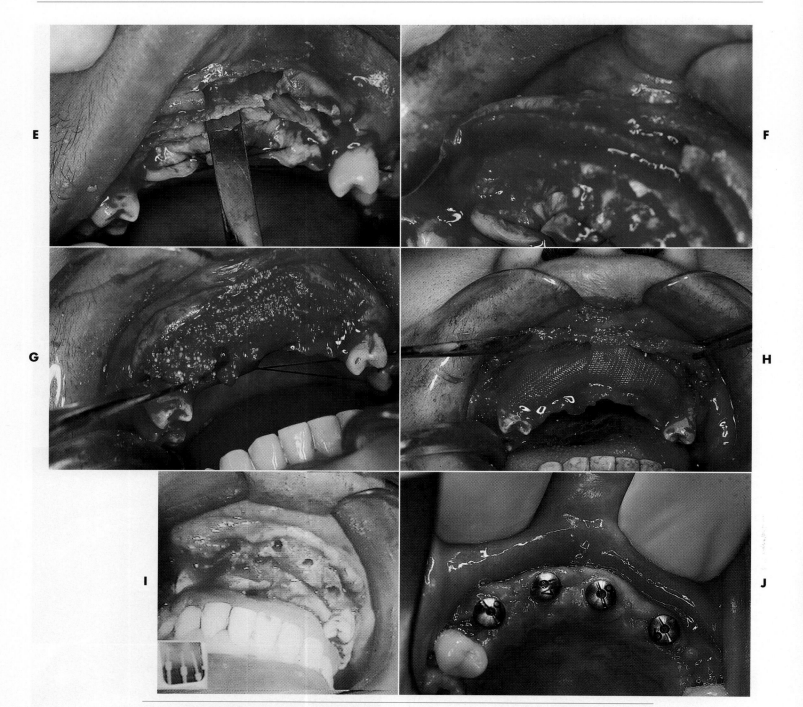

Fig. 8-103, cont'd   **E,** A spatula osteotomy tapped with a mallet, makes the osteotomy regular in depth and then is used as a lever to create microfracture expansion that must be made to occur beneath attached periosteum. **F,** The separated labial and palatal plates demonstrate a significant enhancement of ridge width. **G** and **H,** Firmly tamp particulate DFDB graft material, mixed with a patient's marrow-derived blood into the newly created osteotomy. Cover the area with Vicryl mesh, the margins of which have been tucked beneath the flaps. **I,** Six months later, upon reexposure of the grafted area, its expanded dimensions are clearly evident. The new width permits comfortable placement of implant osteotomies. **J,** An additional 6 months has elapsed, and these osseointegrated implants are now undergoing the restorative phases. Of note is the excellent level of gingival health and the presence of a functional, deep vestibule.

Since threaded implants have sharp flutes, microfractures of bone may occur as they self-tap their pathways to the planned apical levels. Therefore, in procedures of implant placement in altered ridges, press-fit implants such as the Calcitek (3.25 mm) or IMZ (3.3 mm) diameters will enter the osteotomies with fewer complications. In addition, these implants, as well as the Steri-Oss press-fit design, are supplied with smooth-sided metal try-in devices, which further prepare such operative sites in a predictable manner. When the implants reach their full depths, there will be voids between them represented by the bone groove. These defects must be filled with particulate graft material, preferably autogenous bone or DFDB.

If placement of implants is contraindicated after the expansion because of a lack of spongiosa or a fracture, then graft the osteotomy (with widened ridge) within the cortical plates and observe a maturation period of 6 months before implantation (Fig. 8-103, *F-J*).

Make a closure in either case with 4-0 Vicryl or Polysorb suture material used in a horizontal mattress configuration. Inadequate tissue coverage requires undermining and liberation of the labial mucosa from the underlying orbicularis oris muscle. A subsequent vestibuloplasty will have to be performed.

Osteotomes (Steri-Oss and Others)

Steri-Oss osteotomes are available in a set consisting of four diameters: 2, 2.7, 3.25, and 3.8 mm. The dramatic incremental change between 2 and 2.7 and 2.7 and 3.25 threaten the sanctity of the bone. In order to solve this problem, two additional osteotomes were custom machined (at 2.35 and 3 mm) in order to make the gradients more moderate (Fig. 8-104, *A*).

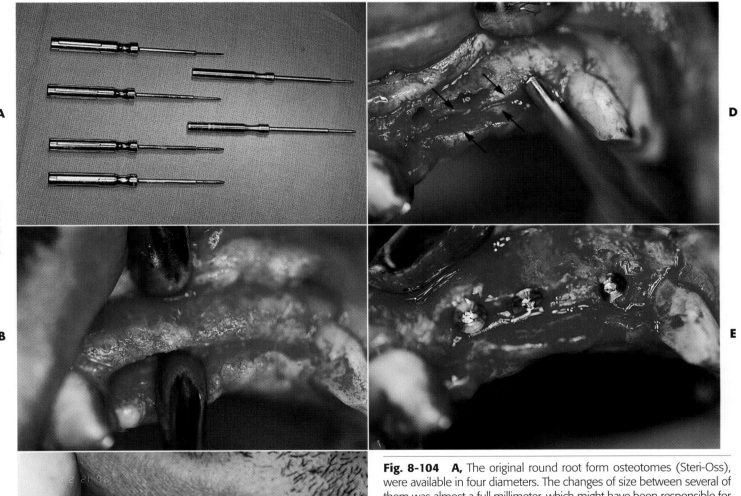

Fig. 8-104   A, The original round root form osteotomes (Steri-Oss), were available in four diameters. The changes of size between several of them was almost a full millimeter, which might have been responsible for cortical plate fractures. In order to ameliorate this morbid possibility, two additional custom-designed instruments of intermediate diameter were added to the set. **B** and **C,** After exposure of the deficient ridge demonstrates that its width will not permit implant surgery, drill the planned sites for implantation to diameters of 2 mm *(right),* which is the size of the smallest osteotome *(left).* Rock this osteotome in circular fashion to create slight additional enlargement. **D,** Increasingly larger osteotomes are hand or mallet-induced. When the ridge is inordinately thin and fracture is threatening, osteotome introduction is abetted by making a full-length, grooved osteotomy *(arrows),* which permits maximal bone elasticity. **E,** The expanded ridge readily permits the placement of root form implants.

If other systems are chosen, the differences in diameters should never exceed 0.4 mm.

The osteotomes, which have blunted and smooth leading tips, may be used in instances when the ridge is only slightly too narrow (i.e., 2.3 to 3.3 mm). In these cases, after the classical incision and reflection is made (Fig. 8-104, *B*), place No. 2 round bur holes at each projected implant site (following the generic technique described in Chapter 9), and enlarge and deepen each using a Brasseler 1.6 × 11 mm internally irrigated drill. After radiographic verification for position and length, enlarge each osteotomy to 2 mm. From this point on, use the osteotomes for graduated expansion (Fig. 8-104, *C*). Push each of the six in the set in an apical direction to the planned depths using firm hand pressure (rotating and forcing upward) or gentle mallet taps. When each osteotome has reached its full depth, gently rock its handle in circular fashion to create slight additional expansion, as well as facilitating smoother exit and entry of the next size. The exceptional compliance and elasticity of most anterior maxillae permit enlargement of the osteotomies to the final size before use of the try-in device for press-fit implants or the final sizing drill for threaded designs (Fig. 8-104, *D*). Total concentration must be devoted to visual and tactile observation of the labial and palatal plates in order to anticipate and avoid fracture. Use threaded implants as self-tapping devices (Fig. 8-104, *E*). After implant placement, make a closure without creating tension of the soft tissues. Undermining may be required.

Anterior Maxillary Height Deficiencies

Block Grafting

A block graft may be performed as described in previous paragraphs for width deficiencies. In the presence of ridges of inadequate height, block grafts make dramatic dimensional changes (Fig. 8-105, *A-C*). After being removed from the symphysis or another donor site selected by the surgeon, hollow the graft specimen so that it is accurately accommodated by the residual ridge and fits atop it, saddle-style. Depending on its width, a single lag screw can serve for fixation (Fig. 8-105, *D*). Combinations of height and width augmentation can be achieved in this fashion with the use of single contoured block grafts and added alloplastic particles (Fig. 8-105, *E*).

Nasal Floor Elevation

Height deficiencies are correctable by grafting superiorly in anterior maxillae. The pyriform apertures can be exposed by means of an intraoral approach. The floor of the nose, either unilaterally or bilaterally, may be grafted for up to 10 mm so that the apical extensions of implants of sufficient length can be enclosed in bone with only modest impingement of the nasal floor.

Make an incision at the crest of the ridge from one premolar area around to the other. Make a relieving incision at either end to permit the elevation of the mucoperiosteum to the level of the anterior nasal spine. Continued elevation of the tissues presents less challenge because they are nonkeratinized. Lateral to the nasal spine, the gentle manipulation of the periosteal elevator permits disclosure of the sharp cortical rims of the pyriform apertures (Fig. 8-106, *A*).

Now change the direction of the elevator to horizontal, and hugging the nasal floor, lift the nasal mucosa (Fig. 8-106, *B*). Because the floor drops precipitously behind the rims, use a Kerrison forceps to reduce the rims in height so that direct access to the floor is attained.

With baby Parker retractors placed at each corner of the upper lip, aggressive elevation facilitates direct visualization of the nasal floor and permits observation of the preparation of each of the planned implant osteotomies from the crest of the ridge. The classical generic technique (Chapter 9) permits the placement of each implant, none of which should be less than 15 mm in length. Bone blocks harvested from the chin are almost impossible for tapping threaded implants because their planned pathways through maxilla and graft cannot be coordinated as a result of an inability to stabilize the blocks. Press-fit implants, however, permit this maneuver (Fig. 8-106, *C, D*). On entering the predrilled blocks, cylinders serve to pin them into position. Threaded implants on the other hand, require that the bone be particulated and packed around their apices after the implants have been placed.

Since the width of most pyriform apertures is between 9 and 11 mm despite the great variation of facial dimensions, it may be predicted with consistency that 8 ml of graft material is required for each side. The donor site therefore must be able to yield 16 ml of bone. The average symphysis from a bilateral approach yields between 8 and 13 cc of material. Therefore in most cases, bone expanders are required. To begin with, the bone excised from the nasal rims increases the volume. This can be followed by the addition of DFDB particles.

After placement of the graft slurry around threaded implant apices, do not initiate closure until the incipient signs of graft stability, fostered by fibrin, are noted. A resorbable membrane may be required if the reliability of graft fixation is questionable.

Closure, which must include replacement of the nasal mucosa, does not present problems because the ridge was not subjected to dimensional change. Continuous horizontal mattress sutures of Biosyn or Vicryl complete the procedure. Allow 9 months for osseointegration and graft consolidation. Patients will not complain of a diminished airway.

Posterior Maxillary Width Deficiencies

Ridge Splitting

Ridge splitting and the use of osteotomies offer the same benefit to the posterior maxillary region as they do for the anterior maxilla.

Monocortical Block Grafting

Width deficiency, although less frequently found in posterior maxillae than in the other quadrants, profits by autogenous

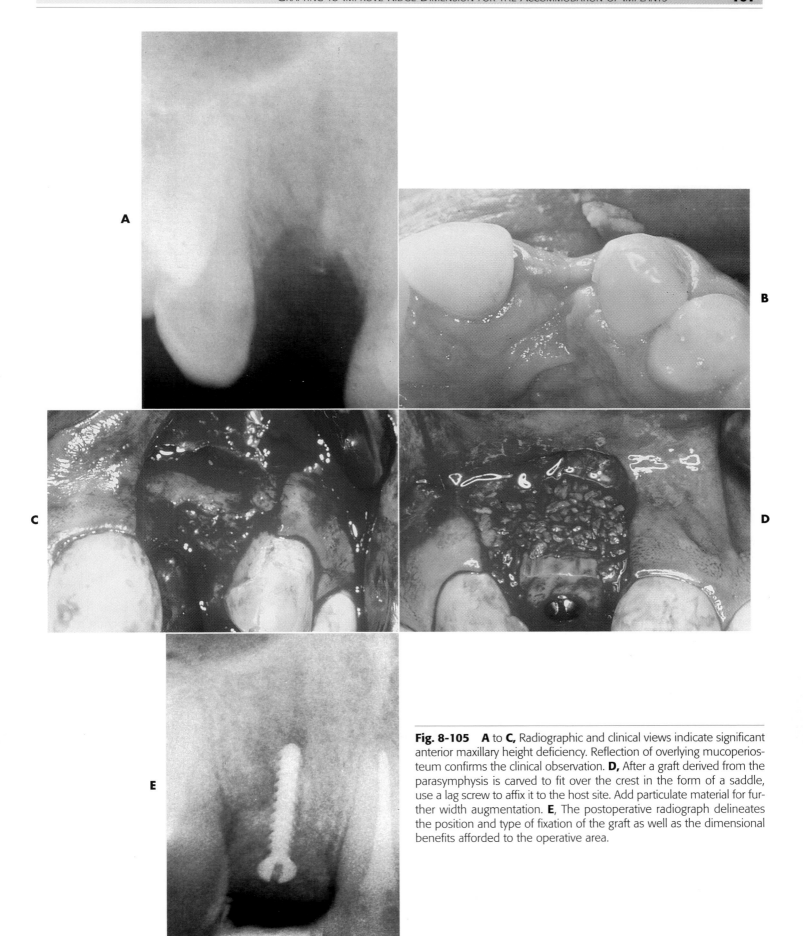

Fig. 8-105 **A** to **C,** Radiographic and clinical views indicate significant anterior maxillary height deficiency. Reflection of overlying mucoperiosteum confirms the clinical observation. **D,** After a graft derived from the parasymphysis is carved to fit over the crest in the form of a saddle, use a lag screw to affix it to the host site. Add particulate material for further width augmentation. **E,** The postoperative radiograph delineates the position and type of fixation of the graft as well as the dimensional benefits afforded to the operative area.

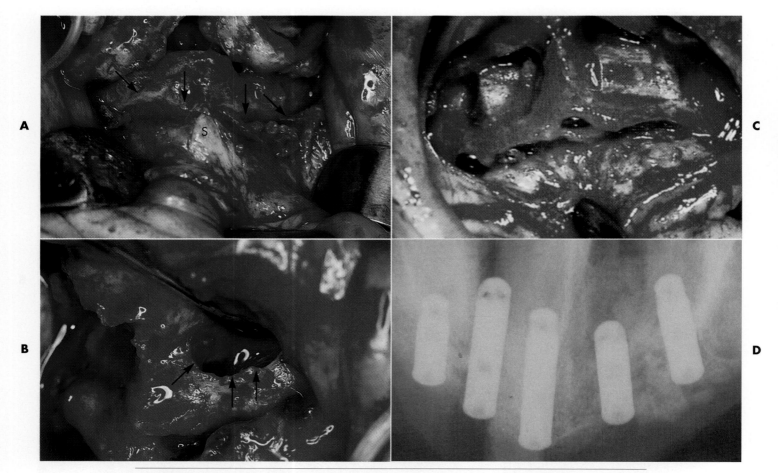

Fig. 8-106   A, Make a crestal incision and elevate the tissue to reveal the inferior borders of the pyriform apertures *(arrows)* as well as the anterior nasal spine. **B,** Continued reflection with a Freer elevator reveals the nasal floors *(arrows).* **C** and **D,** Take bone grafts from the chin and place them into the nasal floor bilaterally, thereby offering increased depth for placement of the implants. The postoperative radiograph reveals the extended implant positions and the locations of the bone grafts into which the implants protrude.

monocortical block grafting when needed. Such defects are caused on occasion by failed plate form implants (Fig. 8-107). There may be some space limitation in the posterior maxilla because of the proximity of the mandibular ramus, which might make fixation screw placement an awkward procedure. Offset screwdrivers are not effective in such situations.

Posterior Maxillary Height Deficiencies

Sinus Floor Elevation, Closed Techniques

CLASSIC METHOD   Often when the posterior maxilla is evaluated for endosteal implants, adequate bone height is not available. An enlarging maxillary sinus causes this. As teeth are lost, pneumatization of the sinuses occurs, thereby decreasing the distance between the floor of the sinus and the crest of the maxillary alveolar ridge. If insufficient vertical bone height for endosteal implants is noted, consider placement of a subperiosteal implant. Even in these cases, it is strongly suggested that opposing sinus floors be augmented to discourage implant struts from settling into them. If utilization of root form en-

dosteal implants is chosen, augment alveolar height using osteotome techniques or by performing a sinus floor elevation. This open operation requires grafting to the antral floor.

When the height of bone falls short of the surgeon's need by a few millimeters, the classical generic root form osteotomy technique may be completed up to but not through the bony floor. Select an implant that has a smooth rounded apical end and a length that is up to 3 mm longer than the host site. Devices such as IMZ and Calcitek press-fit implants particularly satisfy this requirement. On completion of the preliminary operative steps, gently tap into place the implant try-in device, thereby in-fracturing the floor of the antrum and, without lacerating it, elevating the membrane to within its elastic limits (Fig. 8-108).

Of course there is only modest benefit to the use of this method because the implant-support mechanism is restricted to the length of bone adjacent to its sides. However, it permits introduction of a longer implant, encourages secondary periapical bone formation, and avoids complex manipulation.

SUMMERS METHOD   A second more sophisticated, closed technique was developed by Dr. Robert Summers. Using the

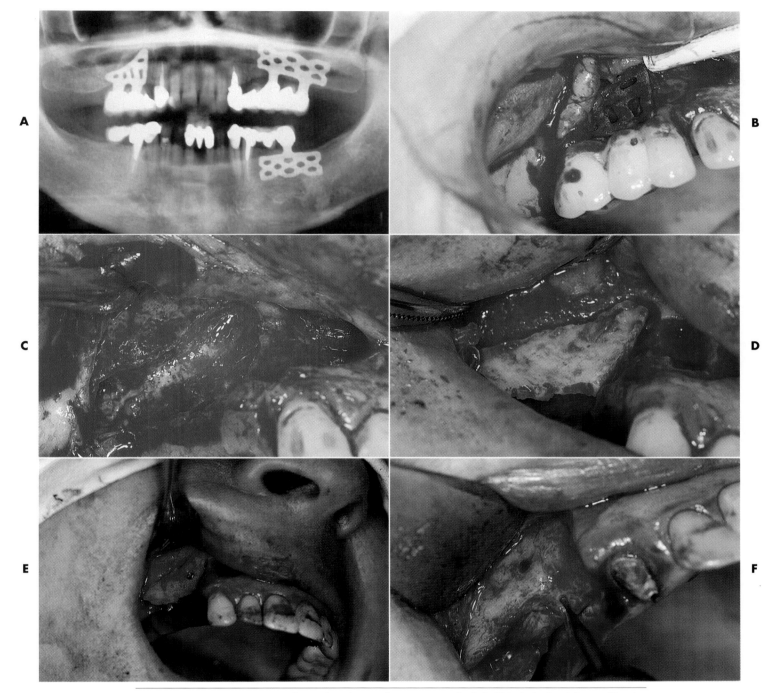

Fig. 8-107   A, A panoramic radiograph indicates the presence of a failed blade in the right maxilla. The obvious etiology is the violation of a basic tenet of blade superstructure construction: the prostheses must always be splinted to natural teeth. **B,** After reflection of overlying tissues, the recently placed implant is picked out easily with a hemostatic forceps. **C,** The defect mimics the outline of the removed blade after the granulomata are excised. **D,** Using the lead-foil template method of graft-shape transfer (noted on p. 145) an accurately shaped bone graft, harvested from the mandibular parasymphysis, is being transferred to the deficient site. The remarkable similarity of the graft to the removed implant's infrastructure is a result of the accuracy of the lead foil template technique. **E,** The monocortical block is affixed to the deficient maxillary host site with a lag screw. A significant addition to dimension may be noted. **F,** The tissues are opened after 6 months of healing. The screw is backed out revealing firm consolidation of the graft. The initial steps for root form insertion in this generously augmented ridge are being undertaken.

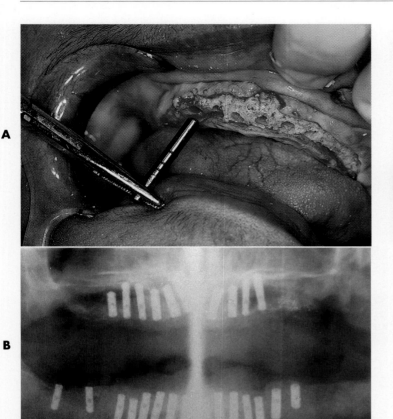

Fig. 8-108 A, Gentle tapping with a press-fit implant try-in, in-fractures the antral floor and, because of its rounded end, protects the membrane from injury. **B,** Using this method, implants slightly longer than the available bone can be inserted without causing harm to the maxillary sinus.

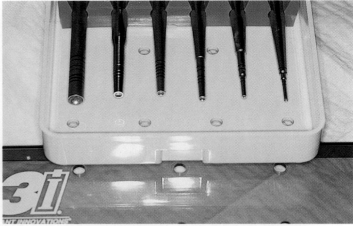

Fig. 8-109 The Summers osteotomes (made by 3i) are of increasing diameter and have sharpened, cupped ends designed to shave the bone and carry it through the antral floor and positioning it under the sinus membrane that they have elevated.

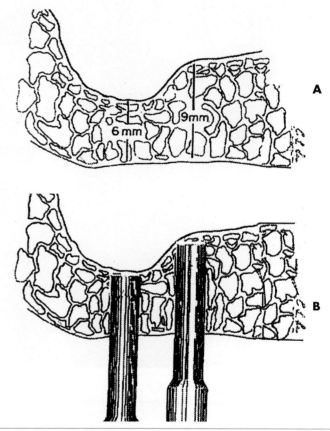

Fig. 8-110 A, Preoperative bone dimensions beneath the sinus floor suitable for the Summers technique. A 6-mm site can be altered to support a 10-mm implant. A 9-mm location can be deepened to accept a 13-mm implant. **B,** In soft bone, insert a small diameter osteotome (Summers Osteotome No. 1) with hand pressure or light malleting to the sinus boundary. In harder bone, use a drill with care to penetrate to this depth. The goal is to stay short of the membrane with the initial osteotomy.

antroplasty methods described earlier and desirous of embodying the protruding implant apices in bone, he developed a system that encourages this osseous augmentation to occur (Fig. 8-109).

Several conditions may be dealt with when using the Summers osteotomes. For all techniques, 4 to 5 mm of residual subantral bone are required.

The first technique uses a 6-mm-diameter trephine malleted at selected sites, each 6 mm apart, in ridges wide enough to accommodate it to its full depth. The plugs produced by the trephine are pushed up through the antral floor, thereby elevating the sinus membrane. If the bone is resistant to this pressure, tapping with a mallet works effectively. Place a graft material of choice into the depressions made in the ridge before suturing. A lapse of 6 months is permitted before implant placement.

A second technique permits immediate implant placement. For this, make an incision at the crest of the ridge and, using a surgical template, mark each of the implant sites with a No. 2 round bur. In cases that offer soft, compliant bone, the floor elevation uses the osteotomes alone. Each, larger than its predecessor, has a concave tip. Enter the established sites using the smallest diameter first. The osteotomy so produced is completed 2 mm short of the antral floor. Enlarge each site until its diameter is equal to the size of the intended implant. Then, placing small quantities of bone taken from adjacent sites (i.e., tuberosity) in the concave tip of the last osteotome that had

been used, further gentle tapping permits in-fracture of the antral floor (2 to 3 mm), elevation of the intact membrane, and introduction of the local bone with the addition of the autogenous graft. Continue this process during subsequent stages of the operation for up to three gentle bony additions. Placement of an implant again with bone being propelled by its apex serves as the final osteotome before suturing (Fig. 8-110).

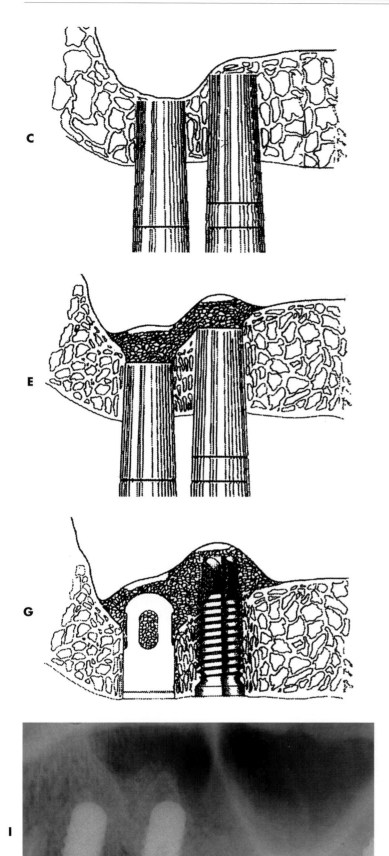

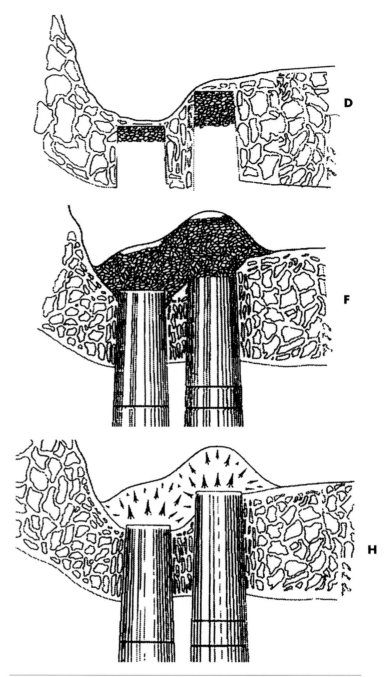

Fig. 8-110, cont'd   C, Widen the osteotomy with the No. 2 and No. 3 Summers osteotomes. The No. 3 instrument prepares a slightly under-sized osteotomy for a 3.75-diameter implant. **D,** Add a prepared bone graft mix into the osteotomy with a sterile carrier before any attempt is made to elevate the sinus floor. The mix should contain 25% autogenous bone obtained from the tuberosity of the same quadrant. A variety of graft materials can be added to the autogenous particles. **E,** Reinsert the largest osteotome used previously to the sinus floor. Pressure from the instru-ment causes the added materials and trapped fluids to exert pressure on the sinus membrane. **F,** Add additional small quantities of bone and re-turn the osteotome to the sinus floor. Each increment of material elevates the membrane by 1 to 1.5 mm. **G,** When the antral floor is displaced, the graft will move freely, elevating the membrane without the osteotome entering the sinus. The implant becomes the final osteotome pushing up the membrane to its ultimate height. **H,** The concave osteotome tip traps bone and fluids as the instrument moves superiorly. Hydraulic force is created, exerting pressure in all directions (Pascal's law). This force ele-vates the membrane over an area wider than the osteotomy. **I,** A radi-ograph demonstrates bone formation in the maxillary sinus graft region around the implant apices using the Summers osteotome technique.

There are cases in which the bone is too dense to yield to the simple use of the osteotomes. For these situations, create each potential host site with a 1.6-mm diameter, internally irrigated bone drill carried to the level of the antral floor. Enlargement is continued with the Summers 3i osteotome set to enlarge each osteotomy to its requisite diameter. The primary purpose of these instruments is vested in their capability, when tapped, to in-fracture and expand the antral floor upward for distances up to 6 mm. The tips are sharp and concave, which permits them to carry small quantities of bone (retrieved from adjacent edentulous sites) as well as to transport shaved lateral bone into the newly made periapical concavities.

Implants, either threaded or press-fit, now may be introduced in the conventional manner to the newly increased depths. Routine closure completes these procedures.

Sinus Floor Elevation, Open Techniques

When a more dramatic improvement of subantral height is required, considerable quantities of graft material are required. This may be obtained from autogenous bone harvested from the ramus of the mandible, the symphysis, the anterior iliac crest, the tibial plateau, a rib, or the calvarium. Autogenous bone can be mixed with allogeneic material (50% autogenous bone with 50% DFDB by volume).

Some clinicians elevate the sinus floor using only synthetic graft materials. However, the chances for success are amplified if autogenous bone is added to the composite. Grind the harvested bone into fine particles with the rongeur forceps. When less than the amount of autogenous bone needed is harvested, mix it with an acceptable expander in accordance with Table 8-1 and store it in the patient's marrow-derived blood. Perform the antroplasty by anesthetizing the area to be grafted from tuberosity to midline with infiltrations, infraorbital, posterosuperior alveolar, and greater palatine (second division) blocks (Fig. 8-111). Make a full-thickness incision along the crest of the maxillary ridge from behind the tuberosity forward

to the canine area (Fig. 8-112). A vertical releasing incision at the anterior end is necessary. Reflect the flap with the periosteal elevator to allow access to the canine fossa just below the infraorbital foramen, to the buttress of the zygomatic arch, and to the lateral maxillary wall posterior to it. Using a No. 8 round diamond stone in a high-speed Impactair handpiece, make a horizontal line parallel to and at the level of the antral floor in the lateral cortex of the maxilla. Create the groove by gentle brushing of the bone so that it barely penetrates the cortical plate. Some experience is required before the surgeon's tactile skills permit this to be done without injuring the sinus membrane. The groove should run the full anteroposterior dimension of the antrum. Place a second line parallel to the first one, 15 mm above it. Be careful to avoid injuring the infraorbital foramen or its contents. Connect these two horizontal lines with vertical ones at either end, again using the diamond in a gentle brushing motion. At this juncture, the outline of a rectangle is plainly visible. Round the two lower corners so that they will not tear the sinus membrane (Fig. 8-113).

After full bony perforation with the diamond drill, use a

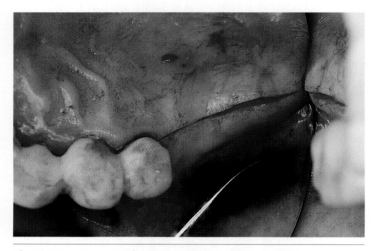

Fig. 8-112 Access to the sinus is achieved by a crestal incision.

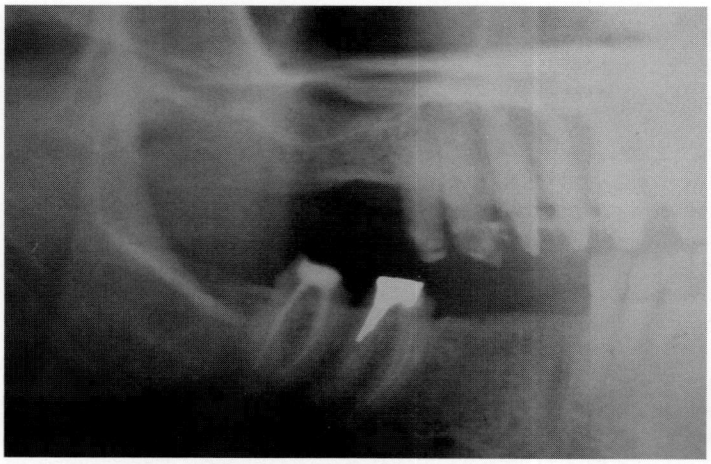

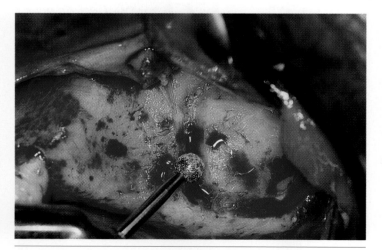

Fig. 8-111 The panoramic radiograph indicates a clear sinus, free of septa. There is inadequate bone for placement of implants. Sinus floor elevation with ramus bone and synthetic grafting materials is indicated.

Fig. 8-113 After reflection of the mucoperiosteum, the lateral maxillary wall is exposed almost to the level of the infraorbital foramen. Use a No. 8 diamond round bur to create an oblong window. Its inferior perimeter is at the level of the antral floor.

mallet and the blunt end of an orangewood stick to gently mobilize the plate of bone inward. As this is done, the superior line with its remaining attachment to the flap becomes a hinge. Take care not to pierce the membrane during any one of the steps in this procedure. After the door is pressed inward for 4 to 5 mm, reflect the membrane from the bony floor of the sinus using the backs of Tatum's elevating instruments (Fig. 8-114). Elevate the lining ahead of the bone trapdoor as it is moved further inwardly. In such a manner, the rotated maxillary wall, when elevated to a horizontal position, becomes the new floor of the sinus, and the antral membrane is advanced in folds above it (Fig. 8-115). If the antral floor has septa (which may be seen on the preoperative Panorex film), contiguous membrane elevation is not possible. Under such circumstances, attempt to remove septa with a thin curved osteotome or a Kerrison forceps. If that effort fails, perform the elevations in sections, gently teasing the membrane from the thin bony partitions as if they were separate sinuses.

Membrane lacerations occur on occasion. In such instances, repair the membrane using 4-0 Vicryl suture on an SH tapered needle. An extremely effective technique is to make tiny No. 2 round bur holes in the bony wall just above the trapdoor hinge. The sinus membrane, which is plentiful because it was elevated in folds, may be sutured to the bone using these bur holes as sites of fixation. This effectively ablates any lacerations (Fig. 8-116). If suturing is not undertaken, Colla tape, which serves as an adhesive on being moistened with blood, can serve as a repair device. Healing is not affected because of the abundance of overfolded, accordion-like tissues and the rapidity of epithelial proliferation.

If less than 4 mm of original crestal bone height is present, place implants only if they are offered a transitional support mechanism such as a miniplate. A description of this technique is found in the last section of this chapter.

On the other hand, if 5 mm or more of bone height exists, place root form implants in routine fashion at the time of antroplasty. However, since primary retention of root form im-

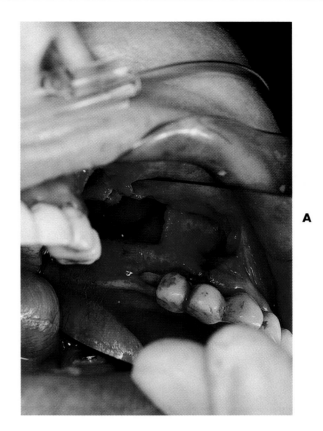

A

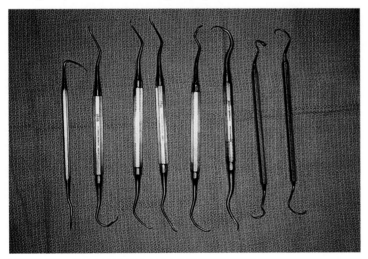

Fig. 8-114 Use Tatum membrane elevators, which are available in a number of sizes and angulations, to tease the sinus lining from the floor.

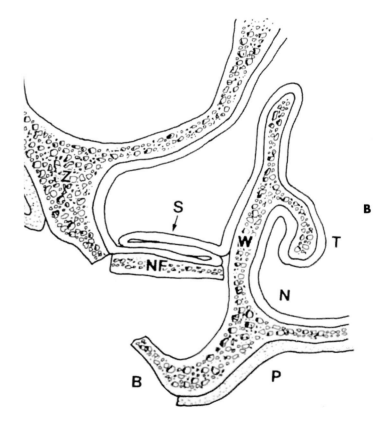

B

Fig. 8-115 Gentle tapping causes a medial translation of the bony window. Rotate the window upward and inward into a horizontal posture with the folded membrane gathered above it. *B*, Buccal surface of ridge; *M*, elevated buccal mucosa; *N*, nasal cavity; *NF*, new antral floor; *P*, palate, *S*, folded sinus membrane; *T*, turbinate; *W*, medial sinus wall.

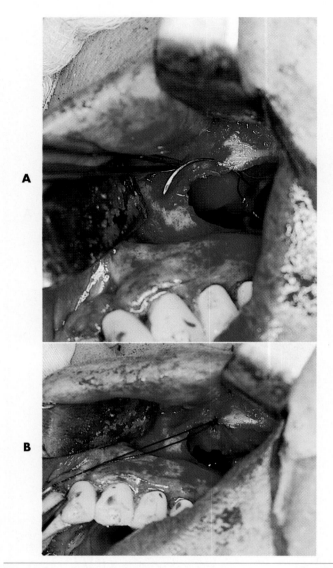

Fig. 8-116   A, If a laceration of the membrane occurs, repair it by suturing the plentiful folds laterally to the bone just above the hinge through tiny bur holes. If the cortex is not fragile enough to permit penetration by the suture needle, it may be passed through a small hole made with a No. 2 round bur. **B,** The membrane then is drawn horizontally to the bone to which it is sutured, thus eliminating the perforation. An alternative technique advocates the use of a collagen sheet against the torn membrane.

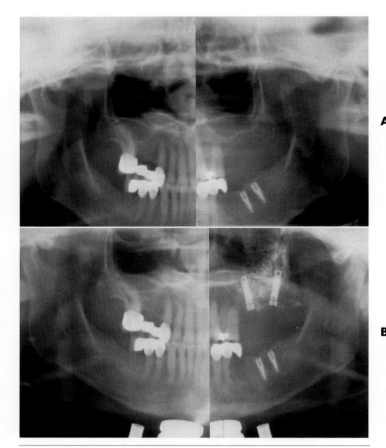

Fig. 8-117   A, This radiograph indicates a sufficient quantity of bone to allow for placement of endosteal implants at the time of grafting. **B,** The postoperative Panorex film shows the acceptance of a combination of autogenous and synthetic graft materials, which have embodied two 15-mm-long Steri-Oss implants.

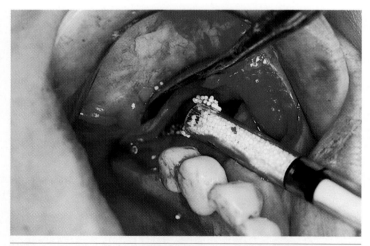

Fig. 8-118   After the antral floor has been made available for grafting, use a syringe to deliver the graft complex.

plants is necessary, threaded rather than press-fit submergible designs are best (Fig. 8-117). Select an implant system that has the greatest number of threads near the cervix, since this is where the bone is found, rather than implants with a wide zone of polished collar. Nobelcare, Steri-Oss, 3I, Lifecore, and Swede-Vent are good choices.

Whether implants have been placed or not, the next step is to fill the floor with the graft material (prepared with antibiotics, saline, and/or blood) to the upper level of the fenestration. This will stabilize the trapdoor in its new horizontal position (Fig. 8-118). Gently push the antral membrane upward ahead of and above it so that its integrity continues to be protected (Fig. 8-119). When the floor is filled completely with graft material totally surrounding the implants (if placed), tuck a resorbable membrane superiorly beneath the mucosal flap

and bring it down to cover the antral window and graft completely, and then crosses over the crest of the ridge. Finally, wedge it beneath the residual palatal mucoperiosteum, which is elevated to receive it. Return the buccal flap to its original presurgical position and close it with a continuous horizontal mattress suture.

Instruct the patient not to blow his or her nose for 2 weeks

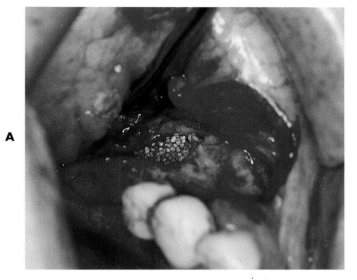

A

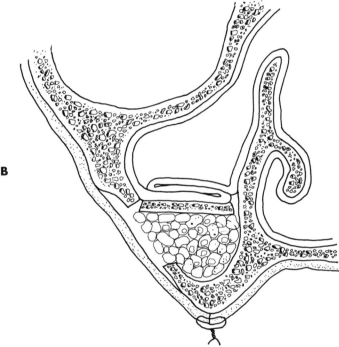

B

Fig. 8-119   A, Use the particulate graft material, moistened in an antibiotic-blood slurry, in a quantity sufficient to fill the antrum to the level of the horizontal window. This will support the newly repositioned antral floor and serve as a matrix for osteogenesis. **B,** Perform closure at the crest of the ridge, after placement of a large square of Vicryl mesh membrane using a continuous horizontal mattress suture.

following this procedure. The standard sinus regimen must be prescribed, as noted in the Appendix G. Emphasize expectations of moderate swelling, pain, and ecchymosis, which are found mostly at the donor site in the mandibular symphysis. In addition, some nasal bleeding may occur during the first day. After the standard postoperative visits, it is recommended that the patient be evaluated at 9 months. At this point make a clinical determination, using radiographs, as to whether the area has matured sufficiently to permit classic root form endosteal implantation. If implantations had already been placed, patients are evaluated to see whether they seem ready for exposure and healing collar placement (Fig. 8-120 through 8-122).

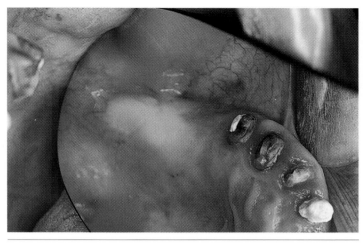

Fig. 8-120   Six months after antroplasty, healing at the alveolar site has been completed.

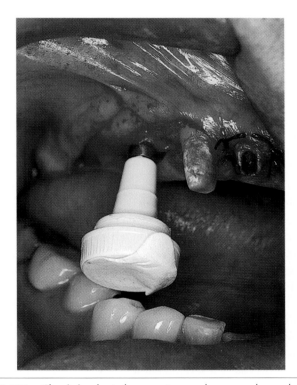

Fig. 8-121   Classic implant placement procedures may be undertaken after sinus floor maturation.

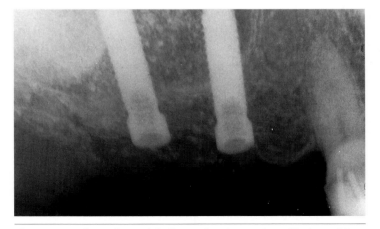

Fig. 8-122   This radiograph indicates that the newly ossified antral floor has accommodated two Steri-Oss root form implants.

Earlier or even immediate surgery may be performed after antroplasty if a subperiosteal implant is the treatment choice.

Posterior Maxillary Deficiency and Miniplate

Generally the absence of adequate alveolar bone (4 mm or less) beneath the maxillary sinus prevents placement of endosteal root form implants at the same time as antroplasty. A technique has been devised that permits implantation simultaneously with sinus floor elevation. This has been made possible by the use of titanium fracture miniplates, which serve as transitional fixation devices until mineralization of the graft material creates implant osseointegration.

This technique uses a miniplate, 2-mm-diameter self-tapping screws, 3.8 × 16 mm threaded, root form implants (i.e., Steri-Oss or ScrewVents), the armamentarium to place them, and titanium healing screws with 3.8-mm diameter heads. In addition, the classic antroplasty instruments are required. The patient is managed by means of regional anesthesia; infraorbital, posterosuperior alveolar, and second division blocks with or without sedation; or general anesthesia.

Make an incision at the crest of the alveolar ridge, with relieving incisions extending distally from the base of the tuberosity and mesially in a vertical-oblique direction to the midline. Reflection of the mucoperiosteum is made to the base of the ridge palatally and to a region just below the infraorbital foramen on the buccal side.

The assistant surgeon must protect the identified infraorbital neurovascular bundle while reflecting the investing tissues so that the lateral antral wall can be exposed aggressively.

Use a No. 8 round diamond in a high-speed, water-cooled Impactair handpiece for sketching the outlines of a fenestration designed to enter the antral environment. Make it oblong, with its inferior border at the level of the antral floor, the superior outline 4 mm beneath the infraorbital foramen, and the anterior and posterior vertical components at the most practicable accessible locations but certainly more mesially and more distally than the planned zone of implantation in precisely the same manner as is described earlier. Use the well-irrigated diamond with gentle brushing motions until the appearance of the antral membrane is seen at all of the osteotomies. The blue, translucent appearance of the membrane is appreciated as the maxillary cortex dissipates beneath the diamond.

At this juncture, the window can be in-fractured by tapping it with an orangewood stick and elevated inwardly by using a periosteal elevator as a lever. Medial retraction permits separation of the membrane from the inferior, internal surface of the sinus using the Tatum curettes. As the membrane is lifted away from the floor and inferior walls, push the trapdoor inward farther by gentle pressure of tapping, and lift it on its membrane hinge to a horizontal posture. The membrane curettes are used to complete the separation of the membrane from the bony floor and lateral walls and lift it in an upward direction above the trapdoor.

At this juncture, place a sponge, moistened in saline, beneath the elevated window with the gathered membrane maintained above it.

Attention is turned to the alveolar crest. Select and cut a strip of Synthes, Osteomed, or similar titanium CP miniplate with 2-mm-diameter holes. Bend it to fit the length and configuration of the ridge from a point just distal to the last tooth in position extending posteriorly to the tuberosity (Fig. 8-123).

With the assistant surgeon maintaining the plate in position, tap holes with a fine tapered diamond in the high-speed handpiece at two appropriate screw sites, and place 1.5-mm diameter short (4 mm) self-tapping screws, fastening the device into position (Fig. 8-124).

Score the bone sites selected for implantation with a No. 2 round bur made in the centers of the selected holes in the miniplate, and then remove the plate by backing out the short fixation screws.

Develop and enlarge each osteotomy by use of the generic technique described in Chapter 9 to a diameter of 3.5 mm (Fig. 8-125). Then, affix 16-mm-long, 3.8-mm diameter Steri-Oss threaded implants (or similarly compatible designs) to the matching holes of the plate by means of their large-head healing screws (Fig. 8-126). Carry the plate-implant assembly to the bone, guide the apical ends of the implants into their re-

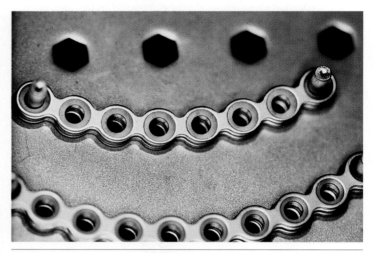

Fig. 8-123 These Synthes titanium miniplates are available in curved and straight designs. Their countersunk holes accept Steri-Oss and Screw-Vent screw heads with precision. These plates can be cut and bent to conform to the shape of the crest of the ridge.

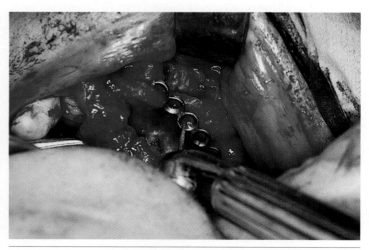

Fig. 8-124 After bone tapping, affix the miniplate to the crest of the ridge with 4-mm-long titanium screws. Place them in holes that will not be used as implant sites.

spective osteotomies, and seat the complex by gentle mallet-tapping with an orangewood stick (Fig. 8-127). When the plate comes to rest at the ridge crest, wider (2-mm-diameter), insert 6-mm-long, plate-holding screws into the original fixation sites in the ridge (Fig. 8-128).

With the implants now securely affixed to the ridge and

protruding into the antrum, remove the sponge, and complete the grafting of synthetic and autogenous bone to the sinus floor and around the implant. Mixtures of HA and DFDB mixed with the patient's own parasymphyseal bone and consolidated with blood and gentamicin (80 mg) serve as a reliable combination (Fig. 8-129).

On complete filling (usually about 16 ml) of the newly occupied implant zone with the window in a horizontal posture and the antral membrane pushed and gathered above it in loose folds, place a square of resorbable Vicryl mesh or laminar bone beneath the periosteum on the bone rim above the fenestration and bring it down over the mass of graft material. From this point, curve the GTRM down over the ridge and then carry it across the crest, thereby covering the implants and their stabilizing plate, to be wedged finally beneath the palatal flap (Fig. 8-130).

Take radiographs to affirm the position of the implants and the location and density of the graft material (Fig. 8-131). Then bring together the flaps (with buccal undermining when necessary) and close them with a 4-0 polyglactic acid continuous horizontal mattress suture (Fig. 8-132).

When only a portion of the floor is thin and the remainder

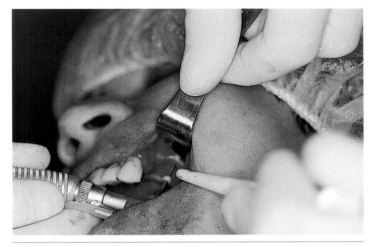

Fig. 8-125 After the ridge is marked through the miniplate holes at each planned implant site, remove the plate and complete the osteotomies to 3.5-mm diameters.

A

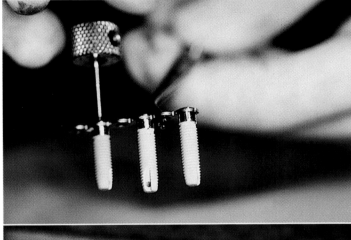

B

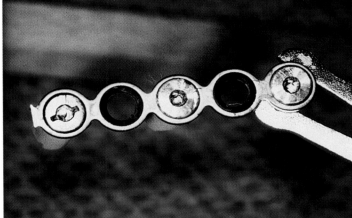

Fig. 8-126 **A,** On completion of the osteotomies, attach each 16-mm long, 3.8-mm-diameter, threaded implant to its corresponding site in the miniplate using the healing screws for fixation. **B,** Note the perfect relationships between the screw heads and the plate.

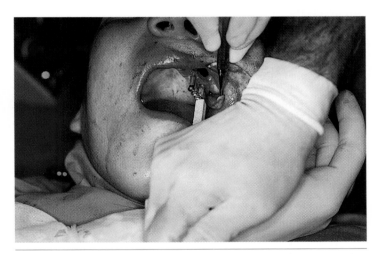

Fig. 8-127 Guide the miniplate-implant complex into the osteotomies, and, using an orangewood stick and mallet, tap it into place.

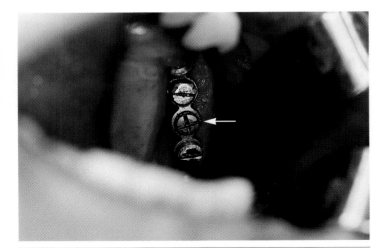

Fig. 8-128 Stabilize the miniplate, which is bracing the implants in the extremely shallow bone, with 6-mm, short, compatible titanium screws, each placed into one of the original 4-mm fixation sites *(arrow).*

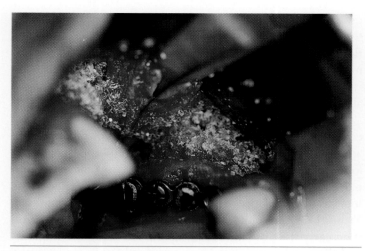

Fig. 8-129 After firm stabilization of the plate, assess the position of the protruding 16-mm-long implants and affirm the posture of the bone trapdoor and the overlying folded sinus lining. This is followed by the placement of the graft material, which consists of parasymphyseal autogenous bone, expanded with TCP and DFDB.

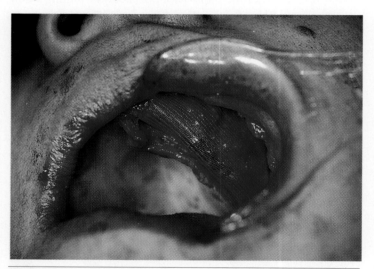

Fig. 8-130 Trim Vicryl mesh to fit over the entire osseous wound. It should be wider than the antrostomy so that it will rest on cortical bone mesially and distally. Tuck it is beneath the flap just below the infraorbital foramen, bring it down over the graft, contour it across the ridge crest and miniplate and, finally, tuck it beneath the palatal flap. Closure follows, which completes the procedure.

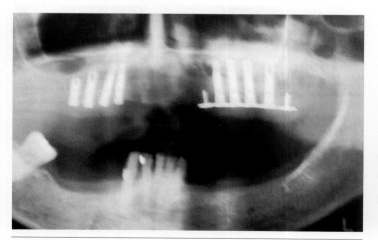

Fig. 8-131 A postoperative Panorex demonstrates a well-placed miniplate with its fixation screws and the implants inserted into a grafted antral floor. Note the 6-mm long fixation screws at either end.

is thick enough to require the use of a conventional osteotomy technique with a bone-tapping drill, the vertical seating of a threaded implant assembled to the plate would become impossible because that implant could not be turned. In such instances, a press-fit implant is substituted to allow seating of the entire complex by tapping (see Fig. 8-126).

As an alternative, the plate can be shortened, allowing the seating of a conventional threaded implant before placement of the plate. After maturation of the graft in 9 months, the healing and fixation screws are backed out at second-stage surgery, the miniplate is removed, and the requisite prosthetic steps are undertaken and completed (Fig. 8-133).

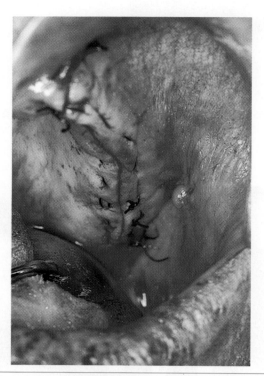

Fig. 8-132 Use violet-dyed Vicryl sutures to create a tight continuous horizontal mattress closure.

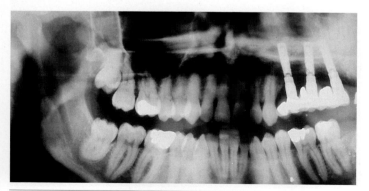

Fig. 8-133 This radiograph shows the satisfactory results of a restoration in the left maxilla that is supported by implants supported by a miniplate that had been placed inot a grafted sinus floor.

Suggested Readings

Adell R, Lekholm U, Rockler B et al: A 15-year study of osseointegrated implants in the treatment of edentulous jaw, *Int J Oral Surg* 10:387-416, 1981.

Avera S, Stampley W, McAllister B: Histologic and clinical observations of resorbable and nonresorbable barrier membranes used in maxillary sinus graft containment, *Int J of Oral Maxillofac Implants* 12:88-95, 1991.

Bahat O: Osseointegrated implants the maxillary tuberosity: report on 45 consecutive patients, *Int J Oral Maxillofac Implants* 7:459-467, 1992.

Bahat O: Surgical planning for optimal aesthetic and functional results of osseointegrated implants in the partially edentulous mouth, *J Calif Dent Assoc* 20(5):31-46, 1992.

Bahat O: Treatment planning and placement of implants in the posterior maxillae: report of 732 consecutive Nobelpharma implants, *Int J Oral Maxillofac Implants* 2:151-161, 1993.

Barzilav E et al: Immediate implantation of pure titanium into extraction sockets of macaca fascicularis. Part II: histologic observations, *Int J Oral Maxillofac Implants* 11:489-498, 1996.

Basu S et al: Comparative study of biological glues: cryoprecipitate glue, two-component fibrin sealant, and "French" glue, *Ann Thorac Surg* 60(5):1255-1262, 1995.

Blitzer A, Lawson W, Friedman W: Surgery of the paranasal sinuses, Philadelphia, 1985, WB Saunders.

Blomqvist J, Alberilus P, Isaksson S: Retrospective analysis of one stage maxillary sinus augmentation with endosseous implants, *Int J Oral Maxillofac Implants* 11:512-520, 1996.

Block MS, Kent JN: Maxillary sinus grafting for totally and partially edentulous patients, *J Am Dent Assoc* 124:139-143, 1993.

Boyne PJ: Comparison of porous and nonporous hydroxylapatite and xenografts in the restoration of alveolar ridges. Proceedings of ASTM Symposium on Implants, Nashville, 1987, pp 359-369.

Boyne PJ, James RA: Grafting of the maxillary sinus floor with autogenous marrow and bone, *J Oral Surg* 38:613-616, 1980.

Brånemark P-I, Zarb GA, Albrektsson T: Tissue integrated prosthesis: osseointegration in clinical dentistry, *Quintessence* 11(77):211-233, 1985.

Brook IM, Lamb DJ: Two stage combined vestibuloplasty and partial mandibular ridge augmentation with hydroxyapatite, *J Oral Maxillofac Surg* 38:613-617, 1980.

Busch et al: Guided tissue regeneration and local delivery of insulin-like growth factor I by bioerodible polyorthoester membranes in rat calvarial defects, *Int J Oral Maxillofac Implants* 11:498-505, 1996.

Buser D et al: Regeneration and enlargement of jaw bone using guided tissue regeneration, *Clin Oral Implant Res* 1:22-32, 1986.

Caplanis N et al: Effect of allogenic, freeze dried, demineralized bone matrix on guided bone regeneration in supra-alveolar peri-implant defects dogs, *Int J Oral Maxillofac Implants* 12:634-643, 1997.

Chanavaz M: Maxillary sinus: anatomy, physiology, surgery, and bone grafting related to implantology – 11 years of surgical experience (1979-1990), *J Oral Implantol* 1:199-209, 1990.

Clinical Results at 36 Months After Loading With Fixed Partial Dentures, *Int J Oral Maxillofac Implants* 11(6)743-749, 1996.

Converse JM, editors: *Reconstructive plastic surgery principles and procedures in correction, reconstruction and transplantation,* ed 2, Philadelphia, 1977, WB Saunders.

Corsair A: A clinical evaluation of resorbable hydroxyapatite for the repair of human intra-osseous defects, *J Oral Implantol* 16:125-129, 1990.

Cranin AN et al: Applications of hydroxyapatite in oral and maxillofacial surgery. Part I. *Compendium* 8:254-262, 1987.

Cranin AN et al: Applications of hydroxyapatite in oral and maxillofacial surgery. Part II. *Compendium* 8:334-344, 1987.

Cranin AN et al: Hydroxyapatite for alveolar ridge augmentation: a clinical study, *J Prosthet Dent* 56:592-599, 1986.

Dahlin C et al: Generation of new bone around titanium implants using a membrane technique: an experimental study in rabbits, *Int J Oral Maxillofac Implants* 4:19-25, 1989.

Deeb ME: Comparison of three methods of stabilization of particulate hydroxyapatite for augmentation of the mandibular ridge, *J Oral Maxillofac Surg* 46:758-766, 1988.

Deeb ME, Hosny M, Sharawy M: Osteogenesis in composite grafts of allogenic demineralized bone powder and porous hydroxylapatite, *Int J Oral Maxillofac Surg* 47:50-56, 1989.

Dufresne CR, Carson BS, Zinreich SJ: *Rib grafts. Complex craniofacial problems: a guide to analysis and treatment,* New York, Churchill Livingstone.

Duncan J, Westwood M: Ridge widening of the thin maxilla: a clinical report, *Int J Oral Maxillofac Implants* 12:221-228, 1997.

Engelke W et al: Alveolar reconstruction with splitting osteotomy and microfixation of implants, *Int J Oral Maxillofac Implants* 12:310-319, 1997.

Fonseca RJ, Frost D, Zeitler D et al: Reconstruction of edentulous bone loss. In Fonseca RJ, Davis WH, editors: *Reconstructive preprosthetic oral and maxillofacial surgery,* Philadelphia, 1986, WB Saunders.

Fonseca RJ, Walker RV: Reconstruction of avulsive maxillofacial injuries, *Oral and Maxillofacial Trauma* 2:1062-1063, 1991.

Frame JW, Brady CL: Augmentation of an atrophic endentuolous mandible by interpositional grafting with hydroxypatite, *J Oral Maxillofac Surg* 42:89-92, 1984.

Friberg B, Jemt T, Lekholm U: Early failures of 4641 consecutively placed Brånemark dental implants: a study from stage I surgery to the connection of completed prosthesis, *Int J Oral Maxillofac Implants* 6:142-146, 1991.

Fugazzotto P: Success and failure rates of osseointegrated implants in function in regenerated bone for 6 to 51 months: a preliminary report, *Int J Oral Maxillofac Implants* 12:17-25, 1997.

Fugazzotto P: The use of demineralized laminar bone sheets in guided bone regeneration procedures: report of three cases, *Int J Oral Maxillofac Implants* 11(2):239-244, 1996.

Gouvoussis J, Sindhusake D, Yeung S: Cross-infection from periodontitis sites to failing implant sites in the same mouth, *Int J Oral Maxillofac Implants* 12:666-673, 1997.

Gramm CT: Implantation of foreign objects in the maxilla, *Dent Dig* 4:832, 1988.

Gross C et al: In vitro changes of hydroxyapatite coatings, *Int J Oral Maxillofac Implants* 12:589-598, 1997.

Hanisch O et al: Bone formation and reosseointegration in peri-implantitis defects following surgical implantation of rhBMP-2, *Int J Oral Maxillofac Implants* 12:604-610, 1997.

Hanisch O et al: Bone formation and osseointegration stimulated by rhBMP-2 following subantral augmentation procedures in nonhuman primates, *Int J Oral Maxillofac Implants* 12:785-793, 1997.

Henry P et al: Tissue regeneration in bony defects adjacent to immediately loaded titanium implants placed into extraction sockets: a study in dogs.

Hollinger JO, Battistone GC: Biodegradable bone repair materials, *Clin Orthop Rel Res* 20:290-305, 1986.

Hupp JR, McKenna SJ: Use of porous hydroxyapatite blocks for augmentation of atrophic mandibles, *J Oral Maxillofac Surg* 46:538-545, 1988.

Hurt WC: Freeze-dried bone homografts in periodontal lesions in dogs, *J Periodont Dent* 39:89, 1968.

Hurzeler L et al: Reconstruction of the severely resorbed maxilla with dental implants in the augmented maxillary sinus: a 5-year clinical investigation, *Int J Oral Maxillofac Implants* 11:466-476, 1996.

Hurzeler M et al: Treatment of peri-implantitis using guided bone regeneration and bone grafts, alone or in combination, in Beagle dogs. Part II: Histologic findings, *Int J Oral Maxillofac Implants* 12:168-175, 1997.

Hute G et al: Does titanium surface treatment influence the bone-implant interface? SEM and histomorphometry in a 6-month sheep study, *Int J Oral Maxillofac Implants* 11:506-511, 1996.

Isaacson G et al: Autologous plasma fibrin glue: rapid preparation and selective use, *Am J Otolaryngol* 17(2):92-94, 1996.

Jaffin RA, Berman CL: The excessive loss of Brånemark fixtures in type IV bone: a 5-year analysis, *J Periodontol* 62:204, 1991.

Jensen J: Reconstruction of the atrophic alveolar ridge with mandibular bone grafts and implants (abstract), *J Oral Maxillofac Surg* 7:116-118, 1988.

Jensen S et al: Tissue reaction and material characteristics of four bone substitutes, *Int J Oral Maxillofac Implants* 11:55-67, 1996.

Johnson M et al: Regeneration of peri-implant infrabony defects using perioglas: a pilot study in rabbits. *Int J Oral Maxillofac Implants* 12:835-840, 1997.

Judy WK: Multiple uses of resorbable tricalcium phosphate, *NY Dent J* 53:1983.

Kahnberg KE et al: Combined use of bone grafts and Brånemark fixtures in the treatment of severely resorbed maxillae, *J Oral Maxillofac Implants* 4:297-304, 1989.

Kan J et al: Mandibular fracture after endosseous implant placement in conjunction with inferior alveolar nerve transposition: a patient treatment report, *Int J Oral Maxillofac Implants* 12:655-660, 1997.

Keller EE et al: Prosthetic surgical reconstruction of the severely resorbed maxilla with illiac bone grafting and tissue integrated prostheses, *Int J Oral Maxillofac Implants* 2:155-165, 1987.

Keller EE, Triplett WW: Iliac bone grafting: review of 160 consecutive cases, *J Oral Maxillofac Surg* 45:11-14, 1987.

Kent J et al: Augmentation of deficient edentulous alveolar ridge with dense polycrystalline hydroxylapatite (abstract 3.8.2). Final programme and book of abstracts, first world biomaterials congress, Society for Biomaterials, Vienna, Austria, 1980.

Kent JN, Block MS: Simultaneous maxillary sinus floor bone grafting and placement of hydroxyapatite-coated implant, *J Oral Maxillofac Surg* 47:238-242, 1989.

Kent JN, Quinn JH, Zide MF et al: Alveolar ridge augmentation using nonresorbable hydroxylapatite with or without autogenous cancellous bone, *J Oral Maxillofac Surg* 41:629-642, 1983.

Kent JN et al: Hydroxyapatite alveolar ridge reconstruction: clinical experiences, complications, and technical modifications, *J Oral Maxillofac Surg* 44:37-49, 1986.

Kirker-Head C et al: A new animal model for maxillary sinus floor augmentation: evaluation parameters, *Int J Oral Maxillofac Implants* 12:403-415, 1997.

Kurita K et al: Osteoplasty of the mandibular condyle with preservation of the articular soft tissue cover: comparison of fibrin sealant and sutures for fixation of the articular soft tissue cover in rabbits, *Oral Surg Oral Med Oral Pathol* 69(6):661-667, 1990.

Langer B, Langer L: The overlapped flap: a surgical modification for implant fixture installation, *Int J Perio Restor Dent* 10:209, 1990.

Lazzara RJ: *Sinus lift for treatment of the posterior maxilla.* Lecture presented to the American Academy of Periodontology Implant Conference, Chicago, July 16, 1994.

Lee DR, Lemons J, LeGeros RZ: Dissolution characterization of commercially available hydroxylapatite particulate, *Trans Soc Biomater* 12:161, 1989.

Leghissa G, Botticelli A: Resistance to bacterial aggression involving exposed nonresorbable membranes in the oral cavity, *Int J Oral Maxillofac Implants* 11(2):210-215, 1996.

Linkow LI: Bone transplants using the symphysis, the iliac crest and synthetic bone materials, *J Oral Implant* 11:211-247, 1983.

Listrom RD, Symington JM: Osseointegrated dental implants in conjunction with bone grafts, *J Oral Maxillofac Surg* 17:116-118, 1988.

Lozada JL et al: Surgical repair of peri-implant defects, *J Oral Implantol* 16:42-46, 1990.

Lundgren S et al: Augmentation of the maxillary sinus floor with particulated mandible: a histologic and histomorphometric study, *Int J Oral Maxillofac Implants* 11(6):760-766, 1996.

Martinowitz U et al: Dental extraction for patients on oral anticoagulant therapy.

Marx RE et al: The use of freeze-dried allogenic bone in oral and maxillofacial surgery, *J Oral Surg* 39:264-274, 1981.

Marx RE: Principles of hard/and soft tissue reconstruction of the jaws, Abstract ML 315, American Association of Oral and Maxillofacial Surgeons, New Orleans, 1990.

Mehlisch DR et al: Evaluation of collagen/hydroxyapatite for augmenting deficient alveolar ridges: a preliminary report, *J Oral Maxillofac Surg* 45:408-413, 1987.

Mercier P et al: Long-term results of mandibular ridge augmentation by visor steotomy with bone graft, *J Oral Maxillofac Surg* 45:997-1003, 1987.

Misch C: *Alveolar ridge augmentations,* American Academy of Implant Dentistry, Western District, Las Vegas, Nevada, March 29, 1985.

Misch C: Comparison of intraoral donor sites for onlay grafting prior to implant placement, *Int J Oral Maxillofac Implants* 12:767-77, 1997.

Misch C: Density of bone: effect on treatment plan, surgical approach, healing, and progressive bone loading, *Int J Oral Implantol* 6:23-31, 1990.

Misch CE: Maxillary sinus augmentation for endosteal implants. Organized alternative treatment plants, *Int J Oral Maxillofac Implants* 4:49-58, 1987.

Misch CM, Misch CE, Resnick RR et al: Reconstruction of maxillary alveolar defects with mandibular symphysis grafts for dental implants: a preliminary procedural report, *Int J Oral Maxillofac Implants* 7:360-366, 1992.

Misch CM, Misch CE: Mandibular symphysis bone grafts for placement of endosteal implant, in press.

Misch CM: The pharmacologic management of maxillary sinus elevation surgery, *J Oral Implant* 18:15-23, 1992.

Mulliken JB et al: Use of demineralized anogenic bone implants for the correction of maxillocraniofacial deformities, *Ann Surg* 194:366-372, 1981.

Nique T et al: Particulate allogenic bone grafts into maxillary alveolar clefts in humans: a preliminary report, *Int J Oral Maxillofac Surg* 45:386-392, 1987.

Novaes Jr A, Novaes B: Soft tissue management for primary closure in guided bone regeneration: surgical technique and case report, *Int J Oral Maxillofac Implants* 12:84-87, 1997.

Nyman et al: Bone regeneration adjacent to titanium dental implants using guided tissue regeneration: a report of two cases, *Int J Oral Maxillofac Implants* 5:9-14, 1990.

Oberg S, Kahnberg KE: Combined use of hydroxyapatite and Tisseel in experimental bone defects in the rabbit, *Swed Dent J* 17(4):147-153, 1993.

Palmqvist S et al: Marginal bone levels around maxillary implants supporting overdentures or fixed prostheses: a comparative study using detailed narrow-beam radiographs, *Int J Oral Maxillofac Implants* 11(2):223-227, 1996.

Picton DC: In Melcher AH, Bown WH, editors: *Biology of the periodontum,* New York, 1969, Academic Press, pp 363-419.

Pietrowkowski J, Massler M: Alveolar ridge resorption following tooth extraction, *J Prosthet Dent* 17:21-27, 1967.

Plattelli A et al: Histologic analysis of the interface of a titanium implant retrieved from a nonvascularized mandibular block graft after a 10-month loading period, *Int J Oral Maxillofac Implants* 12:840-844, 1997.

Raborn GW et al: Tisseel, a two component fibrin tissue sealant system: report of a trial involving anticoagulated dental patients, *J Can Dent Assoc* 56(8):779-781, 1990.

Rakocz M et al: Dental extractions in patients with bleeding disorders. The use of fibrin glue, *Oral Surg Oral Med Oral Pathol* 75(3):280-282, 1993.

Rejda BV, Peelen JCJ, Grot K: Tricalcium phosphate as a bone substitute, *Bioengineering* 1:93, 1977.

Roberts WE et al: Bone physiology and metabolism, *J Calif Dent Assoc* 15:54-61, 1987.

Roberts WE: Bone tissue interface, *J Dent Educ* 52:804-809, 1988.

Sabiston Jr DC, Spencer FC: Thoracic incisions, *Surgery of the Chest* 1:213-214, W.B. Saunders Company, Sixth Edition.

Sawaki Y et al: Mandibular lengthening by intraoral distraction using osseointegrated implants, *Int J Oral Maxillofac Implants* 11(2):186-193, 1996.

Schliephake H: Vertical ridge augmentation using polyactic membranes in conjunction with immediate implants in periodontally compromised extraction sites: an experimental study in dogs, *Int J Oral Maxillofac Implants* 12:325-335, 1997.

Schon R et al: Peri-implant tissue reaction in bone irradiated the fifth day after implantation in rabbits: histologic and histomorphometric measurements, *Int J Oral Maxillofac Implants* 11(2):228-238, 1996.

Schwarz N et al: Early osteoinduction in rats is not altered by fibrin sealant, *Clin Orthop* 293:353-359, 1993.

Sharawy M: *Altografts and bone formation,* International Congress of Oral Implant, World Meeting, London, May 1991.

Sierra DH: Fibrin sealant adhesive systems: a review of their chemistry, material properties and clinical applications, *J Biomater Appl* 7(4):309-352, 1993.

Simion M et al: Treatment of dehiscences and fenestrations around dental implants using resorbable and nonresorbable membranes associated with bone autografts: a comparative clinical study, *Int J Oral Maxillofac Implants* 12:159-165, 1997.

Simion M et al: Guided bone regeneration using resorbable and nonresorbable membranes: a comparative histologic study in humans, *Int J Oral Maxillofac Implants* 11(6):735-742, 1996.

Sindet-Pederson S, Enemark H: Mandibular bone grafts for reconstruction of alveolar clefts, *J Oral Maxillofac Surg* 46:533-537, 1988.

Smiler DG, Johnson PW, Lozada JL: Sinus lift grafts and endosseous implants, *Dent Clin North Am* 36(1):151-186, 1992.

Stanley H et al: Using 45S5 bioglass cones as endosseous ridge maintenance implants to prevent alveolar ridge resorption: a 5-year evaluation, *Int J Oral Maxillofac Implants* 95:1-5, 1997.

Summers RB: A new concept in maxillary implant surgery: the osteotome technique, *Compend Cont Educ Dent* 15:152-160, 1994.

Summers RB: The osteotome technique. II. The ridge expansion osteotomy (REO) procedure, *Compend Cont Educ Dent* 15:422-434, 1994.

Summers RB: The osteotome technique. III. Less invasive methods of elevating the sinus floor, *Compend Cont Educ Dent* 15:698-708, 1994.

Summers RB: The osteotome technique. IV. Future site development, *Comp Cont Educ Dent* 15:1090-1099, 1995.

Swart JN, Allard RHB: Subperiosteal onlay augmentation of the mandible: a clinical and radiographic survey, *J Oral Maxillofac Surg* 43:183-187, 1985.

Tatum H: Maxillary and sinus implant reconstructions, *Dent Clin North Am* 30:207-229, 1986.

Tatum OH Jr: Lecture presented to Alabama Implant Study Group, 1977.

Tatum OH Jr: Maxillary and sinus implant reconstructions, *Dent Clin North Am* 30:207-229, 1986.

Trombelli L et al: Combined guided tissue regeneration, root conditioning, and fibrin-fibronectin system application in the treatment of gingival recession. A 15-case report, *J Periodontol* 65(8):796-803, 1994.

Urist MR et al: The bone induction principle, *Clin Orthop* 53:243-283, 1967.

Vaillancourt H, Pilliar R, McCammond D: Factors affecting crestal bone loss with dental implants partially covered with a porous coating: a finite element analysis, *Int J Oral Maxillofac Implants* 11:351-360, 1996.

Von Arx T, Hardt N, Wallkamm B: The TIME Technique: a new method for localized alveolar ridge augmentation prior to placement of dental implants, *Int J Oral Maxillofac Implants* 11:387-395, 1996.

Wagner JR: A clinical and histological case study using resorbable hydroxyapatite for the repair of osseous defects prior to endossesous implant surgery, *J Oral Implantol* 15:186-193, 1989.

Wheeler S, Holmes R, Calhoun C: Six-year clinical and histologic study of sinus-lift grafts, *Int J Oral Maxillofac Implants* 11:26-34, 1996.

Whittaker JM et al: Histological response and clinical evaluation of heterograft and allograft materials in the elevation of the maxillary sinus for the preparation of endosteal dental implant sites. Simultaneous sinus elevation and root form implantation: an eight-month autopsy report, *J Oral Implantol* 15:141-144, 1989.

Williams PL, Warwick R: *Gray's anatomy,* ed 36, Philadelphia, 1980, WB Saunders.

Williamson R: Rehabilitation of the resorbed maxilla and mandible using autogenous bone grafts and osseointegrated implants, *Int J Oral Maxillofac Implants* 11:476-489, 1996.

Wood RM, Moore DL: Grafting of the maxillary sinus with intraorally harvested autogenous bone prior to implant placement, *J Oral Maxillofac Implants* 3:209-213, 1988.

Youse T, Brooks SL: The appearance of mental foramina on panoramic and periapical radiographs, *Oral Surg Oral Med Oral Pathol* 68:488-492, 1989.

Zitzmann N, Naef R, Scharer P: Resorbable versus nonresorbable membranes in combination with Bio-Oss for guided bone regeneration, *Int J Oral Maxillofac Implants* 12:844-855, 1997.

Zohar Y et al: Human fibrin glue in head and neck surgery, *Harefuah* 126(10):567-570, May 1994. Hebrew.

Zusman SP et al: Postextraction hemostasis in patients on anticoagulant therapy: the use of a fibrin sealant, *Quintessence* 23(10):713-716, 1992.

9

Root Form Implant Surgery: Generic

ARMAMENTARIUM

Boley gauge
Bougies, whalebone, olive-tipped, or lacrimal probes
Bur extender, mandrel (internal irrigation) (to be used when
    adjacent teeth prevent direct access to bone)
Calipers
Colla Cote
Colla Plug
Console, motor, and handpiece
Depth gauge
Disposable bur length markers, Disposaboots (yellow)
Implant system of choice with bone taps (if implant is not self-
    tapping), counter-sink (if required), final sizing drills, and
    try-ins
Millimeter rule
Paralleling pins (double-ended), small and large (Brasseler/Cranin)
Pilot drill (1.6 × 11 mm) with internal irrigation
    (Brasseler/Cranin): 1.6, 2, 2.5, 3, and 3.5 mm, bispade drills,
    16 mm long, each with internal irrigation (Brasseler/Cranin)
    All drills over 3.5 mm in diameter should be selected in relation to
    the specific system selected
Starter burs (No. 2 round)
Surgical instrument set
Surgical template (guide for implant placement)

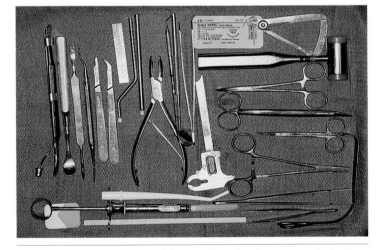

The armamentarium required for root form implant surgery includes a
standard set of instruments in addition to calipers, gauge, mallet, and
implant-seating devices.

Before undertaking the placement of any type of root form
implant, read this section in its entirety. It lists the introductory techniques of insertion for all types of root forms. In addition, recommendations are found in the tables of Chapter 4 for
the selection of a wide variety of implant designs. Techniques
for the placement of the specific proprietary designs follow in
Chapters 10 and 11. First in this section is the generic step-by-
step technique for root form implant insertion. The illustrations and explanatory notes demonstrate the procedure in a se-

quence that starts with gingival incision and ends at a point that
satisfies the introductory requirements for all systems. The final
osteotomies and techniques for specific implant insertions are
described in the following sections. If the instructions in this
chapter are followed, a "generic" root form implant can be
inserted and uncovered. That is, these steps are identical for
most root form systems. After acquiring an understanding
of each maneuver refer to Chapter 4. Its charts describe most
of today's implant varieties, their general grouping, material

CAVEATS

All endosteal implant procedures demand that care be exercised to avoid impairing vital structures. The use of infiltration anesthesia in the mandible helps guide drilling depths when approaching the mandibular canal, since the patient will report lip tingling. Slow drilling keeps intraosseous temperatures at safe levels. Saline irrigants can be chilled preoperatively to contribute to temperature control. Plan implant placement with impeccable care; direct drills accurately as assisted by using paralleling pins and intraoperative radiographs. Avoid perforations of cortical plates. Systems that supply backup (or larger) implant diameters are of value in case an oversized osteotomy is made (see Chapter 28 for specifics). Mark burs and drills with the number of times used and discarded when dull. Pump bone drills vertically (not in an arc) in order to introduce copious irrigant and to encourage straight osteotomies. Do not use pressure when preparing osteotomies, but rather allow the drills to find their own way. In systems that require bone tapping, the use of a ratchet wrench by hand is preferable. Avoid this step completely if the bone is compliant enough to permit the implant to tap itself to place (e.g., Nobel Biocare, 3i, Paragon). This level of pliability is found most frequently in maxillae. In the planning stages, prepare a surgical template for implant placement (see Chapter 4 and the following paragraphs in this chapter). Sometimes even the most careful planning does not yield satisfactory results because the bony ridge is not found directly below the soft tissues. The surgeon must be versatile enough to alter the positions and angles of the implants at the time of surgery. Review root form selection procedures (see Chapter 4) for information on manufacturers' drilling speeds recommended for different implant systems. Particularly in maxillae but in less dense mandibles as well, some of the preparatory steps (i.e., tapping or "threading" the bone and use of the final sizing drill and the counter-sink drill) may be eliminated. The implant can serve to seat itself and to thread and counter-sink the host-site bone.

and design characteristics, surface finishes, methods of primary retention (during the "integration" period), and basic restorative options. There are several systems that offer implants with diameters of 3.25 and 3.3 mm (small diameter). Especially in the maxillae, such implants often may be inserted after use of the 3-mm drill without the formality of tapping, enlarging, or counter-sinking. Diameters of drills should be increased in increments of 0.5 mm only (Brookdale Generic System). Bone density is a determining factor, as are internal irrigation, drill speed, torque, and bur sharpness. The smaller each gradua-tion of bur size, the less heat and trauma is generated to the host site and the more accurate the osteotomy. Not all systems supply all drill sizes. Different manufacturers supply a variety of sizes that may be selected to complete an entire generic set. For example, Nobelbiocare does not manufacture burs or a console that supply internal irrigation; Calcitek recommends a round starter bur (the rosette); and Brasseler supplies graduated-diameter, internally irrigated spade drills. Unless a computed tomography (CT) scan is available, the actual bone dimensions are known only at the time of flap reflection, and they dictate where the implants can be placed and what sizes should be chosen. However, significant benefit accrues to the surgeon who uses a surgical guide or template so that the ideal locations for all implants are presented clearly where bone dimensions can accommodate them.

Surgical Templates

As more experience is gained, it is found that the same template may be used not only for radiographic diagnosis (Chapter 4), but also for surgical placement and even for uncovering the implants. Surgical template fabrication is a necessary step in the planning and placement of implants. Its design is based on the anatomic, prosthetic, and esthetic situations with which the surgeon is confronted. If, as discussed in Chapter 4, a diagnostic, 5-mm ball-imbedded Omnivac template is available and each ball has been processed at a potential implant site, the simple removing of the balls permits the device to be used as an implant site locator. However, one may fabricate a template to be used specifically for intraoperative guidance. One of three possible template types can be made: these include single tooth replacement or edentulous spans between natural teeth, free-end saddle edentulous areas, and completely edentulous sites.

Single Tooth Replacement or Edentulous Spans Between Natural Teeth

Begin the process of single tooth replacement by marking a cast at the ideal location for the implant. Sticky-wax a denture tooth into place. Then make an Omnivac shell using 0.02-inch clear material. After the material has cooled, trim the plastic to include at least two teeth on either side of the operative area. In the edentulous area, shorten those parts of the appliance that extend buccally and lingually beyond the points of flap retraction (approximately 6 mm). Remove the denture tooth and snip away the occlusal and lingual surfaces of the denture teeth area with a fine shears. The device should be cold sterilized and placed into position over the bone after flap retraction. The teeth on either side of the host site will stabilize it, and it serves as an efficient surgical guide (Fig. 9-1).

Free-end Saddle Edentulous Areas

Make a free-end saddle template in the same way as the single tooth design with the following minor changes. Include four or more teeth anterior to the edentulous area in the Omnivac, and extend the shell margin posteriorly past the anticipated distal extent of the incision line. This allows it to be stabilized by a large number of anterior teeth and by its position on the soft tissues posteriorly, which are not to be elevated (e.g., tuberosity retromolar pad) even after flap reflection.

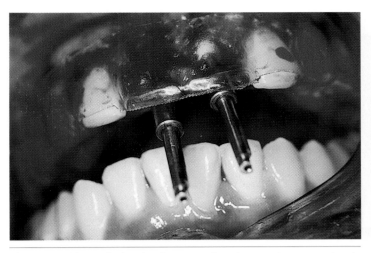

Fig. 9-1 When placing implants as pier abutments, use a simple Omnivac guidance device.

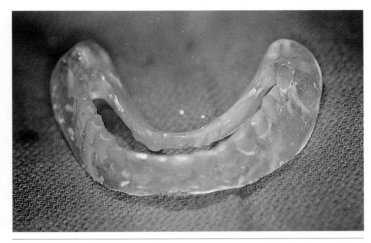

Fig. 9-2 The processed acrylic resin surgical template has its occlusal surface and lingual flange opened and the proposed implant sites exposed. The labial tooth surfaces remain as guides to the surgeon.

Completely Edentulous Sites

For completely edentulous sites, fabricate a new denture at least to the wax try-in stage. If an existing removable denture is being converted or an original full denture is to be used, reline it with a chairside material such as Viscogel. Next, flask the denture using Kentosil in a denture duplicator with petroleum jelly (Vaseline) as a lubricant. Remove the denture and pour clear acrylic resin into its place. Close the flask, and permit the resin to polymerize. On removing it from the elastomer, it is found to be a duplicate of the original denture, made of clear acrylic. Trim and polish the borders. In the areas to be implanted, cut away the lingual and occlusal aspects of the teeth with a bur in the form of a U-shaped trough; leave

the incisal and facial surfaces intact. The fenestrated area denotes the sites at which the implants are to be placed in order to satisfy the reconstructive and aesthetic needs of the case. Individual holes can be made, although this may prove to be too restrictive. The clear labial surfaces permit direct viewing during the preparation for osteotomies (Fig. 9-2). This not only ensures proper angulations, but also presents evidence that the transepithelial abutments (TEAs) emerge from the most optimal areas, such as the cingula of incisors and the occlusal surfaces of molars. After this use, these templates are subsequently of value. They can be used again to point out the site of each implant at the time of uncovering so that there will be no additional need to perform a major reflection of the overlying gingivae.

Surgical Techniques

Anesthetize the patient using an infiltration technique. Make a crestal incision directly to bone with adequate relief at either end and reflect the mucoperiosteum, exposing the bony operative site (Fig. 9-3, *A, B*). Assess the bone. If the ridge is too narrow (i.e., knife-edged), determine if it can be flattened to an acceptable width and still have sufficient depth to accommodate an implant. If so, use the side-cutting rongeur forceps, followed by a small, round vulcanite bur or a fissure type with irrigation (Fig. 9-3, *C*). Perform final smoothing with a bone file (Fig. 9-3, *D*). If the narrow ridge cannot be corrected but enough depth exists, consider ridge augmentation (see Chapter 8) or placement of a blade implant (see Chapter 12). When the ridge is prepared and measurements indicate adequate width (i.e., at least 5.25 mm) (Fig. 9-3, *E*), make the osteotomies. As an alternative, ridge-widening procedures may be undertaken (see Chapter 8). (It must be kept in mind that implants must be spaced one full width apart.) Place a colored sleeve on the shaft of each drill at the level of the planned depth of each osteotomy (Fig. 9-4). Yellow Disposaboots currently are used. The drill tip is made to pierce the rounded

end and the sleeve slid up the shaft to mark the proper length. Place the sterilized clear acrylic or Omnivac surgical template into the patient's mouth. Trim its flanges so that they will nestle comfortably beneath the reflected flaps of tissue. In this position they keep the flaps reflected. Stabilize the template with the host bone appearing directly beneath the U-shaped window. Set the starter bur (No. 2 round) in the center of each proposed implant site and rotate it into the cortex only. Use copious coolant despite the fact that most starter burs are not equipped for internal irrigation. For each planned implant, make a similar starter hole and then deepen it just through the cortex (Fig. 9-5, *A*). Follow the starter bur with the pilot drill, which is 1.6 mm in diameter and internally irrigated, to its full depth of 11 mm unless a shorter implant length is planned (Fig. 9-5, *B*). In such cases, place a colored sleeve on the drill shank to mark the appropriate length. The proper angulation must be achieved in the first osteotomy. It is imperative to check on the accuracy of dimension and location by taking an intraoperative radiograph of the first pilot drill in position (Fig. 9-5, *C-E*). If satisfactory, place another bur or a 1.6-mm-

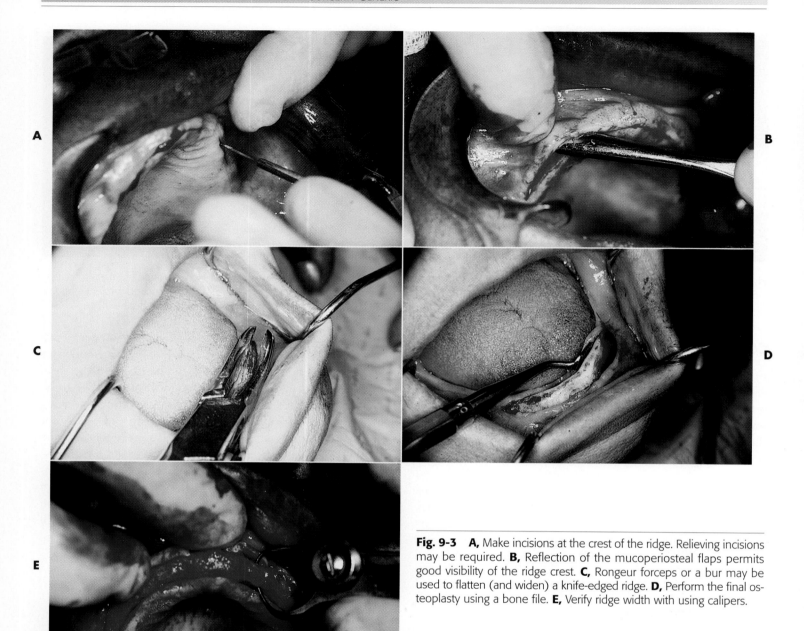

Fig. 9-3 **A,** Make incisions at the crest of the ridge. Relieving incisions may be required. **B,** Reflection of the mucoperiosteal flaps permits good visibility of the ridge crest. **C,** Rongeur forceps or a bur may be used to flatten (and widen) a knife-edged ridge. **D,** Perform the final osteoplasty using a bone file. **E,** Verify ridge width with using calipers.

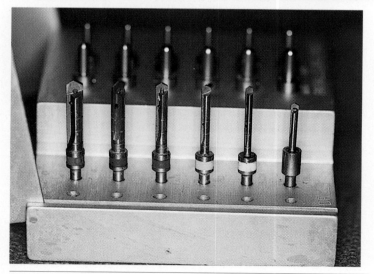

Fig. 9-4 Brasseler bispade drills, internally irrigated, with colored depth markers. They are: 1.6 x 11 mm; 1.6 x 16 mm; 2.0 x 16 mm; 2.5 x 16 mm; 3.0 x 16 mm; 3.5 x 16 mm.

diameter paralleling pin in the first osteotomy as a directional guide. If the pin demonstrates a proper orientation to the eye, leave it in position and with the guidance of the template, make the osteotomy for the second implant with the pilot drill. Parallelism should be created between the two osteotomies. Place a second bur or paralleling pin in this hole (Fig. 9-5, *F*). In this fashion make all the osteotomies at 1.6-mm diameters to the 11-mm (or appropriate) depth, striving for continued parallelism and acceptable angulation. By use of this system, which includes internal irrigation throughout, complete the entire series of pilot holes and verify by placing a paralleling pin into each. Use the template throughout to verify the location and accuracy of each site (Fig. 9-6). Each osteotomy may require deepening, which is done by removing the first bur (which was being used as a guide pin) and using a 1.6-mm hollow core, 16-mm long spade drill (with a yellow Disposaboot depth marker placed on its shank if necessary). Attach it to the

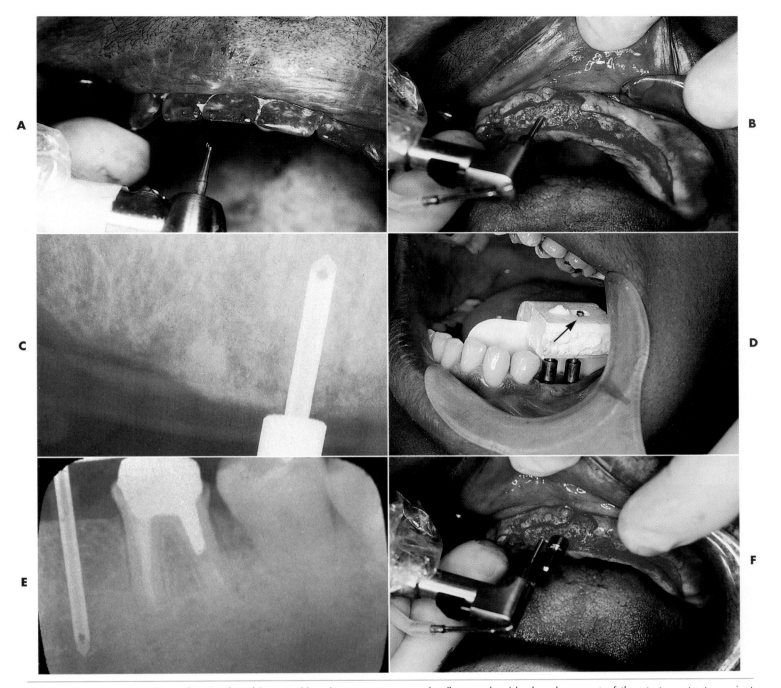

Fig. 9-5 **A,** The surgical template is placed into position; it serves to retract the flaps and guide the placement of the starter osteotomy, just through the cortex. **B,** Make the second step with the 1.6-mm pilot drill at the proper angulation and site, for distances of up to 11 mm. **C,** Take an intraoperative radiograph to confirm length and location of the pilot drill. **D,** Use intraoperative radiographs in all instances when nerves are in the vicinity of host sites. A simple technique, which maintains sterililty and keeps the patient's hand out of the field, uses a gas-sterilized Styrofoam film holder, maintained in position by paralleling pins or burs that pierce its soft block *(arrow)*. **E,** The resulting film offers evidence of safe progress during the operation, as well as accuracy of distances, parallelism, and positioning. The first 1.6-mm diameter drill, if satisfactory, facilitates a simple and flawless operation. **F,** Place pins into each osteotomy to preserve continuing parallelism of adjacent bone cuts.

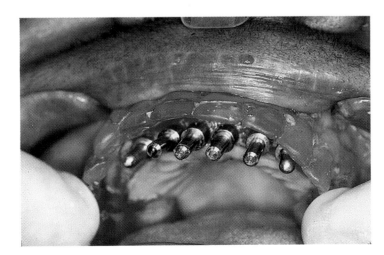

Fig. 9-6 Ascertain final positioning of the 1.6-mm-diameter osteotomies by placing all pins, which should lie within the confines of the template.

internal/external irrigation supply and rotate it at the lowest speed that permits it to cut. Observe care during this step because it is still remotely possible to deviate from the direction of the starter osteotomies. Enter the bone with the drill already turning. Requisite speeds vary depending on the torque of the motor, the bone density, the sharpness of the flutes or spades, and the pressure applied by the surgeon's hand. Maintain parallelism to the remaining pins. Drive this 16-mm-long drill to the full depth of the planned implant. When drilling, use a gentle vertical pumping action to permit maximum coolant effect and minimal bone trauma. However, do not allow the wrist to move in an arc, although there is a natural tendency for most clinicians to do so early in their experience. Each gentle application of force must be strictly vertical. Keep the wrist rigid, and generate movements from the elbow. Withdraw drills from the bone while rotating, not after they have stopped. When the planned number of osteotomies has been completed, each parallel to the others, and all to the proper depth using the 1.6-mm-diameter spade drill, repeat the cycle exactly in the same manner using the 2-, 2.5-, and 3-mm drills. Use paralleling pins at each step for continued verification. There are systems that suggest the use of guide drills (3i, Nobel Biocare, and Steri-Oss). These types of drills have protruding 2-mm-diameter guide pins that discourage deviations from the starting angulations (Fig. 9-7, *A*). If used at the 2-mm osteotomy size, the smooth end enters flawlessly and guides the drill's direction, permitting its cutting portion to enlarge the superficial half of the osteotomy to a diameter of 3 mm. Follow this with a full-length 3-mm drill, which quite naturally finds its path to the full depth. This incremental change, however, exceeds a safe increase of 0.5 mm, so its use is to be discouraged. Rather, if one moves from a starter drill of 1.6 mm to the larger diameters at 0.5-mm increments (Fig. 9-7, *B*), it becomes virtually impossible to deviate from the direction of the pilot hole, so that the counterbore is not necessary. In addition to this safety feature, small increments cause less bone damage and maintain bur sharpness for longer periods of time. For systems that have larger-diameter implants, the same scheme should continue to 3.5 and 4-mm-diameter generic drills. The final diameter of the planned implants determines the largest-diameter drills to use (Fig. 9-8, *A*). They should be from 0.25 to 0.5 mm smaller than the implants so that the final proprietary sizing drill for the selected implant may be used to complete the osteotomy. The drills for the standard generic set are available from companies like Brasseler and Imcor. Although most are identified on their shanks as to diameter, always use a sterile Boley gauge for verifying the measurement of each drill before its use. This ensures that an oversized cut is not made inadvertently (Fig. 9-8, *B*). At this point, initiate the specific steps necessary for the

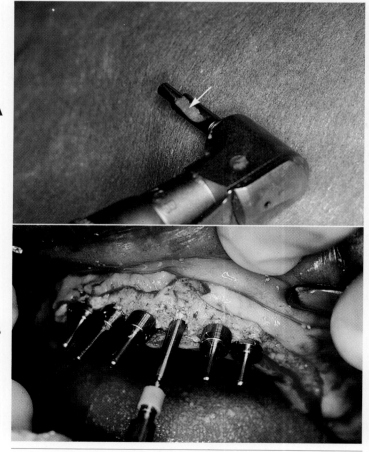

Fig. 9-7 **A,** The guide drill has a smooth end that permits its atraumatic entry into the 1.6-mm diameter osteotomy and allows a fail-safe enlargement to 2 mm. Note bone *(arrow)* embedded in drill flute. This debris, when saved, serves as a source of osteogenic graft material. **B,** Increments of 0.5-mm-diameter spade drills at each step preserve accuracy and enlarge the bone slowly and safely.

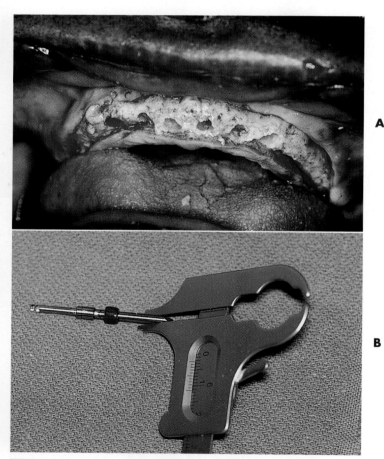

Fig. 9-8 **A,** The last generic step before creating the manufacturer-specific osteotomy is the completion of 3- or 3.5-mm-diameter implant sites of the appropriate depth. **B,** Double-check drill diameters with a Boley gauge.

seating of one of the three major types of root form implants. After reading the following paragraphs, refer to chapters 10 and 11, which describe the specific steps required to place the various implants, starting with the first step after the use of the generic system.

Threaded Pre-tapping Implants

Threaded pre-tapping implant systems (e.g., Steri-Oss, Nobel Biocare, 3i, Paragon, Lifecore) supply the user with taps or threaders, which, if the bone is hard, should be used once and then discarded. After completing the use of a generic drill of a diameter of 0.25 to 0.5 mm less than the planned implant, insert the tap into the osteotomy and rotate it, when possible, with a handheld ratchet, wheel, or wrench (Fig. 9-9, A). If the

progress becomes too difficult, use an ultra low tapping speed (i.e., 5 to 10 rpm) motor drive (Fig. 9-9, B). Conversely, if the progress appears to be too easy, remove the tap and substitute the implant itself as its own bone tap. The same rule applies for the counter-sink drill (Fig. 9-9, C). If the bone is compliant, do not use the counter-sink. Instead, permit the implant to fully seat itself (Fig. 9-9, D). After the threading is completed, carefully back out the tap with great care. Hand pressure should be minimal. The hand is used only to guide the direction of unthreading the bone tap. The pitch of the threads should be depended on to influence its removal from the bone. Placement of the implant follows, again using the handheld ratchet or the ultra–low-speed motor with irrigation (Fig. 9-9, E). Some of the more finely threaded systems demand the development of an even greater skilled tactile sense,

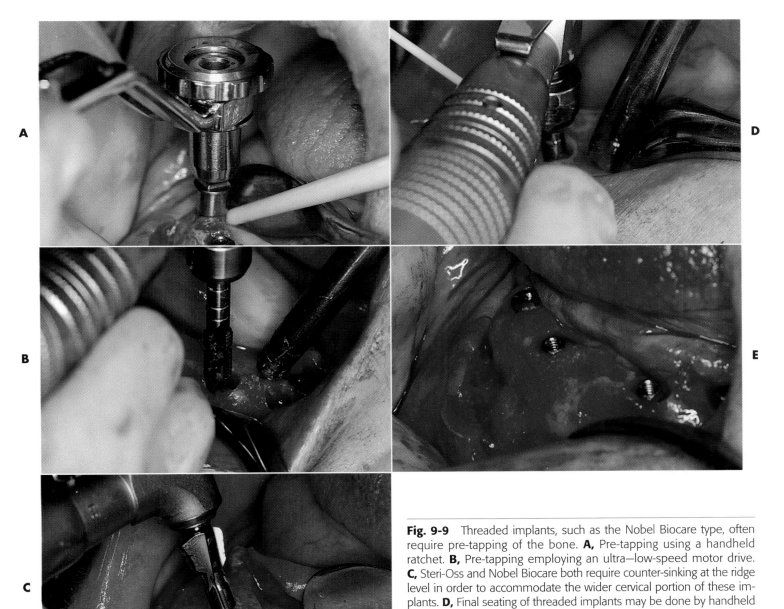

Fig. 9-9 Threaded implants, such as the Nobel Biocare type, often require pre-tapping of the bone. **A,** Pre-tapping using a handheld ratchet. **B,** Pre-tapping employing an ultra–low-speed motor drive. **C,** Steri-Oss and Nobel Biocare both require counter-sinking at the ridge level in order to accommodate the wider cervical portion of these implants. **D,** Final seating of threaded implants may be done by handheld wheel or ratchet wrench, or, as shown, by using an ultra–low-speed handpiece. **E,** Final seating of these implants must demonstrate that they are flush with the surrounding bone.

which requires experience. Early efforts may result in stripping the bone threads. The surgical team must be prepared with larger threaded sizes or press-fit implants to serve as backups. It is wise to start bone tapping using handheld wheels and if resistance is met, ratchet wrenches with lever arms. A much greater sense of touch the procedure is transferred to the surgeon's fingers using the wheel handle as compared with the ratchet wrench. Even less is perceived with the motor and handpiece.

Threaded Self-tapping Implants

Threaded self-tapping implant systems (e.g., Paragon and Nobelbiocare self-tap) are simpler to place than implants requiring pre-tapping. After use of the final bone drill, 0.5 mm smaller in diameter than the implant itself, tap the implant into the unthreaded osteotomy using a handheld ratchet wrench (Fig. 9-10). As an antitorque influence, exert firm pressure in an apical direction with the forefinger of the other hand. Threaded self-tapping implants present a more satisfactory tactile experience to the less initiated practitioner and are recommended to those just entering the field. If the threads become stripped, a number of companies make backup sizes of larger diameters.

Nonthreaded Press-fit Implants

There are several systems (IMZ, Calcitek, Lifecore, and Biovent) of nonthreaded, press-fit implants. The technique is easier and no threading is required, but sometimes the final sizing drill is just slightly too large. Whenever possible, the try-in implant (a stainless steel replica) should be tapped to place

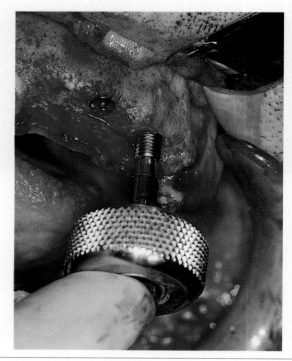

Fig. 9-10 Self-tapping implants, such as this Paragon Screw-vent, find their own way into the bone when a handheld ratchet is used to tighten them.

with a mallet after the next to the final drill has been used (Fig. 9-11, *A*). If the try-in goes to place, eliminate the last manufacturer-recommended step and use light mallet taps to seat the implant itself (Fig. 9-11, *B, C*). Refer to chapters 10 and 11 for the final osteotomy steps required for each system before final implantation (Fig. 9-11, *D*). On completion of each step, verify accuracy with the depth gauge and paralleling pins. After the implants have been fully seated, place healing screws into the implant chambers, which are either smooth or threaded (Fig. 9-12). Some implants are available with healing screws already inserted. Often they require tightening with an Allen wrench. Other brands supply the screws in the hollow caps used to cover the containers in which the implants are delivered. Still others offer them in separate sterile packages.

A valuable maneuver in placing implants in maxillae and softer mandibular areas is to eliminate the final step in the osteotomy preparation recommended by the manufacturers. In less dense bone, the use of the final sizing drill, threadtapper, or counter-sink is not only unnecessary, it frequently creates an oversized osteotomy, causing an unstable implant or necessitating the use of the next largest diameter (or backup sized) implant. It is imperative to have good frictional fit after the implant is seated fully. If the implant is loose as a result of an oversized osteotomy, there are several companies that make larger-diameter implants that can address this problem. Nobel Biocare and 3i make 4-mm-diameter implants in cases when the threads made for the 3.75-mm implants become stripped (Fig. 9-13, *A*). Steri-Oss makes a press-fit implant for the same osteotomy as their threaded (3.9-mm-diameter) implant, should the threads become stripped (Fig. 9-13, *B*). Most root form systems supply implants of varying diameters to serve this emergency function (Fig. 9-13, *C*). Use larger implants if bone dimensions permit it. When selecting a root form implant, allow the benefits of a backup system to influence him or her. If a system does not supply this salutary feature, find a compatible system to serve as backup (see Table 4-2). For stripped bony threads, use a larger threaded implant or a press-fit implant to fit the osteotomy. For a loose press-fit implant, replacement with a larger press-fit or larger threaded implant is advised. Closures are best made using the continuous horizontal mattress suture configuration. Instruct patients in proper postoperative care, which is detailed in Appendix H.

When molars are to be replaced by implants, the ideal goal is to place a long, thin implant for each mandibular root and, when feasible, one for each maxillary buccal root. Although the space is often limited and impression making may present the problems of fitting closely placed copings, the force distribution will be improved when multiple implants are used (Fig. 9-13, *D, E*).

Single implants in such sites present cervical diameters that even at 6 mm, fall far short of the dimensions of the molar being replaced. The result presents the problems of concentrated occlusal forces, exceptionally large and annoying embrasures, and a lack of acceptable esthetics. Even the extra-large esthetic abutments fail to satisfy the anatomic demands made by the molar operative site.

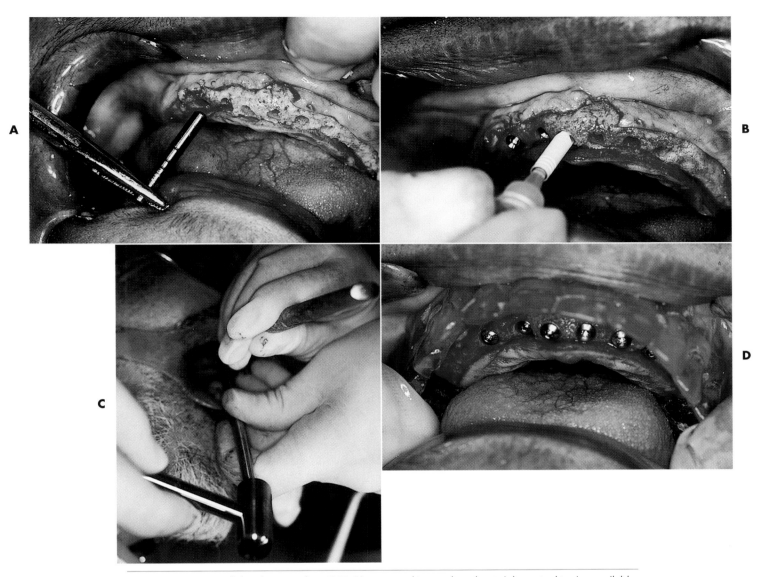

Fig. 9-11   **A,** Press-fit implants, such as IMZ, Biovent, and Integral, make stainless steel try-ins available. When these are tapped into slightly undersized osteotomies, they create very accurate host sites for firm frictional fit. **B,** Some press-fit implants may be removed from their packages by the cover, which also serves as an insertion handle. **C,** After a press-fit can be introduced no farther with finger pressure, it may be inserted more deeply by tapping. **D,** These implants are in position, with the template serving as an indicator of their accurate placement. Healing caps have been placed into the three on the patient's left side.

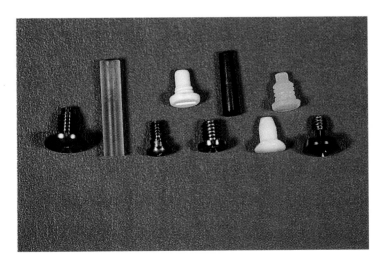

Fig. 9-12   Assorted healing caps and screws made of titanium and polyethylene. Some are threaded, and others snap into position.

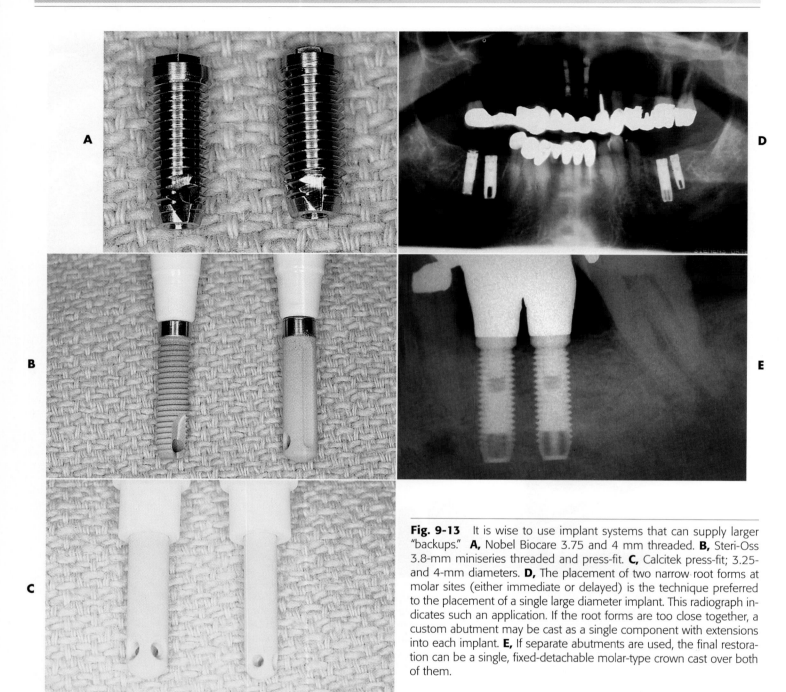

Fig. 9-13 It is wise to use implant systems that can supply larger "backups." **A,** Nobel Biocare 3.75 and 4 mm threaded. **B,** Steri-Oss 3.8-mm miniseries threaded and press-fit. **C,** Calcitek press-fit; 3.25- and 4-mm diameters. **D,** The placement of two narrow root forms at molar sites (either immediate or delayed) is the technique preferred to the placement of a single large diameter implant. This radiograph indicates such an application. If the root forms are too close together, a custom abutment may be cast as a single component with extensions into each implant. **E,** If separate abutments are used, the final restoration can be a single, fixed-detachable molar-type crown cast over both of them.

Immediate Placement of Root Form Implants into Extraction Sites or Former Implant Sites

Although the usual site for implantation of endosteal implants is in well-healed and adequately contoured ridges, there is considerable value in placing them into alveoli immediately after extractions (Fig. 9-14). This offers the following benefits:

1. Combining integration of the implant with mineralization of the socket shortens healing time.
2. Preservation of ridge morphology and dimension is encouraged by the presence of an implant.

3. Position and angulation of the implant is simpler because the recently removed tooth indicates this geometry, and the walls of the alveolus serve as guides in directing the osteotomy.

Certain precautions must be observed. The location and angulation of the tooth to be replaced must be correct. It is difficult to attempt to alter the direction of a socket because of its generally thin cortical plates. Such an alteration may be done, however, even if a buccal or labial cortical plate perforation is created. If part of the implant protrudes through the fenestration, a particulate bone substitute material may be added and covered with a guided tissue regeneration mem-

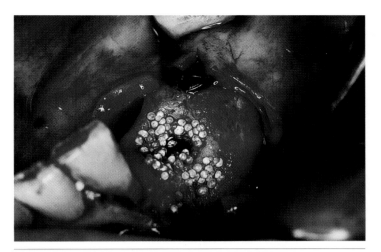

Fig. 9-14 Implants may be placed immediately into extraction sockets, but defects must be augmented with grafting materials and often require coverage with guided tissue membranes.

brane (GTRM). Techniques using membranes and grafting materials are found in Chapter 8.

Ensure total freedom from soft tissue, granulomas, and other infectious debris. This involves thorough use of a No. 15 BP blade, sharp curettes, and small curved mosquito hemostats. Use the scalpel blade to make a 360-degree incision through the periodontal gingivae down to the alveolar bone margins. Curettes then are enabled to undermine the granulomatous lining of the socket, and with the assistance supplied by the traction of a mosquito hemostat, the soft tissue mass comes away cleanly. Make a primary closure of the overlying soft tissues. Verify the adequacy of the flaps before the placement of implants. When necessary, create in advance the appropriate environment for a primary closure. Undermining of the labiobuccal flap from its muscle bed presents the most viable option. As an alternative, interdigitate the facial and lingual papillae. (See Chapter 8.) Adequate apical bone must be present to offer primary retention for at least 40% of the implant length. That would mean that at least 3 to 4 mm of a 10-mm implant would have to reside in newly cut bone. This 40% relationship may be developed from bone beyond the apex or from narrow bone within the extraction site that requires enlargement in order to accommodate the implants. If the socket is wide, choose wider implants. If there is room apically, remove the coronal portions of the alveolus that do not approximate the implant. This permits deeper penetration into virgin bone as well as the elimination of the less predictable, more fragile, and poorly vascularized alveolar margins. It also reduces the diameter of the socket so that a more intimate primary interfacial relationship is encouraged. However, it will increase the final crown-root ratio (Fig. 9-15).

Surgical Technique

Local anesthesia with small quantities of epinephrine by infiltration is the method of choice in implant surgery. Perform the extractions as atraumatically as possible (Fig. 9-16, A). This will contribute to the preservation of a maximum of alveolar

bone. When the availability of adequate soft tissues for closure is ascertained and total freedom from granulomas is achieved, perform the osteotomies. An internally irrigated, 24-mm-long, 1.6-mm-diameter Brasseler spade drill should be marked with a yellow boot. This is to be followed by increasing sizes, as described earlier in this chapter. Often, a bur extender mandrel is required, particularly if adjacent teeth are present (Fig. 9-16, B). Finally, insert the widest and longest implant that can be accommodated (Fig. 9-16, C). In some cases, implantation after extraction of a tooth offers less satisfactory interfacial relationships than when the surgery is performed in healed alveoli. Place a 20-mesh particulate bone substitute material such as HA or DFDB around the implant, which serves as an osteoconductive or inductive medium and encourages a more intimate final osseous interface. When a multirooted tooth has been extracted if implants cannot be inserted into each socket, decide which socket to use for the implant or whether the interseptal bone should be removed. One factor that influences the selection of site is the required angulation of the implant. This can be determined by the insertion of a paralleling pin or implant analog (try-in). Once the appropriate socket has been chosen, complete the osteotomy and place the implant. Fill the operative and adjacent alveoli with a bone substitute material as required, fasten a GTRM into position, and complete the closure. If the separate alveoli are too small to accommodate individual implants, a second factor must govern the management of the host site. Remove one or several septa and use the newly enlarged area for implant placement. Again, a particulate bone substitute material is of value to complement the portions of the osteotomy that fail to have contact with the implant. If the altered host-site dimensions are greater than the selected implant, and primary retention is dependent on the several millimeters of subapical bone into which the osteotomy was extended, consider using a threaded implant. Using an implant that has threads extending to the apical end offers greater primary retention and a more favorable prognosis. Vital structures must be avoided and perforations of the cortical plates create hazards that must be treated with grafting materials and membranes. The benefits of immediate implantation are considerable, and the operative procedures often are simpler because of the guidance offered by the existing extraction socket. Bone grafting materials are generally required (see Chapter 8).

If a single tooth is being replaced by an implant and adjacent teeth are present, maintenance of alveolar height and gingival contour are of great aesthetic importance. In such cases, if inadequate gingiva presents a problem for primary closure and undermining (see Chapter 7), the use of a GTRM is of great benefit. Tailor the material to a size that permits it to extend at least 2 mm beyond the extraction site and onto the surrounding bone in all directions. Then secure the membrane into position by using a crisscross suture pattern over the operative site. This discourages epithelial down-growth by presenting a barrier. Then cover the complex with periodontal pack. Permit such implants to integrate for at least 6 months before carrying out the second-stage surgery.

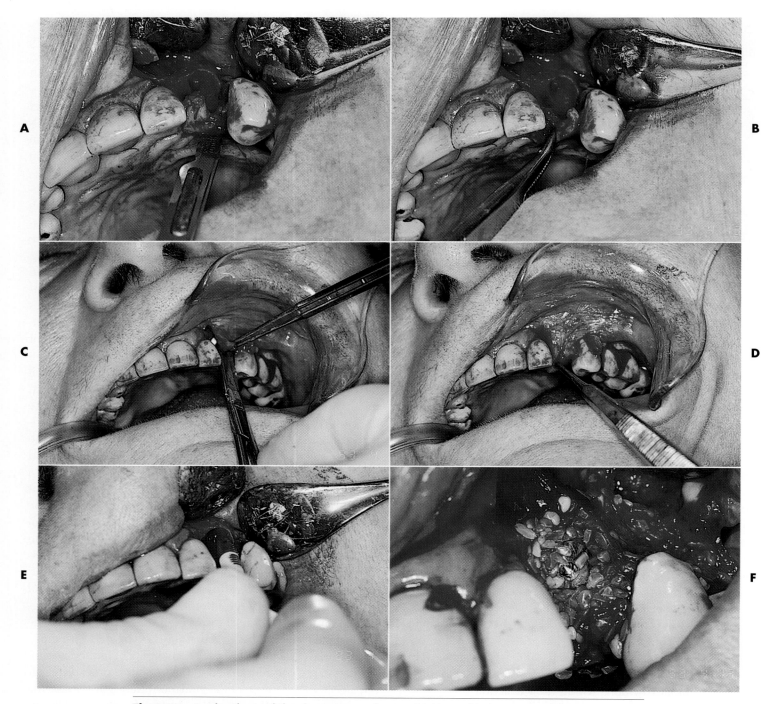

Fig. 9-15 **A,** After the tooth has been removed, use a BP No. 15 blade to excise the invaginated epithelium in a 360-degree incision down to the bone margins. **B,** After the back of a small curette is used to elevate the granulomatous lining of the socket, use a mosquito hemostat for traction and to assist in total soft tissue removal. **C,** In order to create tissue sufficient to permit primary closure, undermine and lift away the facial mucoperiosteal flap from its underlying muscle bed. **D,** The flap is brought across the defect to test its ability to cover the site without tension. **E,** After host-site preparation, place the implant into at least 40% newly cut bone. **F,** Use graft material to fill the periimplant space before suturing the pedicle flap over the graft.

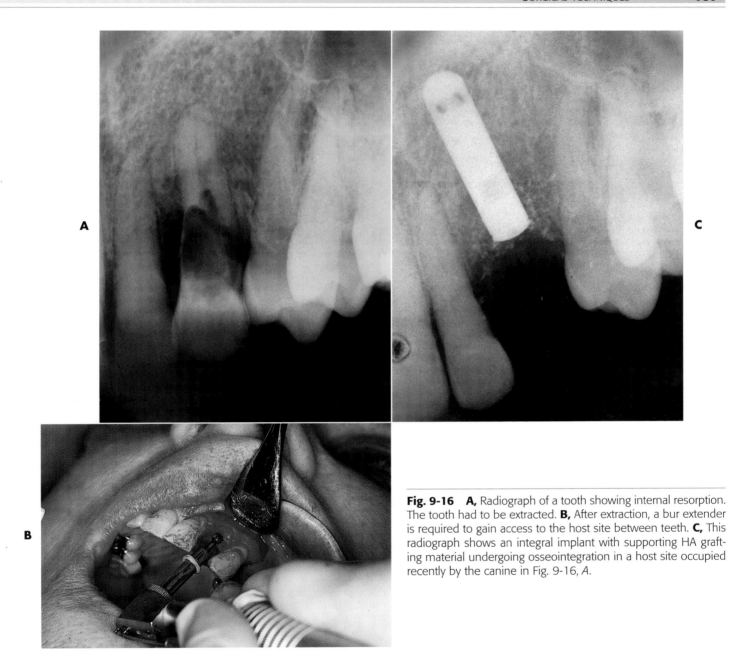

Fig. 9-16 A, Radiograph of a tooth showing internal resorption. The tooth had to be extracted. **B,** After extraction, a bur extender is required to gain access to the host site between teeth. **C,** This radiograph shows an integral implant with supporting HA grafting material undergoing osseointegration in a host site occupied recently by the canine in Fig. 9-16, *A.*

Uncovering Submergible Implants

When the implants have become integrated (3 to 6 months), they are ready for the uncovering, or second-stage procedure. Perform radiographic analysis of the sites before beginning. This examination should consist of panoramic and standardized periapical films. The x-ray films should determine that the bone has healed immediately adjacent to the implants with no intervening radiolucent areas (Fig. 9-17). Once healing appears to be complete, schedule the appointment for uncovering. Before the actual surgical procedure, gather information concerning the type and number of implants placed, the location of each, the kinds of healing caps or screws used, the bone augmentation materials and/or GTRMs employed, and any operative complications that had been encountered at the time of placement. A well-kept chart offers this information.

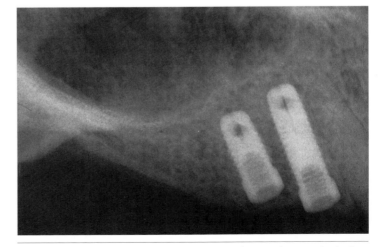

Fig. 9-17 Before uncovering root form implants, take a periapical radiograph to determine the state of mineralization of the host bone.

Review the prosthetic treatment plan so that the proper pregingival, temporary, healing collars are available as well as the final TEAs. The appropriate final abutments, as an option, may be placed at the time of uncovering. However, it is generally recommended that temporary collars be used until the soft tissues mature and can be properly measured for final abutment sizes. Healing collars are of several designs and lengths per implant type, are inexpensive, and are often interchangeable from system to system (Fig. 9-18). They may be used repeatedly simply by being ultrasonically cleaned and autoclaved. Their best feature, however is that some are designed to assist in the creation of a neat, geometric gingival cuff. By using the proper shape and length of collar, the correct emergence profile can be established for the final restoration. Different healing screws necessitate different screwdriver types (i.e., Allen, hex, hooded, modified Phillips). Also, certain abutments require special instruments for seating, countertorquing, and bending. Some gingival punches are also system specific.

Before anesthetizing the area, attempt to visualize the location of the implants. Sometimes the gingivae take on the appearance of small raised circles that may appear blue-gray in color at each site. When such demarcated areas are noted for each implant and these areas are in attached gingiva, use the punch technique. Conversely, if the sites are not identifiable, the sterilized original surgical template may be seated over the intact tissues. Its presence often indicates the location of the implants. Anesthetize these areas with buccal and lingual infiltrations, and press the specific punch for the implant system involved through the tissues and rotate it firmly directly over the site (Fig. 9-19, A, B). After one or two full rotations of the instrument to its full depth, remove the punch. A circle of soft tissue sometimes comes away within the lumen of the instrument. If it does not lift out fully with the punch, grasp it may with a mosquito hemostat and gently dissect it free with a No. 12 BP blade in a scalpel handle. Do not discard these segments of epithelium because they may be used, if necessary, as free grafts to create zones of fixed gingiva adjacent to the newly exposed implants. This may be done simply by pushing the abutting alveolar tissues apically 3 to 4 mm, placing the round free gingival graft over the residual periosteum, and stabilizing it with two crisscross sutures.

In a similar manner, an anterior mandibular vestibuloplasty may be performed at the time of second stage uncovering with a free palatal graft, using a pushback operation, or (as described in Chapter 7) a split-thickness, labial mucosa pedicle graft. Inspect the opening so created to ascertain that the entire surface of each cover screw can be seen along with the full circumference of the implant head (Fig. 9-19, C). It may be necessary to remove more soft tissue at this point, using the scalpel. Also, if bone is seen to be growing over the implant margins, gently remove it using a small sharp osteotome or a saline-cooled No. 2 round bur. Some systems, like the Nobel Biocare, make a cover screw mill specifically for this purpose. Finally, remove the cover or surgical healing screw with a screwdriver and grasp it with a curved hemostatic forceps (Fig. 9-19, D). At this point, the entire superior aspect of the implant should be visible. The area is irrigated gently with sterile saline or a povidone-iodine and saline mixture of 50:50. Confirmation is needed that the implants have become integrated. Confirm this by observing that bone has grown up to and around their most superficial aspects. In addition, a tap on each implant with the back end of a metal mirror handle reveals a solid and resounding response like that made when an ankylosed tooth is tapped. Verify implant rigidity by placing a sterile prosthetic insert into the implant and testing for mobility with the Siemens Periotest. Finally, place the healing collar (Fig. 9-19, E).

In cases in which there is no indication of the exact location of any or all of the implants, make a crestal incision. Anesthesia is administered by infiltration in the same manner as described previously. Then, using a No. 15 BP blade, make a crestal incision directly down to bone and extend it 5 mm mesially and distally to the anticipated implant locations. Next, create a carefully reflected, full-thickness, soft tissue flap facially and lingually until all of the implants are fully exposed (Fig. 9-20). Again, remove any tissue from around the implants with a hemostat or toothed Adson forceps and scalpel. Back out the healing screws and remove any osseous tissues found over the superior aspects of the implants with a bur or mill.

Perform irrigation and verify integration of each implant. After the implants are fully uncovered, measure the soft tissue thickness. Do this with a periodontal probe for each implant. Some systems offer specialized tissue measuring devices that can be used to determine final cuff heights. In nonesthetic areas, a height that extends 1.5 to 2 mm above the gum is proper. Seat the healing collar components completely. Radiographic confirmation of this is important if clinical evidence is unclear (Fig. 9-21, A). Contour the tissues to fit around the cervices of the collars and make a closure using interrupted or mattress sutures (Fig. 9-21, B). Radically relieve and line the existing interim prosthesis with a soft material like Viscogel or Coe Soft. The soft tissue measurements that were made will influence the selection of the final TEAs, which can be placed approximately 2 weeks later. Generally, anesthesia is not required for this step. Reepithelization of the pericervical gingival cuffs should be complete at that time.

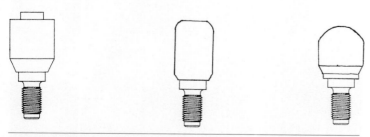

Fig 9-18   Healing collars (center and right) are not available for all systems. Nobel Biocare recommends immediate placement of their final transepithelial abutment (left) in nonesthetic areas.

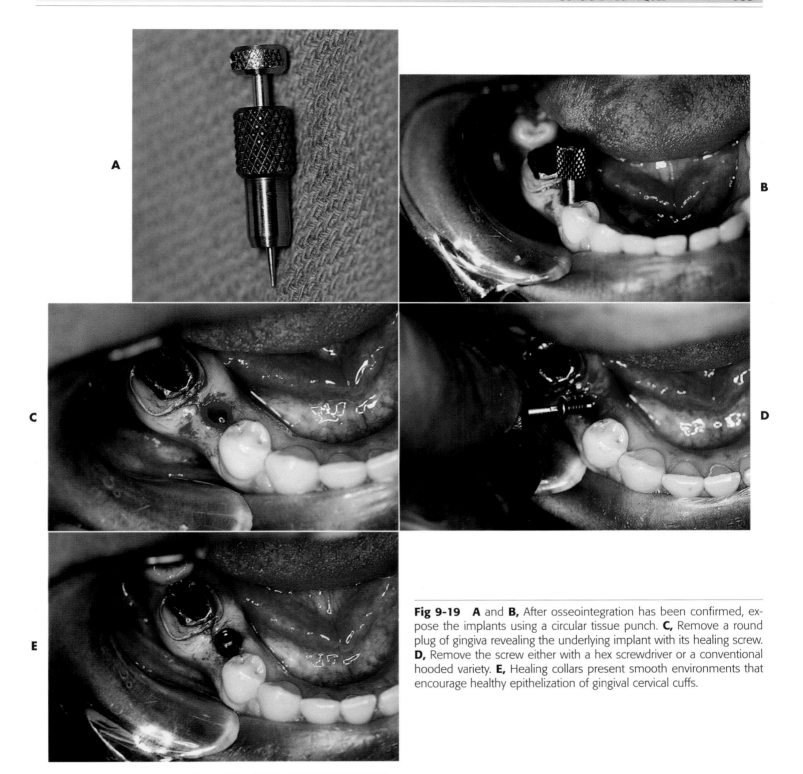

Fig 9-19 **A** and **B,** After osseointegration has been confirmed, expose the implants using a circular tissue punch. **C,** Remove a round plug of gingiva revealing the underlying implant with its healing screw. **D,** Remove the screw either with a hex screwdriver or a conventional hooded variety. **E,** Healing collars present smooth environments that encourage healthy epithelization of gingival cervical cuffs.

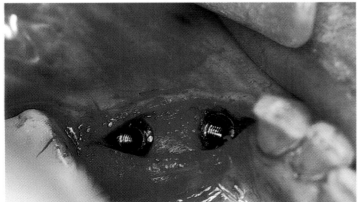

Fig. 9-20 When tissue punches are not practical, a safe way to expose implants is by crestal incision.

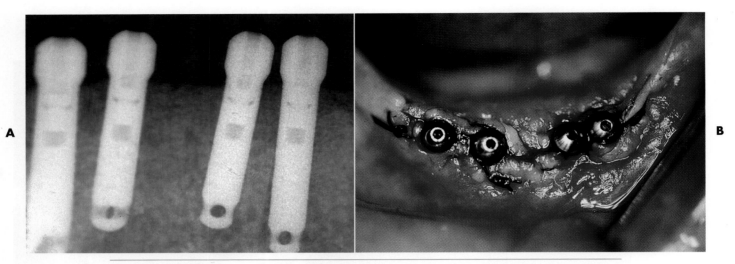

Fig. 9-21   **A,** After healing collars are placed, verify their complete seating by taking a periapical radiograph. **B,** When the position of the collars is assured, scallop the flaps to accommodate the implants, and make a closure with sutures.

Suggested Readings

Abouzgia MB, James DF: Temperature rise during drilling through bone, *Int J Oral Maxillofac Implants* 12:342-353, 1997.

Albrektsson T et al: Osseointegrated oral implants: a Swedish multicenter study of 8,139 consecutively inserted Nobelpharma implants, *J Periodontol* 59:287-296, 1988.

Alling C: Lateral repositioning of the inferior alveolar neurovascular bundle, *J Oral Surg* 35:419, 1977.

Apse P et al: Microbiota and crevicular fluid collagenase activity in the osseointegrated dental implant sulcus: a comparison of sites in edentulous and partially edentulous patients, *J Periodontol Res* 24:96-105, 1989.

Bahat O: Treatment planning and placement of implants in the posterior maxillae: report of 732 consecutive Nobelpharma implants, *Int J Oral Maxillofac Implants* 2:151-161, 1993.

Bahat O: Surgical planning for optimal asesthetic and functional results of osseointegrated implants in the partially edentulous mouth *J Calif Dent Assoc,* 20(5):31-46, 1992.

Babbush C: *Dental implants: principles and practice,* Philadelphia, 1991, WB Saunders.

Babbush C: ITI endosteal hollow cylinder implant systems, *Dent Clin North Am* 30:133-149, 1986.

Bain CA: Smoking and implant failure-benefits of a smoking cessation protocol, *Int J Oral Maxillofac Implants* 11:756-759, 1996.

Balshi TJ, Garver DG: Surgical guidestents for placement of implants, *J Oral Maxillofac Surg* 45:463-465, 1987.

Becker W et al: One-step surgical placement of Branemark implants: a prospective multicenter clinical study, *Int J Oral Maxillofac Implants* 12:454-462, 1997.

Bidez MW, Stephens BJ, Lemons JE: An investigation into the effect of blade dental implant length on interfacial tissue stress profiles. In Spilker RL, Simon MR, editors: *Computational methods in bioengineering,* Proceedings of the American Society of Mechanical Engineers, Winter Annual Meeting, Chicago, November 1988.

Branemark PI et al: Tissue-integrated prostheses, *Quintessence* 214-232, 1985.

Casino AJ, Harrison P, Tarnow DP et al: Influence of type of incision on the success rate of implant integration at stage II uncovering surgery, *J Oral Maxillofac Surg* 55:31, 1997.

Chiche GJ et al: Implant surgical template for partially edentulous patients, *J Oral Maxillofac Implants* 4:289-292, 1989.

Cranin AN, Klein M, Sirakian A et al: Comparison of incisions made for the placement of dental implants, *J Dent Res* 70:279, 1991 (abstract 109).

Crossetti H, Graves S, Gonshor A et al: Experience with multiple endosseous implant systems in private practice, *Int J Oral Maxillofac Implants* 9:10, 1994.

Davis DM, Rogers SJ, Packer ME: The extent of maintenance required by implant-retained mandibular overdentures: a 3-year report, *Int J Oral Maxillofac Implants* 11:767-774, 1996.

Davis TS et al: A histologic comparison of the bone-implant interface utilizing the Integral and three surface variations of the Micro-Vent implant. Submitted for publication.

Donovan TE, Chee WWL: ADA acceptance program for endosseous implants, *J Calif Dent Assoc* 20:60, 1992.

Edge MJ: Surgical placement guide for use with osseointegrated implants, *J Prosthet Dent* 57:719-722, 1987.

English CE: An overview of implant hardware, *J Am Dent Assoc* 121:360, 1990.

English CE: Cylindrical Implants, *J Calif Dent Assoc* 16:17-20, 834-838, 1988.

Eriksson RA, Albrektsson T: Temperature threshold levels for heat-induced bone tissue injury, *J Prosthet Dent* 50:101-107, 1983.

Fagan MJ et al: *Implant prosthodontics,* 1990, Chicago, Year Book Medical Publishers.

Finger IM, Guerra LR: Integral implant-prosthodontic considerations, *Dent Clin North Am* 33:793-819, 1989.

Fishel D et al: Roentgenologic study of the mental foramen, *Oral Surg Med Oral Pathol* 41:682-686, 1976.

Fonseca RJ, Davis W: *Reconstructive preprosthodontic oral and maxillofacial surgery,* Philadelphia, 1986, WB Saunders.

Fox SC, Moriarty JD, Kusy RP: The effects of scaling a titanium implant surface with metal and plastic instruments; an in vitro study, *J Periodontol* 61:485-490, 1990.

Friberg B, Grondahl K, Lekholm U: A new self-tapping Branemark implant: clinical and radiographic evaluation, *Int J Oral Maxillofac Implants* 7:80, 1992.

Hahn JA: *The Steri-Oss implant system: endosteal dental implants,* St Louis, 1991, Mosby.

Heller AL: Blade implants, *Can Dent Assoc J* 16:78-86, 1988.

Ismael JYH: A comparison of current root form implants: biomechanical design and prosthodontic applications, *NY State Dent J* 55:34, 1989.

James RA, Kellin E: A histopathological report on the nature of the epithelium and underlining connective tissue which surrounds implant posts, *J Biomed Mat Res* 5:373, 1974.

James RA, Schultz RL: Hemidesmosomes and the adhesion of junctional epithelial cells to metal implants: a preliminary report, *J Oral Implant* 4:294-302, 1974.

Jansen JA: Ultrastructural study of epithelial cell attachment to implant materials, *J Dent Res* 65:5, 1985.

Jensen OT, Brownd C, DeLorimier J: Esthetic maxillary arch vertical location for the osseointegrated cylinder implant, *J Am Dent Assoc* 119:735-736, 1989.

Johansson C, Albrektsson T: Integration of screw implants in the rabbit: a 1-year follow-up of removal torque of titanium implants, *Int J Maxillofacial Surg* 2:69, 1987.

Kasten FH, Soileau K, Meffert RM: Quantitative evaluation of human gingival epithelial cell attachment to implant surfaces in vitro, *Int J Periodont Restor Dent* 10:69-79, 1990.

Kirsch A, Ackerman KL: The IMZ osteointegrated implant system, *Dent Clin North Am* 33:733-791, 1989.

Kirsch A: The two-phase implantation method using IMZ intramobile cylinder implants, *J Oral Implant* 11:197-210, 1983.

Kirsch A, Mentag P: The IMZ endosseous two-phase implant system, *J Oral Implant* 12:494-498, 1986.

Koth DL, McKinney RV, Steflik DE: Microscopic study of hygiene effect on peri-implant gingival tissues, *J Dent Res* 66(special issue) 186(abstract 639), 1986.

Kwan JY, Zablotsky MH, Meffert RM: Implant maintenance using a modified ultrasonic instrument, *J Dent Hyg* 64:422-430, 1990.

Lambert P, Morris HF, Ochi S et al: Relationship between implant surgical experience and second-stage failures: DICRG interim report no. 2, *Implant Dent* 3:97, 1994.

Langer B, Langer L: The overlapped flap: a surgical modification for implant fixture installation, *Int J Perio Rest Dent* 10:209-215, 1990.

Lavelle CLB: Mucosal seal around endosseous dental implants, *J Oral Implant* 9:357-371, 1981.

Lazzarra RJ: Immediate implant placement into extraction sites: surgical and restorative advantages, *Int J Periodont Rest Dent* 9:333-342, 1989.

Lekholm U, Jemt T: Principles for single tooth replacement, *Quintessence* 117-126, 1989.

Lekholm U et al: The condition of soft tissue at tooth and fixture abutments supporting fixed bridges: a microbiological and histological study, *J Clin Periodontol* 13:558, 1986.

Levy D et al: A comparison of radiographic bone height and probing attachment level measurements adjacent to porous-coated dental implants in humans, *Int J Oral Maxillofac Implants* 12:544-546, 1997.

Lindhe J et al: Experimental breakdown of peri-implant and periodontal tissues: a study in the Beagle dog, *Clin Oral Implants Res* 3:9-16, 1992.

Linkow LJ, Donath K, Lemons JE: Retrieval analysis of a blade implant after 231 months of clinical function, *Implant Dent* 1:37-43, 1992.

Lozada JL: Eight-year clinical evaluation of HA-coated implants: clinical performance of HA-coated titanium screws in Type IV bone, *J Dent Symp* 1 67:8, 1993.

Malmqvist JP, Sennerby L: Clinical report on the success of 47 consecutively placed Core-Vent implants followed from 3 months to 4 years, *Int J Oral Maxillofac Implants* 5:390, 1990.

Misch CE: Density of bone: effect on treatment plan, surgical approach, healing, and progressive bone healing, *Int J Oral Implantol* 6:23-31, 1990.

Misch CE: Osseointegration and the submerged Blade implant, *J Houston Dist Dent Assoc,* January 1988, pp. 12-16.

Misch CE: *The Core-Vent implant system: endosteal dental implants,* St Louis, 1991, Mosby.

Misch CE, Crawford E: Predictable mandibular nerve location: a clinical zone of safety, *Int J Oral Implant* 7(1) 37-40, 1990.

Mombelli A et al: The microbiota associated with successful or failing osseointegrated titanium implants, *Oral Microbiol Immunol* 2:145, 1987.

Niznick G, Misch CE: The Core-Vent System of osseointegrated implants. In Clark JW, editor: *Clinical Dentistry,* Philadelphia, 1987, Harper & Row.

Olive J, Aparicio C: The Periotest method as a measure of osseointegrated oral implant stability, *Int J Oral Maxillofac Implants* 12:487, 1992.

Parham PL et al: Effects of an air powder abrasive system on plasma-sprayed titanium implant surfaces: an in vitro evaluation, *J Oral Implantol* 15:78-86, 1989.

Pietrokovski J: The bony residual ridge in man, *J Prosthet Dent* 34:456-462, 1975.

Rams T et al: The subgingival microbial flora associated with human dental implants, *J Prosthet Dent* 51:529, 1984.

Rams T, Link C Jr: Microbiology of failing implants in humans: electron microscopic observations, *J Oral Implant* 11:93, 1983.

Rapley JW et al: The surface characteristics produced by various oral hygiene instruments and materials on titanium implant abutments, *Int J Oral Maxillofac Implants* 5:47-52, 1990.

Roberts EW et al: Interface histology of rigid endosseous implants, *J Oral Implantol* 12:406-416, 1986.

Rosenquist B: A comparison of various methods of soft tissue management following the immediate placement of implants into extraction sockets, *Int J Oral Maxillofac Implants* 12:43-51, 1997.

Rosenquist B: Immediate placement of implants into extraction sockets: implant survival, *Int J Oral Maxillofac Implants* 11:205-209, 1996.

Saadoun AP, LeGall ML: Clinical results and guidelines on Steri-Oss endosseous implants, *Int J Periodont Restor Dent* 12:487, 1992.

Sabiston DC: *Textbook of surgery,* ed 14, Philadelphia, 1991, WB Saunders, p. 222.

Scharf DR, Tarnow DP: The effect of crestal versus mucobuccal incisions on the success rate of implant osseointegration, *Int J Oral Maxillofac Implants* 8:187, 1993.

Schnitman P et al: Three-year survival rates, blade implants vs. cantilever clinical trials, *J Dent Res* 67(special issue) 347, 1988.

Smithlof J, Fritz ME: The use of blade implants in a selected population of partially edentulous adults: a 15-year report, *J Periodontol* 58:589-593, 1987.

Spiekermann H, Jansen VK, Richter EJ: A 10-year follow-up study of IMZ and TPS implants in the edentulous mandible using bar-retained overdentures, *Int J Oral Maxillofacial Implant* 10:231, 1995.

Stefani LA: The care and maintenance of the dental implant patient, *J Dent Hygiene* 10:447-466, 1988.

Stultz ER, Lofland R, Sendax VI et al: A multicenter 5-year retrospective survival analysis of 6200 integral implants, *Compend Contin Educ Dent* 14:478, 1993.

Sullivan DY et al: The reverse torque test: a clinical report, *Int J Oral Maxillofac Implants* 11:179-185, 1996.

Thomas-Neal D, Evans GH, Meffert RM: Effects of various prophylactic treatments on titanium, sapphire, and hydroxylapatite-coated implants: an SEM study, *Int J Periodont Restor Dent* 9:301-311, 1989.

Tolman DE Keller EE: Endosseous implant placement immediately following dental extraction and alveoplasty: preliminary report with 6-year follow-up, *J Oral Maxillofac Implants* 6:24-28, 1991.

Valeron JF, Velasquez JF: Placement of screw-type implants in the pterygomaxillary-pyramidal region: surgical procedure and preliminary results, *Int J Oral Maxillofac Implants* 12:814-819, 1997.

Viscido A: The submerged blade implant-a dog histologic study, *J Oral Implant* 5(2):195-209, 1974.

Walker L, Morris HF, Ochi S et al: Periotest values of dental implants in the first 2 years after second-stage surgery: DICRG interim report no. 8, *Implant Dent* 6:207, 1997.

Weber SP: A mucobuccal fold extension for implant and other surgical procedures, *J Prosthet Dent* 27:423, 1972.

10

Root Form Implant Surgery: Proprietary I

CAVEATS

The generic steps leading to the definitive procedures described in this section may be found in Chapter 9. Note that not all the systems described in this chapter begin after the use of the 3-mm spade drill. For example, small-diameter implants require that the sequence stop at 2.5- or 2.7-mm drills. If the surgeon uses the 3-mm spade drill for these systems, the host sites will be too wide. Therefore, read each section carefully before beginning. Although this section may not mention all available implant sizes, Table 4-2 lists dimensions for each type and style. If the practitioner does not wish to use the generic system to begin the osteotomy for the chosen implant system, as described in Chapter 9, the illustrations start their instructive patterns with the full spectrum of drills starting with the smallest diameter offered by the specific manufacturer.

EXTERNAL HEX, THREADED IMPLANTS

External hex, threaded implants have an antirotational design for their abutments in the form of an external hexagon protruding from the top of the device as shown in Fig. 10-1.

Manufacturer	System
BioHorizons	Maestro system
Calcitek	Threadloc system
Imtec	
LifeCore	Restore
Nobelbiocare	Branemark system
Osteomed	Hextrac
Paragon	Swede-Vent
Park Dental Research	Star-Vent
Sargon	
Steri-Oss	Replace
	Hex Lock Series
3i	Standard system
	Microminiplant
	Miniplant

INTERNAL HEX THREADED IMPLANTS

Manufacturer	System
Paragon	Screw-Vent
	Micro-Vent
Friatec	Frialit (two stepped)

EXTERNAL HEX PRESS-FIT IMPLANTS

Manufacturer	System
Calcitek	Omniloc
3i	
Duo-dent	
Imtec	
Innova	
Lifecore	Restore
	Sustain
Osteomed	
Steri-Oss	IMZ

SPLINE AND SIMILAR

Manufacturer	System
Calcitek	Spline
Park	Star★Lock

MORSE TAPER

Astra (with screw fixation)
Sustain (with screw fixation), internal bevel
Bicon (without screw fixation)

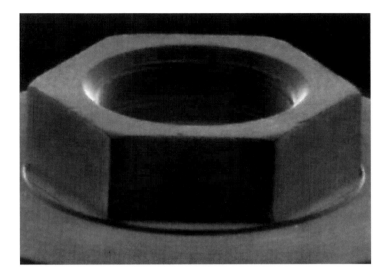

Fig. 10-1 The external hexagon is the most frequently used antirotational device.

Noble Biocare and 3i Systems

Although these systems are quite similar, they are packaged differently. For example, Noble Biocare is available in a scored glass tube that snaps in half on finger pressure. 3i comes in a blister pack that includes the surgical cover screw. Some of the designs are manufactured as self-tapping implants in wide and small diameters. Various coatings (i.e., hydroxyapatite [HA] and titanium plasma spray [TPS]) are available for some as well. The directions for placement are similar for each system (i.e., 3i, Swede-Vent, Restore), but instruments are given different names. In the directions that follow, Nobel Biocare's Brånemark instrument names are used. These implants are available in diameters of 3.75, 4, 4.5, 5, and 5.5 mm. The insertion techniques vary slightly with each size.

The 3-mm twist drill described in the generic system in Chapter 9 will have been used to its final depth.

1. For dense bone, use the 3.5-mm twist drill next. Proceed with care, particularly if internal cooling is not available.
2. Place the compatible (3 mm) end of a paralleling pin into the osteotomy. This verifies the angulation of the preparation.
3. Employ the appropriate counter-sink at the top of the osteotomy. The short counter-sink is recommended for implants that are 10 mm or shorter in length; use the long counter-sink for implants that are greater than 10 mm in length.
4. Measure the osteotomy using the depth gauge, and make corrections if required.
5. Attach the handpiece connector to the ultra–low-speed handpiece, and set the console to its lowest speed.
6. Unless self-tapping implants are being used or the bone is of a compliant density, perform bone tapping. Snap the appropriate bone tap into the handpiece connector (fixture mount) while it is stabilized in the fixture rack with the titanium-tipped hemostat. Do not handle the bone taps and implants with fingers, gloved or otherwise. Use the rack and forceps for mounting and removal. Some manufacturers prepare each implant with its own fix-

ture mount (e.g., Paragon, Steri-Oss). Others (e.g., 3i) prepare some of their implants with a fixture mount and some require the attachment of a mount at the time of surgery.

7. Tap the bone using the low-speed handpiece (8 to 18 rpm) in a forward or clockwise direction. Copious saline irrigant should accompany this maneuver.
8. When the tap has arrived at a point 3 mm short of the full depth, stop the motor and complete the tapping with the handheld wheel or the handheld ratchet.
9. Remove the tap by hand using counterclockwise turning of the wheel or the ratchet wrench in reverse mode.
10. Snap open the glass container and allow the chosen implant to fall gently into the small square container marked "T" (for titanium). Use the titanium-tipped forceps to transfer the implant into a hole of proper diameter in the rack, and attach the implant to the fixture mount with the closed blade screwdriver, stabilizing it with the notched-beak, curved hemostatic forceps.
11. The ultra—low-speed handpiece rotates the implant into its prepared site at less than 20 rpm, until it is 3 mm short of its full seating. Although most motors usually stop when the implant is fully seated, the potential hazard of stripping the bone threads does exist. Therefore it is safest to seat the implant for its last 3 mm using the handheld wheel or, if necessary, the ratchet device. Detach the handpiece from the fixture mount, leaving it attached to the implant. Hold the ratchet handle as close to the implant as possible to enhance tactile sensitivity and to minimize excessive distracting movements that the long handle can exert.
12. Ensure the implant's stability by tightening with the wheel or ratchet wrench. If the operative site demonstrates stripped internal bony threads, the Nobel Biocare system offers 4-mm backup implants of commensurate lengths. They should be introduced into their sites directly without pre-tapping.

13. The closed blade screwdriver backs off the fixation screw while using the open-end wrench to offer countertorque to the implant.

14. Irrigate the wounds and then place the cover screw. A throat pack always should be in place when using small instruments and fittings such as cover screws. Other choices are listed as follows:

   a. Place the capscrew using a special screwdriver in a low-speed handpiece. Tighten it with either the short or long blade screwdriver.

   b. Seat the flat-top cover screw with the hexagonal screwdriver (Fig. 10-2).

The flap may now be sutured (see Chapter 6).

The uncovering procedure is described in Chapter 9, and the appropriate healing collar or cuff or an abutment is placed depending on the thickness of the tissue and its esthetic needs. Healing cuffs should protrude approximately 2 mm above the free gingival margin. Special abutments are found that are similar to the contour and diameter of the anticipated restoration. Keep these abutments in position until the tissues have sufficiently matured to permit the impression procedures. Generally, this takes 2 weeks.

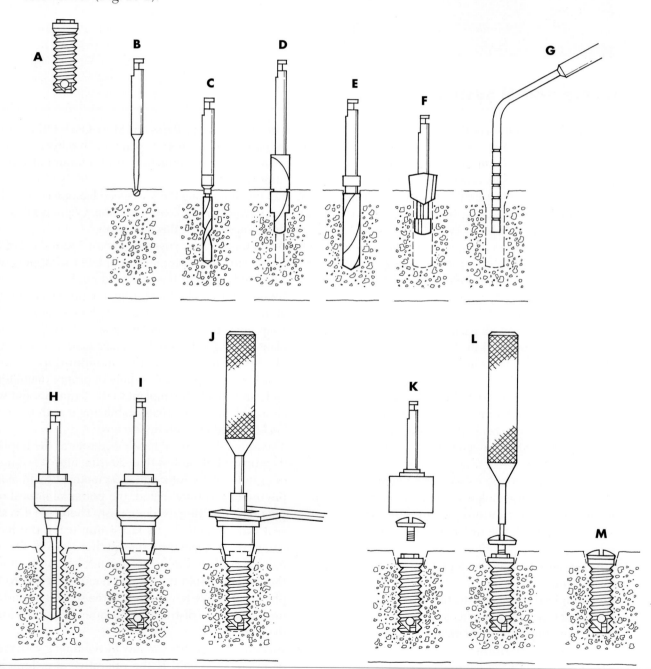

Fig. 10-2 **A,** Nobel Biocare implant. **B,** The manufacturer's recommended procedure begins with using the guide drill to half its diameter to penetrate the cortical plate at the proposed implant site. **C,** Use the 2-mm twist drill to the final implant depth. **D,** Use the counterbore to enlarge the coronal portion of the osteotomy in preparation for the 3-mm twist drill. **E,** The 3-mm twist drill. **F,** Counter-sink drill. **G,** Depth gauge. **H,** Screw tap. **I,** Insert the implant attached to the fixture mount. **J,** The open-ended wrench stabilizes the fixture mount, while its fixation screw is removed from the implant. **K,** Cover screw inserter. **L,** Cover screw placement with the small hexagon screwdriver. **M,** Seat the Nobel Biocare implant so that its cover screw is flush with the crest of bone.

Sulzer-Calcitek Implant System
Spline Cylinders (Groove and Slot Abutment Connection System)
Integral System (Non-hexed)
Omniloc System (Externally hexed)

Calcitek press-fit implants are available in 3.25-, 4-, and 5-mm diameters. Each is available with its own instrumentation, including final sizing drills. These systems suggest the use of a rosette bur at the outset. By creating a dimple to half its diameter on the surface of the bone before the first osteotomy, subsequent bur stabilization during initial cutting is encouraged. This is a technique that may be used for all systems. The 3-mm generic spade drill will have been used to its final depth.

1. Complete the final osteotomy with the full diameter spade drill (final sizing drill) corresponding to the length and diameter of the selected implant. They are available with all lengths marked clearly on spade drills of each diameter.
2. Confirm the accuracy of the preparation by placing or tapping by mallet the appropriate implant body try-in into the osteotomy. The line on the try-in that corresponds to the implant depth must be level with the crest of the ridge.
3. When this requirement is satisfied, open the implant container. The implant will be found attached to the plastic cap. Place the implant into the bone preparation by using the plastic cap as a handle. Use firm finger pressure until it is firmly seated. Remove the plastic cap by rocking and twisting it mesial to distal. Do not draw it in the long axis of the osteotomy or the implant may become dislodged.
4. Place the nylon-tipped tapper on the head of the implant and strike it gently with a mallet until the implant is completely seated. Exercise great care not to drive the implant beyond the bone level (i.e., into the antrum, nasal floor, or mandibular canal). This can be avoided if the tip of the implant driver is larger than the diameter of the head of the implant. As an alternative, an orangewood stick serves as a safe, gentle, and satisfactory disposable seating instrument.
5. After each implant has been seated, tighten its healing screw, which is in place from the package, with the hex screwdriver (Fig. 10-3). Press-fit implants should never be tapped without their healing screws in place because of the hazard of distorting the internally threaded environment.

The flap may now be sutured. Uncovering follows the same techniques previously described.

Calcitek makes a complete spectrum of titanium and coated threaded implants as well as their HA-coated press-fit designs. These are inserted in the same manner as the Sterioss, screw-vent and Brånemark implants.

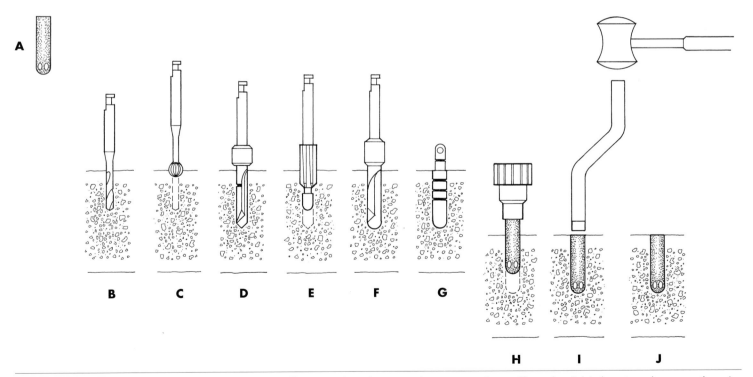

Fig. 10-3 **A,** Calcitek, Integral, and Omniloc. **B,** The following series of steps and part names is specific to the Calcitek system; however, the principles may be applied to other press-fit endosseous cylindrical implants. The manufacturer recommended procedure begins by using the pilot drill to a depth of 8 mm at the appropriate angulation. **C,** Use the rosette bur to half its diameter over the pilot osteotomy. **D,** Use the intermediate spade drill to enlarge the pilot osteotomy. It deepens the osteotomy to its final depth, which is 1 mm longer than the implant. **E,** A counterbore drill enlarges the coronal portion of the osteotomy. **F,** Final spade drill. **G,** Implant body try-in. **H,** Seat the implant with its plastic cap. **I,** Tap the implant into position. **J.** Seat Calcitek implants (Integral, SD [small-diameter] Omniloc) flush with the crest of bone.

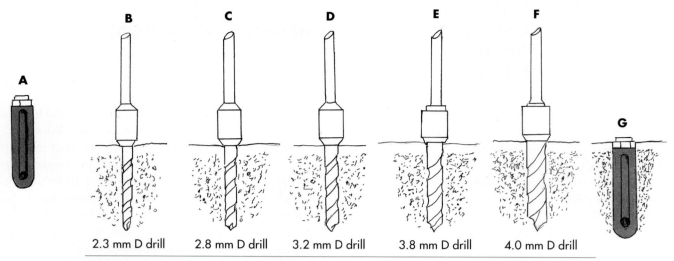

| 2.3 mm D drill | 2.8 mm D drill | 3.2 mm D drill | 3.8 mm D drill | 4.0 mm D drill |

Fig. 10-4 A-G, These six steps depicted for the Paragon Biovent System are described in Fig. 10-3. The technique for cylindrical press-fit implant placement varies very little from one system to another. There are three diameters for these HA coated designs: 3.3, 3.7, and 4.7 mm of four different lengths.

Paragon Implant Systems

Bio-Vent

The 3-mm, internally irrigated generic spade drill will have been used to the planned depth.

1. Take the 3.2-mm internally irrigated spade drill to its final depth and use the Bio-Vent finishing drill to complete the osteotomy (SVD) for 3.3-mm diameter implant and (BVD) for the 3.7-mm diameter implant. Note that when placing the 4.7-mm diameter implant, the wide Bio-Vent finishing drill (BVDW) is used to complete the osteotomy.
2. Remove the implant from the package and place it into its osteotomy.
3. Tap it into place using a mallet and the point-seating instrument. The nylon tip must be of a greater diameter than the implant to avoid accidental overdriving of the implant. The implant should be level with the bone. Use the hex driver to make certain that the healing screw is tight. Suturing the flaps completes the operation (Fig. 10-4).

Screw-Vent

The generic 2.5-mm internally irrigated spade drill will have been used to the planned depth.

1. The 2.8-mm spade drill serves as the final sizing drill for the 3.3-mm diameter implant. Use the 3.2-mm drill serves as final sizing for the 3.7-mm diameter Screw-Vent, and use the 4.2-mm drill as the final sizing drill for the 4.7-mm diameter implant body.
2. If the bone is dense, it may require the use of a bone tap at 15 to 30 rpm to the final depth. If possible, however, complete tapping by hand.
3. Convey the implant to the osteotomy with its prepackaged fixture mount. Before seating, loosen the fixture mount screw by turning the hex driver a half turn counterclockwise. Seat the implant to its final depth by using the hand ratchet in a clockwise direction until the implant is seated flush with the crest of bone.
4. Back out the fixture mount with the hex tool, and place the healing screw using the same driver. Suture the flaps. (Fig. 10-5).

Perform the uncovering of these implants using the standard technique.

Taper-Lock Screw-Vent

The Paragon Company has added a Taper-Lock design to its product line. The method of insertion is the same as for the standard Screw-Lock, and the three available diameters are 3.3, 4, and 4.7 mm. One of the main purposes of this design is that it permits the immediate attachment of an abutment for one-stage utilization (see Chapter 21).

Micro-Vent

The 3-mm internally irrigated, generic drill will have been used to the planned final depth of the osteotomy.

1. Use the MTD drill as the final drill for the 3.7-mm system. Note that the apex of the drill is only 2.5 mm in diameter. The MTDW is the final drill required when the wider diameter 4.7-mm system has been selected. Note that the apex of the MTDW drill is only 3 mm.
2. Carry the implant to the osteotomy with its prepackaged fixture mount, which should be loosened before use and seat the implant completely by using the ratchet wrench in a clockwise direction.
3. Remove the implant mount with the hex tool and replace it with the cover screw.

The flap is now sutured. Uncovering follows the standard techniques described previously.

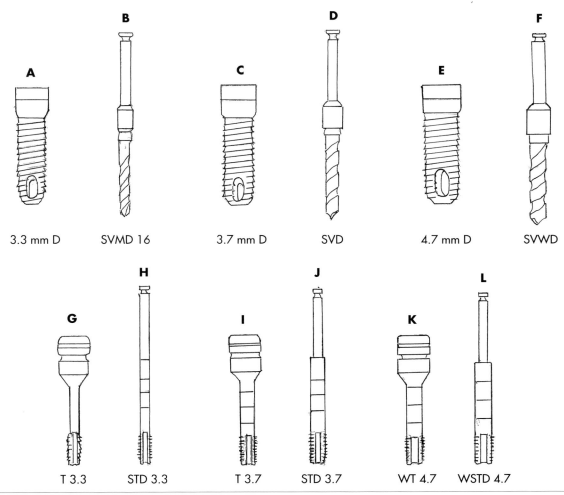

B	D	F
A	C	E
3.3 mm D	SVMD 16	3.7 mm D	SVD	4.7 mm D	SVWD

H	J	L
G	I	K
T 3.3	STD 3.3	T 3.7	STD 3.7	WT 4.7	WSTD 4.7

Fig. 10-5 **A, C,** and **E,** The Paragon Screw-Vent design bears the unique antirotational characteristic of an internal hex. It is available in the following lengths: 8, 10, 13, and 16 mm, and three diameters 3.3, 3.7, and 4.7 mm. Unlike may other threaded implants (e.g., Swede-Vent the polished cervix of this system has the same diameter as the remainder of the implant body. **B, D,** and **F,** Osteotomy with a series of properly measured twist drills of the SV series; place the 3.3-mm diameter implant with the SVMD drill, place the 3.7-mm implant with the SVD after widening with the SVMD drill, and place the 4.7-mm implant with the SVMD drill after going through the previous two stages. **G-L,** In cases of dense bone, as is found particularly in the anterior mandible, a more refined host preparation can be made by prethreading with bone taps. These taps, available in all three diameters, may be turned with the hand wheel, the ratchet handled wheel, or at tapping speeds (20 RPM) with the handpiece.

Steri-Oss

Steri-Oss Threaded Implants

The 3-mm generic spade drill will have been used to its final depth.

1. Steri-Oss supplies anterior and posterior drills, which vary only in the length of their shanks. Select whichever length is most easily accommodated.
2. Rotate the counterbore drill in the cervical few millimeters of the osteotomy. (This may not be necessary in the maxilla.)
3. Tap the implant osteotomy with the threadformer at 15 to 25 rpm. In most cases the maxilla do not require a separate tapping procedure. This can be performed manually with the wheel ratchet wrench with or without its handle.
4. The implant comes packaged with a container cover in which the implant is mounted. Place the implant into the osteotomy using this carrier. Rotate it clockwise with firm finger pressure until it can no longer be turned.

5. Remove the cover by backing off its internal screw with a hexdriver, and place the hex insertion mandrel into the implant. Place the round, knurled handle over it, which permits further manual rotation of the implant. When it is no longer possible to turn this device digitally, place the hand-ratchet on the wrench mandrel and turn it clockwise until the implant locks into place. If the operator prefers the use of an ultra–low-speed handpiece for seating, set the console at tapping speed, place the adaptor into the latched end, and seat the implant to its full extent. If 3.8-mm implants (mini series) are being used and the threads have lost their integrity, remove the implant. The Steri-Oss 3.8-mm cylindrical press-fit implants fit firmly as backup devices. Place them into the osteotomy with hand pressure. The carriers, which are the container covers, may be removed by bending them to one side at a 90-degree angle. This implant may now be tapped

gently into its final position (level with the alveolar crest) by placing the tip of the implant-seating instrument and tapping it with a surgical mallet.

6. Whichever of the two implants has been inserted, the same wrenches can be used to screw the healing cap into place within it. These screws are to be found by lifting the exterior label of the hollow plastic container cap. Suturing the flap completes these procedures.

After uncovering the implant (Chapter 9), place the temporary healing collar by threading it into the implant using a hexdriver. Following a 2-week healing period, the prosthetic treatment may be initiated.

Steri-Oss makes threaded implants with and without external hexes. The hex threaded group includes implants with diameters of 3.25, 3.8, 4.5, 5, and 6 mm with lengths from 8 to 18 mm. The 6-mm-diameter implant, however, is available in lengths up to only 14 mm. The nonhexed, threaded group is available in 3.25- and 3.8-mm diameters with lengths up to 18 mm.

The techniques for insertion of these six designs follow the same pattern as may be noted in Fig. 10-6.

The healing screws are designed with housings to permit them to fit over the external hex configurations. This causes them to extend 1 mm over the bone level.

Steri-Oss Replace System

Steri-Oss Replace implants are made particularly for use in immediate extraction sites and other areas that require an apical taper. They are available in the larger diameters of 4.3, 5, and 6 mm of three lengths: 10, 13, and 16 mm.

The technique of insertion is somewhat simplified because the starting point is within an extraction socket; therefore, begin with a 2.7-mm depth drill and jump to a 4.3-mm tapered drill.

For the larger diameters, the next step is the final drill and the threadformer (when needed in denser jaws) (Fig. 10-7).

Of note in these diagrams is that there is a separate threadformer for each of the three diameters and that the process of bone preparation and enlargement simply continues from the 4.3-mm diameter with the larger threadformers (5 and 6 mm) as required.

Steri-Oss Cylindrical Press-Fit Implants

3.25, 3.25 Hex, 3.8, 3.8 Hex, 5 Hex

The 3-mm generic spade drill osteotomy will have been completed to its final depth.

1. As with all endosseous implants, keep the drill to the minimum speed that cuts effectively.
2. Use the 3.25-mm diameter depth drill to the desired depth. This is the final drill for the 3.25-mm diameter implant. It serves as well, as an intermediate drill for the 3.8-mm diameter implant.
3. If a 3.8-mm diameter implant is planned, use the 3.8-mm diameter depth drill to the final depth. However, use our generic 3.5-mm drill as an intermediate gradient before employing the final size.
4. Verify correct depth of the 3.8-mm drill by inserting the depth gauge into the osteotomy. If satisfactory, tap the steel try-in to its full depth.
5. Place the implant, which is attached to the container cap, into the osteotomy with finger pressure. Remove the carrier by bending it to one side at a 90-degree angle.
6. After implant placement, gently tap the end of the implant-seating instrument with a surgical mallet. Examine the healing screw, which is already in position, for tightness by testing with the Allen wrench. The flap is now sutured.

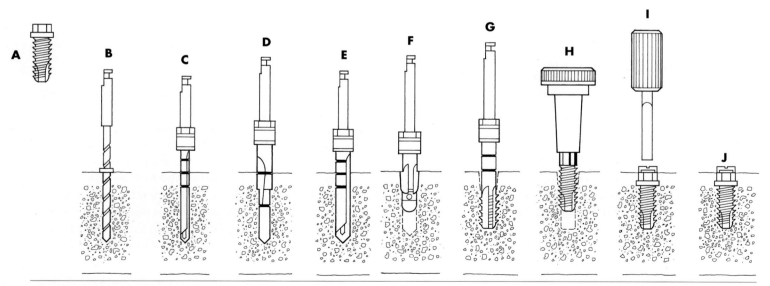

Fig. 10-6 **A,** Steri-Oss miniseries implant. **B,** The manufacturer recommended procedure begins by using the 1.5-mm pilot drill to the final osteotomy depth, which is 1 mm longer than the implant length. **C,** Widen the osteotomy for its full depth with the 2-mm drill. **D,** The guide drill widens the coronal portion of the osteotomy to its final width. **E,** Use the depth drill to its final depth. **F,** Counterbore. **G,** Thread-former. **H,** Remove the implant from its container and then screw it into place with the plastic carrier. **I,** Screw down the healing cap with the flat blade screwdriver. **J,** Seat the Steri-Oss miniseries implant flush with the crest of bone. The healing cap is hollow to permit it to fit over the external hex. This usually results in its 1 mm protrusion above the alveolus.

7. For implants of the 5-mm diameter, use a 5-mm depth drill before tapping the try-in to place (see Fig. 10-3, *A-G*).

Uncovering follows the same rules as outlined for the Steri-Oss threaded implants.

Steri-Oss IMZ Implants

Steri-Oss IMZ implants are of the press-fit design. The 3-mm generic spade drill had been used to create its planned depth.

1. Use the IMZ round drill is used in the osteotomy to a depth of half its diameter, which aids in seating the next drill.
2. Rotate the 3.3-mm cannon drill to its final depth. (Cannon drills do not cut as predictably as spade drills.)
3. Select our 3.5-mm generic drill for the next step.
4. Follow this with a 4-mm cannon drill to the final depth of the planned implant.
5. Remove the implant from its package and attach it to the implant placement head using the Teflon-coated forceps. (As an alternative, use the IMZ implant package with placement heads in position.) Position the implant by its placement head into the osteotomy and seat it with finger pressure.
6. Using the implant tapper and mallet, seat the implant gently into place so that it is level with the alveolar crest.

7. Remove the implant placement head using the hand screwdriver or the contra-angle reduction handpiece with attached screwdriver.
8. Irrigate the inner core of the implant body with saline and fill it with antibiotic ointment (Mycolog, Bacitracin, or Terra-Cortril).
9. Make the IMZ implant available with an IME or internal plastic sleeve that is interposed between its walls and the abutment screw. This is designed to serve as a stress-breaking device and can be inserted at this juncture or at the time of abutment placement. As an alternative, a titanium IME is available.
10. Place the titanium surgical healing screw into the implant using the hand or reduction handpiece screwdriver. If the handpiece is being used, make the final two to three turns with the hand screwdriver. The flap now may be closed (see Fig. 10-3, *A-G*).

After uncovering the implants, attach the appropriately sized transmucosal implant extension to the implant with a sealing screw. This system has a temporary healing collar, which is similar to Calcitek's. Following a 2-week healing period, the final abutments may be inserted with Teflon or titanium IMEs and prosthetic treatment undertaken. In addition, an antirotational external hex feature is available with IMZ implants.

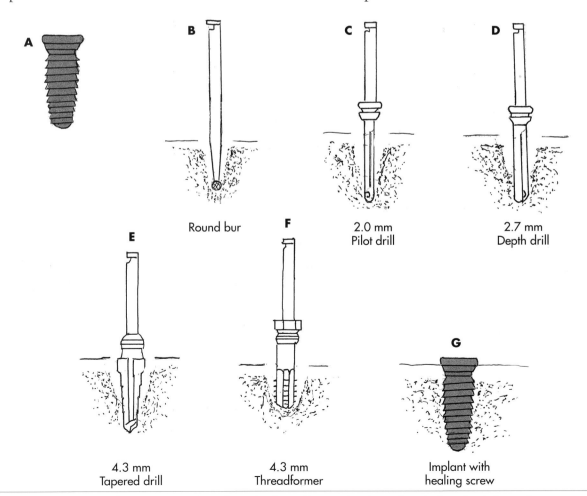

A

B Round bur

C 2.0 mm Pilot drill

D 2.7 mm Depth drill

E 4.3 mm Tapered drill

F 4.3 mm Threadformer

G Implant with healing screw

Fig 10-7 **A-G,** The Steri-Oss Replace system consists of tapering large-diameter implants of particular value in immediate or recent extraction sites. In the illustrations, the alveolus is deepened by 30% and widened to permit precise access of the replace implant as well as to ensure a minimum of 40% newly cut bone contact.

Lifecore Biomedical

Lifecore makes four designs of threaded implants called *Restore* and *Sustain* plus a series of press-fit cylinders.

Threaded Implants

Sustain Design

The Sustain design is HA coated, has an external hex (as do all of the threaded models), and may be obtained in lengths of 8 to 20 mm and the following diameters: 3.3, 3.75, 4, 4.5, and 5 mm.

Restore Design

The three other threaded series of Lifecore Biomedical implants are called *Restore* and are available in a versatile number of lengths and widths. Depending on the surface design (CP titanium, Ti-RBM [distressed surface] [resorbable blast media], or Ti-TPS [irregular surface] [titanium plasma spray]) the diameters vary from 3.3 to 6 mm, and the lengths from 8 to 20 mm. Of particular interest is the RBM, which is a hybrid design, having textured threads apically and, depending on diameter, machined threads (from two to four) beneath the cervices.

The technique of insertion for Sustain and Restore follows the general outline shown in Fig. 10-8.

Press-Fit Cylinders

The Press-Fit cylinder system (like IMZ, Calcitek, and Bio-Vent) is of the smooth-surface design. The 3-mm generic spade drill will have been used to its final depth (1 mm deeper than the length of the chosen implant, which is always a good rule to follow).

1. For the 3.3-mm implant, use the appropriate length trispade finishing drill (10, 13, or 15 mm) to complete the osteotomy.

Threaded Implants

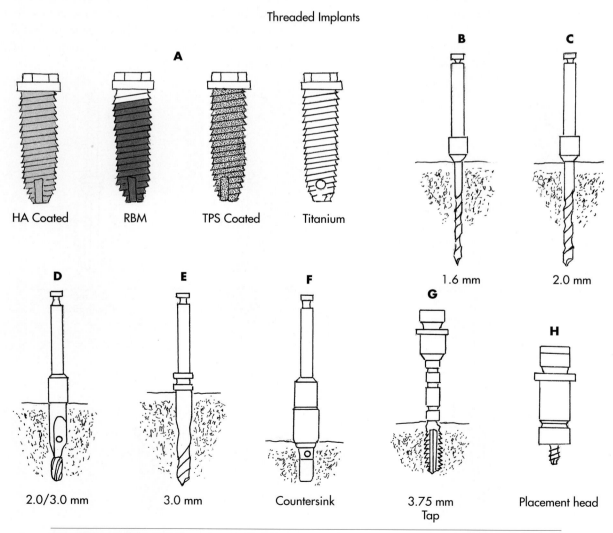

HA Coated   RBM   TPS Coated   Titanium

1.6 mm   2.0 mm

2.0/3.0 mm   3.0 mm   Countersink   3.75 mm Tap   Placement head

Fig. 10-8   A-H, The LifeCore threaded implant system is present with four universally acceptable designs. For implants of 3.3-mm diameters, use a 1.6-mm drill followed by a 2-mm twist drill. This is followed by the pilot drill and the 3-mm twist drill, and finally, the finishing drill. For the three larger dimensions, this diagram should be followed with increasing twist drill and bone tap diameters as needed.

2. If the 4-mm implant is planned, use the matching-diameter trispade finishing drill (available in 8-, 10-, 13-, or 15-mm lengths) to the planned depth, but only after a generic 3.5-mm diameter drill had been used as an interim device.

3. If a 4.7-mm implant is selected, use a 4.5-mm drill followed by the 4.7-mm trispade finishing drill (again in 8-, 10-, 13, or 15-mm lengths) to its final depth.

4. The system supplies steel try-ins in 3.3-, 4-, and 4.7-mm diameters. Use the proper one to confirm proper depth and width.

5. Place the implant into the preparation with firm finger pressure using the package cover, which is the carrying implement. Then twist off the head. Final implant seating is done with a Biocare mallet supplied by the manufacturer and the anterior straight or the posterior bayonet tapper.

The tapper has been designed with a wide diameter plastic tip, which prevents implant overdriving. When properly seated, the implant should be at rest level with the alveolar crest.

6. Place the appropriate healing screw into the implant. In addition to the conventional design, Orthomatrix also makes flanged healing screws. They are intended for use in areas where there is the possibility that the implant may be seated too deeply (e.g., into the maxillary sinus or nasal floor). The flanged screws have a lip that extends beyond the implant circumference that serves as a stop against the bone, thereby preventing the implant from being impelled into an undesirable zone. Their placement into the implant is mandated before it is seated (Fig. 10-9).

Flap closure now may be performed.

Cylindrical Implants

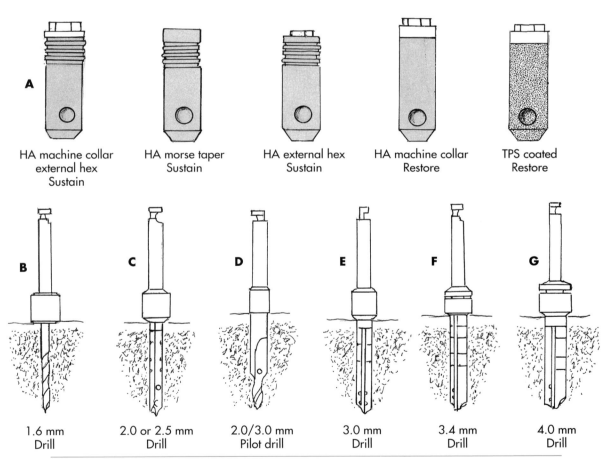

Fig. 10-9 **A-G,** Lifecore makes five press-fit implants. They are available with an external hex and are either hydroxyapatite (HA) or titanium plasma spray (TPS) coated. Under the Restore name there is a TPS and an HA design, each hexed, and with diameters of from 3.4 to 5 mm. Presented in the Sustain product line, are three versions, each with the same dimensional choices. These are all HA coated, two of which are plasma-sprayed over the entire implant, leaving a machined titanium collar. Of interest as well is the use of a screw-in Morse taper abutment for the Sustain design without the exposed metal collar. The Sustain group is further distinguished from the Restore implants by three concentric grooves made below the cervix. This figure presents the classical steps used to seat any of these five designs. Drills of appropriate width must be coordinated with implants of matching diameters. Not shown is the mandatory steel implant try-ins for each design, nor the step using the bayonet tapping instrument with its nylon tip. (Refer to Fig. 10-3 for these steps.)

Implant Innovations Incorporated

The 3i company began its product line by supplying universal abutments for a wide variety of implants. In recent years they have introduced a series of clones that cover the entire spectrum of external hex implants available commercially.

In addition, 3i has made a unique implant design called the *Osseotite* available. It is a hybrid, threaded implant in which the apical threads up to the fourth level are TPS coated and the three most cervical threads are machine finished. The purpose of this design is to incorporate the most desirable features embodied by similar products into one implant (i.e., greater retention apically, less irritating finish cervically).

In addition to Osseotite, the company sells a Brånemark clone as well as models similar to currently available press-fit implants (Fig. 10-10).

These implants are available in the usual lengths of from 7 mm to 20 mm for the standard designs. There are four major categories that are termed *micro, mini, standard,* and *wide* and that vary from 3.25 mm to 6 mm in diameter. The difference between micro and mini is the emerging cervical area.

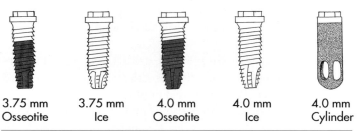

| 3.75 mm | 3.75 mm | 4.0 mm | 4.0 mm | 4.0 mm |
| Osseotite | Ice | Osseotite | Ice | Cylinder |

Fig 10-10   Implant Innovations, Inc. (3i) is a company that manufactures a large variety of implant designs suitable for virtually any application. All of these designs have the external hex configuration, and each is placed following the standard techniques described in this chapter and Chapter 11.

The former is offered with a diameter of 3.4 mm, and the latter, for purposes of improved cosmesis and emergence profile, is available in a diameter of 4.1 mm.

Each of these implant systems is inserted in the fashion described for the same designs of other companies.

Straumann ITI

Hollow Cylinder, Hollow Screw Implants

All implants from the Straumann system are of the single-stage category. The implant neck or abutment-receiving position remains exposed after suturing. The healing screw, therefore, is exteriorized (Fig. 10-11, *A, B*).

Hollow Cylinder, Hollow Screw

ITI hollow cylinder and hollow screw implants are available in 3.5-mm diameters. In addition, they come in both straight and 15-degree angulations.

The principles outlined in Chapter 9 may be followed, but the generic osteotomy steps do not apply to this system.

1. After reflecting the flaps, use the 3-mm diameter spherical bur to make a depression on the ridges at the planned osteotomy site (Fig. 10-11, *C*).
2. Following this, use the appropriate-diameter twist drill (it corresponds to the diameter of the implant that has been chosen) to prepare a 4-mm-deep osteotomy (Fig. 10-11, *D*).
3. Place the matching-diameter trephine mill in the handpiece and, at a fixed low speed, rotate it from this 4-mm level to the final depth. The trephine mill has depth markings indicated by colored rings on the shaft. These rings correspond to the color coding on the implants, each indicating a different length (Fig. 10-11, *E*).
4. The depth gauge, when placed into the osteotomy, will verify the proper depth and is marked with the same color codes (Fig. 10-11, *F*).
5. Place the cylinder implant into the osteotomy with firm finger pressure. Light tapping using an orangewood stick and mallet seats it properly (Fig. 10-11, *G, H*).

6. Before seating the hollow screw implant, use the tap to create a thread pattern within the osteotomy (Fig. 10-11, *I*).
7. Seat the hollow screw with the insertion instrument and is then ratchet wrench it to its final position (Fig. 10-11, *J*).

The flaps now are ready to be closed with sutures placed in purse string fashion around the exposed neck (see Chapter 6).

Solid Screw

ITI solid screw implants are available in 3.3-, 4.1-, and 4.8-mm diameters. For the 3.3-mm-diameter implant, the initial osteotomy should be completed to a 2.5-mm diameter using the generic, internally irrigated burs described in Chapter 9. The final ITI sizing bur is the 2.8-mm twist drill. When selecting the wide diameter (4.8 mm) implant, the final sizing drill is a 4.2-mm twist drill. For the standard diameter 4.1 mm-implant, the osteotomy may be completed to a 3.6-mm diameter. This technique requires placing of the generic osteotomy of 3-mm diameter as first outlined in Chapter 9.

TPS Screw

1. Drive the 3-mm spade drill to a depth 2 mm deeper than the length of the implant and use it for implants of 3.5-mm diameter.
2. For implants of 4-mm diameter, use the 3.2-mm diameter standardized drill to its final depth.
3. Measure each osteotomy with the depth gauge; make it

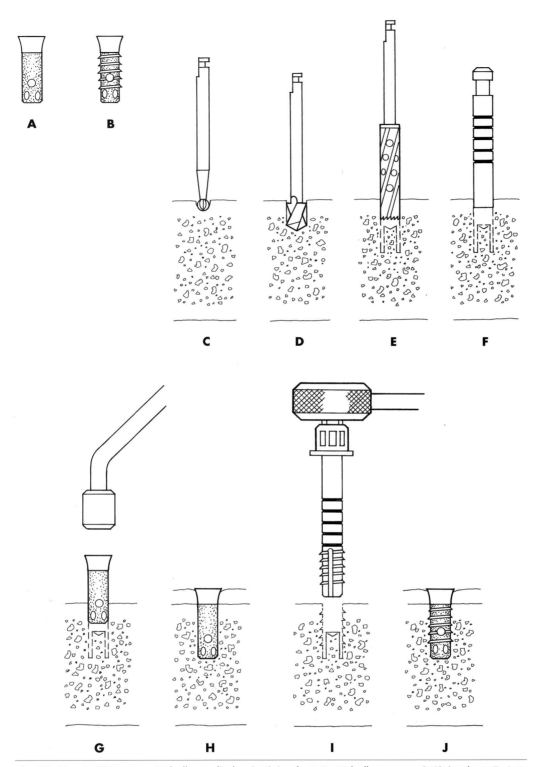

Fig. 10-11 **A,** Straumann ITI hollow cylinder (HC) implant. **B,** ITI hollow screw (HS) implant. **C,** A 3-mm round bur. **D,** A 3.5-mm drill. **E,** Trephine drill. **F,** Depth gauge. **G,** Gently tap the HC implant into position. **H,** Seat the HC implant so that it protrudes through the soft tissue after suturing. **I,** Thread tap with attached ratchet wrench. **J,** Seat the HS implant so that it protrudes through the soft tissue.

1 mm deeper than the length of the chosen implant. This discourages stripping the threads of the osteotomy.
4. Insert these self-tapping, one-stage implants and ratchet them in place with the guide key. Apply gentle apical pressure to the head of the instrument while it is being turned clockwise. Seating is complete when the screw shoulder is found to be lying level with the crest of the ridge (Fig. 10-12).

The flaps now may be closed. The manufacturer suggests that these implants be put into prosthetic service immediately.

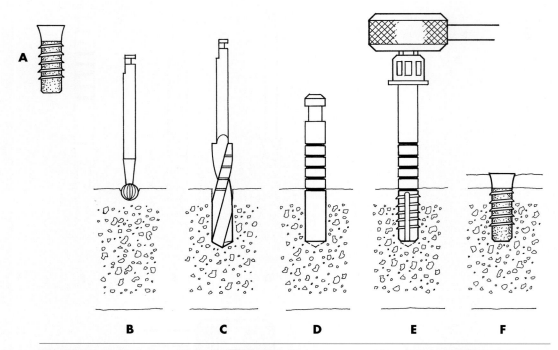

Fig. 10-12 **A,** Straumann ITI Screw (S) implant. **B,** A 3 mm round bur. **C,** Twist drill. **D,** Depth gauge. **E,** Thread tap. **F,** The screw implant is seated so that it protrudes through the soft tissue after suturing.

Suggested Readings

Albrektsson T et al: Osseointegrated oral implants: a Swedish multicenter study of 8,139 consecutively inserted Nobelpharma implants, *J Periodontol* 59:287-296, 1988.

Babbush CA et al: The IMZ endosseous two phase osteointegration system, *Alpha Omegan Scientific* 52-61, 1987.

Becker W et al: One-step surgical placement of Branemark implants: a prospective multicenter clinical study, *Int J Oral Maxillofac Implants* 12:454-462, 1997.

Block MS, Kent JN, Finger IM: Use of the integral implant for overdenture stabilization, *J Oral Maxillofac Implants* 5:140-147, 1990.

David TS et al: A histologic comparison of the bone-implant interface utilizing the Integral (TM) and three surface variations of the Micro-Vent (TM) implant, submitted for publication.

English CE. Part I: Cylindrical implants, Part II: Questions need answering, Part III: An overview (Implants), *Calif Dent* 26-38, 1988.

Friberg B, Grondahl K, Lekholm U: A new self-tapping Branemark implant: clinical and radiographic evaluation, *Int J Oral Maxillofac Implants* 7:80, 1992.

Hahn JA: *The Steri-Oss implant system. Endosteal dental implants* St. Louis, 1991, Mosby.

Kirsch A: The two-phase implantation method using IMZ intramobile cylinder implants, *J Oral Implantol* 11:197-210, 1983.

Kirsch A, Ackerman KL: The IMZ osteointegrated implant system, *Dent Clin North Am* 33:733-791, 1989.

Kirsch A, Mentag P: The IMZ endosseous two phase implant system, *J Oral Implant* 12:494-498, 1986.

Linkow LI, Rinaldi A. Evolution of the Vent-plant osseointegrated compatible implant system, *J Oral Maxillofac Implants* 3:109-122, 1988.

Malmqvist JP, Sennerby L: Clinical report on the success of 47 consecutively placed Core-Vent implants followed from 3 Months to 4 years, *J Oral Maxillofac Implants* 5:53-60, 1990.

Niznick G, Lubar R: The Core-Vent system of osseointegrated implants, *Alpha Omegan Scientific* 62-66, 1987.

Niznick G, Misch CE: The Core-Vent system of osseointegrated implants. In Clark JW, editor: *Clinical dentistry,* Philadelphia, 1987, Harper & Row.

Parel S: Tissue-integrated prosthesis, *J Oral Implantol* 12:435-448, 1986.

Patrick D et al: The longitudinal clinical efficacy of Core-Vent dental implants: a five-year report, *J Oral Implantol* 15:95-103, 1989.

Ross SE et al: The immediate placement of an endosseous implant into an extraction wound: a clinical case report using the *RosTR system, Int J Periodont Rest Dent* 9:35-41, 1989.

Saadoun AP, LeGall ML: Clinical results and guidelines on Steri-Oss endosseous implants, *Int J Periodontics Restorative Dent* 12:487, 1992.

Stultz ER, Lofland R, Sendax VI et al: A multicenter 5 year restropective survival analysis of 6200 Integral implants, *Compend Contin Educ Dent* 14:478, 1993.

Valeron JF, Velasquez JF: Placement of screw-type implants in the pterygomaxillary-pyramidal region: surgical procedure and preliminary results, *Int J Oral Maxillofac Implants* 12:814-819, 1997.

Wozniak WT: Dental implants and ADA acceptance, *J Am Dent Assoc* 13:879, 1986.

Zarb GA. A status report on dental implants, *Can Cent Assoc J* 49:841-843, 1983.

11

Root Form Implant Surgery: Proprietary II

BioHorizons Maestro System

The BioHorizons Maestro System consists of four basically styled, titanium alloy–threaded implants (Fig. 11-1, *A*). They have slight tapers from cervix to apex. These implants take variable bone density into account by altering thread design and spacing as well as surface configuration.

A No. 6 round bur is used to start the osteotomy. Twist drills (externally irrigated only) are available in a variety of lengths and in 10 closely graduated diameters. When the appropriately sized osteotomy is completed for either Division A (best to better bone: 4 and 5 mm), Division B (poorer bone: 3.5 mm), or Division CH (compromised height), the crestal or counter-sink drill is used. The D1, D2, or D3 bone tap is then applied (depending on bone quality) to complete the fully threaded osteotomy (Fig. 11-1, *B-E*).

The thread patterns and surfaces of these implants have been designed to serve optimally in the bone for which it is planned. For the poorest bone density (type D4) all the implants are hydroxyapatite (HA) coated; for the next level of bone (type D3), all the implants are titanium plasma spray (TPS) coated. When presented with the highest quality of bone (D1, D2), the implants are coated with resorbable blast media (RBM). In addition, the implants designed for the densest types of bone have the fewest number of threads, which are wider, thicker, and have sharper angles to facilitate their entry.

Bicon

In accordance with the manufacturer's instructions for using a Bicon implant, create a depth 2 mm greater than the planned implant length with the 2.5-mm spade drill (Fig. 11-2, *A-C*).

The remaining steps may be performed by hand reaming or by the use of a cooled spade drill.

1. Advance the 3-mm drill to a depth of 2 mm greater than the implant length. The markings on the drills are actual distances and represent the real implant length (Fig. 11-2, *D*). Collect the bone chips, grindings, and osseous coagulum produced in a bone filter (Ace Surgical; see Chapter 8) and place in a saline solution. Some particles will cling to the reamers or must be harvested from the suction filter.
2. The procedure should be repeated using the 3.5-, 4-, and then 5-mm VLS drills, depending on the implant diameter that corresponds with them (Fig. 11-2, *E*).
3. When the osteotomy is complete, place the depth gauge into the implant osteotomy for corroboration. The markings on this instrument correspond to measurements that are 2 mm greater than this system's implant lengths. The proper line on the gauge should be level with the crest of the ridge, which ensures that the implant rests 2 mm below the crest of bone (Fig. 11-2, *F*).
4. The implant inserter is connected to the implant with finger pressure.
5. Push the implant into the osteotomy, and then rotate clockwise with finger pressure, approximately 180 degrees (Fig. 11-2, *G*).
6. Remove the implant inserter by rotating its lower knob counterclockwise while stabilizing the top knob with the other hand (Fig. 11-2, *H*).

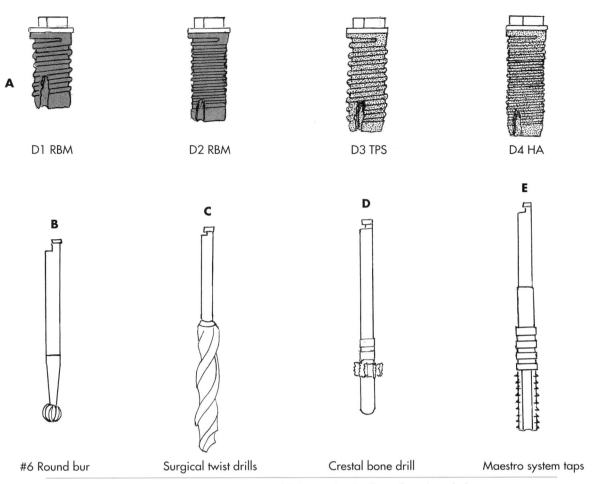

D1 RBM   D2 RBM   D3 TPS   D4 HA

#6 Round bur   Surgical twist drills   Crestal bone drill   Maestro system taps

Fig. 11-1 BioHorizons Maestro System. **A-E,** This innovative titanium alloy–threaded system uses varying thread designs and surface configurations for bone of different density. *A* indicates implant designs for bone of decreasing density. Note that D4 bone calls for tight threads and hydroxyapatite coating. The methods of osteotomy follow classic techniques with drills of increasing diameter.

7. Place the black plastic healing plug into the implant with finger pressure. It should extend approximately 4 mm above the implant (Fig. 11-2, *I*).
8. The bone chips and grindings that were harvested should be packed around the cervix of the implant (Fig. 11-2, *J*).

9. The healing plug should be cut flush with the level of the bone with a fine diamond stone in a water-cooled, high-speed handpiece or with sharp scissors (Fig. 11-2, *K, L*).

   The flap may now be sutured.

Park Dental Startanius, Starvent

When using the Park Dental Startanius, Starvent, the 3-mm generic spade drill is used to its planned depth.

1. The osteotomy is enlarged with the 3.17-mm spade drill to the predetermined depth.
2. Continue the steps of enlargement with the finger-held, final sizing reamer (3.3 mm).
3. Using gentle finger pressure to form the counter-sink, complete the osteotomy by hand and by using the counterbore reamer in a clockwise direction.
4. The millimeter-calibrated depth gauge should be placed into the osteotomy to confirm its depth.

5. Screw the one-piece StarVent insertion instrument to the implant.
6. Seat the implant and start to thread it into the surgical preparation using the StarVent hand wrench. Complete the seating by using the ratchet wrench turned in a clockwise direction.
7. When the implant is fully seated, place the healing closure plug using the plug socket-and-hexhead wrench.

   The flaps should now be sutured.

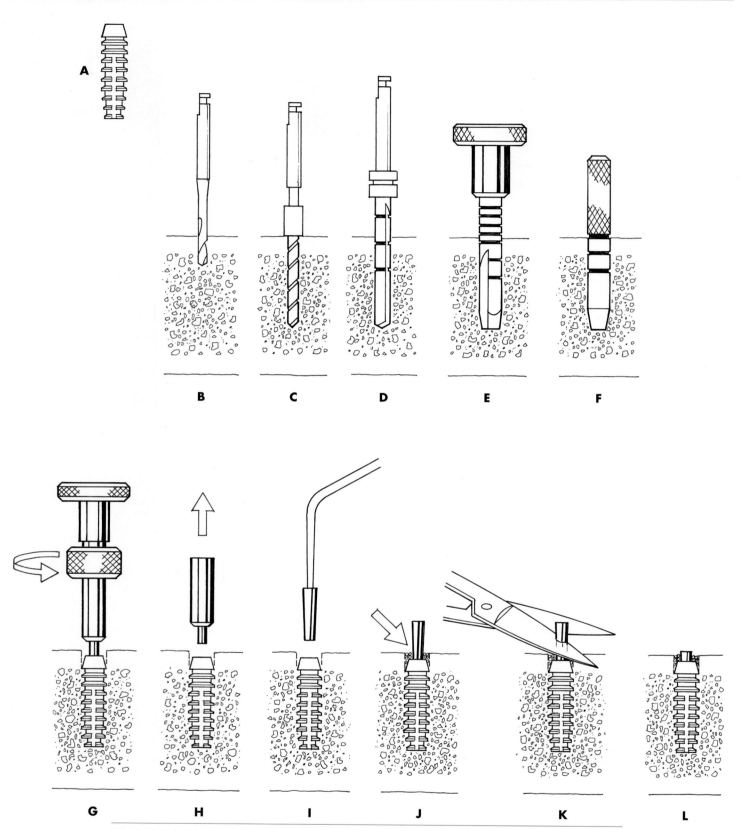

Fig. 11-2 **A,** Bicon precision fit implant. **B,** The manufacturer's recommended procedure begins by penetrating the cortical bone at the planned implant site with a 700 XL bur. **C,** The 2.5-mm spade drill. **D,** The 3-mm spade drill. **E,** The 3.5-mm hand reamer. **F,** Depth gauge. **G,** Seat the implant. **H,** Remove the implant inserter. **I,** Plastic healing plug. **J,** Pack bone chips around the implant. **K,** Cut the plastic healing plug flush with the bone. **L,** Seat the Bicon implant 2 mm below the crest of bone with the plastic healing plug flush with the bone.

Oratronics Spiral

When using the Oratronics Spiral implant, the 3-mm generic spade drill is used to the final, preplanned depth.

1. The spiral tap that corresponds to the appropriate implant width (3.5 or 5 mm) and length (No. 2, 3, or 4) is selected and attached to the hand ratchet.
2. Enlarge the osteotomy to the chosen length and width in a clockwise direction. Apply apical pressure to the head of the ratchet wrench with the forefinger of the other hand for purposes of exerting countertorquing influences.
3. On completion of the osteotomy, the implant should be attached to the titanium inserter, placed in the hand wrench, and rotated to its final seating position. The implant, when fully seated, has its Periohead in place.

The flaps are sutured to complete the insertion of the Spiral.

Omni-R

When using the Omni-R, complete the 3-mm generic spade drill to its predetermined depth (Fig. 11-3, *A-C*).

1. Rotate the Omni intermediate drill to its final depth (Fig. 11-3, *D*).
2. Insert the R2 hand auger into the osteotomy and rotate counterclockwise while applying firm apical pressure. This is continued to the final depth. If greater torque is needed, the straight handle may be used with the hand auger (Fig. 11-3, *E*).
3. The R2 hand auger grants the requisite width for the 3.5-mm-diameter implant.
4. For the 4.5-mm implant, flush the osteotomy with sterile saline and repeat step 3 using the R8 hand auger.
5. The 5.5-mm implant requires the use of the R2, the R8, and the R10 hand augurs. The osteotomy must be flushed with sterile saline between auger applications.
6. Place these implants into the bone with finger pressure.
7. Follow the placement with gentle tapping with a mallet and a titanium- or a Delrin-tipped seating instrument. The implant should be driven to a position level with the alveolar crest (Fig. 11-3, *F*).

Suturing the flaps completes the procedure.

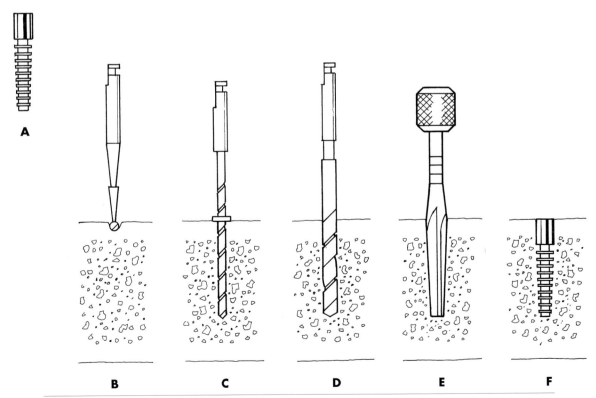

A   **B**   **C**   **D**   **E**   **F**

Fig. 11-3   A, Omni-R series implant. **B,** The manufacturer recommended procedure begins by penetrating the cortical plate at the proposed site with a No. 4 round bur. **C,** Use the pilot drill to the full implant depth. **D,** Intermediate drill. **E,** R2 hand auger. **F,** Seat the Omni-R series implant so that it is flush with the crest of the bone.

Kyocera Bioceram

Before using the Kyocera Bioceram implant, the osteotomy is performed to the determined depth using the 2.5-mm generic spade drill. (The minimum recommended depth is 11 mm for the short implants and 14 mm for the long implants.) The porous portion of each implant should ideally be 5 mm below the alveolar crest, although the minimum acceptable depth is 3 mm.

1. Enlarge the generic osteotomy with the cannon drill to the final diameter.
2. In dense bone, the osteotomy is enlarged and refined with the expand reamer. If the bone is not dense, the bone harvested from the surgery may be packed into the osteotomy before implant insertion to create a firmer receptor site. Surgically produced bone (osseous coagulum) can be collected and retrieved by using an in-line bone filter in the surgical evacuation tip (Gelman Sciences, product 4320). The finger driver (marked EX[pos] or EX[ant]) is attached

to the expand reamer and turned one full revolution. At this time, parallelism must be rechecked using the large end of a paralleling pin. The osteotomy depth should be checked, as well, with the depth markings on the pin.
3. Place the implant with firm finger pressure.
4. Attach a finger driver to the implant. For the 42 [pos] (L) implant, the 37 to 42 [ant] or [pos] driver should be used. For the 48 [pos] (L) implant, the 48 [ant] or [pos] driver is recommended. Rotate the finger driver clockwise with firm finger pressure until the implant is fully seated.

Suturing now may be performed. This is a one-stage implant. If it interferes with the occlusion after placement and suturing, the coronal portion must be reduced using a water-cooled, high-speed diamond. While trimming the implant, stabilize it firmly with a notched hemostat that has its beaks covered with polyethylene tubing.

Innova Endopore Implant

The first stage surgical procedure for the Endopore dental implant system is completed in four basic steps.

1. Expose the crestal bone by an appropriate incision and reduce the ridge if necessary using a tapered irrigated carbide bur at 2000 to 3000 rpm. Dimple the crest at the pilot drill site with a No. 6 round bur at 1800 to 2000 rpm. Use the pilot drill at 1000 rpm to create a bone passage for the implant bur. Drilling is recommended in short bursts and

only to the indicated depth corresponding to the chosen implant length. Remove bone chips with frequent irrigation (Fig. 11-4, *A*).
2. Select an implant bur that corresponds to the implant length. This bur deepens the osteotomy. Operating the bur at 700 rpm with constant irrigation minimizes heat (Fig. 11-4, *B*).
3. The appropriately sized trial-fit gauge should be placed into the site. All aspects of the gauge must be inspected visually

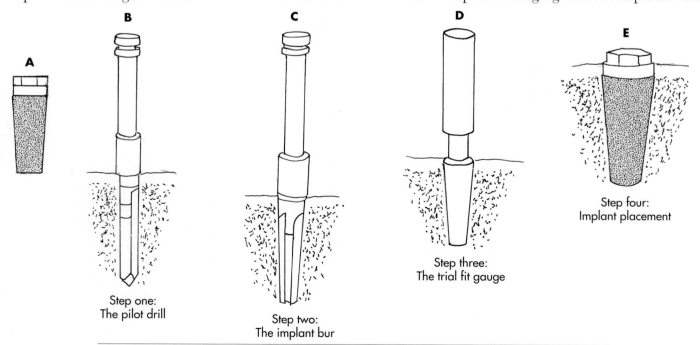

Step one:
The pilot drill

Step two:
The implant bur

Step three:
The trial fit gauge

Step four:
Implant placement

Fig. 11-4   A-E, The Endopore implant has a surface macrostructure of sintered titanium beads. Such a design greatly increases the surface area and encourages high levels of intraosseous retention. The technique for seating uses the classic bone enlargement drill, a steel try-in, and placement of the implant in the press-fit mode.

to confirm that its shoulder is 1 to 2 mm below the bone surface. This will ensure that the implant is placed deeply enough in crestal bone to help prevent micromovement during the healing phase. If the shoulder margin is visible, the implant bur should be reintroduced to deepen the host site. A final rechecking with the trial-fit gauge should precede the implant placement (Fig. 11-4, *C*).

Friatec and Frialit 2

The manufacturer describes the Friatec and Frialit 2 implants as stepped screw or press-fit TPS-coated implants designed to increase primary stability in poor-quality bone. Place them into a tapered, stepped osteotomy first with finger pressure and then, for final seating, ratchet them into a deeper threaded environment. The nonthreaded designs are accompanied by a plastic-tipped seating instrument, which is used to tap the implant fully into place in its incrementally shaped infrabony site. The implants are available in 3.8-, 4.5-, and 5.5-mm diameters.

1. Prepare a primary purchase point at the planned osteotomy site with a 3.8-mm round drill (Fig. 11-5, *A*).
2. The 3-mm generic spade drill has already been used to create the final depth of the osteotomy.
3. Enlarge the receptor site to its final diameter using the 3.8-mm stepped drill. It should be noted that when placing the 4.5-mm and 5.5-mm diameter implants, the successive use of the 4.5- and 5.5-mm stepped drills is required (Fig. 11-5, *B*).

4. Aseptically transfer the implant to the prepared bone site. A gentle rocking motion will disengage the implant delivery tool. The plastic tip of the seating punch should be set on the implant cap. Several sharp taps of the mallet on the punch firmly and completely seat the implant into the site. Close the gingiva with interrupted 4-0 Vicryl mattress sutures moving from the distal anteriorly (Fig. 11-4, *D,E*).

4. Press the implant into the receptor site. It is important that one of the vertical grooves on the implant be placed toward the facial aspect to properly align the internal hex (Fig. 11-5, *C*).
5. Tap the placement head with the seating instrument and a surgical mallet to position the implant in its primary location.
6. Remove the placement head. Insert the stepped screw implant driver into the internal hex of the implant and place the ratchet on the other end of the driver. Three full turns are sufficient to place the implant in its final position (Fig. 11-5, *D*). (The press-fit design requires nothing but simple tapping.)
7. Then remove the ratchet and stepped screw implant driver. Thread the sealing screw into position with a screwdriver (Fig. 11-5, *E*).

The flaps are sutured to place. The uncovering of these implants is performed in standard fashion.

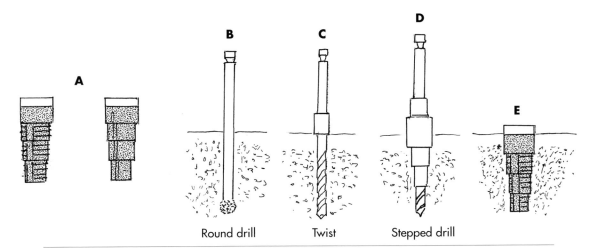

Round drill   Twist   Stepped drill

Fig. 11-5 **A-E,** The Frialit 2 implant has a worthy ancestor, the polycrystalline Al_2O_3 Tubingen Frialit 1 implant. This early press-fit design produced excellent results in Tubingen University, and its titanium offspring present an attractive entry into the marketplace. Its metallic construction has permitted the addition of a threaded version described in **A,** *left,* as well as the traditional press-fit (**A,** *right*). The threaded implant is supplied with a ratchet wrench for purposes of self-tapping.

Sargon

The manufacturer describes the Sargon implant as having an apical expansion design that allows the immediate placement of a functional restoration. The implant is activated at the time of surgery so that it expands, molly bolt–like, into the surgical site. The implant is 3.8 mm in diameter with a collar diameter of 4.1 mm (Fig. 11-6, *A*).

Use the 3-mm twist drill to create the generic width and the final selected implant length.

1. To prepare the superior portion of the osteotomy for the collar of the implant, rotate the counterbore drill 1 mm, the height of the implant collar (Fig. 11-6, *B*).
2. Initiate the tap and set the direction of the threads with the pilot tap (Fig. 11-6, *C*).
3. Thread the surgical site to the desired depth with the final tap. In order to avoid binding while threading the site, the tap should be periodically reversed a few turns, before completion of final threading to the appropriate line. Sargon implants are not designed to be self-tapping.
4. Screw the implant into the surgical site by hand with the im-

plant driver assembly until it bottoms out in the site; then remove the assembly driver with a quick turn (Fig. 11-6, *D*).
5. Insert the screwdriver into the head of the implant's slotted screw and turn clockwise to draw the expansion mechanism up into the implant. As the mechanism rises, the body of the implant expands into the walls of the surgical site. When the screw no longer turns, the implant is completely expanded and seated (Fig. 11-6, *E*).
6. Strike the implant lightly with a metal instrument. The sound should be that of a fully integrated implant. If the sound does not represent full integration, or if the implant is mobile, retightening the internal screw will further expand the implant. As an alternative criterion, the Periotest can be applied. Readings of −2 or lower should be reached (Fig. 11-6, *F*).
7. A healing collar of appropriate length or an immediate fixed abutment can be placed (Fig. 11-6, *G*).

The flaps are then sutured to place around the abutment neck in the same fashion as for a blade or ITI implant.

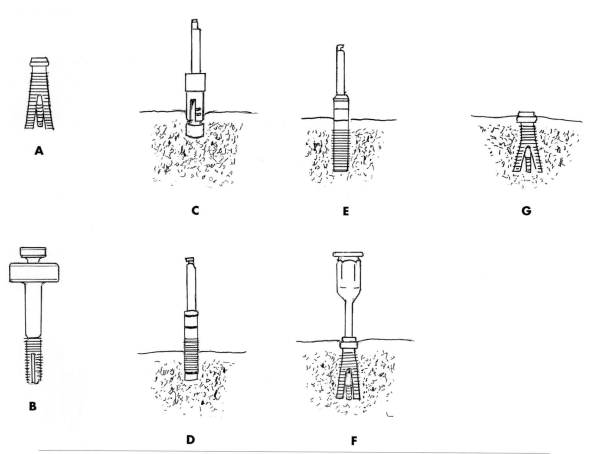

Fig. 11-6   A-G, Seat the Sargon expandable implant designed for extraction sites using the technique pictured in these six **(B-G)** illustrations. Considerable interest has been elicited by this design because of the immediate high levels of stability exhibited after activation of the expansion mechanism. Previous designs similar to this were described by Leger-Dorez in 1920 and Lehmans in 1959 . After pilot drilling, enlarge and tap the osteotomy. Finally, fully seat the implant into deep virgin bone, and open its legs with the wrench.

Astra Tech Dental Implant

The Astra Tech Dental Implant is described by the manufacturer as being a self-tapping, parallel-sided implant having a conical seal design (Morse taper; see Chapter 2) that allows for simple, self-guiding seating of the abutment. The implant is available in 3.5- and 4-mm diameters (Fig. 11-7, *A*). The implant sites are prepared in a step-by-step procedure using Tiger drills of different diameters with indicators revealing a direct reading of the correct depth (Fig. 11-7, B, *C*).

The procedure ensures an efficient and gentle widening of the host site. The Tiger drills should be replaced when they become less efficient, normally after preparation of 50 to 60 fixture sites, or when judged necessary by the surgeon (Fig. 11-7, *D-G*).

All preparation of the bone tissue is carried out under profuse irrigation with room-temperature saline and with an intermittent drilling technique. This prevents over-heating of the bone and creates a pumping effect for efficient removal of ground tissue debris. After completion of the osteotomy, the implants are placed employing the following protocol.

The implants are packaged in glass ampules. Snap open the ampule and drop the implant into a saline-filled titanium bowl. Pick up the implant with the titanium forceps and screw the adapter into the implant while holding the implant by the smooth cylindrical part. Grip the lock nut with the forceps and turn the adapter clockwise. Install the implant by fastening it with a few turns manually. Turn the self-tapping implant further with the contra-angle, and use the ratchet to finalize the placement. Release the adapter by turning the lock nut clockwise and unscrewing it completely. Place the cover screw with the hexagonal screwdriver. The flaps are then sutured to place in the usual fashion (Fig. 11-7, *H*).

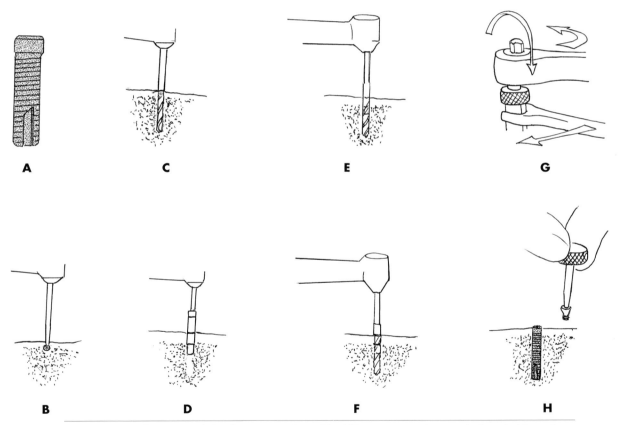

Fig. 11-7   **A,** The Astra Tech implant. **B,** Use the guide drill to penetrate the marginal cortical bone layer and the underlying spongy bone. During the initial preparation, the guide drill should be tilted to allow more precise and efficient cutting. **C,** Initially, the fixture site is prepared with the 2.5-mm Tiger drill (red). Careful positioning of the drill ensures a correct depth and inclination of the holes. The objective is to level or slightly submerge the fixture in relation to adjacent marginal bone. Direction indicators (paralleling pins) may be placed in the sites to facilitate the inclination of the subsequent drilling. **D,** Use the pilot drill as an intermediate step in spongy bone. Guide the pilot drill for the 3.5-mm fixture into the 2.5-mm holes and create a 3.2-mm osteotomy. **E,** As a standard procedure, drill all fixture sites to full depth with the 3.2-mm Tiger drill (green). **F,** Widen the 3.2-mm hole with the 3.7-mm Tiger drill (black) for the 4-mm fixture. **G,** Use cortical drills when the marginal bone layer is thick and dense. The cortical drills create a hole of the same diameter as the smooth neck of the fixtures (3.55 and 4 mm, respectively). **H,** Use the 3.35-mm Tiger drill (1.106) for the 3.5-mm fixture, and use the 3.85-mm Tiger drill (brown) for the 4-mm fixture when the quality of the medullary bone is dense (i.e., at the symphysis of the mandible). The final step before suturing is placement of the healing screw.

Osteomed Hextrac Fixture

The Osteomed Hextrac Fixture is a titanium Brånemark-like implant that is placed in the classical fashion. It is an external hex implant available in 3.75- and 5.2-mm diameters and in lengths of from 8 to 20 mm. The maximum length of the 5.2-mm design however, is 13 mm. The smaller diameter is available with an HA coating (see Fig. 10-2, p. 194).

The company manufactures press-fit cylinders to complete its implant line. They are available as 3.3-mm diameter implants, varying in length from 8 to 15 mm, and they are coated with TPS as well as HA over TPS. The technique of placing them follows the instruction for insertion of the Calcitek press-fit implant group (see Fig. 10-3, p. 195).

Suggested Readings

Babbush CA, Robbins AM: The titanium plasma spray (TPS) screw implant system, *Alpha Omegan Scientific* 80-85, 1987.

Babbush CA: ITI endosteal hollow cylinder implant systems, *Dent Clin North Am* 30:133-149, 1986.

Buser D et al: The treatment of partially edentulous patients with ITI hollow-screw implants: presurgical evaluation and surgical procedures, *J Oral Maxillofac Implants* 5:165-174, 1990.

Hashimoto M et al: Single-crystal sapphire endosseous dental implant loaded with functional stress clinical and histological evaluation of per-implant tissues, *J Oral Rehabil* 15:65-76, 1988.

Lefovke MD, Beals RP: Immediate loading of cylinder implants with overdentures in the mandibular symphysis: the titanium plasma-sprayed screw technique, *J Oral Implantol* 16:265-271, 1990.

McKinney RV et al: The single-crystal sapphire endosseous dental implant, *J Oral Implantol* 10:487-503, 1982.

Misch CE: Density of bone: effect on treatment plans, surgical approach, healing and progressive bone loading, *Int J Oral Implant* 6:23-31, 1990.

Muhlbradt L et al: The sensitivity to touch of the Tubingen immediate implantations, *Dtsch Zahnarztl Z* 35:334-338, 1980.

Pietrokovski J: The bony residual ridge in man, *J Prosthet Dent* 34:456-462, 1975.

Quayle AA et al: The immediate or delayed replacement of teeth by permucosal intraosseous implants: the Tubingen implant system. Part I. Implant design, rationale for use and preoperative assessment, *Br Dent J* 166:365-370, 1989.

Roberts R: *History of the Ramus frame implant,* Alabama Implant Congress, Birmingham, Alabama, May 1985.

Schroeder A et al: ITI double hollow cylinder implant, *Schweiz Montatsschr Zahnmed* 94:503-510, 1984.

Sutter F et al: The new concept of ITI hollow-cylinder and hollow-screw implants. Part I. Engineering and design, *J Oral Maxillofac Implants* 3:161-172, 1988.

Weiss MB: Titanium fiber-mesh metal implant, *J Oral Implantol* 12:498-507, 1986.

12

Blade and Plate-Form Implant Surgery

ARMAMENTARIUM

Amalgam carrier, nylon-tipped plunger type
Blades: No. 12, No. 15 (BP)
Bone substitute materials
Burs: No. 1, 700 XL and XXL
Curettes, surgical
Diamond, pear-shaped (SFX-30/L)
Forceps, Gerald or Adson (toothed) pickup
Handpieces: high-speed friction grip (FG), Impactair, low-speed
     (laboratory type)
Hemostat: titanium or plastic-tipped, small, curved (mosquito)
Implant sham or try-in (when available)
Low-speed, channel cutting wheels
Mallet, nylon-headed
Metal cutter, broad blade, heavy-duty
Periodontal probe
Periosteal elevators

Pliers, titanium-tipped, cone-socket (for bending, when needed)
Polishing wheels, aluminum oxide impregnated (⅝ inch) and
     mandrel for mounting
Retractors (Henahan, beaver tail, Seldin)
Retractors, blunt Mathieu
Syringe, irrigating
Sterile saline
Suction (Frazier No. 12) tips (plastic)
Seating instruments (straight and bayonet) for abutment and
     shoulder seating
Suture with FS2 needles or C12, 4-0 dyed Vicryl, Polysorb, or
     Biosyn
Scissors, tissue and suture
Sterilizer, glass bead
Sterile glass beaker filled with sterile saline
Scalpels, handles

CAVEATS

The surgeon must have completed each of the steps described in Chapter 4. Establish the thickness and depth of the prospective host site. If the ridge is less than 3 mm in width, flatten it to the requisite width and then determine the remaining height to ascertain that there is still room for blade placement.

Know the presence, locations, and depth of fossae, depressions, and undercuts (see Chapter 4), and make all osteotomies midway between the buccal and lingual cortices.

Be aware of the floors of the antra and nose, as well as the mandibular and mental neurovascular bundles, which are critical structures. It is possible, however, to reroute bundles as well as to elevate the antral floor (see Chapter 8). Novel S-shaped or visor-type incisions should not be used, or the tissues between the crest of the ridge and the incision might be lost (see Chapter 7).

Unless the mucoperiosteal reflection is restricted, attempts to "spring" thin cortical plates after completing the osteotomy are discouraged, particularly in the mandible, because fracture or devascularization of these bony walls may occur. Before seating an implant, test the depth, patency, and integrity (i.e., absence of perforations) of each osteotomy using a periodontal probe for exploration.

Wash the talc from rubber gloves and handle the implant as little as possible. It should be stored between manipulations and try-ins in a glass beaker of sterile saline, and the bead sterilizer can be used to sterilize it again if handling has caused it to become contaminated. Wash residual glass beads from the interstices using saline.

Select implant systems that come supplied with try-ins. Blades with the anchor-shoulder-cervix configuration are preferable (Fig. 12-1).

If a revision of the infrastructure is required, it should be cut, trimmed, and polished impeccably. If bending or curving of the infrastructure or cervix is needed to permit better fit or alignment, do it slowly and carefully and never at sharp angles. To permit maximal control, the operator's elbows should be braced against his or her body with stiffened wrists while the bending is done. Avoid overbending because further reshaping may cause fractures. Fit the implant gently into the osteotomy after each alteration, using finger pressure only, and store it in saline or a bead sterilizer between steps. Polish all cut ends with an alumna-impregnated wheel, and rinse them carefully with saline.

Use continuous horizontal mattress sutures for closure (see Chapter 6).

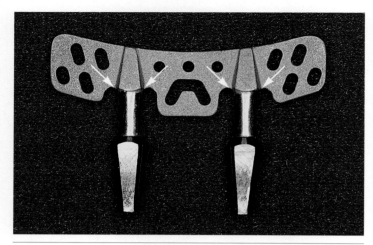

Fig. 12-1   A two-abutment blade implant with an anchor configuration shoulder *(arrows)*. This design discourages complications resulting from the saucerization phenomenon.

Surgical Techniques

Conventional Blade Implants: Single Stage

Incision and Reflection

When possible, anesthesia for the posterior mandible (see Chapter 4) should be made by infiltration only. This permits the lower lip to remain unanesthetized. By infiltrating, the surgeon is granted the built-in protection of having the patient possibly respond as the neurovascular bundle is approached (Fig. 12-2).

Make the incision by placing a No. 15 BP blade against bone using the fine linea alba at the crest as a guide and drawing the scalpel firmly forward. Take care not to deviate from this critical narrow avascular zone. Novel crestal incisions of any design (e.g., "S" visor) that deviate from the crest should be avoided, since areas of gingivae included within them may become necrotic. When it becomes necessary to extend the incision distally beyond the fixed gingiva in the posterior mandible and into the retromolar pad, keep in mind the location of the pterygomandibular space and its contents. To avoid injuring these tissues, the anterior border of the ramus should be palpated and the incision directed over this structure, which is often found about 5 mm laterally.

The incision should be sharp and clean so that it need not be retraced. By retracing the incision, strips of periosteum are created that interfere with the gingival and superficial osseous vascular supply (Fig. 12-3).

The incision needs no buccal or lingual relief posteriorly, but, at the anterior end, extend it buccally and lingually around the most distal tooth in position. These two extensions offer sufficient relief to permit adequate exposure of the host bone. Initiate the reflection of the flaps anteriorly at the mesial papilla of the most distal tooth and complete it by moving the elevator posteriorly (Fig. 12-4). This exposes the ridge to the base of the vestibules buccally and lingually.

The periosteal elevator should be sharp so that it succeeds in incising periosteal fibers rather than tearing them. If these fibers are resistant to the elevator, the full-thickness flap may be lifted with a mouse tooth (Adson) forceps and the periosteal fibers cut with a No. 12 blade (see Chapter 8).

The ideal location for the placement of the osteotomy is at the crest of the ridge. If the ridge is knife-edged, flatten (Fig. 12-5). By placing retractors (beaver tails, blunt rakes, or periosteal elevators) and using a pear-shaped diamond (SFX-30/L) in the high-speed handpiece or Impactair, the crest can be flattened so that a minimal table width of 3 mm is achieved. Inspection of the operative site then should be performed.

1. Identify the location of the mental neurovascular bundle. It should not be exposed or dissected unless its sanctity is potentially threatened by the procedure.
2. Evaluate the external oblique and mylohyoid ridges as well as the configuration of the cortical plates inferior to them. Extreme undercuts or exaggerated concavities such as the submandibular and canine fossae demand redirection or relocation of the osteotomy.
3. Record the width of the ridge not only at the crest, but also at all points apically that correspond with the planned implant depth. If the ridge is less than 4 mm wide at the deepest portion of the planned implant site, conduct the operative plan with great care, detect and treat perforations of bone with grafting materials (see Chapters 7 and 8).
4. Establish the nature and quality of the cortex. Note its color, consistency, and morphology. It offers evidence of good local health (ivory in color, freedom of porosities, properly shaped with minimal irregularities or defects).

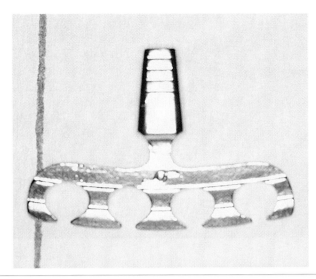

Fig. 12-2 A conventional single-stage mandibular blade implant. Bone, connective tissue, or both will anchor the infrastructure in place by growing through the interstices. Place the shoulder at least 2 mm below the ridge crest. Such titanium implants may be adjusted by bending for abutment parallelism.

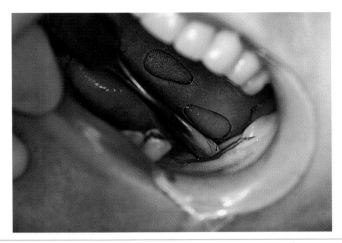

Fig. 12-4 Flap reflection should be made with a sharp periosteal elevator to expose enough bony structure to permit entry of the bur for the osteotomy.

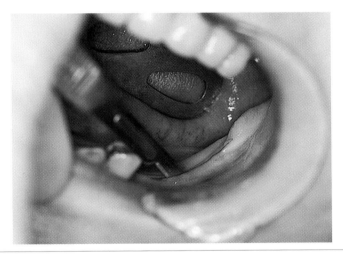

Fig. 12-3 Make incisions for blades in the linea alba at the crest of the ridge.

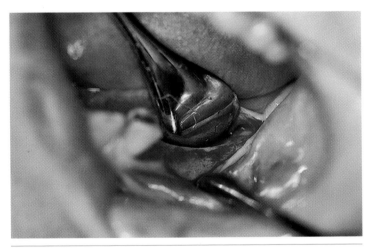

Fig. 12-5 Sufficient retraction is necessary to ascertain ridge morphology. Excessive exposure is to be discouraged. This knife-edged ridge requires flattening with a diamond bur or rongeur forceps.

5. Assess the condition of the newly reflected mucoperiosteal flaps. Record tears, loss of tissue, or ischemic appearance. If the flaps are considered to be irreparable, cancellation or delaying of the surgery is recommended. Chapter 7 offers advice on how to make primary closures when the supply of tissue is absent or the flaps fall short of approximating each other.

Osteotomy

Use of a preoperatively prepared surgical template is of benefit. Fabrication details are given in Chapter 4. Once it has been determined that acceptable ridge height, morphology, and width are available, select the osteotomy site. Place a No. 1 round bur into the high-speed handpiece and, after establishing the anteroposterior length by measuring the chosen implant, make bur holes at the anterior and posterior ends of the planned groove.

Make a series of bur holes just through the cortex between the anterior and posterior witness marks along the crest of the ridge using a saline-cooled No. 1 round bur (Fig. 12-6). On completion, assess their alignment and location. If they are straight and properly located, they can be connected with a 700 XXL fissure bur (Fig. 12-7, A-C). Light brushing motions and copious amounts of coolant are important. Score the shank of the bur at the point that signifies the proper osteotomy depth. Using a firm but light grasp, deepen the host site to the score line on the bur. Since the shoulder should be buried beneath the bone margins to a depth of 2 mm, the osteotomy deep enough to permit this. Flatten any deep irregularities by brushing the bur gently through the bone groove. Test the osteotomy with the periodontal probe to assess depth, smoothness, and lack of cortical plate perforations (Fig. 12-8).

The surgeon may use an osteotomy wheel as an alternative to a high-speed bur. It is designed for a low-speed, water-

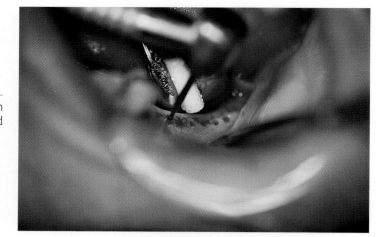

Fig. 12-6 Start the osteotomy for blades and plate-form implants with a series of perforations made about 2 mm apart with a small, No. 1 round bur in the air turbine.

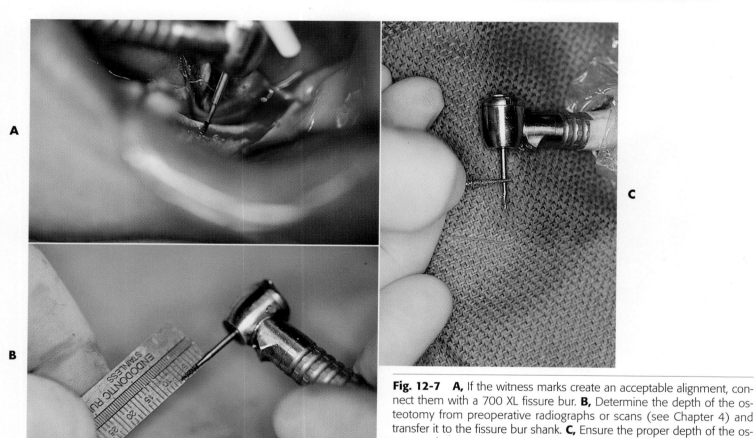

Fig. 12-7 **A,** If the witness marks create an acceptable alignment, connect them with a 700 XL fissure bur. **B,** Determine the depth of the osteotomy from preoperative radiographs or scans (see Chapter 4) and transfer it to the fissure bur shank. **C,** Ensure the proper depth of the osteotomy by scoring the fissure bur shank with a diamond drill. Hold the diamond against the rotating bur in order to make an accurate mark.

Fig. 12-8 After the osteotomy has been completed and is satisfactory in length and depth, test it for integrity (i.e., no perforations) and smoothness, using a periodontal millimeter probe.

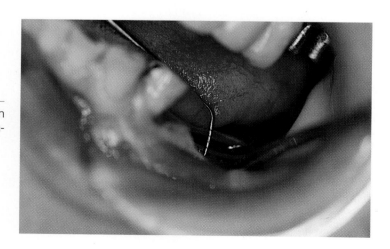

cooled operation and can serve as an excellent groove starter. Final shaping and deepening to accommodate the selected blade or plate-form implant must be completed with burs, however, as described in the previous paragraphs.

Implant Placement

If the manufacturer does not supply the implant as "ready-to-insert," Appendix E offers methods of treating metals. When the implant is ready, place it into the osteotomy and, using strong finger pressure, force it down as far as it will go. Evaluate appropriate length of the groove and parallelism of the abutment (Fig. 12-9). If needed, remove the implant and bend the abutment using two titanium-tipped, cone-socket pliers (Fig. 12-10). When the abutment is properly aligned, replace the implant into the osteotomy and position it by using light mallet taps on the bayonet or a straight seating instru-

ment over the abutment while supporting the patient's mandible (Fig. 12-11). The pointed shoulder-seating instrument assists in tapping the implant to its final position within the osteotomy (Fig. 12-12).

Place the implant at the planned optimal depth. The shoulder must be located 2 mm below the cortical level (Fig. 12-13). If it fails to reach this depth and gentle tapping does not help, remove the implant by grasping it with cone-socket pliers. Place the implant in a sterile glass beaker filled with saline or in a bead sterilizer. Refine the osteotomy until it becomes deep enough or freed from interferences so that the blade implant can be accommodated.

If it is necessary to make a curved osteotomy, reshape the implant so that it, too, becomes curved. To do this, place the implant infrastructure between the beaks of the two titanium-tipped, cone-socket pliers and carefully introduce the bend. Ensure that the curvature is even and equal from shoul-

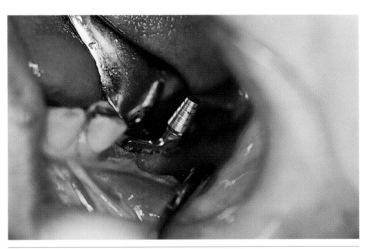

Fig. 12-9 Place the implant using finger pressure only. This verifies osteotomy length and abutment angulation.

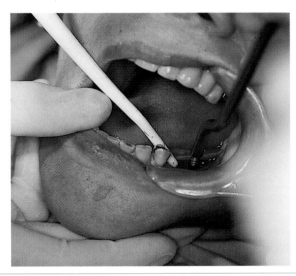

Fig. 12-11 After the alignment of the abutment, place a seating instrument (bayoneted if used for the posterior) over its head. Tapping with a mallet seats the blade shoulder 2 mm beneath the alveolar ridge. The assistant's hand should support the patient's mandible or head.

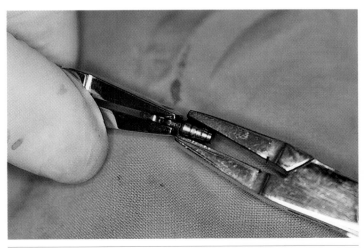

Fig. 12-10 If the abutment is malaligned (Fig. 12-9), it may be bent gently using two titanium-tipped, cone-socket pliers. This may be done safely only when using single-stage blade implants.

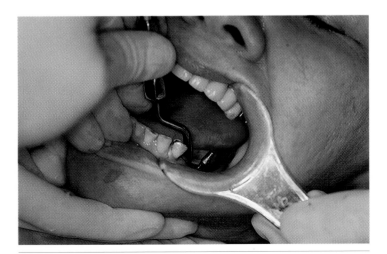

Fig. 12-12 After seating the implant with the abutment bayonet, further positioning usually is required. This is done by using the shoulder-point seating instrument, which snuggles into appropriately shaped dimples in the upper surface of the shoulder.

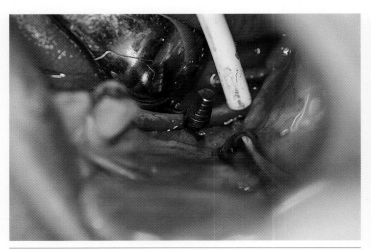

Fig. 12-13 Final position of a plate-form or blade should reveal its shoulder 2 mm evenly, below the ridge crest.

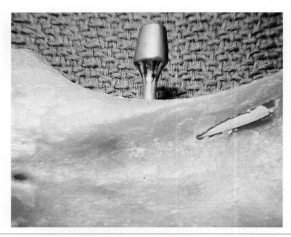

Fig. 12-14 Exercise care, both before and after osteotomies, to respect the mandibular architecture. One common site of perforation is the submandibular fossa, a major convexity beneath the mylohyoid ridge. The best way to avoid this complication is to cant the osteotomy laterally in this region of the jaw.

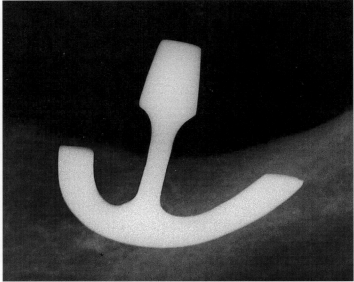

A

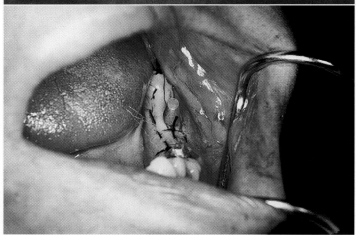

B

Fig. 12-15 **A,** Take an immediate postoperative film to ascertain proper implant position. In this case, an additional osteotomy is indicated to permit deeper positioning of the implant. **B,** The most reliable form of closure for ridge crest incisions is the continuous horizontal mattress suture. Coaptation and primary healing are best ensured using this technique.

der to base, and make frequent pauses to check the accuracy of the contour as it relates to the osteotomy. Particular care is needed when the curve is in the anterior maxillary region (see Anterior Blade and Plate-Form Implants, page 226). The bone cut has not only been made in a curved course, it has also been canted inwardly (in accordance with the anterior maxillary inclination), introducing a second deviation from the vertical direction. Actually, these osteotomies are segments of truncated cones, and shaping and seating of blade implants to fit them present a difficult and critical task.

Before final placement, use a periodontal probe along the depth of the osteotomy. If it falls through a defect in a lateral or inferior wall, this indicates a perforation. In the mandible, these openings occur most often through the lingual cortical plate into the submandibular fossa beneath the mylohyoid ridge or into the mandibular canal itself (Fig. 12-14). In either instance, do not place the implant, but a graft is of benefit to repair the defect. Delay implant insertion at least 6 months, and then use a smaller device.

When the integrity of the osteotomy is ensured (after thorough debridement, irrigation with saline, and inspection of the wound), seat the implant and tap it into its proper position and depth (Fig. 12-15, *A*). Check its position with a periapical film.

Closure

Use a mouse tooth forceps (Gerald) to coapt the flaps. If they appear intact and well vascularized and reach across the implant shoulder without tension, suturing may be undertaken. The use of 4-0 Polysorb with a C13 needle in the continuous horizontal mattress configuration creates a reliable closure (Fig. 12-15, *B*). Ensure that the patient can close into centric occlusion and perform excursions without traumatizing the abutment. If interferences are noted, relieve them with a cooled, high-speed, pear-shaped diamond. During these maneuvers, support the implant firmly. When the occlusion is satisfactory, the patient may be dismissed with an ice pack placed

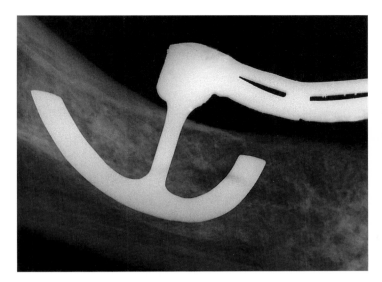

Fig. 12-16 Reconstruction of blade implants may begin after 12 weeks. The soft tissues should be healed firmly around the cervix, and the implant must be firm and comfortable. Routine prosthodontics, as described in Chapter 24, may be completed.

against the check. The patient should follow the routine postoperative regimen given in Appendixes G and H. Subsequent prosthetic reconstruction may be undertaken at the end of the twelfth week (Fig. 12-16).

Alterable Blade Implants

If an alterable blade is selected, refer to Table 4-3. These implants may be somewhat more troublesome, but their use avoids the necessity of keeping a large inventory of fixed or standard designs on hand. Planning and preparation are the same as for standard blade implants. Whether single or double abutments are required and the approximate size of the host site must be determined in advance of surgery. If the implant is a two-stage type, the section below presents the technique of bone preparation that must accommodate the round and enlarged cervix. For one-piece, abutment-bearing blades, select the implant closest to the bone size after cutting the osteotomy to the maximal depth and optimal length. Use a metal cutter to reduce the height and length by snipping, one strut at a time, until the preplanned shape is achieved. Select the shape from one of the plastic templates supplied by many of the implant companies (Fig. 12-17, *A, B*) (see Appendix K for manufacturers). Proceed slowly, washing debris from the infrastructure at each step, and continuing to retry the blade into the osteotomy. When shape and configuration are achieved, polish the altered ends thoroughly with an aluminum oxide wheel, seated into the bead sterilizer for 10 seconds, cooled in saline, and place it into its osteotomy. Before final seating, many implantologists prefer to treat blades and plate-form implants as described in Appendix E. Titanium, unlike the chrome alloys, is self-passivating (air causes an almost instant surface oxide layer to be formed), so that this step may be eliminated. Follow gentle tapping with the seating instrument and mallet by suturing.

Submergible Blade and Plate-Form Implants

The benefit of a submergible blade is that it can be semiburied to permit a trauma-free period of integration (Fig. 12-18). The disadvantages of a submergible blade are that the cervix is quite large, requiring a large accommodation for it at the ridge crest, and that corrections in abutment angulation or alignment are much more difficult, if not impossible, to achieve. However, some companies do make adjustable angled abutments.

Make all corrective manipulations on submergible blade implants only with the prosthetic abutment screwed or placed firmly into position. If this is not accomplished, it is likely that the threaded socket will become distorted, thus destroying the implant. After the osteotomy is completed successfully, mark the site that corresponds to the abutment location. Use a No. 4 round bur with irrigant to make an ovoid enlargement, half from the buccal, half from the lingual, to accommodate the cervix and permit full seating of the shoulder (Fig. 12-19). Leave the abutment attached so that its angulation and prosthetic acceptability can be ascertained before, during, and immediately after implantation. Remove the abutment and keep it for use with that specific implant at the time of second-stage surgery. Threaded or plastic healing caps are available, depending on implant type. If the bead sterilizer has been used, carefully inspect the abutment receptacle so that any beads that have become entrapped can be removed.

Use Vicryl continuous, horizontal mattress sutures (Fig. 12-20) for closure. Try to suture over the cervix, thereby enclosing the entire implant. Reentry for purposes of transepithelial abutment placement should take place from 3 (if mandibular) to 4 (if maxillary) months later. This surgery may be performed by placing the clear surgical template into place (if one had been used), thus identifying the buried cervical site

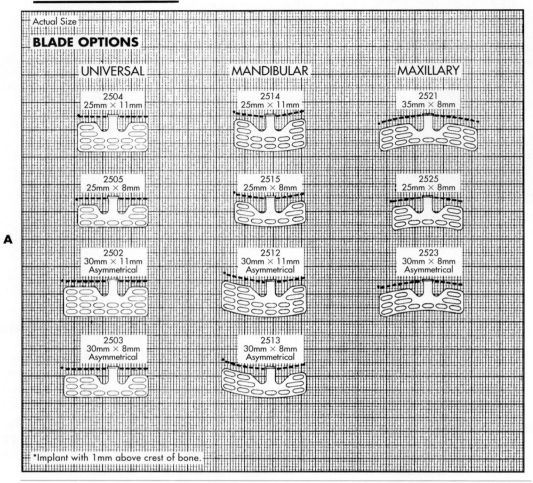

Fig. 12-17   Current blade and plate-form manufacturers are listed in Table 4-3. Most of these companies produce templates that are designed to be held against radiographs. **A** and **B,** Such a maneuver enables the doctor to choose a design of the most favorable size and configuration. Templates with 25% enlargements are available for use with panoramic x-rays; however, this is not a reliable technique for final selection.

A Courtesy Steri-Oss. **B** Courtesy Ultimatics, Inc.

directly beneath the implant locator hole. Particularly with blade implants, which have more pronounced protrusions, a circular cutting trephine is effective because identification of the cervix is made so readily. In fact, they often become exposed spontaneously. The healing cap should be removed, the receptacle irrigated thoroughly, and a healing collar inserted (Fig. 12-21). Two weeks later, the abutment, which had been set aside at the time of implantation, can be screwed into place

(Fig. 12-22). Its complete seating should be verified with a bitewing radiograph.

Coated Blade and Plate-Form Implants

The use of coated blade or plate-form implants requires several deviations from the methods presented in the preceding sections.

ENDOSSEOUS LINKOW BLADE VENT IMPLANTS - ACTUAL SIZE - MAXILLARY

All Implants Are Shown Actual Size 1:1

Order Toll Free: 800-872-7070

APRIL 1988

ULTIMATICS INC.
P.O. Box 400
SPRINGDALE, AR 72765 U.S.A.
Tel: 501-756-9200

When ordering specify standard or submergible. For purposes of prosthetic alignment, implants are depicted with abutment posts.

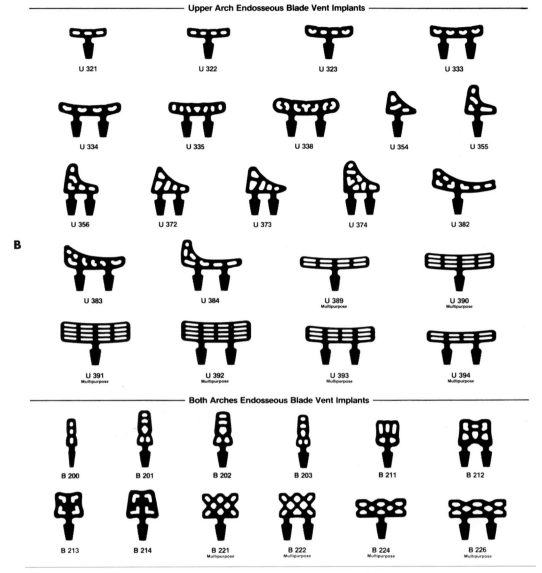

Fig. 12-17, cont'd
For legend, see opposite page.

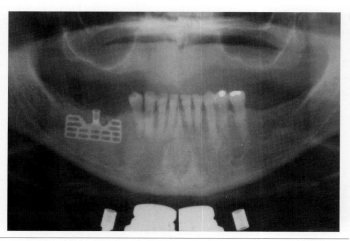

Fig. 12-18 A submergible blade 8 weeks after placement. The major disadvantage is its large cervical diameter. There is no zone of lucency about its infrastructure, and integration appears to be occurring.

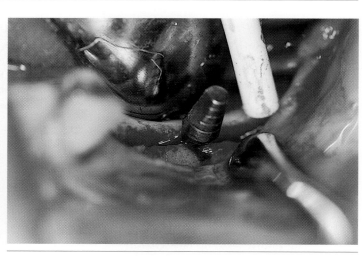

Fig. 12-19 Some crestal bone must be sacrificed to permit seating of the cervix of a two-stage submergible blade implant. Cut the scallops (buccal and lingual) with a saline-cooled No. 4 round bur.

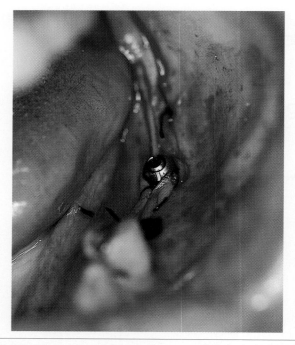

Fig. 12-20 Some submergible blades are not fully buried. Their design creates a need for the cervix to protrude about 2 mm. Use healing screws to seal their threaded interiors.

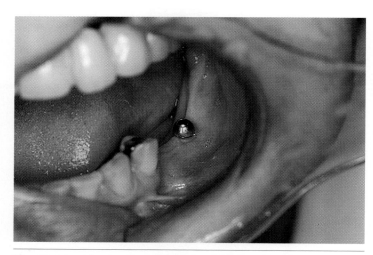

Fig. 12-21 After healing, a firm cicatricial, keratinized cervical collar should be in evidence around the healing cap. Do not probe it.

Fig. 12-22 After integration (8 to 12 weeks), a variety of abutment shapes and angles are available. They are often interchangeable with root form abutments of the same manufacturer. After placement, evaluate the integrity of abutment seating with a periapical x-ray.

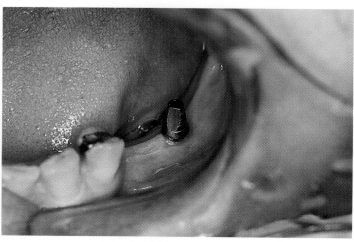

First, they cannot be bent or altered by cutting. Second, these systems must have a metal try-in or sham available for each implant size and shape. Only when the sham fits passively should the coated implant be seated. Once seated, it may not be removed because removal may damage the surfaces or cause delamination of the coating. Third, the use of coated blade implants requires a large inventory (Fig. 12-23). Despite these disadvantages, one advantage if the coating is hydroxyapatite (HA), is the potential creation of a stable interfacial bond.

Custom-Cast Implants

If the preoperative workup (see Chapter 5) results in a decision to place a blade or anchor as the most acceptable device and neither a manufactured nor alterable manufactured design is suitable, a custom casting may be made to suit the requirements of the area.

Place an oriented periapical x-ray with accurate dimensions (as verified with the 5-mm steel ball technique described in Chapter 4) on a viewbox, and outline the available bony host area. Draw the infrastructure of a blade or buttressed anchor design over the available bone, leaving a 2-mm margin at all boundaries. Create a 4-mm shoulderless cervical zone, add an abutment and cervix of appropriate size and extension, and make a titanium or Vitallium casting (Fig. 12-24). As an alternative, a blade may be waxed directly on the patient's periapical x-ray (Fig. 12-25). This may be cast in Vitallium and annealed so that some infrastructural or cervical bending maneuvers can be done, if necessary, at the time of seating.

The finish should be matte for the abutment and infrastructure as well as for the lower half of the cervix. The upper half or permucosal portion of the cervix must be highly polished.

Before implantation, these custom anchors should be handled by properly treating and sterilizing the metal (see Appendix E).

Maxillary Posterior Blade and Plate-Form Implants

In planning for the maxilla, the same principles apply as for the mandible.

In some cases, particularly with females or others with less dense maxillae, the osteotomy need not be made to its full depth. The blade itself can be used as an osteotome. When tapped, it seats itself firmly and snugly into an environment that has not been subjected to the trauma of bone drilling. A few simple taps with the mallet will offer advice regarding the feasibility of seating the implant without a full-depth bur cut. If the implant does not continue to seat, it should be removed with the cone-socket pliers while being careful not to stress or snap the cervix. The osteotomy is completed with an irrigated 700 XXL bur. The implant then may be seated fully (Fig. 12-26).

Before seating a posterior maxillary blade test the osteotomy with a millimeter probe. If a defect is encountered, it

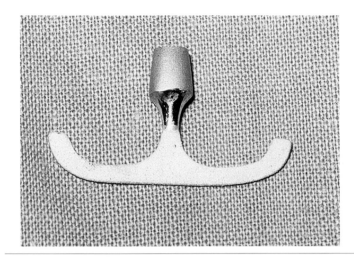

Fig. 12-23 Hydroxyapatite-coated blade implants such as this anchor design encourage a firm osseointegrated interface. Classic design characteristics, such as a highly polished cervix, must be incorporated.

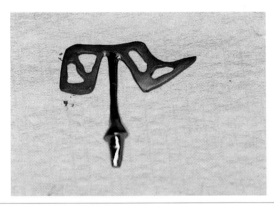

Fig. 12-24 Custom-cast blades are popular. This buttressed anchor (designed and produced by Dr. Robert James) was fabricated to fit a specific maxillary host site.

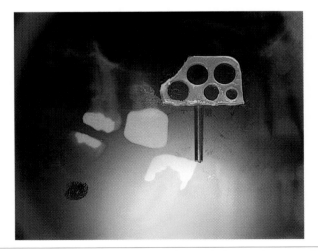

Fig. 12-25 Plate-form implants may be made by creating a wax base pattern directly against a nondistorted apical x-ray.

is probably the maxillary sinus. Request that the patient exhale, and gently obturate his or her nares. If air bubbles emanate from the groove, this is confirming evidence of a communication. In such an instance, tuck a strip of Colla Cote into the depth of the groove with a periosteal elevator, fill the osteotomy with tricalcium phosphate (TCP) grafting material, and close the wound. In 4 to 6 months a shallower blade may be placed, and an aggressive, watertight closure is made. The antral regimen (see Appendix G) should be prescribed postoperatively.

Anterior Blade and Plate-Form Implants

In the areas anterior to the antrum in the maxilla and the mental foramina in the mandible, there is less of an anatomic challenge in placing implants. Often, however, the ridge is thin, and labial plate fracture represents a significant hazard. Fracture is possible because of the curved nature of the anterior ridges, which dictate that the osteotomy follow their contour. An additional difficulty, particularly in the maxilla, is its 30- to 45-degree labial inclination, which means that the bur must be canted at the proper angle to keep it midway between the labial and palatal cortical plates. This added geometric complexity puts the bone in jeopardy as the implant is being tapped to place. The implant must be prepared by curving it with the contouring pliers so that it fits into the osteotomy passively. Because the arc at the base of the osteotomy is smaller than that at the crest of the ridge, the implant must be curved in a similar manner. It must be contoured like a truncated cone because, if it is not, the labial plate may fracture as the implant is driven to its full depth. As the plate-form is tapped into position, the seating instrument must be angled in the long axis of the infrastructure so that the host bone is subjected to minimal torquing forces. On the positive side, however, maxillary bone is sufficiently compliant so that a thin, modest, gently made osteotomy suffices and the implant may be seated fully, serving to make its own pathway (Fig. 12-27).

The mandible is denser and requires a sense of feel, judgment, and experience to serve as a guide in these matters. It is not as procumbent as the maxilla, which presents a less difficult approach. The surgeon's capability to comprehend and behave manually in a three-dimensional geometric field is of significant value.

Suturing and postoperative care should follow the general guidelines outlined in Chapter 6. Despite the fact that using newly placed single-stage blades in the posterior regions is not recommended, it is a requisite that temporary splints be made in the anterior portions of the mouth. They should be constructed in a manner that permits following hygienic measures and that does not place excessive masticatory stresses on the implant during the integration period.

Immediate Placement of Blade Implants into Extraction Sites

Immediate placement of endosteal implants into sites of recent extraction is a valuable alternative to the traditional method of waiting for socket mineralization.

Situations exist in which a potential implant site is unsuitable for root form implants. In such cases or in cases in which the implantologist prefers blades and plate forms, they may be used immediately after an extraction.

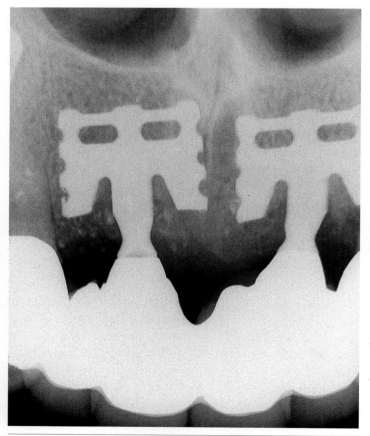

Fig. 12-27 Manufactured blades may be customized by trimming their infrastructures and polishing the edges with an aluminum oxide impregnated wheel. These implants may be two-stage submergible or one-stage. Pay particular attention to contouring them for anterior maxillary placement.

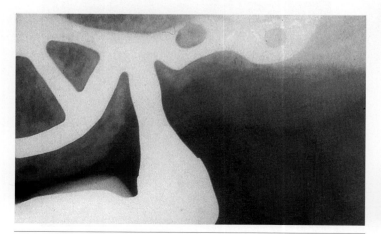

Fig. 12-26 Restore a buttressed anchor in the maxilla with a fixed bridge prosthesis. The implant design promotes vital structures to be avoided.

Because blade implants extend mesiodistally, freshly cut osteotomies, both anterior and posterior to the extraction socket, offer greater stability. Blades may be placed into sites that have had several extractions or sites where the vacated alveolus is not located in the center of the edentulous zone, but some portion of the blade infrastructure must extend into healthy, intact ridge areas, preferably both mesially and distally to the extraction sockets.

To insert a blade implant into an area requiring an extraction, use a No. 15 Bard Parker blade at the crest of the ridge at a distance from the planned extraction adequate to accommodate the blade. Carry the incision from the distal end anteriorly to the tooth, around it buccally and lingually, and continue it on the crest forward to a point that allows the blade to be placed (Fig. 12-28, *A*). Vertical releasing incisions are necessary to allow adequate exposure of bone. Use a sharp periodontal elevator to reflect the gingivae.

Extract the tooth in the most atraumatic fashion, with an effort to preserve the integrity of the alveolar walls as well as

the interseptal bone (if a molar). Curette the socket or sockets thoroughly.

Check the adequacy of the flaps for primary closure over the extraction site before beginning the osteotomy. If necessary, undermine the buccal flap as described in Chapter 6. The position of the osteotomy must be planned, and some modification of the socket area may be necessary. The ridge, mesial and distal to the extraction site, often has to be flattened to achieve adequate width and to create a homogeneous level for blade placement.

Use a No. 1 round bur in a high-speed handpiece to mark the anteroposterior boundaries of the osteotomy, which are determined by the length of the blade selected. Make a series of holes crestally through the cortex, marking the location of the osteotomy. The osteotomy will be disrupted by the presence of the extraction socket, and extra care should be taken to ensure the bony groove's proper alignment (Fig. 12-28, *B*).

Connect the holes into a slot with a 700 XXL fissure bur. When the osteotomy is complete, seat the implant following

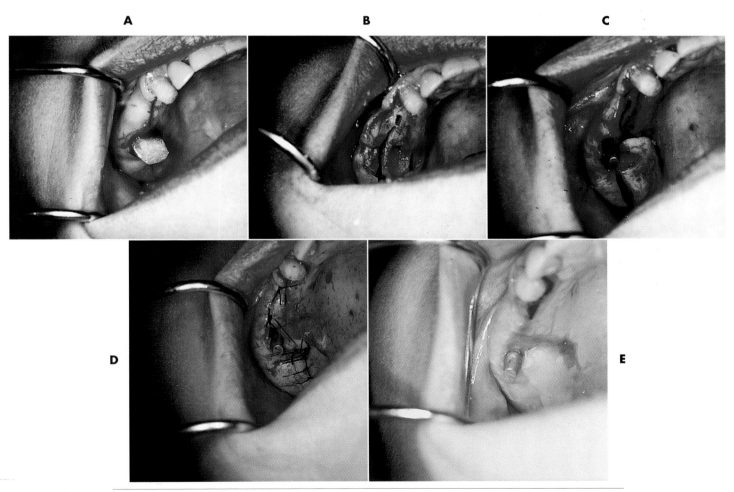

Fig. 12-28   **A,** Make the incision for blade placement at the crest of the ridge, both anterior and posterior to an upper molar with a hopeless prognosis. **B,** After extraction, cut the osteotomy. Because of a trifurcation involvement, intact bone actually exists at the ridge crest. **C,** Seat the blade in the completed osteotomy; it is now surrounded by bone. Repair the recently vacated alveoli with a synthetic bone substitute material. Closure can be effected only by creating a buccal or, as in this case, a palatal pedicle flap. **D,** Mobilize the palatal pedicle over the osteotomy and suture it. **E,** Two weeks postoperatively, healing has taken place at both donor and host sites.

the steps described earlier in this chapter. After the final placement of the implant, the shoulder should be at least 2 mm beneath all borders of the osteotomy (Fig. 12-28, *C*). Use a graft material such as demineralized freeze-dried bone (DFDB) to fill in voids adjacent to the implant and in the recently vacated socket. After removal of granulomatous tissue and invaginated epithelium from the undersurface of the flaps, a resorbable guided tissue regeneration membrane (GTRM) can be prepared with a poncho design to fit intimately around the implant cervix. It must overlay surrounding healthy bone for at least 2 mm circumferentially and be applied in a smooth, wrinkle-free fashion. Membrane stabilization often is necessary, and this can be done with 4-0 dyed Vicryl applied to the deep periosteum, which is at the base of the flaps or by membrane tacks (see Chapter 8). Complete the closure using the horizontal mattress suture. The use of submergible blade implants for immediate implantation into extraction sites is strongly recommended. Immediate loading of implants disturb the regeneration of bone in the socket area and should be avoided whenever possible. More details on grafting are given in Chapter 8.

Blade Implants

Single-stage blade implants are not recommended for use with overdentures and should not be incorporated into such appliances unless four or more of them have been employed and connected by a bar for a full-arch reconstruction.

Two-stage blades, which can achieve osseointegration, may be substituted for root forms if there is enough ridge length for their use, but overdentures are rarely used in such reconstructions. Abutments are available for blades (as described in Chapter 19) of the same dimensions and design as for root forms made by the same manufacturer.

Suggested Readings

Apse P et al: Microbiota and crevicular fluid collagenase activity in the osseointegrated dental implant sulcus: a comparison of sites in edentulous and partially edentulous patients, *J Periodontol Res* 24:96-105, 1989.

Babbush CA: Endosteal blade-vent implants. Reconstructive implant surgery and implant prosthodontics, *Dent Clin North Am* 30:97-115, 1986.

Babbush CA: Endosseous blade-vent implants: a research review, *J Oral Surg* 30:168-175, 1972.

Bain CA: Smoking and implant failure - benefits of a smoking cessation protocol, *Int J Oral Maxillofac Implants* 11:756-759, 1996.

Bidez MW, Staphens BJ, Lemons JE: An investigation into the effect of blade dental implant length on interfacial tissue stress profiles. In Spilker RL, Simon MR, editors: *Computational methods in bioengineering*, Proceedings of the American Society of Mechanical Engineers Winter Annual Meeting, Chicago, Nov. 17-Dec. 2, 1988.

Cranin NA: The Anchor oral endosteal implant, *J Biomed Mater Res* 235 (suppl 4), 1973.

Cranin NA: *Oral Implantology*, Springfield, 1970 *Charles C. Thomas*, pp. 161-178.

Dahl GS: Mechanical analysis of Linkow blade bent implants, *J Oral Implantol* 11:89-92, 1983.

Dahler C: Endosseous blade implants, *Schweiz Monatsschr Zahnmed* 879-888, 1985.

Fazili M: Blade implants, *J Biomed Eng* 5:141-142, 1983.

Fishel D et al: Roentgenologic study of the mental foramen, *Oral Surg Med Oral Pathol* 41:682-686, 1976.

Fonseca RJ, Davis W: *Reconstructive preprosthetic oral and maxillofacial surgery*, Philadelphia, 1986, WB Saunders.

Fox SC, Moriarty JD, Kusy RP: The effects of scaling a titanium implant surface with metal and plastic instruments: an in vitro study, *J Periodontol* 61:485-490, 1990.

Heller AL: Blade implants, *Calif Dent J* January:78-86, 1988.

Hoexter DL: Endosteal blade implants, *NYDental J* 56:214-220, 1986.

James RA, Kellin E: A histopathological report on the nature of the epithelium and underlining connective tissue which surrounds implant posts, *J Biomed Mat Res* 5:373, 1974.

James RA, Schultz RL: Hemidesmosomes and the adhesion of junctional epithelial cells to metal implants: a preliminary report, *J Oral Implant* 4:294-302, 1974.

Jansen JA: Ultrastructural study of epithelial cell attachment to implant materials, *J Dent Res* 65:5, 1985.

Kasten FH, Soileau K, Meffert RM: Quantive evaluation of human gingival epithelial cell attachment to implant surfaces in vitro, *Int J Periodont Restor Dent* 10:69-79, 1990.

Koth DL, McKinney RV, Steflik DE: Microscopic study of hygiene effect on peri-implant gingival tissues, *J Dent Res* 66 (Spec. Issue) 186 (abstr. 639), 1986.

Kwan JY, Zablotsky MH, Meffert RM: Implant maintenance using a modified ultrasonic instrument, *J Dent Hyg* 64:422-430, 1990.

Lavelle CLB: Mucosal seal around endosseous dental implants, *J Oral Implant* 9:357-371, 1981.

Leger-Dorez H: *Implantation de racines extensibles*. Paris, 1920 Ash Sons e Co.

Lehmans J: Contribution a l'etude des implants endo-osseus. Implant a arceau extensible, *Rev Stomatolog*, 415:224, 1959.

Lekholm U et al: The condition of soft tissue at tooth and fixture abutments supporting fixed bridges: a microbiological and histological study, *J Clin Periodontol* 13:558, 1986.

Levy D et al: A comparison of radiographic bone height and probing attachment level measurements adjacent to porous-coated dental implants in humans, *Int J Oral Maxillofac Implants* 12:544-546, 1997.

Lindhe J et al: Experimental breakdown of peri-implant and periodontal tissues: a study in the beagle dog, *Clin Oral Implants Res* 3:9-16, 1992.

Linkow LJ, Donath K, Lemons JE: Retrieval analysis of a blade implant after 231 months of clinical function, *Implant Dent* 1:37-43, 1992.

Linkow LI: The endosseous blade-vent: twenty years of clinical applications, *Alpha Omegan Scientific* 36-44, 1987.

Linkow L: Mandibular implants: a dynamic approach to oral implantology, New Haven, Conn, 1978, Glarus, pp 10-12.

Linkow LI: The multipurpose blade. A three-year progress report, *J Oral Implantol* 9:509-529, 1981.

Linkow L: The multipurpose Blade-Vent implant, *Dent Dig* 1967.

McGivney GP et al: A comparison of computer-assisted tomography and data gathering modalities in prosthodontics, *Int J Oral Maxillofac Implants* 1:55-68, 1968.

Misch CE, Crawford E: Predictable mandibular nerve location: a clinical zone of safety, *Int J Oral Implant* 7(1):37-40, 1990.

Misch CE: Density of bone: effect on treatment plans, surgical approach, healing and progressive bone loading, *Int J Oral Implant* 6:23-31, 1990.

Misch CE: Osteointegration and the submerged blade implant, *J Houston District Dent Assoc* January 1988, pp. 12-16.

Mombelli A et al: The microbiota associated with successful or failing osseointegrated titanium implants, *Oral Microbiol Immunol* 2:145, 1987.

Parham PL et al: Effects of an air powder abrasive system on plasma-sprayed titanium implant surfaces: an in vitro evaluation, *J Oral Implantol* 15:78-86, 1989.

Pietrokovski J: The bony residual ridge in man, *J Prosthet Dent* 34:456-462, 1975.

Rams T, Link C Jr: Microbiology of failing implants in humans: electron microscopic observations, *J Oral Implant* 11:93, 1983.

Rams TE et al: The subgingival microflora associated with human dental implants, *J Prosthet Dent* 5:529-539, 1984.

Rapley JW et al: The surface characteristics produced by various oral hygiene instruments and materials on titanium implant abutments, *Int J Oral Maxillofac Implants* 5:47-52, 1990.

Root D: Laboratory techniques and implant dentistry, *American Academy of Implant Dentistry*, Washington D.C., 1988.

Schnitman P et al: Implant prostheses. Blade vs. cantilever—clinical trial, *J Oral Implantol* 12:449-459, 1986.

Schnitman P et al: Three-year survival rates, blade implants vs. cantilever clinical trials (abstract), *J Dent Res* 67(special issue):347, 1988.

Smithlof J, Fritz ME: The use of blade implants in a selected population of partially edentulous adults: a fifteen-year report, *J Periodontol* 58:589-593, 1987.

Smithlof M, Fritz ME: The use of blade implants in a selected population of partially endentulous adults: a ten-year report, *J Periodontol* 53:413-415, 1981.

Smithlof M: Blades—15 year clinical trial report, *J Oral Implantol* 12:460-466, 1986.

Stefani LA: The care and maintenance of the dental implant patient, *J Dent Hygiene* 447-466, 1988.

Tallgren A: The reduction in face height of edentulous and partially edentulous subjects during long-term denture wear: a longitudinal roentgenographic cephalometric study, *Acta Odontol Scand* 24:195-239, 1966.

Thomas-Neal D, Evans GH, Meffert RM: Effects of various prophylactic treatments on titanium, sapphire, and hydroxylapatite—coated implants: an SEM study, *Int J Periodont Restor Dent* 9:301-311, 1989.

Valen M: The relationship between endosteal implant design and function, *J Oral Implantol* 11:49-71, 1983.

Viscido A: The submerged blade implant—a dog histologic study, *J Oral Implant* 5(2):195-209, 1974.

Yosue T, Brooks SL: The appearance of mental foramina on panoramic and periapical radiographs, *Oral Surg Oral Med Oral Pathol* 68:488-492, 1989.

Yurkstas AA: The effect of missing teeth on masticatory performance and efficiency, *J Prosthet Dent* 4:120-123, 1954.

13

Ramus Frame and Ramus Blade Implant Surgery

ARMAMENTARIUM

Burs: 2 L, 557 L, 700 L, 701 L, and 702 L
Chisel: long seating or bayonet instrument (titanium-tipped)
Handpiece: high-speed
Handpieces: Impactair high-speed, contra-angle
Implants: ramus type
Jig: bending
Mallet: surgical
Pliers: Roberts anterior bending
Pliers: Titanium-tipped bending
Templates: trial (implant try-ins)

CAVEATS

In order to keep incisions to minimal lengths, make careful measurements preoperatively. Keep burs cool and change them frequently. A 135-degree angled handpiece (Impactair) facilitates the creation of the ramus osteotomy. The mandibular canal must be avoided. Bend the anterior foot of the ramus frame carefully so that it enters the symphysis evenly between the cortical plates and directly into the medullary bone. This discourages fracture of the labial cortical plate. The ramus osteotomies must also be cut with care so that perforations are not made laterally, medially, or posteriorly. Make every effort to insert the implant passively so that it is not the cause of compressive forces on the host bone.

RA-2 Ramus Frame (Pacific Implant Company)

The RA-2 implant may be used to support an overdenture for patients with atrophied mandibles (Fig. 13-1). This implant was originally made of 316 L surgical stainless steel, but more recently, it is made of grade 2 surgical titanium. It is a one-piece tripodal design device and is available in only one size.

The RA-2 model requires that the anterior incision and osteotomy be made first. The posterior components of this surgery should be performed after satisfactory completion of the anterior portion.

Surgery

Anesthetize the patient with bilateral mandibular and long buccal blocks and local infiltration. Make a full-thickness incision along the crest of the ridge in the anterior region of the mandible. Start the incision at the area just distal to the mental foramen and proceed around to the opposite side. It will be approximately 25 mm in length (Fig. 13-2).

Reflect the flaps lingually and labially, including an anterior vertical relieving incision just lateral to the labial frenulum to facilitate this procedure (Fig. 13-3). Explore the bony site for lingual and labial concavities as well as for adequate height. The mental nerve should be protected; the safest way to ensure this is to expose the superior halves of the foramina as described in Chapter 8, Nerve Repositioning.

Level and flatten the alveolar crest by using rongeur forceps followed by bone files and burs.

Place the anterior try-in template at the crest of the ridge and use it as a guide for making the osteotomy (Fig. 13-4). Create this cut with a 557 L surgical bur in a high-speed handpiece in the same manner as for conventional blade or plateform implants. First, sketching perforations are made with a No. 2 round bur. If they are well aligned, they should be converted into a continuous groove with the 557 L fissure bur (Fig. 13-5). The osteotomy is deepened to 6 mm if the vertical bone height is 10 mm or less. If, however, 10 to 20 mm of

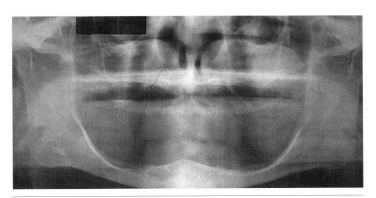

Fig. 13-1 Panoramic radiograph of a mandible suitable for a ramus frame implant. There must be adequate dimensions for the anterior component (foot) as well as the posterior or ramus segments.

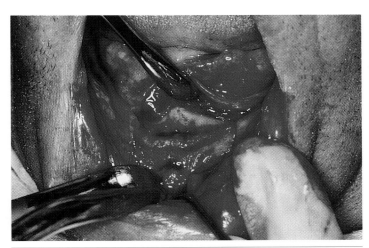

Fig. 13-3 Perform reflection of the symphyseal flaps with care. The exposed anterior ridge should demonstrate the crest, its curvature, and the angle of anterior inclination.

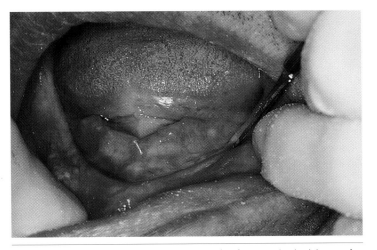

Fig. 13-2 For the RA-2 ramus frame, make the anterior incision at the crest of the ridge from mental foramen to mental foramen.

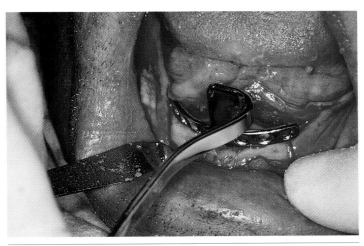

Fig. 13-4 After the flaps have been reflected, hold the template with its large curved border over the bony ridge in order to outline the shape of the osteotomy for the anterior component (foot). The template must be bent to conform to the ridge shape.

height is available, make the osteotomy 8 mm deep. Cant the osteotomy labially and place its base in a slightly more anterior position than at the crest. Angling the bur in an anterior direction keeps it parallel to the ideal host site in a midcortical posture.

The anterior template now should be tried in. Its shape may require modification using the Roberts anterior bending pliers. This instrument adapts the template more closely to the shape of the osteotomy. When seating of the template is satisfactory, make these same bending modifications to the implant.

Make a full-thickness incision beginning at a point 10 mm above the retromolar pad and just lateral to it, which is approximately at the level of the sigmoid notch. Continue the incision downward and forward from the anterior border of the ramus along the external oblique ridge. As the anterior incision is approached, direct the scalpel medially to the crest of

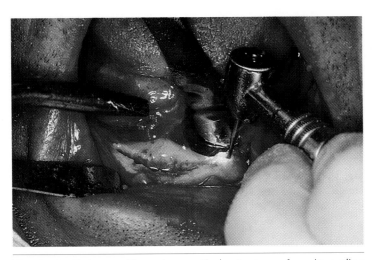

Fig. 13-5 Before making a transcortical osteotomy, form its outline with a small, saline-cooled round bur in the high-speed handpiece. Construct the initial effort in the form of shallow perforations, each separated by 3 mm.

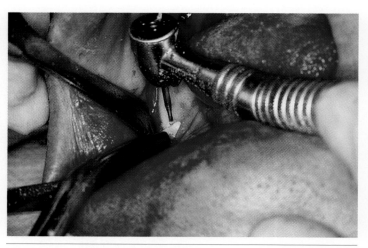

Fig. 13-6 Make an alveolar crestal incision in each ramus retromolar area into fixed gingivae and then carry it forward to meet the anterior incisions. Exposure of the ridge must be made from the ramus anteriorly to the mental foramen. The posterior (ramus) osteotomies are made most easily with a straight (Hall) handpiece or an obtusely angled Impactair, although a conventional handpiece may be used if the patient is capable of opening sufficiently. The osteotomies should be made by first initiating transcortical bur holes in a perforated pattern.

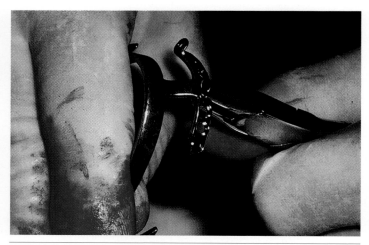

Fig. 13-8 The anterior foot must be bent into a pattern replicating the template. Roberts pliers assist in achieving this.

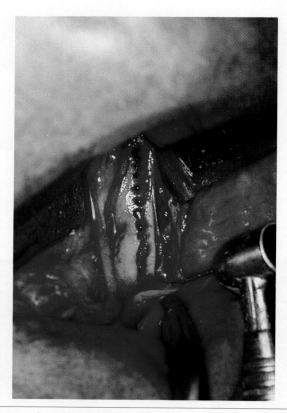

Fig. 13-7 When the perforations are aligned satisfactorily, use a long tapered 701 fissure bur to connect them at a depth capable of accommodating the posterior components of the ramus frame.

the ridge so that the two incisions meet. Repeat on the contralateral side. Reflect the posterior flaps buccally to expose the external oblique ridges and lingually just to the mylohyoid ridge.

Measure and mark a point 18 mm distal from the end of the anterior osteotomy. This is the site at which the posterior osteotomy begins (Fig. 13-6). It should be noted that the posterior try-in template has two marks on it—at 18 mm and at 30 mm.

Place the posterior template on the crest of the ridge with its 30-mm mark on the ramus at the posterior end of the projected osteotomy and its anterior mark at the 18-mm point. Place the template at the angulation of the long axis of the ramus and 2 mm medial to the lateral cortical plate. It acts as a guide for making the osteotomy, which should be as close to a straight line as is possible.

With a No. 1 round bur just through the cortical plate, make a series of perforations. They should be 1.5 to 2 mm apart along this line, beginning at 30 mm and working forward to 18 mm (Fig. 13-7). The surgeon's tactile sense indicates when the cortex has been perforated and the marrow cavity reached. The template must guide the placement of the dots. When they have been completed, survey their alignment and accuracy. Make corrections, if necessary, and then connect and deepen the dots using a 701 L surgical bur. The resultant groove is completed when it reaches a depth of 6 mm, which is 1 mm deeper than the flutes of the bur.

Place the distal end of the template in the posterior part of the osteotomy and force it under the anterior cortical plate of the ascending ramus. Bring the foot down into place anteriorly. If the osteotomy requires a curve because of ramus anatomy, the shape of the template demands a matching modification, with the bending jig and pliers. Once the template fits satisfactorily, transfer these modifications immediately to the implant while the reshaping procedure is fresh in the surgeon's mind (Fig. 13-8 and 13-9, A, B).

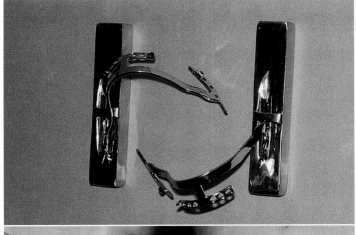

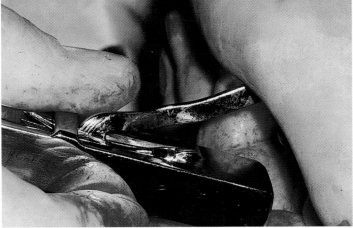

Fig. 13-9 A, The posterior components of the RA-2 often need to be bent. Bending jigs facilitate these maneuvers. **B,** These handheld devices allow the surgeon to make precise adjustments of angle or inclination.

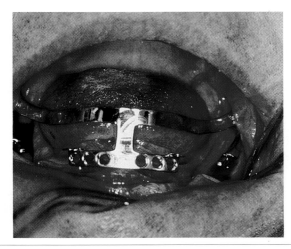

Fig. 13-10 Place the posterior components and seat them first, which should be followed by tapping the anterior foot into its osteotomy.

After the completion of one side, perform these same steps for the contralateral side. If the patient has a class II (retrusive) or a class III (protrusive) mandible, modify the shape of the implant. For the class II mandible, bend the anterior center post posteriorly up to 4 mm. For the class III mandible, bend the center post up to 4 mm anteriorly.

Seat the implant at this point. First, place its distal ends into the posterior extents of the osteotomies. The implant is 2 mm too long for the anterior ramus border; therefore, the distal ends of the implant must be placed posteriorly into the rami grooves with firm finger pressure until the 2-mm extensions are accommodated and the ramus frame fits passively into the osteotomies (Fig. 13-10).

Rotate the anterior foot of the implant downward toward the symphyseal osteotomy. Using hand pressure first and then a surgical mallet, tap the implant into the anterior groove. Make additional bending adjustments for more accurate accommodations if necessary.

The three infrastructures of these implants have seating tabs. When seating the anterior foot, inspect the posterior tabs on the posterior feet. If they are already seated, then the anterior foot will not seat unless tension is placed on the arc of the implant. To rectify this, remove the implant and open

or close its arc by using the bending instrument as may be required.

Then reseat the implant and check it for accurate passive seating of the posterior tabs. If they continue to go into place before the seating of the anterior foot, remove 2 mm of additional bone from beneath the sites of the posterior tabs. Some anterior bone removal from beneath the tab site may have to be done at this time as well.

Only reasonable force should be used to seat these implants. When excessive force is required, it indicates that the osteotomies are inadequate or nonconforming or the implant is improperly aligned in relationship to them.

When alignment and osteotomy sizes appear to be correct, tap the anterior and then the posterior feet of the implant into place. When bone height permits, bury the shoulder of the anterior foot 2 mm below the crest of the ridge. This can be accomplished by removing 2 mm of bone from beneath the anterior seating tabs (Fig. 13-11). Perform seating with the bayonet instrument, which should be tapped with a mallet over the anterior center post. Then place the seating instrument on the posterior tabs and tap to deliver the posterior feet to place. Finally, bend the anterior tabs by placing the seating chisel into their small holes and tapping down until they hug the bone.

Irrigate all areas and make a closure with a continuous horizontal mattress suture using purple dyed 4-0 Vicryl (Fig. 13-12). Complete the procedure with a panoramic radiograph (Fig. 13-13).

The patient's denture may be relined with soft, self-curing Durabase Soft, Coe Conditioner or Viscogel, and it may be worn immediately. Normal postoperative recommendations for analgesics, antibiotics, antiinflammatory agents, and postoperative care as described in Appendixes G through J are to be followed. After a healing period of 6 weeks, a new overdenture may be made for the patient, as described in Chapter 25 (Fig. 13-14).

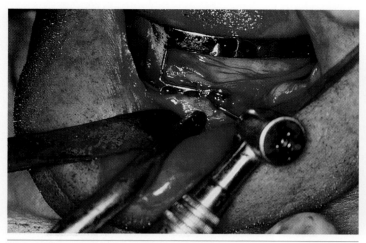

Fig. 13-11 Cut small grooves into the cortex in order to accommodate the seating tabs.

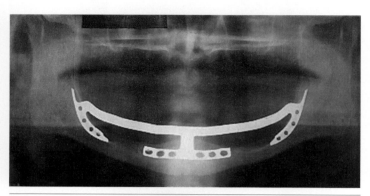

Fig. 13-13 The postoperative panoramic x-ray should show complete seating in bone of the three components of the ramus frame. There should be evidence of canal clearance as well as generous use of anterior osseous structure.

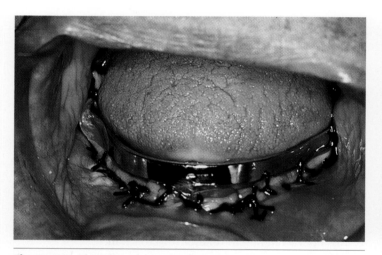

Fig. 13-12 Complete closure by mattress or interrupted sutures.

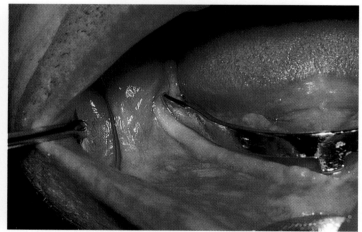

Fig. 13-14 Healing should show a high level of tissue health, good keratinization, and emergence of the posterior components through fixed gingivae.

RA-1 Ramus Frame (Pacific Implant Company)

The RA-1 implant is available in four sizes, depending on the dimensions of the patient's jaw. The implant is selected by measuring from the midline of the mandible to the posterior entry site into the ramus. Then, depending on the measurement, one of the following four sizes is chosen.

No.	Size
4	45 to 52 mm
5	53 to 55 mm
6	56 to 62 mm
7	63 to 68 mm

Most patients require the No. 5 size.

Surgery

Start the first incision 5 mm lateral and 5 to 8 mm superior to the retromolar pad and against the anterior border of the coro-noid process. Continue the incision anteriorly against the bone, passing the retromolar pad on its lateral side and up to the crest of the ridge in the first molar area. From this point, extend the incision on the crest anteriorly to the first premolar region. Reflect the buccal and lingual flaps, exercising care not to disturb the mental neurovascular bundles.

Determine the appropriate position for the posterior rail. Place the rail at the superior portion of the retromolar pad and midway between the inner and outer borders of the ascending ramus.

Using a high-speed, water-cooled Impactair handpiece with a No. 2 L round surgical bur at this site, perforate the cortical plate and make a series of separate transcortical holes that ascend the ramus 6 to 7 mm to the predetermined site. If the perforations appear to be located correctly, they may be connected into a groove using a No. 700 XL bur. Widen this groove to 2 mm with a No. 701 XL bur and then a No. 702 XL bur.

Place the trial template into the osteotomy and force it back through the cancellous bone to a depth of 11 mm. In many cases the handpiece has to be used to deepen the osteotomy to the required dimension.

When the first trial template fits properly, make a horizontal osteotomy from the anterior base of the vertical groove laterally just to the external oblique ridge using the 702 XL fissure bur. Do not permit the bur to pass through this hard cortical layer.

The second posterior try-in template, which contains a wing on its side, is fitted into the osteotomy. When seated properly, completely submerge the winged portion of the template.

Repeat these steps for the contralateral side. Finally, prepare the anterior incision and osteotomy as described for the RA-2 model.

When all three osteotomies have been completed, fit the implant first into the ramus areas. Compress the frame toward the midline if needed, in order to align the posterior extensions so that they are permitted to slip passively into the osteotomies.

Coax the implant into place posteriorly by gentle rocking. When it is seated, rotate the foot downward into the anterior osteotomy.

At this point, remove 2 mm of bone from beneath the anterior seating tabs using a 557 XL bur that allows the foot to be seated below the crest of the ridge.

In order to complete the operation, place the long bayonet seating instrument over the implant center post and tap gently with a surgical mallet. Then insert the seating instrument or chisel into the holes in the anterior tabs and gently tap, bending them over the crest. If the accommodation of the implant to its host site is not satisfactory, make one or two alterations to aid in seating it.

1. The center post of the implant may need to be bent more labially or lingually in order to seat the anterior foot successfully. If so, this may be accomplished using a Roberts anterior bending pliers.
2. If one or both of the lateral posterior tabs do not fit within the confines of the patient's rami, one or several of them may be removed to allow the posterior components to become buried.

Before final seating of the ramus frame, all bony and other debris must be irrigated from beneath flaps and within the bone grooves. Suture the three wounds using a continuous horizontal mattress closure and take a postoperative panoramic radiograph.

The patient's denture should be reamed and relined with a soft, self-curing liner. The patient may be dismissed with it in position. After a healing period of 6 weeks, a new denture superstructure is constructed, which may be used with a soft liner (i.e., Durabase) to grant it a "sloppy fit."

Follow postoperative recommendations for analgesics, antibiotics, antiinflammatory agents and follow-up care as described in Appendixes G through J.

Ramus Blade

The ramus blade has been designed to serve as a distal abutment for fixed bridge prostheses in atrophic mandibles in which insufficient bone is available in the more anterior conventional areas. It may be used with as little as 5 mm of bone available above the inferior alveolar canal.

The ramus blade is available in both standard (Fig. 13-15) and relief (Fig. 13-16) designs. The latter is for use when minimal bone above the inferior alveolar canal is present. Ramus blades are made of commercially pure titanium and are placed in the second molar areas with their infrastructures extending upward and backward into the ramus. In addition, they are available in several lengths as well as three different abutment angulations.

Implant designs are selected by superimposing a ramus blade clear plastic template over a periapical x-ray of the area to be implanted. The head of the implant template must be aligned so that it is parallel to the long axes of the more anterior natural teeth with which it shares the roles of abutments. Each template design should be tested until the correctly angled implant is discovered. Ideally it should occupy all of the usable bony space.

Surgery

When possible, use only local infiltration to anesthetize the patient. Start a full-thickness incision 3 mm lateral to and 8 to 10 mm above the retromolar pad against bone. Palpate the external oblique ridge to offer guidance in making the incision directly on it (Fig. 13-17). Continue the incision downward and forward, lateral to the retromolar pad and then anteriorly to the premolar area. After the retromolar pad has been passed, direct the incision onto the crest of the ridge.

Reflect the buccal and lingual flaps to expose the external oblique ridge and the anterior border of the ramus. Protect the mental bundles.

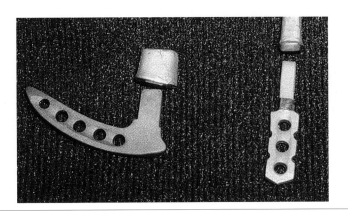

Fig. 13-15   The standard ramus blade is available with three different angles of their abutment heads. Copings must be custom-cast.

Locate the desired position of the implant abutment, which should emerge through keratinized epithelium, and place a bone dot at this site with a No. 2 round bur. Make a mental image as to the projected position of the implant. The posterior extension of the osteotomy must be directed along the center of the exposed anterior ramus or slightly lateral to it, using the lateral cortical plate as a guide. The anterior, or abutment end, should emerge from a zone of fixed gingiva on the ridge at the spot previously marked.

With these requirements in mind, start at the anterior dot using a high-speed, water-cooled Impactair handpiece with a No. 1 round bur to penetrate the cortical plate. Make repeated penetrations 3 mm apart for 15 to 18 mm distal to the starting point until the full length of the selected implant is accommodated. Place the implant over the outline and, if conforming, connect the dots to create a grooved osteotomy. Change the

bur to a No. 701 XL and then to a 702 XL, if necessary, in order to widen the osteotomy to 2 mm and deepen it to between 4 and 6 mm, depending on the dimensions of the selected implant design (Fig. 13-18).

Place the posterior point of the implant in the distal end of the osteotomy and place the bayonet seating instrument on top of the anteriorly located abutment. Seat the implant's infrastructure by gentle tapping with a mallet. When correctly seated, the implant should be firm and its shoulder 1 mm below the cortex of bone. If either labial or lingual inclination of implant abutment is required, do this before final seating by using the slot of the bending jig to hold the implant while angling the abutment with the Roberts pliers.

After acceptable parallelism, tap the implant firmly into place by mallet taps directly to its shoulder (Fig. 13-19) and close the wound with 4-0 Polysorb continuous horizontal mat-

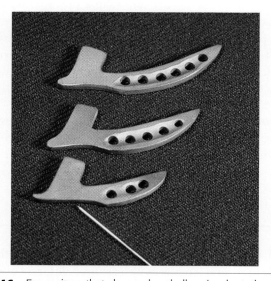

Fig. 13-16 For regions that demand a shallow implant, these relief-designed ramus blades may be placed without injuring the mandibular neurovascular bundle.

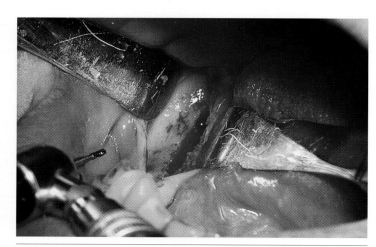

Fig. 13-18 The posterior osteotomy should be long enough to accommodate the ramus blade infrastructure and be located centrally so that neither cortex is perforated and the implant is located within the marrow cavity.

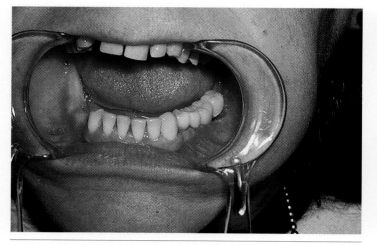

Fig. 13-17 A suitable operative site for a ramus blade must be evaluated by thorough palpation and confirmed by radiography.

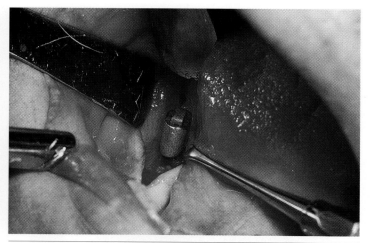

Fig. 13-19 The technique of seating requires slipping the posterior end into the osteotomy until the anterior abutment portion of the blade can be tapped inferiorly, where it will be surrounded completely by bone.

tress sutures. The postoperative regimen as described in Appendixes G and J is recommended. Three months should elapse before beginning prosthodontic rehabilitation using a classic fixed bridge technique. Sanitary pontics are recommended whenever possible.

Suggested Readings

Bodine RL: Implant denture bone impression: preparations and technique, *J Implant Dent* 4:22-31, 1957.

Byrd DL: Mandibular ramus frame, *Calif Dent J* 1:40-46, 1988.

Chamoun EK, Lemons JE: Clinical longevities of ramus frame implants, *J Oral Implantol* 16(2):121-124, 1990.

Collings GJ: Insertion of a ramus frame implant, *Dent Clin North Am* 24:571-583, 1980.

Craig RG: A review of properties of rubber impression materials, *Mich Dent Assoc J* 59:254, 1977.

Kerley TR et al: The ramus frame implant, *J Oral Surg* 39:415-420, 1981.

Linkow LI: The horizontal ramus frame assembly system, *J Oral Implantology* 10:55-99, 1982.

McGivney GP et al: A comparison of computer-assisted tomography and data gathering modalities in prosthodontics, *Int J Oral Maxillofac Implants* 1:55-68, 1968.

Misch CE: Design modification of the ramus frame implant, *J Oral Implantol* 9:178-186, 1980.

Pietrokovski J: The bony residual ridge in man, *J Prosthet Dent* 34:456-462, 1975.

Robert HD, Roberts RA: The ramus endosseous implant, *Oral Implantol* 6:202-209, 1975.

Roberts R: *History of the ramus frame implant,* Alabama Implant Congress, Birmingham Alabama, May 1985.

Root D: *Laboratory techniques and implant dentistry,* American Academy of Implant Dentistry, Washington, D.C., 1988.

Schnell RJ, Phillips RW: Dimensional stability of rubber base impressions and certain other factors affecting accuracy, *J Am Dent Assoc* 57:39, 1958.

14

Mandibular Subperiosteal Implant Surgery

ARMAMENTARIUM

Acrylic: self-curing (Formatray)
Diamond drill: Atwood 473 diamond for the straight (Hall)
    handpiece
Drill: Hall
EZ Tray material
Forceps: Gerald (toothed)
Hemostats: long curved hemostats (i.e., tonsillar)
Hemostats: mosquito
Impression material and adhesive: Surgident Neoplex regular body
    polysulfide
Mortise mesh: titanium (TiMesh)
Needles: hypodermic 20G, 1½ inch
Orangewood sticks
Pliers, crimping
Retractors: beaver tails (Henahan), Army-Navy
Scissors: Mayo
Screwdriver: Vitallium, titanium tipped
Screws: Vitallium 5 or 7 mm, titanium, 5 and 6 mm
Scalpel: long handle
Surveyor
Suture: 2-0 black silk
Suture: 4-0 dyed Vicryl
Tissue conditioner: Coe Comfort, Viscogel
Tubes: 0.045-inch orthodontic, ID
Water: thermostatically controlled bath (to 178° F)

CAVEATS

The exposed operative site demands the absolute respect of the surgeon. The bone that supports the subperiosteal implant must be treated with the highest levels of care, and its response to the simple trauma of mucoperiosteal reflection is responsible for some level of resorption, as evidenced by radiographic signs of change about 3 months after insertion.

Some clinicians say that the crest of the ridge can be grooved (with "witness marks") to permit the counter-sinking of primary struts, but this is a poor suggestion, which may threaten the prognosis of the implant. Bone has plastic memory, and if it is altered by cutting a groove or mortise form for the purpose of seating a component of the infrastructure, it almost immediately begins to undergo resorption. What might begin as an intimate metal-to-bone relationship can, within weeks, become a growing, rounded radiolucency. Since this phenomenon takes place beneath the abutments, it can be the initiating steps in the cascade of events leading to failure (Fig. 14-1).

Completely Edentulous Designs

It is important to avoid injury to mental or dehiscent mandibular nerves. Select implant designs with discerning skill in advance (Fig. 14-2), and if any question of dehiscence exists, plan a tripodal infrastructure (See Edentulous Tripodal Design: Brookdale bar, p. 244).

Make the more complex impressions in several parts and have the materials and capabilities on hand to make an index to assemble the segments of the impression accurately. Make

tissue thickness measurements so that the laboratory is able to construct a casting with abutments that have accurate cervical height.

The laboratory must receive a good surgical centric recording relating the bony mandible to the cranial base, or the implant abutments may be placed in incorrect and unusable positions. Do not make complete mandibular implants in opposition to natural maxillary dentitions.

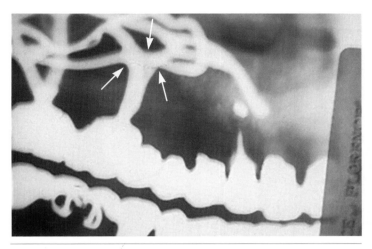

Fig. 14-1 Witness marks are grooves cut across the crest of the ridge to permit the flush seating of the primary struts of subperiosteal implants. Such a maneuver should never be performed, because geometric patterns cut into bone will not retain their sharp line angles. This radiograph demonstrates the pathologic downfall of an implant under which such grooves had been cut and subsequently resorbed into rounded troughs *(arrows).*

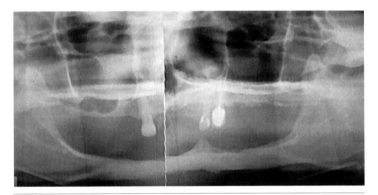

Fig. 14-2 Severe mandibular atrophy is a problem that is managed well with the subperiosteal implant. Dehiscence of the neurovascular bundle contributes a significant complication.

Procedure

Before beginning surgery, examine the intact mucosa that covers the mandible. Palpate the sublingual adnexae (sublingual glands, mylohyoid and genioglossus muscles, plicae sublinguales, Wharton's ducts). These adnexae usually lie above the ridge crest. The vestibules often ill defined, and a mucosal linea alba is seen at the ridge crest (Fig. 14-3).

The linea alba is a fine white scar resulting from the trauma caused by past extractions and denture wearing. At the four to six potential permucosal sites (points of implant after emergence), use a sharpened periodontal millimeter probe to measure and record the thickness of the mucoperiosteum on a chart. Do this after administration of bilateral mandibular block anesthesia but before incision. Local infiltrations in the form of long buccal blocks and infiltrations deeply in the anterior area should be used as well. These infiltrations create profound anesthesia so that aggressively made flaps may be reflected fully for properly designed implants. Eight ampules of 2% lidocaine for the first hour are the limit for the average adult. Give subsequent injections only after absorption of the solutions that were given at the outset.

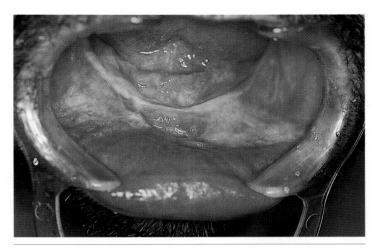

Fig. 14-3 Absence of vestibular morphology and knife-edged ridges are aspects of the atrophied ridge that respond positively to the mandibular subperiosteal implant.

Incision

Use a No. 15 BP blade to trace the linea alba. Start the incision at one retromolar pad and proceed around the arch to the contralateral side (Fig. 14-4). If the radiograph shows that the mental foramina are at or near the crest of the ridge, slightly curve the incisions lingually to avoid injuring the emerging neurovascular bundles. In addition, make a vertical relieving incision just lateral to the labial frenulum. Make incisions directly to bone so that they need not be retraced.

Reflection

Use a sharp periosteal elevator to reflect the mucoperiosteum. Carefully elevate full-thickness flaps. If the flaps are resistant to reflection, use a No. 12 BP blade hugging the bone to cut scar adhesions. The following structures must be exposed and visualized:

1. The external oblique ridges and beyond, inferiorly to the angle, anteriorly to the inferior border for the full width of the ramus.
2. The mental foramina, superior rims only (the neurovascular bundles should not be dissected from their fibrous sheaths).
3. The symphysis to the inferior border of the mandible for a width from canine to canine.
4. The genial tubercles, superior surfaces only (the genioglossus muscle attachments must not be released).
5. The lingual cortex from the anterior ends of the mylohyoid ridges forward to the genial tubercles; carry the reflections down lingually to the inferior borders in the canine areas. Often finger dissection presents the simplest and least traumatic manner in which to perform this procedure. Extend the implant periphery into these areas to compensate for the potential facial structural weakness caused by the scallops designed to circumvent the mental foramina. Do not elevate the mylohyoid muscles from their attachments.

After exposing these vital anatomic structures, suture the two lingual flaps to each other with a 2-0 black silk suture,

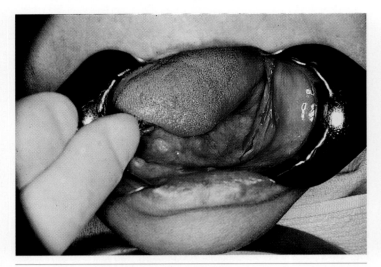

Fig. 14-4 Surgery begins with a crestal incision. It should be made from retromolar pad to retromolar pad. An anterior vertical relieving incision is required.

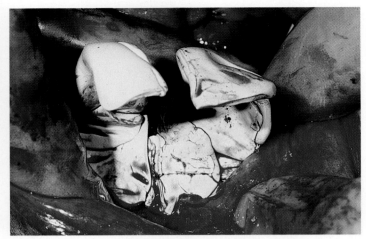

Fig. 14-6 Shaping thermolabile EZTray segments directly on the bone aids impression making because, when necessary, they can be seated separately.

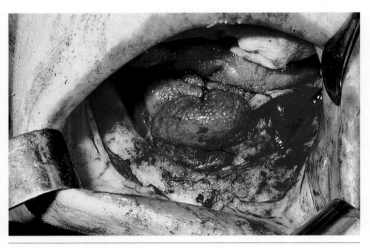

Fig. 14-5 Suturing the lingual flaps to each other across the dorsum of the tongue facilitates complete exposure of host bone. The genial tubercles, mylohoid muscles, external oblique ridges, mental foramina, and symphysis should be in evidence.

bringing it across the dorsum of the tongue. If the tongue slips from beneath these shoestring ties, include its lateral border on either side in the suturing process. Tie these sutures tightly so that the tongue, floor of mouth, and lingual flaps are bundled compactly together in the midline and the mandible is well exposed for impression making (Fig. 14-5).

Protect the exposed bone with saline-moistened sponges. This creates hemostasis and prevents dehydration of the tissues.

Impression Making

1. Heat EZ Tray material to 178° F in an electric water bath. When it is soft, remove one cake and compress it over the bone immediately after the surgical assistant removes the sponges. Mold it so that it extends to all significant peripheral regions (Fig. 14-6).
2. After irrigating the tray until it becomes hardened, fashion an extra piece of the material as a handle and attach it to

the tray. Drying is not necessary; the material is quite cohesive. Remove the tray and, if it is shy in any area, augment it with newly softened material until the entire planned bony host site is covered. The surgical assistant should use a beaver tail (Henahan) retractor beneath one buccal flap, and the operator should retract the other in order to perform enough rehearsal seatings to ensure efficient and rapid tray placement at the time of the final impression. If buccal flap manipulation presents problems, pass several 2-0 black silk sutures through them. The ends of the sutures can be tied in loops after removing the needle, and they can be used as retractor handles. Repack the wound with moistened sponges while applying adhesive to the tray.

3. Mix impression material (Surgident Neoplex Regular) (Fig. 14-7, *A, B*) thoroughly, load the tray with the material, and seat the implant per rehearsal. Hold it firmly in position for 8 minutes. One of the valuable handling characteristics of this material is that it need not be used until after it passes through its sticky or stringy stages. A puttylike consistency is proper for manipulation.

4. Remove the impression and examine it for the following landmarks:
   a. The mylohyoid muscle in the form of ruffled borders
   b. The genial tubercles as two indentations
   c. The symphysis, which is smooth and curved inwardly as it represents the inferior border of the mandible
   d. The mental foramina, which may be seen only as semilunar indications of their superior borders, along with the fan-shaped representations of the neurovascular bundles
   e. The external oblique ridges, which should be clearly demarcated with extensions beneath them down to the inferior borders, when possible (Fig. 14-8)

If the impression is accurate and its texture is smooth, set it aside while irrigating and thoroughly debriding the host site using copious saline. Making a new impression best solves the problem of an unsatisfactory effort, attempts to correct existing impressions are to be discouraged. A panoramic radiograph should be taken postoperatively to seek the presence of fragments of residual impression material, which are radiopaque. These fragments may be removed during second-stage surgery.

Surgical Jaw Relationship: Centric Recording

Place the patient's acceptable maxillary denture prosthesis or a prefabricated, properly adjusted wax rim on a base-plate, and use a thick roll of Optosil putty or a prefabricated bite rim to establish centric and vertical relationships. Press the elastomer and mold it to the bone while guiding the patient to closure in a natural mandibular position (Fig. 14-9). Remove the Optosil after setting, reinspect the wound, irrigate it again with saline, and remove the retraction sutures from the tongue and buccal flaps. An impression of the upper denture, which should have been made previously, serves as a countermodel.

Closure

1. Coapt the flaps and compress them firmly with the thumb and forefinger using a surgical sponge.
2. Grasp the buccal flap at the right posterior end of the incision with a Gerald forceps and make a closure with a continuous box-lock suture using 3-0 black silk suture on a FS 2 or C-13 cutting needle (Fig. 14-10) (see Chapter 6, Surgical Principles, p. 75). Employ the routine postoperative regimen (see Appendix G). The patient's original mandibular denture may be adapted for use as a transitional appliance after it is lined with a tissue conditioner such as Coe Comfort or Viscogel.

Implant Design

1. Box and pour the model in pink Velmix stone.
2. Separate it after setting and check for the landmarks listed in the preceding paragraphs (Fig. 14-11). Then articulate it with the countercast.
3. Mark the designated places for primary, secondary, and peripheral struts with a sharp pencil. Use an "x" to delineate placement of permucosal cervices or posts. Place the peripheral struts to the fullest extent of dissection, but respect undercuts. Undercuts can be established by surveying the cast before design. Primary struts (the ones bearing the abutments) are the only ones that should cross the ridge crest. Each must contain only one cervix. The secondary struts should be plentiful in order to incorporate strength and rigidity, but they must never be placed less than 7 mm apart because doing so discourages strong periosteal reattachment to bone.

Place three screw holes in each casting and delineate them as small circles. The casting, which is waxed slightly below some of the undercuts, still may not achieve primary reten-

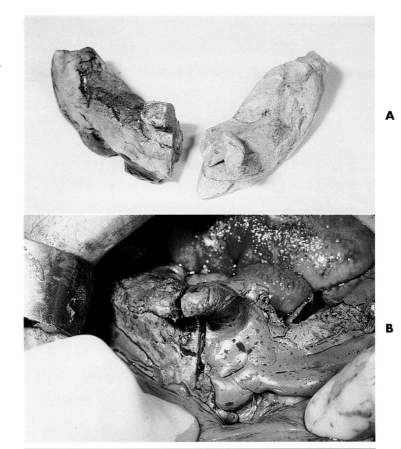

Fig. 14-7 **A,** When there are undercuts in the rami area and a tripodal implant is planned, the tray can be made in two or three segments. **B,** Each tray portion is filled with an elastomeric impression material and may be seated and removed separately if there is no satisfactory path of insertion. An index, made while the tray halves are in position, is used after removal for reassembly.

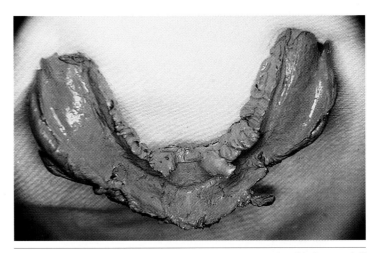

Fig. 14-8 The completed rubber base impression should show a dull homogeneous surface, mental bundles, genial tubercles, the turned border of the symphysis, both external oblique ridges, and the ruffled border of the mylohyoid muscles.

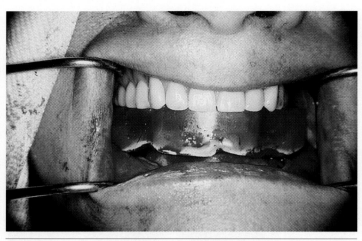

Fig. 14-9 After impression making, vertical and centric relationships are established with an Optosil-lined wax rim resting directly on the bony surface of the mandible.

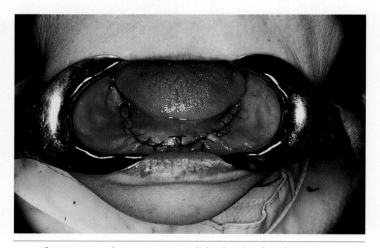

Fig. 14-10 Closure is accomplished with a box-lock suture.

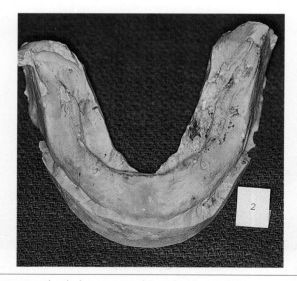

Fig. 14-11 Check the separated cast for the vital structures listed in Fig. 14-8.

tion. If this is experienced and the implant fails to snap into position, one to three screws will be required. Make one hole just lateral to the symphysis (which is too dense to permit entry directly into the midline), and make the other two holes, if needed, facing anteriorly (to permit direct screwdriver use) entering the lateral oblique ridges.

Add 3 mm to tissue thickness measurements to establish cervical lengths and the height of the bar over the mucosa. Permit sufficient space for cleansing, placement of retention clips or devices, and some implant settling and soft tissue hypertrophy (Fig. 14-12). Instruct the laboratory to articulate the models and wax and cast an implant of surgical Vitallium in accordance with the outlined design. Bar configurations to accommodate internal clips, Hader clips, O-rings, or other retentive devices must be requested at the time of casting (see Chapter 26, Overdentures, p. 385). Individual abutments, rather than a bar, may be used if the patient's prosthetic requirements are best suited by this approach. In such cases, a sturdier infrastructure must be designed to substitute for the rigidity offered by the Brookdale bar.

Recall the patient for second-stage surgery either after 36 hours or in 4 to 6 weeks. Any period between these times portends poorly for healing.

Implant Insertion

If a two-stage "immediate" 12- to 24-hour insertion is planned, regional anesthesia is more difficult to achieve. When the silk sutures are removed, the tissues will fall open with ease (which is an advantage of the 1-day procedure). Irrigate the host site with care and remove all residual clots and debris. Use a Poole or Frazier plastic suction tip rather than a metal one. Seat the sterilized, passivated implant (see Appendix E) in the host site. Tap it firmly into place with an orangewood stick and a mallet,

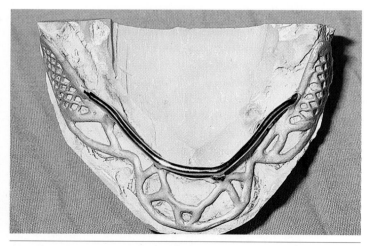

Fig. 14-12 Vitallium casting of the lateral ramus design of Dr. Robert James. The peripheral struts should avoid the mental foramina and extend to the symphysis. The Brookdale bar, which is highly polished, has six points of permucosal penetration, and the ramus extensions should curve laterally to permit their exits from fixed gingivae. Bar height is determined by tissue thickness measurements, with additional consideration given for hygiene measures, hypertrophy of the mucosa and manipulation of clip or other extension devices.

while ensuring that the flaps have not been caught beneath the peripheral struts. Accurate adaptation and primary retention must be verified (Fig. 14-13). If retention is not positive, use the anterior or all three of the fixation screws in order to establish primary retention. With the assistant holding the implant firmly in place, use an Atwood 473, tapered diamond drill in a Hall handpiece in the anterior receptacle to make a concentrically placed screw hole to its full depth. Bevel the most superficial 5 mm to the 2-mm diameter of the casting's hole. Introduce a 7-mm length Vitallium screw and turn it with a Vitallium screwdriver, one revolution clockwise followed by a half revolution counterclockwise (to permit the blood to act as a lubricant) until the screw is seated fully (Fig. 14-14). If three screws are required, none should be fully placed until all are within two turns of complete seating. However, each screw hole must be drilled and the screw partially seated before making the subsequent holes.

The final fastening should take place in the same way that lugs on a spare tire are tightened: half a turn of each until all three are fully in place and all are resting passively in their counter-sunk holes. If there are places of improper fit of metal to bone but the implant is stable (does not rock), these deficiencies may be managed by the use of 20-mesh hydroxyapatite (HA) particles, which are tamped beneath and around the errant strut with a moistened cotton applicator (Fig. 14-15). After thorough irrigation, make a closure with horizontal mattress sutures using 3-0 violet-dyed Vicryl material (Fig. 14-16). In addition, tie a single pursestring suture around each cervix. Dismiss the patient with the routine postoperative regimen (see Appendix G). The postoperative course should be less complex than after the first stage of surgery. Sutures need not be removed, since they are resorbable, and the existing denture may be hollow ground and lined with tissue conditioner immediately after inserting the implant. Postoperative appearance 6 weeks after insertion should indicate maturation of the supporting tissues (Figs. 14-17 and 14-18).

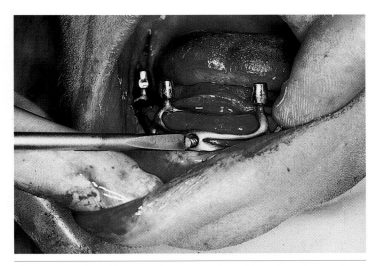

Fig. 14-14 If positive retention cannot be achieved by simple placement of the infrastructure, screw fixation is recommended. Introduce this anterior screw into the bone just lateral to the midline.

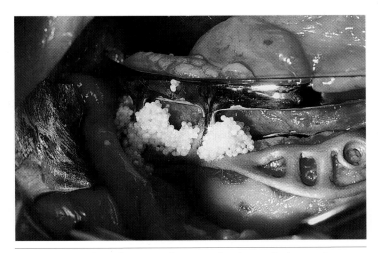

Fig. 14-15 When there are discrepancies beneath the casting, synthetic particulate bone substitutes, such as hydroxyapatite or hard tissue replacement (HTR), may be used as a grout.

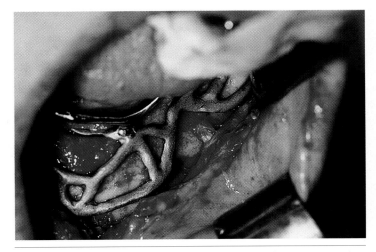

Fig. 14-13 The second-stage operation involves a soft tissue reflection that can be somewhat less aggressive than the first. Protection of the mental neurovascular bundle must be an integral part of the operation and the implant design.

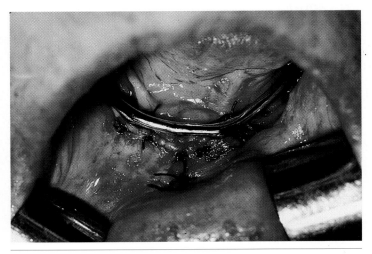

Fig. 14-16 Closure with a resorbable suture (dyed Vicryl) is completed with a continuous horizontal mattress configuration.

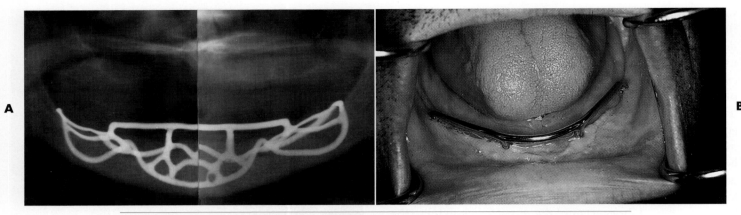

Fig. 14-17 **A,** The Panorex radiograph of a completed implant shows good extension, a Brookdale bar configuration, and proper adaptation. **B,** Six weeks after insertion, the implant is firm, and the gingival cuffs are pink and well keratinized. Impression making may begin at this interval.

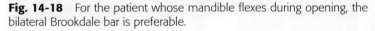

Fig. 14-18 For the patient whose mandible flexes during opening, the bilateral Brookdale bar is preferable.

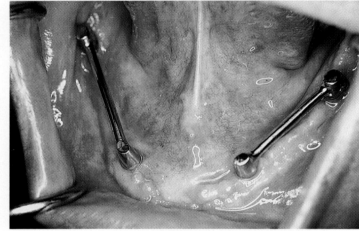

Edentulous Tripodal Design: Brookdale Bar

Procedure

Incisions

The tripodal implant requires three incisions. Make the first anteriorly in the linea alba at the crest of the ridge from a point just anterior to one mental foramen and around to the same position on the contralateral side with an additional parafrenular vertical relieving incision. Make the second on one side in the region extending from a point halfway down the ramus and forward to a second point 1 cm posterior to the mental foramen. Make the third in a like manner on the contralateral side. Make incisions through mucosa and directly down to bone. When planning and making the ramus components, palpation of its anterior border is mandatory. (Review Chapter 4, Surgical Anatomy, and Chapter 13, Ramus Frame.) The anterior border of the ramus is quite far laterally from the ridge crest. The surgeon must anticipate its location and flare. At the distal end of each of these posterior incisions, a lateral re-

lieving incision of 1 cm in length is required. Some brisk bleeding is encountered here, but firm tamponade controls it.

Reflection

Using a sharp periosteal elevator, reflect the anterior flaps labially and lingually to expose the entire symphysis to its inferior border. Reveal the crest of the ridge almost to the mental foraminal areas and the superolingual aspect to the genial tubercles. On either side of the tubercles, use blunt dissection by finger to approach the inferior border. Pack these exposed bone areas with saline-moistened sponges. The posterior reflections take more time and patience to complete. Start the elevation anteriorly at the ridge crest and lift the keratinized gingivae away to the buccal and lingual sides. Once the eleva-

CAVEATS

The same precautions apply for this section as those listed for the first section of this chapter.

If an estimation of the host site indicates a dehiscent neurovascular bundle, either mandibular or mental, a three-islet (tripodal) implant may be planned. The basic armamentarium, principles of surgery, placement, closure, and postoperative care are the same as for those of the traditional design, which should be referred to first before proceeding.

The only connection of the three-islet components that coordinates the infrastructure of a tripodal implant is the Brookdale Bar (either complete or in bilateral segments). Such bars may be designed to accept the superstructure retentive devices of choice. (See Chapter 26, Overdentures, p. 385). The bar therefore is a structural element that serves as a mandatory portion of the planned device.

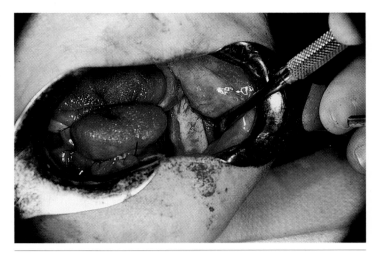

Fig. 14-19 The tripodal implant design preserves the mentomandibular canal in instances of dehiscence by permitting three separate incisions, one over each anterior ramus and one anterior to the mental foramina.

tor reaches a point below this zone on the buccal side, it slides more easily downward, lifting the investing tissues with ease. A sponge can be used ahead of the elevator, exposing the entire lateral surface of the ramus from the mandibular angle along the inferior border forward to a point just beneath the anterior extent of the incision. Blunt finger dissection is effective as well. Lift the crestal tissues lingually over the crest of the ridge and down to the mylohyoid ridge, and pack these wounds with saline-soaked sponges. The safest sizes are 4 × 4 (2 × 2 sizes should never be used because they may get left behind). Raytex, with built-in radiopaque markers, are preferred (Fig. 14-19).

Cover the zones of bone that have been exposed with the three islets of the tripodal implant. Incisions have not been made in the dangerous premolar and molar areas, which contain mandibular or mental nerve dehiscence.

Impression

Place retraction sutures of 2-0 black silk (see Part I of this chapter) for the buccal and lingual flaps. In order to make a tray, mold three polymethylmethacrylate segments to the bone or heat three pieces of EZ Tray. As each gets soft, cut it with a Mayo scissors to the approximate shape of each of the three exposed bone areas and press it over the cortex while the assistant retracts the flaps. Extend each of the three tray elements to the inferior border of the mandible. The anterior component should extend over the ridge crest to the superior surfaces of the genial tubercles and posteriorly to a point 2 mm anterior to the mental foramina. The posterior components should rise from the inferior border of the rami, over the ridge crests, and extend anteriorly to a point just short of the extent of the incision.

Attach an extended retention device to each of the outside tray surfaces. The device can be 0.059 flanged orthodontic buccal tubes, copper bands, or pieces of right-angled 0.045 SS orthodontic wire staples. After placing and fusing each of these retentive devices to the tray with a hot spatula and then cooling with irrigant, dry and sear them to achieve more reliable retention (Fig. 14-20). Irrigate the host sites, keeping each of

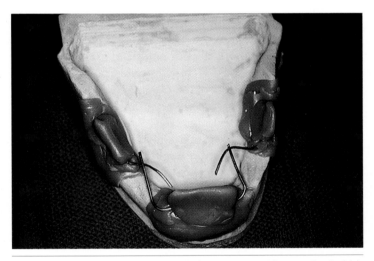

Fig. 14-20 Impression making with three separate islets, each of which is seated individually, will facilitate fabrication of the tripodal implant. The metal loops are used for connecting the segments.

them moist at all times before impression making. Apply adhesive lining to each of the three trays.

Mix the Neoplex polysulfide material separately for each of the three components. Line the first posterior segment with the impression material, seat and hold it (8 minutes) until setting is complete. Keep the other two surgical sites moist. Permit this first islet to remain in place while seating and holding the second, contralateral segment until it sets. Complete the anterior portion last. Prevent the impression material from blocking out the wires or tubes that have been placed as tray assembly devices. After each of the three impressions has set, place a roll of autopolymerizing Formatray acrylic, at least 1 cm in diameter, so that it engages the three tray retention wire loops or tubes. Spray the resin with coolant to counteract exothermic heat as it sets. Lift the entire complex out gently as a unit without dislodging or displacing any of the three components.

Take a surgical centric recording (as described on p. 241) with a polyvinylsiloxane putty and make a counterimpression with alginate. Debride and irrigate the wounds, and remove the transdorsal retention sutures. Make a closure with 3-0 black silk suture. The cast should be boxed, poured in Velmix, separated, and articulated.

Design of Casting

Determine the design of each islet after the cast has been surveyed. Barring undercuts, the peripheral struts of each segment should cover as much area as was included in the impression. Secondary struts should be 7 mm apart and plentiful.

The Brookdale bar, of a shape that serves as an overdenture retainer, should be connected at two points to each islet. This means that the patient has an implant with six sites of permucosal penetration. Two should be placed (by making an "x" on the cast in the designated positions) on the anterior islet in each of the canine positions. On the posterior islets, one each is located at the anterior ends, at the ridge crest. The most posterior cervix on either side should be a horizontal extension of the Brookdale bar directly through the tissues and connecting with the highest extent of the posterior islet's peripheral strut. Because the bar should exit through fixed gingiva, it has to course laterally backward in an "S" configuration to become joined at the lateral aspect of the ramus (Fig. 14-21, A, B).

Insertion

Place tripodal implants by retracing the original incisions. Place the implant, tap it for final seating, and close using the classic suture techniques as previously described in Section I of this chapter (Fig. 14-21, C). If there is rocking or instability of the infrastructure that cannot be solved by firm tapping with an orangewood stick, review Chapter 28, Diagnosis and Treatment of Complications, p. 404.

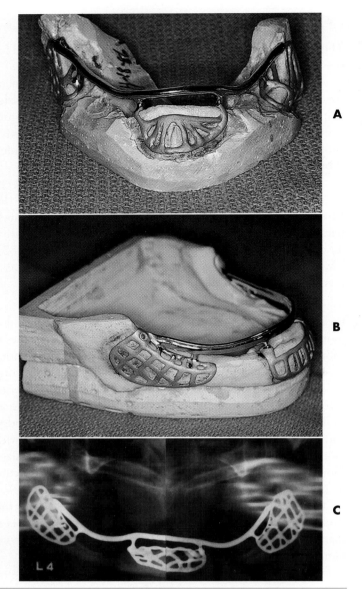

Fig. 14-21   A, The tripodal design has few crestal elements and a significant symphyseal component. **B,** The rami are sites of vital support. As they come closer together during jaw openings, tension that stimulates a dynamic osseous environment and ongoing bone remineralization are created. There are two points of permucosal penetration at each posterior end: the first is horizontal to the ramus, the second is vertical to the retromolar pad. Either one of these may be resected if the need arises. **C,** The Panorex demonstrates the dramatic extension of the tripodal islets and the bar configuration.

Partially Edentulous Designs

Implants for partially edentulous jaws are rarely used for the atrophied mandible, since ramus blades usually are more appropriate, less costly, and far less complicated to seat. Use them only as posterior abutments for fixed bridge prostheses, and place one or two abutments in the most desirable locations to receive fixed retainers (Fig. 14-22). Their abutments should be shaped like crown preparations.

The impression technique, design, and placement of such implants, either as paired unilaterals or as a universal implant

that circumvents the remaining anterior natural teeth, should follow the steps outlined in PMV of this chapter for the tripodal implant.

The universal implant must be designed with bilateral islets similar to those of the tripodal. It is connected by lingual supragenial tubercle and labial juxtasymphyseal struts, permitting the anterior teeth to remain untouched and allowing them to be connected in a fixed, stress-broken prosthesis or mesostructure bar to the implant's abutments. The steps in

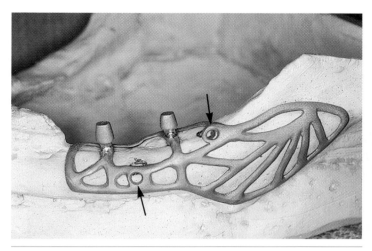

Fig. 14-22 This unilateral subperiosteal implant with two abutments is designed for reception of a fixed bridge prosthesis. Two screw holes will be required to achieve primary retention (arrows).

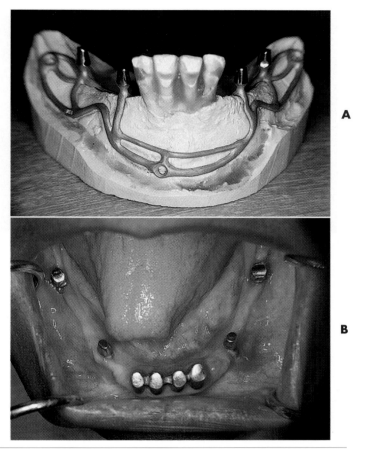

Fig. 14-23 **A,** The universal subperiosteal implant (Samuel Weber design) circumvents natural teeth. The abutments must be made parallel to the natural dentition. **B,** After insertion of the universal subperiosteal implant and the cementation of protective copings on the incisors, an overdenture prosthesis may be made.

making a universal implant are the same as for the classic fully edentulous one. However, the natural teeth must be included in the impression. The design, which does not permit bar construction in the areas of natural teeth, must have stronger peripheral and secondary struts in order to offer better rigidity in these cutout areas. Placement follows standard techniques, and guidance for prosthetic options is given in Chapters 20 and 21 (Fig. 14-23).

Subperiosteal Implant Prosthodontics

Universal and unilateral subperiosteal implants are cast with their abutments attached, and as such, are considered one-stage implants. They may be, and often are, restored with fixed prostheses. Exercise care so that the natural teeth do not become carious as a result of cement failure (caused by the differences of support mechanisms between natural teeth and implants). The implant abutments should have been cast parallel to the natural teeth (Fig. 14-24, A), but if they were not, corrective telescopic castings solve such problems. The abutments should be matte-finished for the creation of a more lasting cement seal. Each natural tooth should have a separate gold coping cemented to it. On completion of this step, make a bridge of high-percentage precious metal alloy using a standard elastomeric impression technique. Follow acceptable crown and bridge procedures, including the use of a custom tray and a syringe. Polyether (e.g., Impregum) or polyvinylsiloxane (e.g., Reprosil) materials are recommended for single-stage implant impression making. Treat implant abutments as if they were natural teeth, including the use of retraction cord. All small fins of impression material that might

have become wedged beneath the gingivae at the implant cervices must be removed after completion of the impression. Crown margins (except in areas that require a high level of esthetics) shouldbe supragingival. Designs should include canine-protected occlusion, free from lateral excursive interferences. The buccolingual occlusal tables over implants should be narrow and approximating the width of premolar teeth. Alaboratory-quality composite restorative material processed to the metal castings completes the process of fabrication (Fig. 14-24, B).

Final prostheses for unilateral and universal implants may be cemented with temporary cement, since the underlying natural teeth have been protected with gold copings. This allows for repairs, hygiene treatments, and simple troubleshooting procedures (see Chapters 27 and 28). In instances when retrievability is sought, or because abutments are short and poorly retentive, the addition of lingual retention screws (Howmedica) may be employed (Fig. 14-25). Final prosthesis construction for complete subperiosteal implants follows the instructions presented in Chapter 26, Overdentures, p. 385.

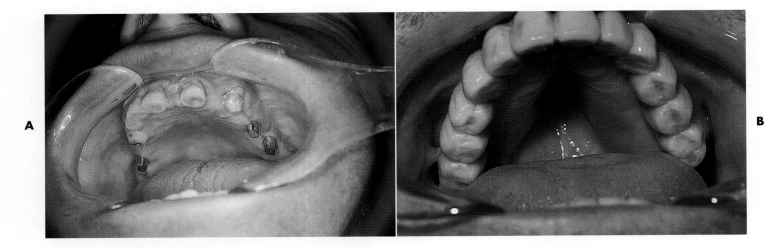

A

B

Fig. 14-24   A, A fixed prosthesis is sometimes desirable for the restoration of a universal subperiosteal implant combined with natural abutments. **B,** This composite veneered gold coping bridge serves both functionally and esthetically as a final prosthesis. If temporary cement is to be used, supply the natural teeth with gold copings.

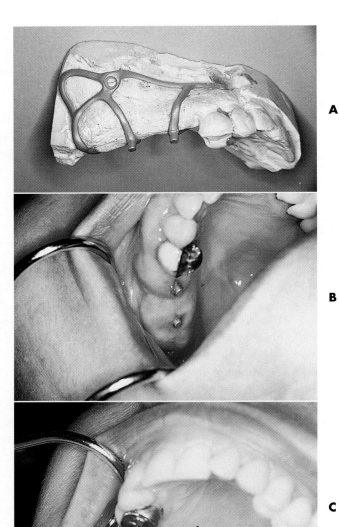

A

B

C

Fig. 14-25   A and **B,** Interocclusal distances do not permit the creation of full-sized abutments for this subperiosteal implant. **C,** Retention of the fixed prosthesis was achieved with the use of lingually placed headless Howmedica screws, which, when tightened, nestle into female recesses placed on the implant abutments *(arrows)*.

Computer Assisted Design-Computer Assisted Manufacture (CAD-CAM) Technique

ARMAMENTARIUM

CAD-CAM company for stereolithographic laser model fabrication
Jaw-positioning splint
Particulate grafting material: 20 mesh
Radiologist with GE 9800 CT scanner or its equivalent

CAVEATS

The implantologist must be experienced with subperiosteal implant bone impression techniques before attempting this method in order to manage situations in which the CAD-CAM–generated casting does not fit and a traditional impression must be taken.

Using an advanced computer can eliminate the first stage bone impression surgery and radiographic technology called *computer assisted design-computer assisted manufacture* (CAD-CAM). If a diagnostic computed tomography (CT) scan had been performed for endosteal implant placement analysis (see Chapter 4), in most instances the head position has not been correct for use by the CAD-CAM company. A new head orientation, depending on the software (but using the same immobilization jigs, without the original gutta percha points), may have to be adapted. Basically, the CT scan data are transferred to a magnetic tape that is subsequently loaded into a computer. The computer then interfaces with a three-point milling machine to generate a model of the bony maxilla or mandible. This model is used as the master cast when designing an implant casting. Recently, technology has been introduced that produces bone models from CT scan magnetic tapes by means of laser sculpture. It is called *stereolithography.* Particular advantages of this method are the excellent accuracy achieved as well as the liberal requirements permitted by the imaging process. Records are acceptable from virtually any scanner, and specific head angulation plays no role in the process.

There are significant benefits to using these techniques. First, the patient is spared the lengthy first stage surgical procedure. Second, since only one surgical procedure is performed, the mucosal tissue is less traumatized and, consequently, heals more readily. Third, greater extension of the implant can be achieved on bearing bone sites than would be possible with a two-stage impression technique.

Since this technique permits design of an implant that can extend much farther peripherally, the dissection for seating has to be more aggressive than is ordinarily required. If the casting is not acceptable at the time of surgery, however, a direct bone impression may be required in order to make a satisfactory implant. As mentioned elsewhere in this chapter, accuracy of fit alone should not cause rejection of an implant.

Stability, on the other hand, is mandatory. If innovative adjustments can achieve three or more point contact stability, screw fixation and particulate 20-mesh HA augmentation proves of value in completing the operation. The patient must always be informed that a two-stage procedure may become necessary (see Appendix F).

The patient should be told as well that the total radiation exposure of the CT scan is about equivalent to that of a chest x-ray and that he or she will be on the gurney for about 20 minutes unless the unit is a helical scanner, which completes the process within 50 seconds. It is necessary for the patient to remove all metal from his or her head and shoulders (e.g., earrings, necklaces, and metal-based dentures) before the scan. Metallic restorations will have to be removed from the jaw to be scanned.

Preparing for the Scan

The following are essentials that must be performed in preparation for the CT scan procedure:

1. Consult the radiologist to acknowledge that he or she has been trained in these techniques. The CT machine must be one of the following: GE 9800, GE 8800, Phillips T-60, Phillips 310, Picker 1200, or Techni-Care 2020. However, the newer laser technology makes no such restrictions.
2. Ensure that there is no metal in the arch to be scanned (it causes an obliteration of adjacent structures). If metal does exist, replace it, at least temporarily, with nonmetallic restorations. Titanium does not cause "starburst" or scatter effect, however, and may be left in position.
3. Provide the patient with an intraoral jig or jaw-stabilizing device to be worn during the scanning process. This prevents jaw movement during the scan. This is accomplished by fabricating base-plates with wax occlusal rims for both arches and using standard prosthodontic techniques, luting them in a proper centric relationship and at the correct vertical dimension. After mounting the casts on a semiadjustable articulator (Hanau or Whipmix), remove all wax and bite paste material and lock the upper and lower baseplates together with self-curing acrylic rims. They should be supraoccluded with 3-mm high shims. One vertically placed No. 50 gutta percha point should be processed into each canine area of the lower rim. On the images this assists in establishing the mental foramina locations. Denture adhesive may be used to help stabilize this jig during the scan procedure. If there is a question about retention, the appliances may be relined with Viscogel (Fig. 14-26). For more details about appliance fabrication, refer to Chapters 4 and 20.
4. A nonmetal saliva ejector and a source of suction must be available in the radiologist's office. It should be operated at minimal force so that it does not injure the tongue or floor of the mouth. An antihistamine, such as diphenhydramine

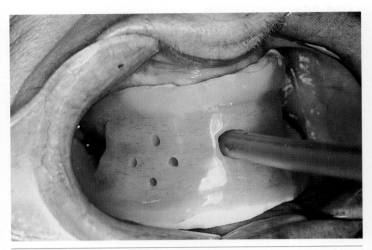

Fig. 14-26   The CT scan intraoral stabilizing device is in position. The four small holes are for breathing, and the metal-free, plastic tube is for saliva aspiration.

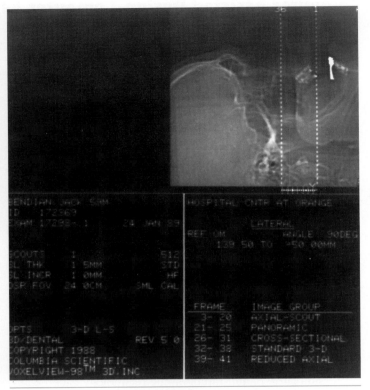

Fig 14-27   The first, or scout, film for preimplant CT scanning has two dotted lines. They indicate the inferior and superior extents of the scan. They must be parallel to the occlusal plane or crest of the ridge.

(Benadryl), 50 mg IV, helps in decreasing salivation and allaying anxiety.

5. Provide the radiologist with a recent panoramic x-ray film of the patient. This assists in explaining the perimeters of the scan field.

6. Calibration rods that are taped to the patient's face over the zygomas should accompany him or her; they are used to detect patient movement. The CAD-CAM company supplies them, and the rods can be reused for subsequent patients.

Role of the Radiologist

The following are essentials for the radiologist in preparation for the CAD-CAM procedure.

1. Review the panoramic x-ray film so that the total area included in the scan is recognized (the perimeters).

2. Minimize patient movement. The x-ray slices must be acquired in rapid sequence from inferior to superior in one direction over a period of about 20 minutes. Instruct the patient not to swallow during the scan. Salivary evacuation and diphenhydramine contribute toward this goal.

3. The technician must take a lateral skull film (scout view) with the maxilla or mandible at a 15- to 20-degree angle to the x-ray beam for the Calcitek protocol or a 0-degree angle to the alveolar crest for the Techmedica protocol (Fig. 14-27). A total of 30 to 50 slices are needed. (See Appendix C, page 453 for scanner settings.) Laser (stereolithographic) fabrication has no such angulation requirements (see Appendix C, page 454).

4. The radiologist should load the image data and image heading into a new magnetic tape in the uncompressed form and label it with the following information: CT scanner used; radiologist's name, address, and telephone number; patient's name; surgeon's name; jaw that was studied; and date.

5. The radiologist must understand that 1 to 2 mm of movement is the maximum that is acceptable. The calibration

rods taped to each of the patient's cheeks parallel to the table top and perpendicular to the x-ray beam indicate by the clarity of their reproduction on the completed images if the results are free from distortion.

6. The first slice should start below the inferior border of the mandible and the last should end at the sigmoid notch level. This will grant a complete mandibular model. For maxillae, the perimetric boundaries should extend from below the residual ridge or occlusal surfaces of the teeth, and extend superiorly to the infraorbital rims.

Stereolithography (Laser-Forming Technology)

As services available for CAD-CAM technology wane, an accurate technique that requires far less rigid protocols on the part of implantologist and radiologist has been introduced.

Innova is one such laboratory that presents a simple protocol. It instructs the radiologist to use a 0-degree gantry tilt and scan the supine patient with the nasomental line at right angles to the table. They recommend 1-mm slices. To ensure that the patient remains still throughout the scan, affix opaque positioning or calibration rods to the patient's face.

The technology for model manufacture is different from the milling machine fabrication formerly used. Stereolithography is an additive process of creating physical replicas from the electronic data produced by CT scanning. The apparatus consists of a computer-guided laser that creates a layer-by-layer augmentation using a photosensitive liquid that solidi-

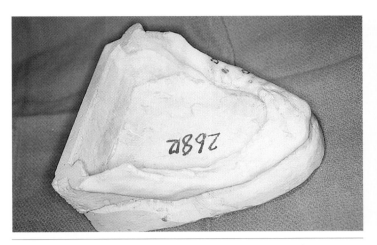

Fig. 14-28 A cast produced by stereolithography shows the extensive exposure of peripheral structures.

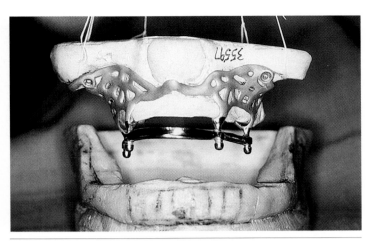

Fig. 14-29 The completed casting cannot be related to the opposing jaw, nor can abutments and bars be placed in appropriate positions. It is essentially "hanging in space."

fies, on completion, into an anatomic model. Other companies that offer similar services are Medical Modeling Corporation and 3D SLA Bio-tec Systems. The protocols for these companies are given in the Appendix C, page 454. These technologies can use magnetic resonance imaging (MRI) as well as CT scans in order to fabricate models and are less demanding about CT scanners and patient head position.

Fabrication of the Cast

Once the CT scan tape has been given to the company of choice, it fabricates a model of the jaw (Fig. 14-28). A detailed laboratory prescription must be written; the implant is designed on the final model following the recommendations made in this chapter. If both maxillary and mandibular subperiosteal implants are planned using this technique, the patient has to be passed through the scanner twice with head orientation altered for each jaw. However, for sterolithography, only one cycle great enough to include cuts for both jaws is required.

Implant Fabrication

Until recently, doctor and laboratory would have had to make an educated guess at abutment or bar locations, since the generated model could not be related to the opposing jaw. Soft tissue occlusal records have been shown to be very inaccurate, causing extreme misplacement of abutments or bars (Fig.14-29). To solve this problem using a cast returned from the CAD-CAM laboratory, employ the steps in the following section.

Tube and Stylus Technique for Establishing Centric Relationships

1. Make a preoperative cast of the ridge to be implanted. An acrylic base-plate and wax rim are used for accurate centric and vertical measurements using a conventional pros-

thetic technique. An alginate counterimpression (of natural teeth or prosthesis) completes this step.
2. At each of five sites in the peripheral flange of the acrylic base-plate (right and left first molars, canines, and in the midline), cut a ¼-inch diameter round hole.
3. Lute an orthodontic tube with a welding flange, 0.045-inch inside diameter, into each of the round holes that have been cut into the base-plate, and lock into place with acrylic (Fig. 14-30, A). Place each in an oblique direction aimed toward the ridge crest. The deep end of each tube must be placed directly against the tissue surface of the rim. Access to each tube must be available from the buccal side when seating the rim and retracting the lips and cheeks.
4. Use five 20-gauge, 1½-inch long, disposable hypodermic needles. They will fit passively but snugly into the orthodontic tubes (Fig. 14-30, B).
5. Place the acrylic rim into the patient's mouth to confirm that a correct occlusal plane has been established and that it offers the proper vertical dimension and centric relationship.
6. Anesthetize the patient in the buccal vestibule at the locations of each of the five tubes.
7. Ask the patient into close into centric occlusion, thereby stabilizing the rim. Place one hypodermic needle through each of the orthodontic tubes. Retracting the lips or cheeks elevates the tissues of the vestibule. Use a needle holder to push each needle through its tube until bone stops it (Fig. 14-30, C). The patient keeps the rim stabilized by continuing to bite while these simple needle-seating procedures are performed (Fig. 14-30, D).
8. In order to stabilize the needles, fix each by crimping the orthodontic tube with a pliers (Fig. 14-30, E). The rim then may be removed by gentle manipulation after opening the patient's mouth.
9. Affix the model of the opposing arch on a simple articulator.
10. Occlude the operative wax rim with needle positioners to the countermodel and lute with sticky wax.

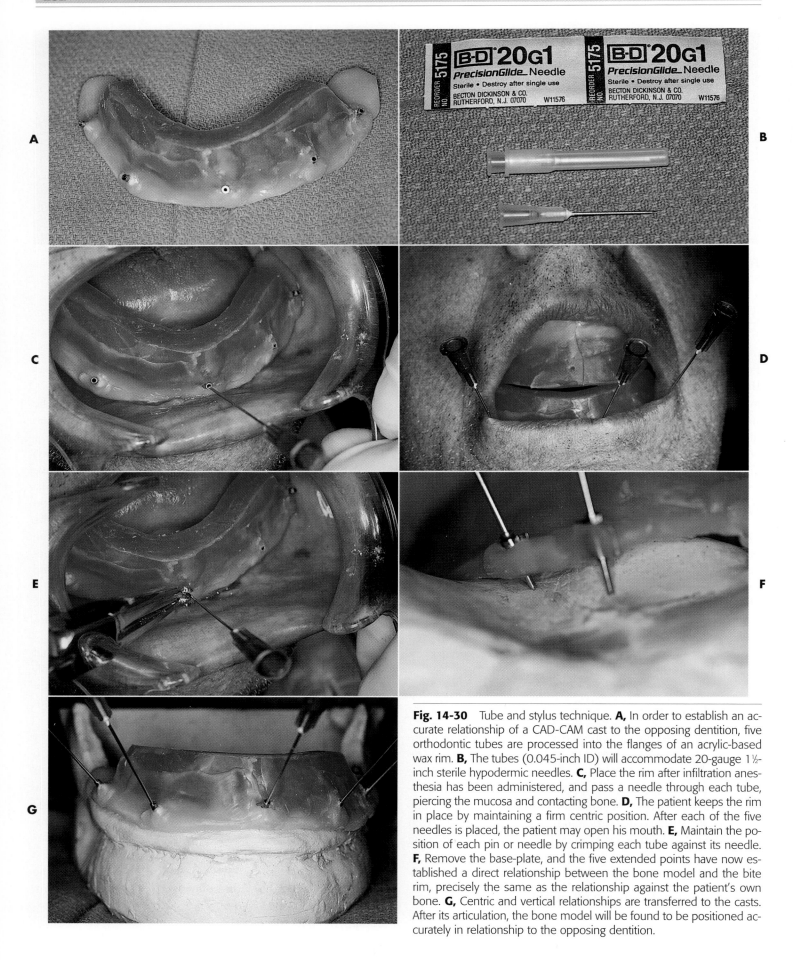

Fig. 14-30 Tube and stylus technique. **A,** In order to establish an accurate relationship of a CAD-CAM cast to the opposing dentition, five orthodontic tubes are processed into the flanges of an acrylic-based wax rim. **B,** The tubes (0.045-inch ID) will accommodate 20-gauge 1½-inch sterile hypodermic needles. **C,** Place the rim after infiltration anesthesia has been administered, and pass a needle through each tube, piercing the mucosa and contacting bone. **D,** The patient keeps the rim in place by maintaining a firm centric position. After each of the five needles is placed, the patient may open his mouth. **E,** Maintain the position of each pin or needle by crimping each tube against its needle. **F,** Remove the base-plate, and the five extended points have now established a direct relationship between the bone model and the bite rim, precisely the same as the relationship against the patient's own bone. **G,** Centric and vertical relationships are transferred to the casts. After its articulation, the bone model will be found to be positioned accurately in relationship to the opposing dentition.

11. Place the CAD-CAM model into the base-plate (Fig. 14-30, *F*). The points of the needle will strike the bone model at the five sites, yielding accurate seating. Fix the model to the articulator with quick-setting plaster, which completes the mounting (Fig. 14-30, *G*).

At this point, the mounted models accurately relate the relationship between the bony operative jaw to its opposing dentition (Fig. 14-31). This permits accurate implant bar or abutment placement and height. In this fashion, an implant may be constructed with accuracy and precision following the designs described in this chapter (Fig. 14-32). After it is returned from the laboratory, the implant should be passivated, treated, and sterilized as described in Appendix C.

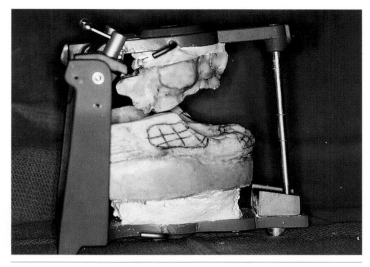

Fig. 14-31 Articulation using the tube and stylus technique accurately relates even the most unusually related bone models.

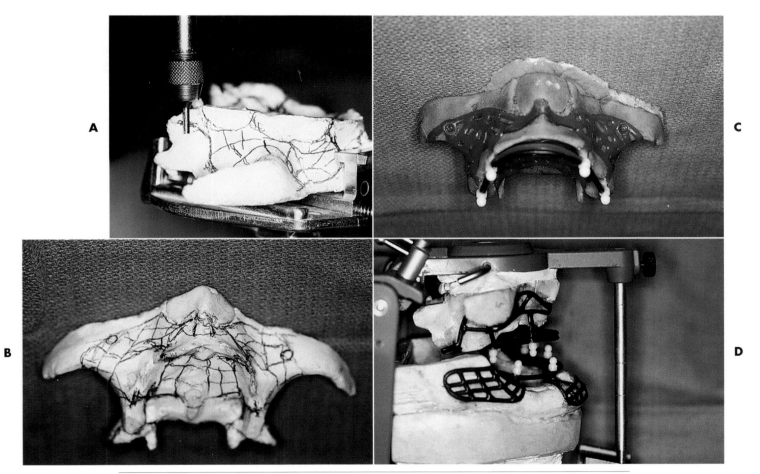

Fig. 14-32 **A,** Positive, screw-free retention can be achieved by surveying a stereolithographic cast and marking the points of widest dimension. **B,** The design of an infrastructure should extend slightly into undercut zones. Screw holes are included for elective use. **C,** The wax-up with bar and O-ring attachments, when cast, will go to place only by tapping with a mallet and orangewood stick. It will then fit quite firmly. **D,** Waxed implants must be related to each other or to the opposing denture so that occlusal forces will be directed optimally through their infrastructures. For the C-T scan technique, these relationships are achieved only by using the tube and stylus technique.

Surgery for Insertion of the Implant

Surgery for placement of the CAD-CAM implant is the same as described in the first part of this chapter. Observe every precaution. The use of regional block anesthesia is more effective for placing CAD-CAM implants than for conventionally made ones because the anesthetic will be given for the first time.

After the bone has been exposed, inspect it carefully. Eliminate minor areas of irregularity, as well as spinous and irregular structures that might not have been detected by the scan. With proper retraction, the implant is seated. The expe-

rienced implantologist may be moderately disappointed in noting the lack of expected accuracy of metal-to-bone adaptation. After several cases, a new set of standards is acquired for acceptability. Instability or rocking, however, is not permissible. If there are three or more points of good bone contact that permit stable or firm seating, liberal quantities of 20-mesh particulate HA graft material should be used under and around all struts that demonstrate deficiencies (Figs. 14-33).

Closure should follow in the routine manner described earlier (Figs. 14-34 and 14-35).

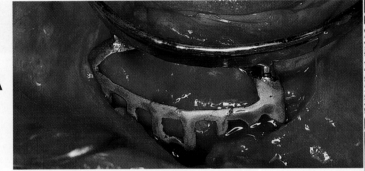
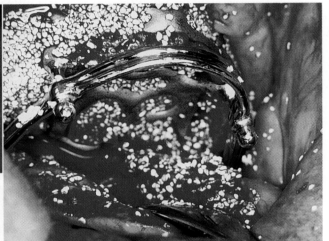

Fig. 14-33 A, After castings are placed, check each strut for accuracy of fit. **B,** In case of inaccurate fit, if the casting is stable, the discrepancies may be managed successfully with the addition of grafting materials.

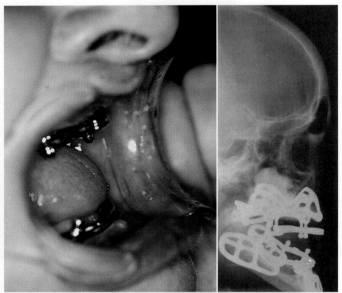
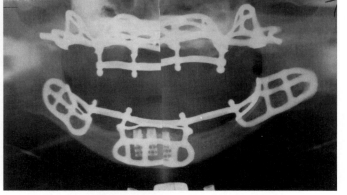

Fig. 14-34 A, Careful presurgical and prosthetic planning eliminates the guesswork of bar and abutment placement. This makes prosthetic techniques simple and accurate. **B,** C-T scan technology allows for the fabrication and placement of two subperiosteal implants in one operative session (under general anesthesia). Because the osseointegrated Core-Vent implants that were permitted to remain in the symphysis are made of titanium, scatter did not blemish the scans. **C,** Direct bone impressions will not permit the kind of peripheral extension that computer generation allows.

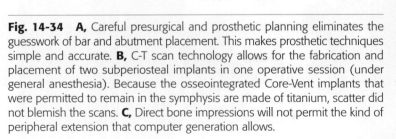

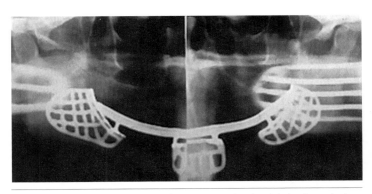

Fig. 14-35 The CAD-CAM technique permits the fabrication of tripodal implants, which allow islet placement in zones best designed to resist stress and sometimes too inaccessible for direct bone impression maneuvers.

Suggested Readings

Berman N: Implant technique for full lower denture, *Wash Dent J* 19:15-17, 1950.

Berman N: Methods for improving implant dentures, *Oral Surg* 8:227-236, 1955.

Berman N: Physiologic and mechanical aspects of the implant technique and its application to practical cases, *Dent Diag* 58:342-347, 1952.

Bodine RL: Construction of the mandibular implant denture superstructure, *J Implant Dent* 1:32-36, 1954.

Bodine RL: Evaluation of 27 mandibular subperiosteal implant dentures after 15 to 22 years, *J Prosthet Dent* 32:188-197, 1974.

Bodine RL: Implant denture, *Bull Nat Dent Assoc* 11:11-21, 1952.

Bodine RL: Implant denture bone impression: preparations and technique, *J Implant Dent* 4:22-31, 1957.

Bodine RL: Prosthodontic essentials and an evaluation of the mandibular subperiosteal implant denture, *J Am Dent Assoc* 51:654-664, 1955.

Bodine RL: Twenty-five years experience with the mandibular subperiosteal implant denture, *J Oral Implant* 8:124-145, 1978.

Bodine RL et al: The subperiosteal implant denture program at the University of Southern California, *J Oral Implantol* 193-209, 1977.

Bodine RL, Kotch RL: Experimental dental implants, *US Armed Forces Med J* 4:441, 1953.

Craig RG: A review of properties of rubber impression materials, *Mich Dent Assoc J* 59:254, 1977.

Cranin NA: The Brookdale bar subperiosteal implant, *Trans Soc Biomater* 2:1978.

Cranin AN, Cranin SL: *The one day subperiosteal implant,* Springfield, 1970, Charles C. Thomas.

Cranin AN et al: Reconstruction of the edentulous mandible with a lower border graft and subperiosteal implant, *J Oral Maxillofac Surg* 46:264-268, 1988.

Cranin AN, Klein M, Sirakan A: A technique for mounting computer-generated models for subperiosteal implants: the Brookdale tube and stylus centric system, *J Oral Implantol* 16:52-56, 1990.

Dahl GSA: Subperiosteal implants and superplants, *Dent Abstr* 2:685, 1957.

Davis DM, Rogers SJ, Packer ME: The extent of maintenance required by implant-retained mandibular overdentures: a 3-year report, *Int J Oral Maxillofac Implants* 11:767-774, 1996.

Fishel D et al: Roentgenologic study of the mental foramen, *Oral Surg Med Oral Pathol* 41:682-686, 1976.

Fonseca RJ, Davis W: *Reconstructive preprosthetic oral and maxillofacial surgery,* Philadelphia, 1986, WB Saunders.

Gershkoff A: *Surgical considerations of the subperiosteal implant,* Springfield, 1970, Charles C. Thomas.

Goldberg NI, Gershkoff A: A six-year progress report on full denture implants, *J Implant Dent* 1:1, 1954.

Goltec TS: CAD-CAM multiplaner diagnostic imaging for subperiosteal implants, *Dent Clin North Am* 30:85-95, 1986.

Goltec TS: The mandibular full subperiosteal implant—a ten year review of 202 cases, *J Oral Implantol* 15:179-185, 1989.

Goltec TS: The use of hydroxylapatite to coat subperiosteal implants, *J Oral Implant* 12:21, 1985.

James RA: *HA coated subperiosteal implants,* 6th Annual Meeting, New Concepts in Prosthetic Surgery and Implant Dentistry, Louisiana State University, New Orleans, 1986.

James RA: Subperiosteal implant design based on peri-implant tissue behavior, *NY J Dent* 53:407-414, 1983.

James RA, Truitt HP: *CT scan models for subperiosteal implants,* Proceedings of the International Congress of Oral Implant, San Diego, 1984.

James RA et al: Subperiosteal implants, *Calif Dent J* 1:10-14, 1988.

Jermyn AC: Implant dentures, *Dent Radio Photog* 3:34, 1961.

Jones SD, Travis C: Load-transfer characteristics of mandibular subperiosteal implants, *J Prosthet Dent* 42:211, 1979.

Judy KWM, Misch CE: Evolution of the mandibular subperiosteal implant, *J Prosthet Dent* 53:9-11, 1983.

Kay JF, Goltec TS, Riley RL: Hydroxylapatite coated subperiosteal dental implants: design rationale and clinical experience, *J Prosthet Dent* 58:343, 1987.

Lee TC, Lattig EJ: Mandibular subperiosteal implant technique, *J Calif Dent Assoc* 34:400-405, 1958.

Linkow LI: Clinical article—some variant designs of the subperiosteal implant, *J Oral Implant* 2:190-205, 1972.

Linkow LI: Evolutionary trends in the mandibular subperiosteal implants. *J Oral Implant* 11:402-438, 1984.

McGivney GP et al: A comparison of computer-assisted tomography and data gathering modalities in prosthodontics, *Int J Oral Maxillofac Implants,* 1:55-68, 1968.

Mentag PJ: Current status of the mandibular subperiosteal implant prosthesis, *Dent Clin North Am* 24:553-563, 1980.

Mentag PJ: Mandibular subperiosteal implant, *J Oral Implant* 9:596-603, 1979.

Misch CE: Density of bone: effect on treatment plans, surgical approach, healing and progressive bone loading, *Int J Oral Implant* 6:23-31, 1990.

Misch CE: *Design consideration of the complete mandibular subperiosteal implant, (workbook),* 1985, Misch Implant Institute, Dearborn, Michigan.

Misch CE: *Direct bone impression—material and techniques,* International Congress of Oral Implant, 1st Subperiosteal Symposium, San Diego, October, 1981.

Pietrokovski J: The bony residual ridge in man, *J Prosthet Dent* 34:456-462, 1975.

Rivera E: *HA castings on the subperiosteal implant,* International Congress of Oral Implant, Puerto Rico, 1983.

Root D: *Laboratory techniques and implant dentistry,* American Academy of Implant Dentistry, Washington, D.C., 1988.

Schnell RJ, Phillips RW: Dimensional stability of rubber base impressions and certain other factors affecting accuracy, *J Am Dent Assoc* 57:39, 1958.

Tallgren A: The reduction in face height of edentulous and partially edentulous subjects during long-term denture wear: a longitudinal entgenographic cephalometric study, *Acta Odontol Scand* 24:195-239, 1966.

Travis CT, Bodine RL: The implant denture mesostructure bar, separate bilateral versus anterior continuous, *J Oral Implantol* 10:233-254, 1982.

Truitt HP et al: Non-invasive technique for mandibular subperiosteal implant: a preliminary report, *J Prosthet Dent* 55:494-497, 1986.

Truitt HP et al: Use of computer tomography in subperiosteal implant therapy, *J Prosthet Dent* 59:474-477, 1988.

Weber SP: Complete bilateral subperiosteal implants for partially edentulous mandibles, *J Prosthet Dent* 20(3):239-241, 1968.

Weiss CM, Judy KWM: Severe mandibular atrophy: biological consideration of routine treatment with complete subperiosteal implants, *J Oral Implant* 4:431-469, 1974.

Whittaker JM et al: The suspension mechanism of subperiosteal implants in baboons, *J Oral Implant* 16:190-197, 1990.

Yosue T, Brooks SL: The appearance of mental foramina on panoramic and periapical radiographs, *Oral Surg Oral Med Oral Pathol* 68:488-492, 1989.

Yurkstas AA: The effect of missing teeth on masticatory performance and efficiency, *J Prosthet Dent* 4:120-123,1954.

15

Maxillary Pterygohamular Subperiosteal Implant Surgery

ARMAMENTARIUM

Acrylic: Self-curing (Formatray)
Articulator, Whipmix
Coe Comfort soft tissue conditioner
Diamond drill: Atwood 347 for the straight handpiece
EZ Tray material
Forceps: Gerald
Hall drill
Hemostats: Long curved (i.e., tonsil hemostats) and mosquito
Impression material and adhesive: Neoplex (regular)
Mallet
Needleholder
Needles: sterile hypodermic, 20 G, 1½ inch

Orangewood sticks
Orthodontic tubes: 0.045-inch (ID)
Pliers, crimping
Scalpel: Long handle
Scissors: Mayo and Dean
Screws: 7-mm Vitallium
Screwdriver: Vitallium
Surveyor
Suture: 2-0, 3-0 black silk
Suture: 4-0 dyed Vicryl
Thermostatically controlled hot water bath (180° F)

CAVEATS

When reflecting the lateral posterior mucoperiosteum either below or just adjacent to the zygomatic buttress, take care not to perforate the maxillary sinus. Some eggshell bone may come away, but if it is permitted to remain attached to the periosteum, it serves in a viable reconstructive role. Protect antral openings from becoming filled with impression materials.

An overenthusiastic periosteal elevator or long needle in the posterior superior area may cause pterygoid plexus hemorrhage. If this should occur, as noted by considerable venous bleeding or rapid swelling of the face, apply firm tamponade with the forefinger upwardly and inwardly in the posterior vestibular area for a full 10 minutes.

A periosteal elevator may injure or tear the infraorbital or greater palatine neurovascular bundles. Exercise care when approaching these foramina.

The buccal pad of fat is always beneath the retractor. If it prolapses (as it often does), it should not be cut or resected. The patient's facial symmetry may change markedly if this is done. When the surgery is completed, tuck it back in and suture the flaps over it.

If the pterygoid plate or raphe dissections are bilateral and are performed vigorously in a susceptible patient, edema from each side may compromise the airway. The surgeon must be aware of the possibilities of this occurrence and be prepared to use steroids (dexamethasone 10 mg orally or 20 mg intravenously followed by 5 mg four times daily) or to institute surgical airway management (e.g., orotracheal or nasopharyngeal tubes or airways, tracheostomy).

Hydroxylapatite (HA) coatings may be of benefit at interface areas, but they do not permit the implant to be flexed or malleted to place, nor do they offer assurance of the classic suspension mechanism required for implant success. Design considerations must play a role in prescribing HA coatings.

In addition, 12- to 36-hour, two-stage subperiosteal implants cannot be performed if HA coatings are ordered, since time considerations will not permit this procedure.

The surgery for pterygohamular subperiosteal implants requires experience and aggressiveness to expose the prospective bone-bearing areas.

Completely Edentulous Designs

Experience over the past 20 years has presented unpredictable prognoses of maxillary unilateral and complete subperiosteal implants. Failure probably resulted from placement of infrastructural components on a bone foundation not well designed to withstand occlusal stresses. The resulting resorption led to a failure of bony support, antral complications, and subsequent exteriorization of these devices. However, a design change took place that was termed the *pterygohamular extension*. With the addition of peripheral struts placed in the pterygohamular areas and on other more reliable basal bone buttresses, a more predictable device was produced. This chapter outlines each step leading to the production of pterygohamular complete, universal, and unilateral maxillary subperiosteal implants. If surgeons are comfortable with other designs, placement techniques are the same.

Procedure

For surgeons experienced in hospital procedures, this operation may best be performed under general anesthesia in the operating room. However, regional block with sedation is an alternate way to proceed.

Routine maxillary infiltration anesthesia is not sufficient. Second division (greater palatine), posterior-superior alveolar, and infraorbital blocks are necessary in addition to considerable deep infiltration into the pterygomandibular raphe. After the tissues are anesthetized, use a sharpened millimeter probe to measure tissue thicknesses at the sites of planned permucosal abutments, each of which should be placed in attached gingiva. Record these measurements on a preoperative study model or chart.

Incision

Make the incision at the crest of the ridge on the linea alba from the distal incline of one tuberosity around the arch to the contralateral side. A midline-relieving incision is required just lateral to the labial frenulum, which extends up to the nasal spine.

Reflection

Using a sharp periosteal elevator, lift the palatal flap cleanly from the bone. Lift it posteriorly as close posteriorly to the junction of the soft palate as can be managed (Fig. 15-1). This cannot be affected without severing the incisive neurovascular bundle, but no significant harm results from doing so. The structures that prevent a complete soft tissue reflection are the greater (anterior) palatine neurovascular bundles bilaterally, and they must be preserved. They may be seen clearly running anteriorly from their foramina (located just medial to the ridge crests in the second molar areas) within the periosteal surface of the reflected palatal flaps. Extend the periosteal elevator behind and lateral to these foramina, and lift the overlying tissues away from the hamulus bilaterally (which is found just at the anterior end of the medial pterygoid plate) (Fig. 15-2).

On the labiobuccal aspects, elevate the mucoperiosteum beginning at the midline and proceeding posteriorly on both sides. In this way, the following structures become exposed and may be identified clearly: anterior nasal spine, pyriform apertures, canine fossae up to the lower rim of the infraorbital foramina, zygomatic buttresses (no less than 3 cm beyond their roots), posterolateral maxillae (to a height that is level with the superior surfaces of the zygomatic arches), and the entire bony tuberosity.

The remainder of the pterygohamular complex is the last structure to be exposed. Use a No. 15 BP blade on a long handle to extend the original incision from the distal end of the tuberosity downward in the mucosa overlying the pterygomandibular raphe. As the mucosa falls open, the gleaming white fibers of the raphe become evident (Fig. 15-3). Blunt

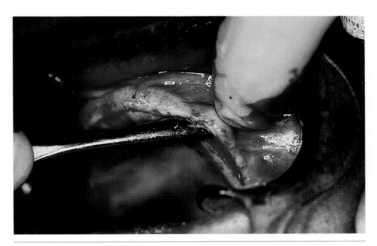

Fig. 15-1 To obtain an impression for a pterygohamular implant, make a crestal incision from the base of the tuberosity forward to the midline of each side. Reflection must be completed with a sharp periosteal elevator.

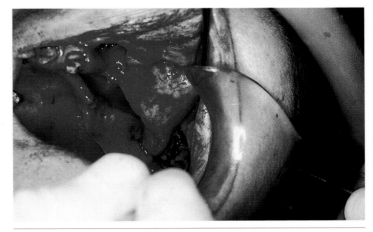

Fig. 15-2 The reflection, when complete, should reveal the zygomatic buttresses, the greater palatine foramina, the canine fossae, the incisive foramen, the anterior nasal spine and the pyriform apertures.

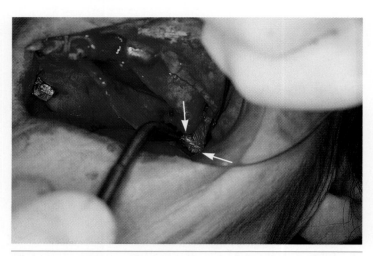

Fig. 15-3 After the primary reflection has been completed, make a second incision from the base of the tuberosity downward over the pytergomadibular raphe for a distance of 2 cm. Blunt and sharp dissection beneath this incision exposes the gleaming white fibers of the raphe *(arrows)*. Dissect these fibers from the lateral and medial pterygoid plates and the hamulus. This can be done only by sharp dissection using pointed, long, curved surgical shears.

dissection on either side of the raphe, using the forefinger, reveals the attachment of these fibers to the pterygoid plates. Stretch the raphe with the periosteal elevator, and using curved or angled long-handled (Dean) scissors, snip away the fibrous attachments, being careful to stay directly against bone. In most cases, the raphe is extensive, and considerable cutting is necessary. When it finally becomes freed, it is intact and easy to identify because of its glistening whiteness. Beneath it are the pterygoid plates; the surgeon uses the fingers of his or her dissecting hand to identify them. Further vigorous blunt dissection of the overlying soft tissues, will push them firmly from both plates. They are clearly palpable despite the fact that they may not be visualized. The probing finger should be able to nestle into the fossa between them. The sharp dissection is complete only when this complex is exposed fully. Pack a saline-soaked sponge into the site to maintain hemostasis and prevent desiccation.

The periosteal elevator should lift the palatal tissues anteromedially from the base of the medial pterygoid plate forward to the hamulus, a small finger of bone. If the tissues are resistant to elevation, use a No. 12 BP blade. Use it as if it were a periosteal elevator, stroking gently but firmly at the bone level until the hamulus is exposed. When the overlying mucosa has been elevated, a tendinous structure will be found at its lateral base. The hamulus serves as a pulley for this structure, the tendon of the levator veli palatini muscle. In order to expose the hamulus for the impression, cut the tendon with a No. 12 blade.

The final bit of exposure is done on the lateral maxilla posterior to the zygomatic root and anterior to the lateral pterygoid plate. Elevate the tissues starting from the distal attachment of the zygoma and proceed posteriorly to the lateral surface of the lateral plate using a periosteal elevator. The raphe fibers are resistant to elevation, and the plate becomes

free of these fibrous encumbrances only if curved, sharp scissors or a No. 12 BP blade is used to separate them. This requires removing the original saline-soaked pack and replacing it with a larger one that encompasses the entire pterygohamular plate complex.

Before making the impression, note the following exposed structures: the anterior nasal spine, the pyriform apertures, the canine fossae up to the infraorbital foramina, the base of the zygomas (including a minimum of 3 cm of exposed arch), the lateral maxillae, the lateral and medial pterygoid plates, the hamuli, the greater (anterior) palatine foramina, the palatal surfaces of the maxillae, and the incisive foramen. Round the sharp spicules of crestal bone and knife-edge ridges with burs, rongeurs forceps, and bone files.

Not all patients have well-defined pterygoid plates and, for them, even the most careful palpation fails to reveal their presence. Therefore, it is possible that only one plate may be palpated, or, rarely, neither may be palpated. There is always some rudiment of a plate at the pterygomaxillary suture, however, so uncover the area because it is important as a site for implant bearing.

Impression Making

Pack the flaps open with saline-soaked sponges, and suture the palate into a midline bundle.

Place an EZ Tray sheet (instructions on the use of this material are given in Chapter 14) into the hot water heater at 178° F until it softens. Lift it from the bath while the assistant removes the saline sponges from the wound. As the assistant retracts the flaps, slip the soft material beneath them and then tease, massage, and push the material peripherally to the fullest extent of the dissection. Use the forefinger to press the compliant material over the pterygohamular structures. Before its total setting, lift it out and seat it several times so that it does not become locked into undercuts.

If there is insufficient working time to fabricate the entire custom tray at once, augment the EZ Tray in its wet state by adding small heated supplementary peripheral pieces These "welds," even when wet, are reliable, as when handles are added to the trays. On each removal of the tray, however, be sure to dry the welded areas and reinforce them by using a heated wax spatula and, when indicated, sticky wax.

If the exposed bone appears to be geometrically complicated and numerous undercuts portend difficulties in creating an acceptable path of removal, make two separate half trays, each with its own handle. Trim them in the midline so that they seat together and fit snugly against each other from the anterior nasal spine all the way back to the posterior palate, as is described for the mandibular implant in Chapter 14. Seat the two halves separately for the final impression; after an index is made using self-curing acrylic, remove them either in one piece or separately and collate them by using the index. If it is necessary to remove the impression in two halves, make indexing structures on the trays' outside surfaces. This may be accomplished by cutting 4-mm cubes of EZ Tray and luting them to the outer surfaces of the tray halves.

When the impressions have been completed in two halves, remove excess impression material from the attached cubes, applying a thin layer of lubricant and placing a U-shaped Formatray (acrylic polymer) index over them (as described in Chapter 14).

If the entire complex can be removed in one piece, this should be done. If it is resistant, remove the index first, then the tray halves separately. Complete their reassembly on the countertop using the indexing cubes for accuracy.

After a satisfactory tray or pair of half trays have been completed, repack the wound with saline-soaked sponges. Elastomeric impression materials such as Optosil, Reprosil, or Neoplex do not displace fluids such as blood, mucus, or saliva, so the importance of creating a clean, dry host site cannot be emphasized sufficiently.

In order to place the trays efficiently after they have been filled with impression material, surgeon and assistant should conduct tray-seating rehearsals with the palatal flap sutured together in the midline. In addition, the surgeon should pass 2-0 black silk sutures through the labiobuccal flap margins and remove the needles. He or she can attach each to a hemostat so that it serves as a retractor. Beaver tails (or Henahans) also work well to lift the flaps.

The path of insertion of each tray should be practiced, elevating and lifting the flaps in the appropriate sequence, and when it becomes evident that this may be done with consistency, make the final impression.

Apply adhesive to the trays and mix even lengths of the white and brown accelerator and base of regular body Neoplex and place them in the tray in modest amounts. If the tray fits accurately, the material serves merely as a wash.

Remove the packing and seat the trays following the rehearsal pattern: one tray and then the next. Vibrate each one into place to eliminate entrapped air. Some impression material should extrude beyond the tray flanges. The handles must be aligned as they had been during the practice seating.

Hold the trays firmly in position for 8 full minutes. Remove any material that may be covering the cubed indexing structures.

Lubricate the retention cubes; mix some autopolymerizing resin, mold it into a sausage-shaped mass, and press it over them. As the acrylic sets, use coolant to control the temperature.

After polymerization, remove the index and seat it once again to be sure that it serves as a reliable assembling device.

Remove each of the hemitrays. Sometimes the rubber from each tray flows along the entire length of the seam, and the two halves can be removed as one. If that happens, they still must be supported by the index.

Examine the impression for all requisite details (Fig. 15-4). If any is missing, repeat the impression. Wash techniques usually are unsuccessful and consume valuable operating time. If the impression is acceptable, bead, box, and pour the implant in Velmix pink die-stone (Fig. 15-5).

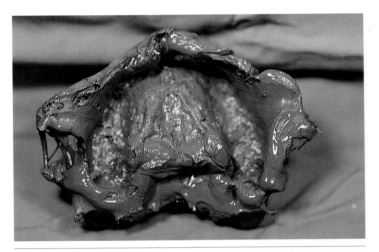

Fig. 15-4 A tray, fabricated from the theromolabile polymeric, EZ tray material and molded directly on the exposed maxillae, pterygoid plates, and hamuli, is coated with adhesive and a Neoplex, polysulfide impression is registered. It should demonstrate all of the vital structures noted in Fig. 15-3 and in the paragraphs of this section.

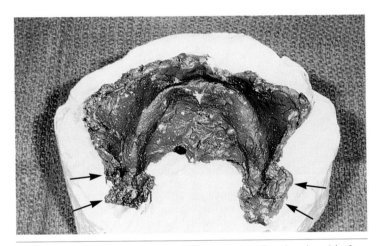

Fig. 15-5 The impression should be boxed and art-bordered before pouring. Note the pterygoid extensions *(arrows)*.

Surgical Jaw Relationship: Centric Recording

Take a counterimpression of the lower teeth or denture using alginate, and following this, use a large roll of Optosil putty to record the centric and vertical relationships between the bony maxillae and the opposing mandibular dentition using classic prosthodontic techniques.

Closure

Retract the flaps widely and inspect the wound. Debride it carefully, irrigate it with saline in a syringe, inspect it again for impression material fragments, and then remove the retraction sutures. Coapt the wound margins, express blood and fluids from beneath the flaps, and make a closure using a 3-0 black silk, continuous, horizontal mattress configuration (see Chapter 6). Begin suturing at the posterior end of the incision on each side and proceed no farther than the premolar area;

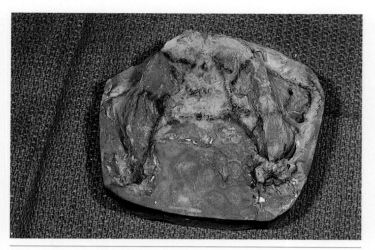

Fig. 15-6 The cast resulting from the poured impression is to have the infrastructural struts and borders outlined for the technician's wax-up.

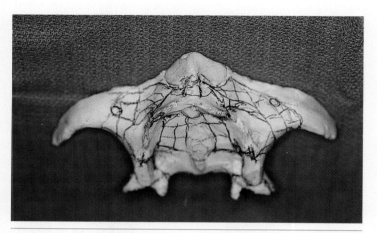

Fig. 15-7 The computer-generated cast will offer a more generous exposure of the prospective implant's support structures. Care must be exercised, when designing implants on these models, not to extend their peripheries beyond a point that would prevent them from being seated. Include strategically placed screw holes. The tube-and-stylus method of articulation (see p. 251) is mandated for casts produced in this manner.

otherwise, there is difficulty in retracting the upper lip, which is necessary in order to close the contralateral side. After closing each posterior half, continue the bilateral sutures anteriorly until they meet in the midline. Tie the right and left sutures together in a final square knot and repair the relieving incision separately.

Immediately insert the patient's denture to avoid hematoma formation or edema beneath the palatal flap. The pooled blood beneath the flap can cause fibrosis and an annoying permanent palatal thickening. Employ a denture adhesive if retention is lacking. Instruct the patient to follow the postoperative regimen given in Appendix G-I.

Implant Design

After separating the trimmed Velmix pink die-stone model, design the implant using a freshly sharpened No. 4 hard lead pencil (Figs. 15-6, 15-7).

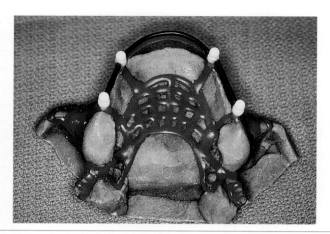

Fig. 15-8 The wax-up is done on a refractory cast and should be checked by the doctor to ensure its conformity to the original prescribed design. Interstices must be made large enough to permit strong periosteal reattachment and viable revascularization. "Trailer-hitch" attachments for O-rings are a viable prosthetic option.

The peripheral struts should rest on the structures noted previously. Only the primary struts should cross the ridge crest. Each of these struts should be in a canine or first molar area. The remaining secondary struts may be left somewhat to the designer's imagination, but there should be ample numbers, although no closer than 7 mm apart, to lend torque resistance to the infrastructure and to distribute stresses more evenly throughout the casting.

The cervices should be long enough to allow for the premeasured tissue thicknesses unless there is a plan to thin it (particularly in the tuberosity areas) by a filleting procedure (see Surgical Principles, Chapter 6, p. 75). Instruct the laboratory to add 2 mm additionally to the length of the cervices so that the Brookdale bar (which may be designed for Hader clips, custom-made clips, Lew attachments, O-ring attachments, or other retention devices) is placed above the mucosa at a distance sufficient to permit performing hygienic measures and to allow for a small degree of implant settling or gingival hypertrophy (Fig. 15-8).

Mark the cast by a surveyor stylus so that the peripheral struts can be placed in locations that lock them into slight undercuts. There need be no concern about this unless an HA coating is planned because the bearing bones are compliant and resilient enough to permit snapping a rigid casting over them. By following this technique, screw fixation does not have to be incorporated into the operative design.

Instruct the laboratory to supply an implant that presents a sandblasted infrastructure and a highly polished Brookdale bar and cervices. Design the shape and size of the bar or abutments that best serves the patient's prosthetic needs (see Chapter 26, Overdentures, p. 385). Note the height required for each cervix on the prescription (Fig. 15-9). Three countersunk screw holes suitable to receive the standard 5- or 7-mm self-tapping Vitallium implant screws should be designed in the peripheral struts of all implants: one just lateral to the midline and one on either side, in the zygomatic buttresses facing anteriorly. As an alternative, one or several vomeral screws

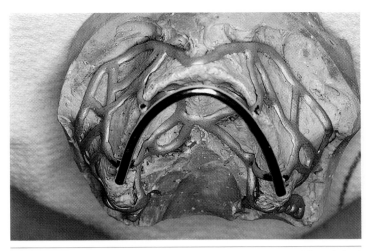

Fig. 15-9 The casting should be matte finished with a highly polished Brookdale bar and cervices. Allow adequate space beneath the bar for the exercise of oral hygiene measures. The centric, vertical dimension and aesthetic demands of the reconstruction must govern bar placement. Peripheral struts extend to the anterior nasal spines, pyriform apertures, infraorbital foramina areas of the canine fossae, zygomatic buttresses, hamuli, greater palatine foramen regions, and pterygoid plates.

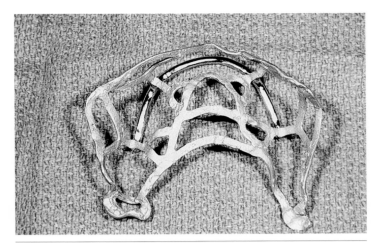

Fig. 15-10 The undersurface of the casting should represent the matte-type host site morphology. Make extensions onto the pterygoids aggressively.

may be placed palatally. Even if screws are not required, their use should be planned at the design stage.

Implant Insertion

If a 12-hour implant procedure is the method selected, the next steps are easier to perform. General anesthesia also makes the second stage simpler for patient and staff. Regional anesthesia may be used, but problems are presented as a result of the changes of pH in the tissues. When the sutures are removed, the flaps almost fall open spontaneously.

If, on the other hand, 4 to 6 weeks are permitted to elapse, the incision and reflection has to be repeated as in the first stage. This is slightly more difficult because the fibrosis of healing has made the tissues more resistant to reflection.

The implant should have been ultrasonically cleaned and passivated if the laboratory has not already done so. (Refer to Appendix E "Treatment of Metals.") It should not be touched by hands or gloves that contain talc. Rinse gloves in sterile saline after they have been donned. Place the implant into a porcelain cup and autoclave it for 20 minutes at 370° F, or treat it with a radiofrequency glow discharge (RFGD) apparatus as an alternative. Appendix E also offers details on the use of this equipment.

After appropriately preparing the implant for insertion, hold the flaps of the wounds with plastic retractors (plastic suction tips should be used as well) and introduce the casting following the same rehearsal pattern as was used for impression making. The flaps or other soft tissues must not become trapped beneath the peripheral struts during the seating procedure. Tap the implant firmly into place using a mallet and orangewood stick unless it is HA coated (Fig 15-10). When seating has been completed, irrigate the wound thoroughly with saline in a syringe. Check each strut and component to verify that the infrastructure is firmly and accurately seated

(Fig. 15-11). In areas of deficiency or inaccuracies of strut-to-bone fit, firmly tamp particulate HA (20 mesh) beneath and around the metal (Fig. 15-12) (see Chapter 8).

On viewing the pterygomandibular portion of the operative sites, the raphe on each side will be seen because of its stark, gleaming whiteness. It is somewhat withdrawn, but nevertheless present and easy to locate. Pass a 3-0 Vicryl suture with a tapered needle beneath the horizontal strut located at the pterygomaxillary junction just before final seating. After full seating, pass the needle into the most anterior portion of the raphe, which is being stabilized with a Gerald forceps. Tie a firm horizontal mattress surgical knot, drawing the raphe to a point close to its original anatomic position. When using screws (either zygomatic [Fig. 15-13] or midline [Fig. 15-14]), place them by pre-tapping with the Atwood 347 tapered diamond and then by self-tapping with a Vitallium screwdriver.

Coapt and close the flaps using 4-0 dyed Vicryl suture material with a cutting needle (FSI) in a horizontal mattress configuration. Start at the tuberosities and move forward to the premolar areas on both sides before proceeding more anteriorly. Then continue the suturing anteriorly beneath the bar. Use the two sutures that come together in the midline for the final knot. With 3 mm of clearance, the suturing is easy to complete once a rhythmic pattern is established. Conclude the closure by making a separate horizontal mattress suture (drawstring type) around each of the four cervices (Fig. 15-15).

Inspect the wound to verify that it is well closed. If not, add more sutures. When the closure is satisfactory and the mattress welt is clearly discernible, heat a piece of EZ Tray in a water bath to 178° F and press it against the palatal tissues to discourage prolapse. When the palate has been compressed firmly against the underlying bone, use a warmed plastic instrument to wedge and stabilize the stent material beneath the Brookdale bar from the palatal side (Fig. 15-16). This discourages the palatal tissues from becoming edematous, and it promotes healing in their normal arched configuration by preventing a pooling of fluids in the subperiosteal compartment.

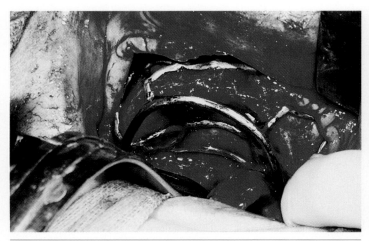

Fig. 15-11   Second-stage surgery should present evidence of accurate fit of metal to bone, stability, positive retention (or the use of screws to achieve retention), and proper room for tissue beneath the bar.

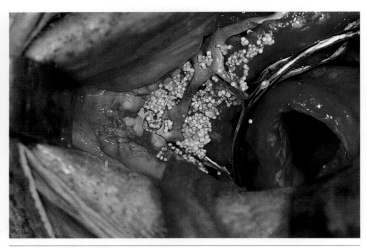

Fig. 15-12   When discrepancies are noted between struts and bone, use grafting materials as a filler to encourage a dense fibrous tissue response.

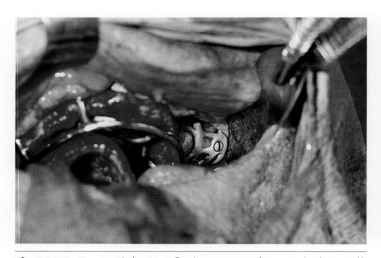

Fig. 15-13   Zygomatic buttress fixation screws, when required, are self-tapping Vitallium and are 7 mm in length.

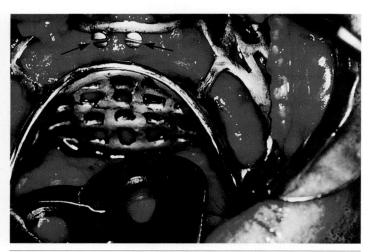

Fig. 15-14   On occasion, midpalatine vomeral or labioalveolar screws *(arrows)* will achieve primary retention. This is of particular value if the malar buttresses are thin and the underlying antra are enlarged.

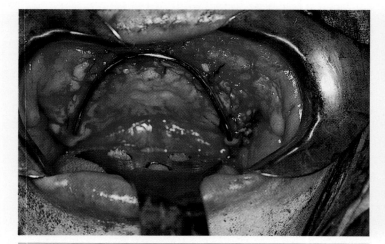

Fig. 15-15   After satisfactory placement of the maxillary pterygohamular subperiosteal implant, a primary closure is effected with a 4-0 dyed Vicryl continuous, horizontal mattress suture. The tissues appear to be pink and well vascularized upon the completion of suturing.

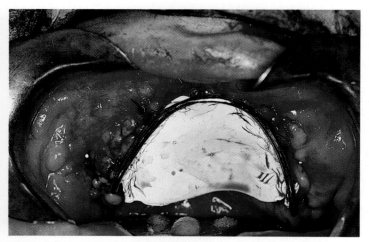

Fig. 15-16   In order to prevent prolapse of the large palatal flap with subsequent permanent thickening of this tissue, place an EZ Tray stent against the palate, and retain it by wedging it beneath the bar. Remove stents after the fourth day to prevent mucosal ischemia.

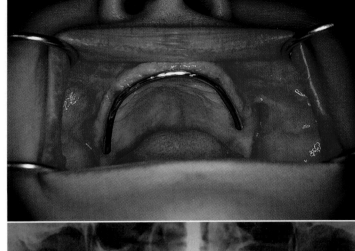

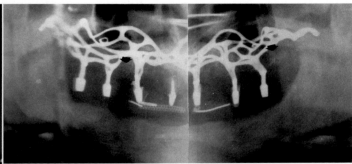

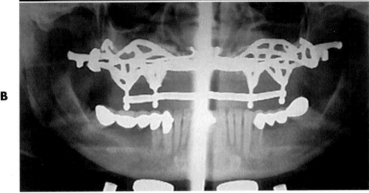

Fig. 15-17 **A,** After 4 weeks, the investing soft tissues have healed well, and keratinization is proceeding satisfactorily. **B,** Postoperative Panorex films show good adaptation of the infrastructure and appropriate alignment of the Brookdale bar and retentive O-ring devices. **C,** Occasionally, individual abutments are desirable. The pterygoid extension constitutes a major component of the design of these implants, (in this case over 35%). Arrows indicate graft material.

The patient, again, should be given the appropriate postoperative regimen.

These sutures resorb, but long ends can be snipped if needed on the seventh postoperative day. After 7 to 10 days, ream the tissue-borne surface of the patient's denture and line it with a chairside soft material (e.g., Viscogel) so that the patient has the benefits of a prosthesis for the remaining 5 weeks. This may be done after the palatal stent has been removed (Fig. 15-17). Sometimes, a heated instrument is necessary to soften the stent facilitating its delivery.

In 6 weeks the prosthodontic phases may be initiated.

Partially Edentulous Universal Designs

Construction of maxillary pterygohamular universal (bilateral) implants should follow the same plan as outlined for the totally edentulous case, except that all natural teeth have to be included in planning, impression making, design, and closure (Fig. 15-18).

Anatomic considerations may play a major role in the design and peripheral strut location of maxillary pterygohamular universal implants because of the maxilla's truncated cone shape. A design feature that permits the implant to pass over anterior teeth and a wide maxilla and come to rest at a superior and narrower location requires the addition of an adjustable labial strut. What otherwise might be an impossible maneuver is made possible by the presence of an anterior hinged strut using Howmedica's DE hinge, which may be closed and ligated with wire using two retention buttons for this purpose.

On the completion of this ligation, using Vitallium wire, the implant will be snug in position (Fig. 15-19).

Most reconstructions using the universal design are planned for fixed crown and bridge-type cementable superstructures. As such, careful surveying is required to ensure that the implant abutments are placed in strategic positions and aligned in parallel relationships to the natural teeth.

Make fixed prostheses by joining subperiosteal to natural abutments, without concern about their different support mechanisms. The design of such prostheses should take hygienic measures into consideration (large embrasures and sanitary pontics).

Protect natural teeth with individually cemented cast gold copings so that temporary cements may be used for long-term superstructure fixation and retrieval.

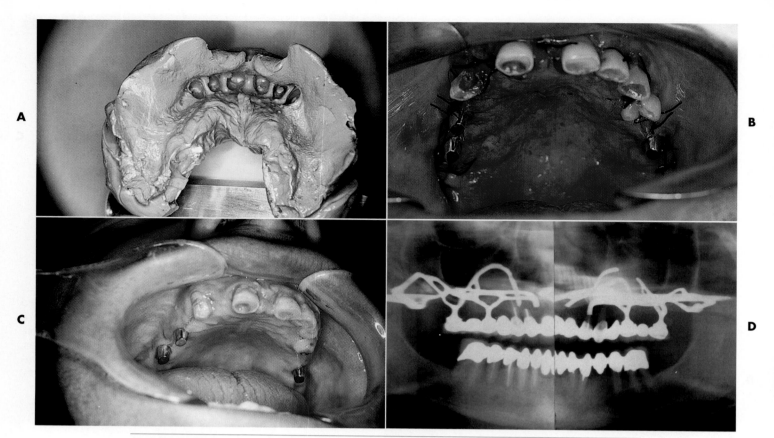

Fig. 15-18 A, Make the universal implant with an impression that must include the natural dentition. **B,** Placement of a universal casting should include abutments made parallel with the patient's natural teeth. Maintain the integrity of the high palatal vault by the use of an EZ Tray stent. **C,** After healing, the implant abutments are seen to emerge from zones of fixed gingivae. After 6 to 8 weeks, undertake prosthodontic reconstruction. **D,** A radiograph of a fully restored maxillary universal pterygohamular subperiosteal implant shows good peripheral extension and a functional relationship between natural and implant abutments.

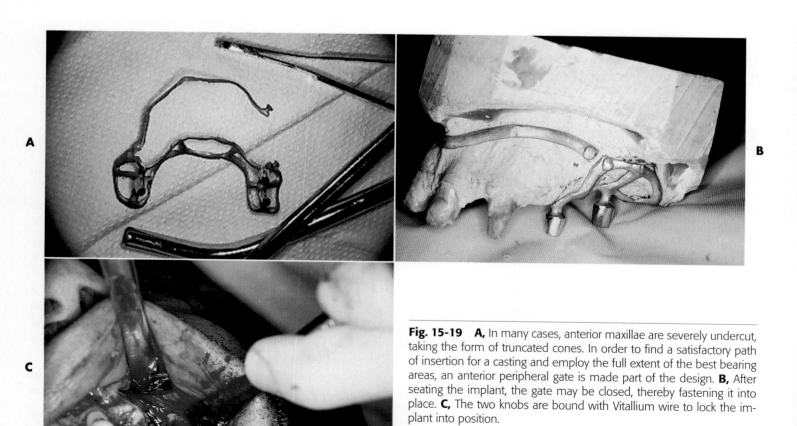

Fig. 15-19 A, In many cases, anterior maxillae are severely undercut, taking the form of truncated cones. In order to find a satisfactory path of insertion for a casting and employ the full extent of the best bearing areas, an anterior peripheral gate is made part of the design. **B,** After seating the implant, the gate may be closed, thereby fastening it into place. **C,** The two knobs are bound with Vitallium wire to lock the implant into position.

Partially Edentulous Unilateral Maxillary Pterygohamular Designs

The preprosthetic workup is extremely important for the unilateral pterygohamular subperiosteal implant. Since the final restoration is to be fixed, predetermine the buccolingual positions of the abutments to ensure that the fixed prosthesis will not be overcontoured buccally or palatally. The positions of the abutments are also important to verify that they are placed in the positions of natural teeth and not in potential embrasure spaces, which would create esthetic and hygienic problems.

The procedures for the fabrication of a unilateral pterygohamular implant are identical to those described in the previous sections, except that only one half of the maxilla need be exposed.

Use Formatray or a self-curing acrylic for impression making (Fig. 15-20). Include all natural teeth in the operative quadrant and extend the recordings at least to the midline (Fig. 15-21). Surgical occlusal registrations with Optosil putty and alginate counter impressions complete the requisite steps for implant fabrication.

Infrastructural design and sites of support follow the same rules as for the complete implant (Fig. 15-22). However, since unilateral implants are placed with the plan of making fixed prostheses, design abutments that will be parallel to natural teeth (Fig. 15-23). This is why the adjacent natural teeth must be included in the impressions.

After healing in 6 to 8 weeks, construct the fixed bridge prostheses following classic techniques (Fig. 15-24).

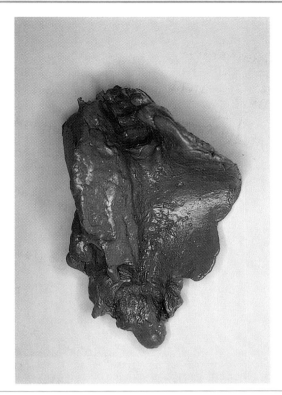

Fig. 15-21 After coating with adhesive, use the tray for a rubber base impression. Inspect it for accuracy in recording the pterygoid plates, the hamuli, foramina, malar buttresses, and natural teeth.

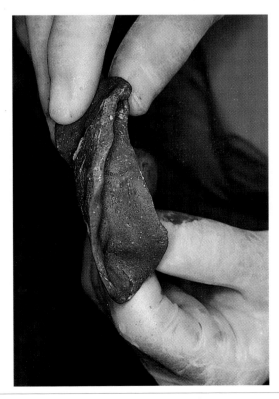

Fig. 15-20 The unilateral pterygohamular implant impression tray may be made directly on the operative site with Formatray.

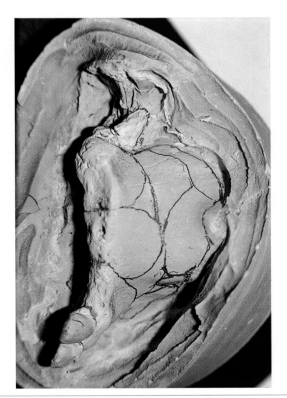

Fig. 15-22 The cast resulting from pouring the rubber base impression is used to design the unilateral implant. Abutment locations should be delineated and tissue height information presented to the technician as a result of studying the articulator relationships.

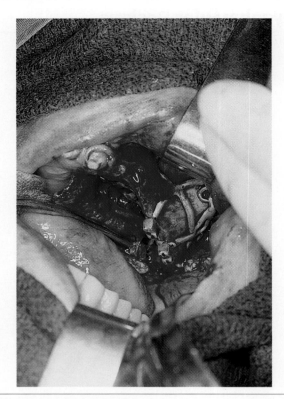

Fig. 15-23 The casting resulting from the poured model should fit accurately. Because of the compliance of the maxilla, slight inaccuracies may be eliminated by malleting the infrastructure into position with an orangewood stick. If positive retention does not occur, use screw fixation.

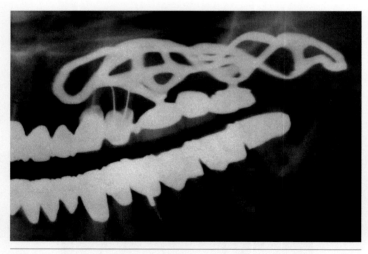

Fig. 15-24 This pterygohamular casting extends over the pterygoid plates for almost 40% of its total length.

Make maxillary unilateral and complete pterygohamular implant castings using the CAD-CAM–generated model system in exactly the same fashion as described for mandibular implants in Chapter 14 (see Fig. 15-7). Remove metal restorations from all maxillary teeth before imaging. Counterimpressions and occlusal records are required as if the models had been generated by direct bone impressions. Record taking for centric and vertical dimension cannot be done for CAD-CAM casts in the classic manner. In order to place the base model in an accurate relationship, follow the tube and stylus technique described in the CAD-CAM section of Chapter 14.

Design considerations include anatomic abutments made parallel to natural teeth so that fixed prostheses can be fabricated. When implants on computer-generated casts are designed, there is a tendency to permit them to extend far more aggressively onto peripheral bone. When such castings are being inserted, the practitioner may find that he or she faces a dissection of greater extent than that with which he or she is comfortable; therefore, conservatism in the extent of placement of peripheral struts should be observed.

Suggested Readings

Cranin AN, Cranin SL: The unilateral pterygohamular subperiosteal implant: evolution of a technique, *J Am Dent Assoc* 110:496-500, 1986.

Flynn HE, Natiella JF et al: The unilateral subperiosteal implant: a clinical technique evolving from experimental studies, *J Prosthet Dent* 48:82-85, 1982.

Linkow LI: Maxillary pterygoid extension implants: the state of the art, *Dent Clin North Am* 24:535-551, 1980.

Natiella JR et al: Unilateral subperiosteal implants in primates, *J Prosthet Dent* 48:68-77, 1982.

16

Intramucosal Insert Surgery and Prosthodontics

ARMAMENTARIUM

Autopolymerizing polymethyl methacrylate powder and liquid
Base-preparing bur
Endodontic explorer, sharpened tip
High-speed water-cooled handpiece with No. 4 and No. 6 round burs
1-0 black silk suture on curved cutting needles
Indelible pencil
Intramucosal inserts
Kerr ball-tipped Dycal applicator
Local anesthesia
Locking college pliers
Long-handled scalpel with No. 11 blade
Millimeter perioprobe
Mosquito hemostats
Needle holder
Pressure indicator paste
Racellet cotton pellets
Sable paintbrush, No. 00
Surgical indicator styli
T-burnisher
Trephine

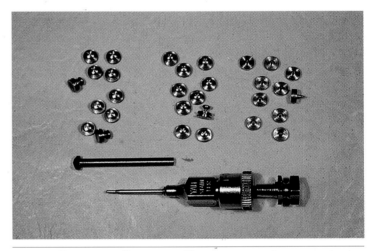

The intramucosal insert armamentarium consists of a base-preparing bur that prepares the denture with holes designed to receive the inserts, a surgical trephine to create the mucosal receptor sites, surgical indicator styli, which transfer the sites from denture to tissue, and the inserts themselves. From 8 to 14 inserts must be used. In addition, a scalpel with No. 11 blade, pressure indicator paste (PIP), and indelible pencil, college pliers, paintbrush, and autopolymerizing resin are required.

CAVEATS

Avoid the greater palatine and incisive neurovascular bundles. Do not penetrate low-dipping antra. Place inserts at least 1 cm apart. Set insert bases in exact continuity with adjacent denture base material (neither too deep nor too shallow) and at absolute right angles to the tissue-borne denture surface at each site. Inserts need not be parallel to each other. It is best, in fact, if they are not parallel, since this offers additional (interhead) clasping. Proper patient selection is a requisite for success. This technique benefits only those who gag or have a lack of retention; it is not meant for patients who reject dentures because they "burn," are "too tight," or cause "pressure."

Intramucosal Insert-Supported Complete Maxillary Dentures

Intramucosal inserts may be used for full upper dentures or unilateral partial dentures in either jaw. They are of value for patients who have problems with maxillary full denture retention. They are not for use with patients who claim that their dentures are "too tight" or for those who say that their tissues "burn" from denture wearing. However, if patients gag from denture wearing, these inserts can assist by shortening postdam areas. U-shaped or palateless dentures, however, work for short periods of time only, and then they slowly lose their retention as the healed receptor sites fill in with secondary intention epithelium, thus gradually reducing denture retention.

Follow the technique carefully by setting the inserts into the denture base exactly flush with and perpendicular to the acrylic. If they are placed too deeply, they fail to develop retention. Shallow placement may cause their protruding bases to create ischemia and necrosis of the opposing mucosa, with subsequent chronic inflammation or loss of receptor sites.

The implantologist must start with a denture that satisfies his or her highest prosthodontic standards. The next step is to eliminate sore spots and decubitus ulcers.

Select 8 to 14 sites on the surface of the maxillary mucosa, depending on insert head design. The newer (Park) flatheads develop superior retentive qualities and succeed with as few as eight inserts. The traditional inserts, more round arrowhead in shape, function best with 14 devices.

Dry the tissues and then, using a Kerr Dycal applicator tipped with pressure indicator paste (Fig. 16-1), mark the spots, which should be evenly placed at the crest. Make the first mark 5 mm lateral to the midline. Make the second mark in the center of the tuberosity, and make the third halfway between them. Divide the distance between these three marks, and place marks four and five at these midway points. Repetition on the opposite side of the arch locates the first 10 marks. This is more than sufficient for the Park-type heads.

For the earlier designs, place the eleventh marks 1 cm palatally from the ridge crest and midway between marks three and four. Place the twelfth mark midway between marks four and five in line with the eleventh mark. Repeat these steps on the opposite side to locate the thirteenth and fourteenth marks. Check the radiographs for low-dipping antra and avoid the regions of major foramina and nerve bundles.

Dry the denture and seat it directly upward. Guide the patient into a firm centric closure. When the denture is removed, the white marks will have transferred to it from the opposing tissues (Fig. 16-2). At the site of each white spot on the denture, use the base-preparing bur to make an opening at an absolute right angle to the acrylic at each of the marks (Fig. 16-3). Sink the bur precisely to the depth of the cutting blade to create holes into which the intramucosal insert bases will find flawless housing, exactly level with the acrylic.

A 30-gauge, short anesthetic needle with lidocaine 2% and 50,000 epinephrine, is used for infiltrating a single drop into each of the 8 to 14 white marks in the tissues, assuming that the patient has no contraindications to the use of these drugs (Fig. 16-4).

Place a single arrowhead surgical indicator stylus into each of the holes in the denture (Fig. 16-5) and tip each with a moistened purple indelible pencil. If the chosen system does not supply indicator styli, a somewhat less exacting technique has to be used. Process the intramucosal inserts into place with self-curing acrylic, and tip them with indelible pencil to transfer their locations to surgical sites in the mucosa. Again, seat the denture aggressively in a directly vertical maneuver so that each of the arrowheads or indelible pencil marks transfers to the tissues exactly opposite the site of its denture hole. Remove the denture with care after placing a gauze throat curtain (to catch any loosened styli).

About half of the styli remain lodged in the tissues, and the other half come away with the denture (Fig. 16-6). The

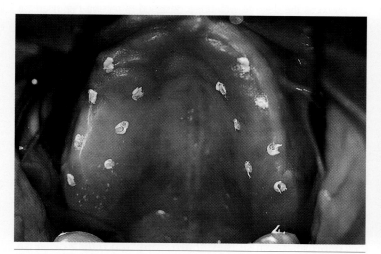

Fig. 16-1 Mark the potential host sites on the mucosa with pressure indicator paste.

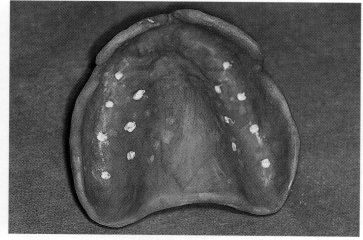

Fig. 16-2 Seat the denture, and transfer the marks to its tissue-borne surface.

A

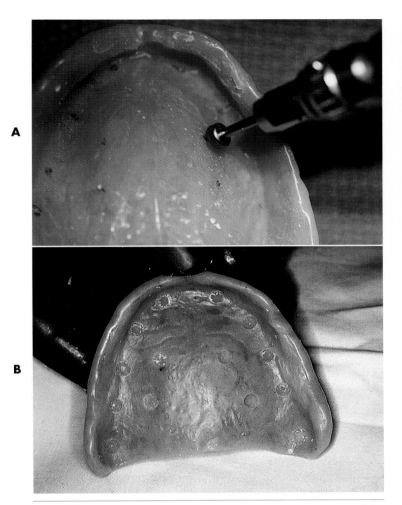

B

A

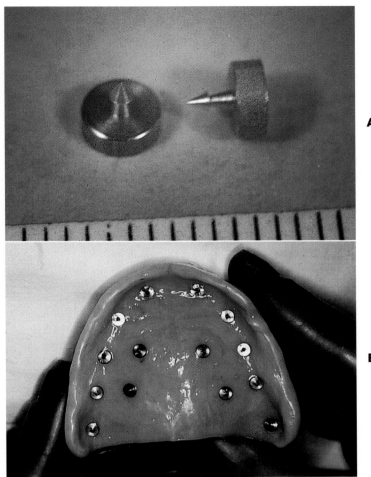

B

Fig. 16-3 **A,** Use the base preparation to make an opening at each location marked by the PIP. Drill these apertures at right angles to the acrylic and to the full depth of the bur's blade. **B,** Completion of the 14 insert recesses has been made with the base-preparing bur.

Fig. 16-5 **A,** Surgical indicator styli have bases of a slightly smaller diameter than the inserts themselves. They are characterized by sharp arrowhead-shaped tips. **B,** A surgical indicator stylus occupies each of the apertures.

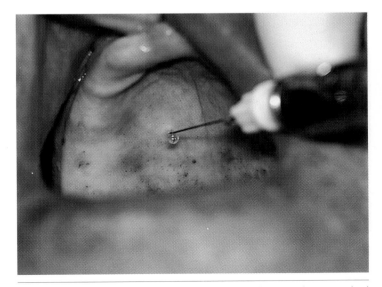

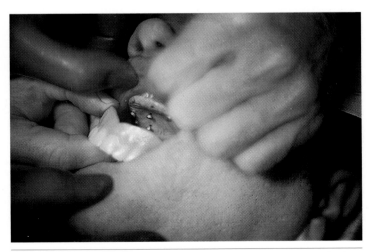

Fig. 16-4 A drop of local anesthetic is infiltrated into each PIP-marked receptor site.

Fig. 16-6 Seat the denture, and check its position for accuracy by having the patient close in centric. On its removal, the styli will remain embedded in the tissues, thereby transferring the exact concentric relationship of each denture aperture to the tissue.

latter group leaves the tissues tattooed with punctate purple spots.

After removing the styli one-by-one, cut a round hole into the tissues with the trephine, which should be forced through the tissues in a perpendicular direction. Push its handle directly to bone and then rotate it clockwise and counterclockwise several times (Fig. 16-7). Exercise care not to press too hard in the premolar and molar areas, or the maxillary sinus may be penetrated. If this should occur, abandon the site until it heals by secondary intention. If it fails to do so, refer to Chapter 28, Diagnosis and Treatment of Complications, p. 404. The trephine is removed and its lumen unplugged by using the stylet. A small core of tissue should be forthcoming. This happens only when the cutting end of the trephine is rotated against bone firmly enough to excise the tissue thoroughly. Create each receptor site in the same fashion. There may be some brisk bleeding, but tamponade solves this problem. Plugging a Racellet cotton pellet into the site will also grant dramatic hemostasis.

There are now 8 to 14 holes, each the diameter of an insert cervix. At this point, none will be wide enough to accommodate the insert head. To permit the entry of these larger components, make a cruciform or "X" incision at each site. Use a No. 11 blade in a long BP handle. Two incisions of 3 mm at right angles to each other with the trephined hole at the center complete this operation (Fig. 16-8).

Measure the depth of each hole with a periodontal probe or with an actual insert that has been soldered to a broken instrument handle so that the measurements can be recorded on an anatomic chart. If any of the sites is less than the full depth of the insert head and cervix (usually 2.2 mm but as much as 2.5 mm, depending on the system being used), the bone that lies at the base of the surgical site has to be deepened. A sterilized No. 6 round bur in the high-speed handpiece should penetrate the bone to the bur head's full depth, thereby creating enough vertical depth to accommodate the head and cervix of the insert (Fig. 16-9). Check the patencies of each "X" incision one last time, and instruct the patient to bite on a roll of saline-moistened surgical sponges.

Wash and dry the denture thoroughly, and using a sable paintbrush, place a drop of monomer in the first receptor site (Fig. 16-10, *A*). Follow this with a thin slurry of acrylic powder and liquid into the retentive groove of the intramucosal insert base. Hold the inserts at their necks with the beaks of locking college pliers forceps and vibrate each into its receptacle in the denture (Fig. 16-10, *B, C*). Exercise care to ensure that its platform is perfectly level with the surrounding acrylic. Use minimal quantities of acrylic to permit total seating of the insert base.

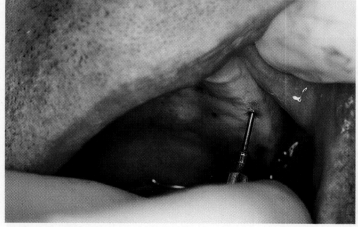

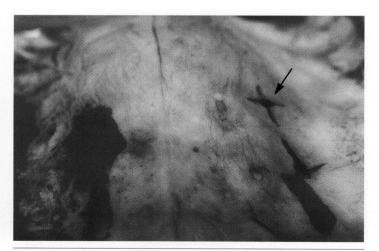

Fig. 16-7   **A,** Use the trephine, a sharpened 18-gauge needle with LuerLok handle and a stylet, to remove a plug of tissue of sufficient diameter to accommodate the cervix of each insert. **B,** Place the trephine at each stylus mark and force it with firm finger pressure into the mucosa until it strikes bone. At this point, rotate it against the bone, which causes a full-thickness plug of tissue to be excised. Use the stylet to empty the lumen of this tissue.

Fig. 16-8   Use a No. 11 blade to create 3-mm cruciform incisions *(arrow)*. This completes the creation of each receptor site by enlarging them to permit entry of the insert head.

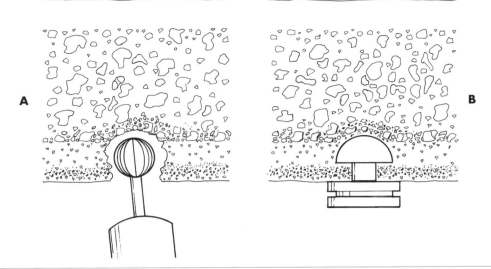

Fig. 16-9   A, In instances of shallow mucosae, ascertained by using a millimeter probe, a No. 6 round bur is used to deepen the bone. Care must be observed not to enter the maxillary sinus. **B,** Within 72 hours, the deepened receptor site becomes lined with secondary intention epithelium.

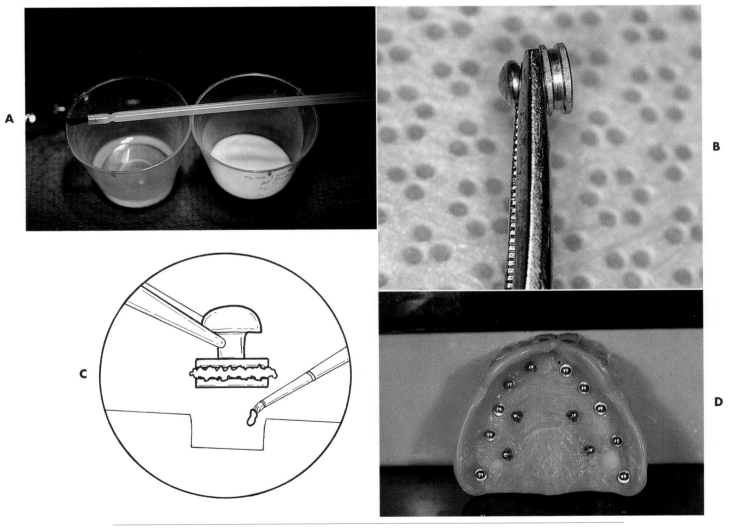

Fig. 16-10   A, Pink autopolymerizing polymethyl methacrylate with a paintbrush is required to seal each two-tiered or textured (see Fig. 16-14) insert base into the denture. **B** and **C,** The inserts are held with the tips of pliers, and small quantities of acrylic are used to lute each into its assigned aperture. **D,** On completion of intramucosal insert placement, the denture is seated and centric occlusion confirmed.

Repeat this operation until all inserts have been processed into the denture base. Wipe any excess acrylic from the areas around the insert bases using a cotton-tipped applicator.

Remove the sponges from the patient's mouth, and seat the denture. The inserts should go completely into place (Fig. 16-10, *D*). This can be verified if centric occlusion is correct and the postdam area is well seated. If this is not the case, each surgical site requires reassessment with a depth gauge as instructed previously, and the offending ones must be deepened.

In theory, the procedure has now been completed. However, practical experience indicates that the 14-day period after surgery, during which the denture must not be removed for even the shortest of times, has the potential of being a disappointing one. Patients, particularly those who gag when uncomfortable, will remove their dentures despite all warnings. Warrant the highest levels of success, it becomes necessary to ligate the denture into place. To do this, perform the following steps:

First, remove the denture. Moisten sponges replaced over the receptor sites, and drill three pairs of holes into the denture flanges using a No. 4 round bur. Place the first pair on either side of the labial frenulum, high in the flange and obliquely inward so that each is aimed at the other. Of the second pair, one is made high in the buccal flange opposite the tuberosity, and its opposing mate is located palatally at a point 25 mm from the ridge crest and aimed obliquely toward the buccal. Finally, the same combination is completed on the contralateral side.

Reseat the denture after sponge removal, and ask the patient to close into position. With the assistant holding the denture securely with a single finger placed on the palatal acrylic, the tissues are tattooed through each of the six new holes with an endodontic explorer that has been tipped with a moistened indelible pencil (Fig. 16-11, *A, B*).

Next, remove the denture and pass a 1-0 black silk suture on an FS1 or C14 cutting needle through the buccal surface of

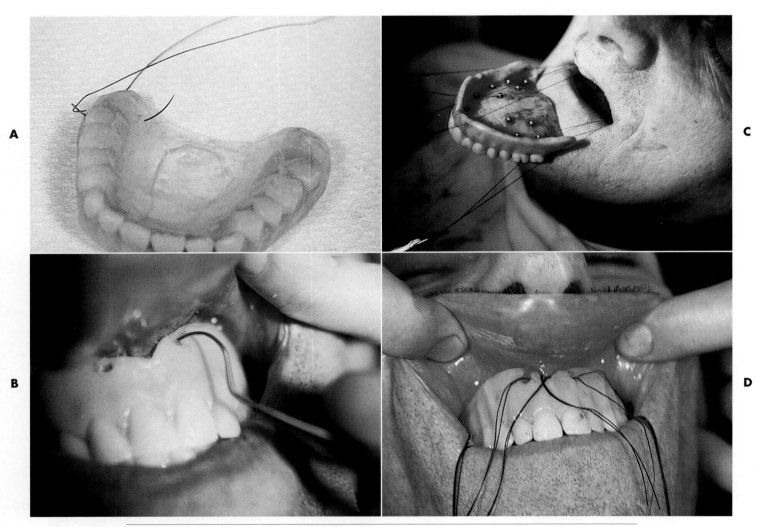

A

B

C

D

Fig. 16-11   **A,** In order to suture a maxillary full-denture prosthesis into place, make six holes in its flanges: buccal and palatal at each tuberosity and on either side of the labial frenulum. **B,** The newly made holes are transferred to the tissues by tattooing them with an indelible pencil–tipped explorer. **C,** Place each of the three 1-0 black silk sutures using the tattoo marks for guidance. The sutures are led out of the mouth and held taut by the assistant while the doctor threads each suture through its matching denture hole. The denture is then trolleyed into position. **D,** On its final seating, centric and vertical relationships are checked again. With the patient in closed position, knots are tied firmly at each site, and each is covered with acrylic.

the tissue covering the tuberosity to the palatal tattoo. Take a deep "bite" of soft tissue, direct both ends of the suture out of the mouth, and clamp the ends with a mosquito hemostat. Manage the opposite side with the same technique. Finally, pass the suture from one anterior mark to the other, making sure that the needle has grasped periosteum, thereby obtaining reliable fixation. There are now three pairs of suture ends protruding from the mouth, each clamped in a mosquito hemostat.

The next step is to thread each suture end through its matching hole in the denture from the tissue-borne side outward. After this step, remove the three needles and replace the hemostats, one to each pair of sutures. With the assistant holding the hemostats straight out, thus stretching the sutures taut, the denture is trolleyed up the sutures and into its final position (Fig. 16-11, C, D). To ascertain that suture material has not been trapped beneath the denture, pull the paired ends back and forth until they slide easily. The patient should close the denture into a firm centric position and maintain it in this fashion. When proper occlusion is established, the anterior hemostat may be removed and this suture tied very tightly. Ask the patient to open his or her mouth, and with the assistant again supporting the denture firmly, knot the right and left posterior sutures behind the second molars and across the tuberosities. The denture now is fixed firmly into position.

Cover each suture with acrylic using a paintbrush, and make a final check to ensure that the occlusion has not been altered.

The patient is dismissed, and if no sore spots occur, the denture should remain ligated in position for 4 to 6 weeks. If a sore spot develops, cut away the offending flange with a round bur without removing the sutures or the denture.

When the postoperative healing period has elapsed, brush away the acrylic overlying the three sutures with a No. 6 round bur, cut the sutures, and remove the denture. Fourteen well-epithelized receptor sites will be noted (Fig. 16-12).

On occasion, the patient may complain of tenderness at a receptor site, and it will be unclear as to which one is the offender. To test for this, the balled-end of a T-burnisher is in-serted into each site (Fig. 16-13). If this pressure causes the pain about which the patient complained, grasp the corresponding intramucosal insert cervix with the well-heated beaks of heavy laboratory pliers and, after the heat diffuses through the insert base, remove it. Fill the hole in the denture with acrylic and allow the receptor site to heal.

After the ligated denture has been removed, repair the suture holes with acrylic, polish them, and reinsert the denture. Ask the patient not to remove the denture for 2 to 4 weeks. Make adjustments as required, and finally, arrange a once-a-week removal and hygiene regimen. The patient should never be without the denture, since at any time (even after years of wearing it) the surgically created receptor sites fill in with epithelium in little more than 24 hours. The instructions presented apply to the intramucosal insert design that looks like a rounded arrowhead (i.e., Denserts). The benefit of these inserts is that soft tissue healing is usually uncomplicated, and removal and reinsertion of the denture are facilitated with ease and comfort. On the other hand, because of their gentle slopes, no fewer than 14 of these devices are required for effective retention.

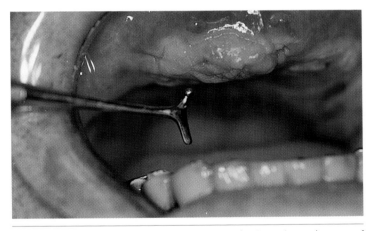

Fig. 16-13 A T-burnisher is used to assess the integrity and status of each receptor site. Gentle pressure may indicate the presence of individual problems of pain.

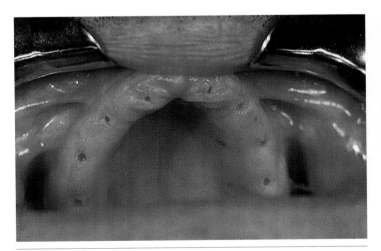

Fig. 16-12 Six weeks postoperatively, the patient returns, the sutures are removed, and the denture is cleansed. The receptor sites will be found to be well epithelized, keratinized, and firm, and positive retention is offered for each nestled insert head.

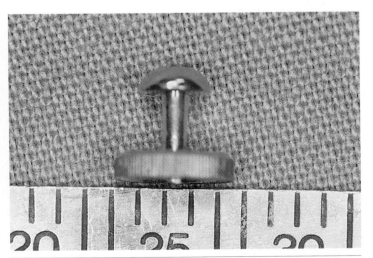

Fig. 16-14 The more recently designed flattened insert heads (Park Dental Research) offer more resistance to removal. Because of their design, as few as eight of these devices may be used.

The newer flattened heads of Park Dental Research Mucosal Inserts (Fig. 16-14) are more acute in their under-surfaces. Although they offer superior retention, their dentures offer more resistance to insertion. In addition, more frequent instances of mucosal receptor site inflammation are noted, and a greater period of postinsertion adjustment time is required to remove, manipulate, and replace such inserts.

Because of their effectiveness, usually only 8 or 10 Park in-serts, all placed at the ridge crest, are required. The steps of placement, postoperative care, and maintenance are the same for both designs. In some instances, patients with less tolerance or poor manual capabilities have difficulty with removal of a denture containing the flattened or Park insert.

For these patients, judicious removal of the small devices must be done one at a time, over a period of weeks, until a balance of retention and comfort has been reached.

Intramucosal Insert-Supported Unilateral Partial Dentures

The value of inserts may be extended to partial lower and upper dentures (but not to full lowers). There are three design features that must be built into such unilateral partials:

1. A stress-broken saddle (e.g., DE hinge, Crismani, or Dalbo attachment)
2. An absolutely reliable retentive (clasping) device at the anterior end (e.g., precision attachment, Tach EZ clasp device, or reciprocating Bonwill clasps)
3. Fenestrations in the saddle casting large enough to permit entry of the base-preparing bur (since it is burdensome to attempt to cut into a metal saddle to seat the insert bases) (Fig. 16-15, A)

The technique and placement of the inserts are similar to those for the full denture. As many inserts as can be used comfortably should be set into the saddle in at least two rows 1 cm apart. They should be located at the ridge crest, buccally in the mandible, and palatally in the maxilla.

The partial denture must have an absolutely reliable clasping system for its retention on the anterior abutment teeth.

The saddle must be stress-broken just distal to the last natural tooth.

The laboratory should have prepared the metal casting of the saddle with sufficiently large, well-distributed spaces at the planned sites of insert placement to permit full entry of the base-preparing bur.

After the surgery has been completed and the inserts have been processed, seat the partial denture and permit it to remain in position, untouched for 1 month. If initial reliable retention is lacking, gain support by placing one transalveolar or circummandibular No. 1 stainless steel ligature wire at the distal end of the saddle, as described earlier in Chapter 6. Sufficiently positive retention occurs after 6 to 8 weeks in a unilateral removable partial denture prosthesis to substitute for palatal or lingual bar, contralateral clasps, or a posterior abutment tooth (Fig. 16-15, B).

Kyocera, a Japanese company, makes a polycrystalline, alumina intramucosal insert that may be used in a manner similar to the techniques described for the devices in this chapter.

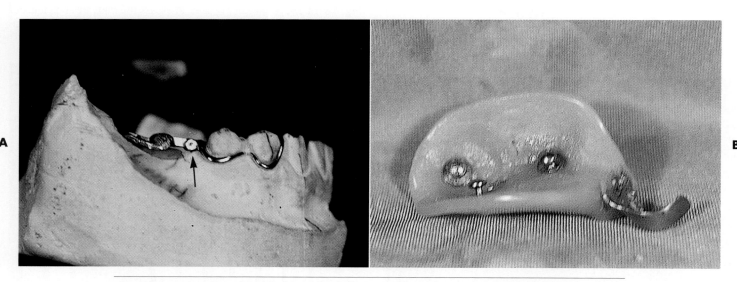

Fig. 16-15   A, Unilateral maxillary or mandibular partial dentures are effective when coupled with in-tramucosal inserts. The integral components of such designs are a DE hinge or another stress breaker *(arrow)*, a reliable anterior clasping system, and a cast saddle with fenestrations of sufficient size to accommodate insert bases. **B,** The unilateral partial denture must be made to accommodate a sufficient number of intramucosal inserts to offer a self-sustaining, highly retentive saddle. This, in conjunction with the reliable clasping system, allows for the successful functioning of unilateral partial dentures.

Relining Full Upper Dentures that Have Lost Retention After Having Had Intramucosal Inserts

If a patient complains of loss of retention of an intramucosal insert denture, examine the tissues supporting the denture. A loss of depth and undercut in some or all of the receptor sites may be noted.

Grasp the mucosal insert cervices one at a time with the beaks of heated heavy laboratory pliers, which will permit their easy withdrawal. First, clean them in an ultrasonic bath and then sterilize them by autoclaving.

Treat the denture with a chairside reline material (Durabase regular, Triad, or similar). Perform muscle molding with care and, after the reline material sets, polish the denture flanges. Opposite each tissue receptor site, a small dimple of acrylic will be found that corresponds to it. At each of these elevations, cut a new site with the base-preparing bur and reset the original insert with acrylic, as was done the first time the denture was so equipped.

Anesthetize each site and perform the surgical steps as described originally. The prosthesis does not have to be sutured into place this time, however, since the patient had achieved comfort as a denture wearer.

Instruct the patient not to remove the denture for 4 weeks, by which time a brand new prosthesis/mucosa relationship will have been established.

Suggested Readings

Babbush CA: Mucosal inserts: a technique for the atrophic alveolar ridge, *J Oral Surg* 34:517-521, 1976.

Cranin AN, Cranin SL: The intramucosal insert: a method of maxillary denture stabilization. *Oral Implantology*, Springfield, 1970, Charles C. Thomas.

Guaccio RA: Intramucosal inserts for retention of removable maxillary prostheses, *Dent Clin North Am* 24:585-592, 1980.

Misch CE: Improved mucosal insert and endodontic implant techniques, *NY J Dent* 53:393-399, 1983.

17

Endodontic Stabilizer Implant Surgery

ARMAMENTARIUM

Cement: carboxylate
Complete endodontic armamentarium, including rubber dam
   and clamps
Diamond: discs, pear-shaped stone
Engine reamers: 28, 31, 40 mm long; in diameters 40, 45, 50, 55, 60,
   70, 80, 90, 100, 110, 120, 130, 140
Hand reamers: 28 and 40 mm long; in diameters 40, 45, 50, 55, 60,
   70, 80, 90, 100, 110, 120, 130, 140
Implants: endodontic, 70, 80, 90, 100, 110, 120, 130, 140
Mandrels
Surgical needle holder

CAVEATS

The tooth or teeth that require treatment must have at least
25% of their alveolar support remaining. There cannot be an
untreatable endodontic-periodontal complication. Consider
mechanically splinting the tooth needing treatment (i.e., "A"
splint, bonding, and ligation) and placing the endodontic stabilizer by means of an open-flap procedure. Complete the operation by performing a periodontoplasty and adding osseous
grafting material (see Chapter 8). Do not attempt these procedures, however, unless sound capabilities in traditional endodontic and periodontal repair procedures have been acquired.

A minimum of 10 mm beyond the apex or apices is necessary unless the implant is being used to manage a root fracture. Treat multirooted teeth either with stabilizers for each
of the canals or in combination with conventional canal ob-
tundents for the canals not chosen for implant placement.

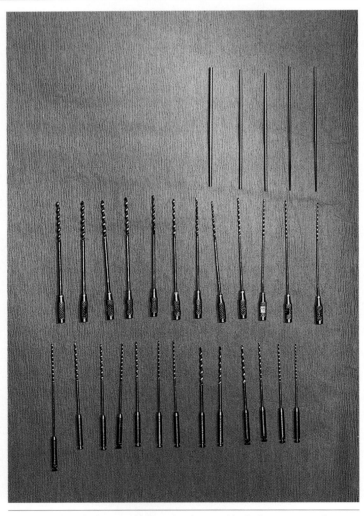

An array of endodontic stabilizer implants with their corresponding engine and hand reamers.

276

If the tooth is nonvital, carry out classic debridement, enlargement, and sterilization procedures until two successive negative cultures or dry, odor-free canals are achieved. If the tooth is vital, a one-visit procedure may be performed. Change and discard implant reamers with frequency to avoid bone injury and instrument breakage. Mark each storage box with the number of uses of the instruments stored within it. Use an instrument no more than five times before discarding it.

Matte-Finished Tapered Implants (Howmedica, Park)

For a vital tooth, using a rubber dam, open the pulp chamber with a No. 4 round bur, and remove all overhanging dentin and enamel (Fig. 17-1). Completely ablate the pulp cornua as well. Gain direct straight-line access to the pulp canal and remove the pulpal tissues with a barbed broach. Use sodium hypochlorite as an irrigant, achieve the apex in gradual stages until a No. 6 rat-tail file can be passed with ease (Fig. 17-2).

Record the distance from the incisal edge of the tooth to the apex. Check the position of the file with a periapical x-ray. Minimize distortion and measure the length of the file on the radiograph.

The following formula presents the amount of bone beyond the apex available for placement of an implant:

$$\frac{fl}{rf} = \frac{x}{rsd}$$

where *fl* is the actual file length, *rf* is the radiographic file length, *rsd* is the radiographic subapical distance and *x* is the actual subapical distance.

When the actual incisal-to-apical length is added to *x* (the apex-intraosseous length), the total length of the endodontic stabilizer will be known.

Using an ultra–low-speed (10:1 reduced gear ratio) latch-type contra-angle, select the No. 40 diameter engine reamer of an appropriate length. (They are available in lengths of 28, 31, and 40 mm from the Union Broach Corporation or Park Dental Research Company.) The diameter of the engine reamer used to begin the procedure, No. 40, represents a diameter of 0.4 mm and is the size of the last hand reamer used. (Each instrument's number indicates its diameter; for example, a No. 100 is 1 mm at its widest diameter.)

Place a sterile rubber marker on the reamer at the sum of the lengths of canal and bone. For purposes of illustration, a total length of 35 mm and a tooth length of 20 mm are planned; this means that the stabilizer will exceed into the subapical bone for a distance of 15 mm.

Use copious amounts of sterile saline or anesthetic that does not contain epinephrine as an irrigant and make sure that the reamer does not bind in the canal. Cut a 15-mm-deep subapical osteotomy using a gentle, pumping vertical motion. This creates a total length of 35 mm. Reverse the engine to remove the reamer, or if possible, back it out by hand. Turning the handpiece wheel counterclockwise helps.

Since a strong, rigid, and inflexible stabilizer is desirable, it is recommended that nothing smaller than a No. 90 implant

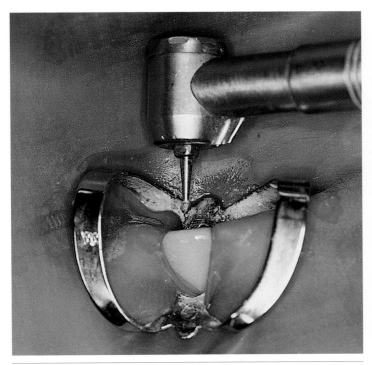

Fig. 17-1 Isolate the tooth or teeth being treated, and if the teeth are vital, remove the pulps.

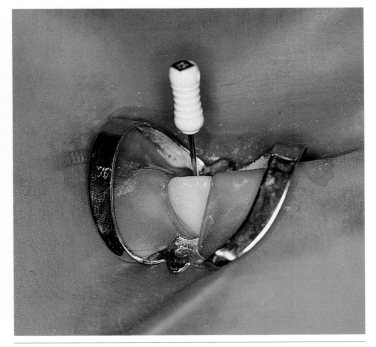

Fig. 17-2 Each canal is instrumented to its apex with K-files and rat tails up to the No. 40 size.

be used. No. 110, 120, or even 140 in fact, are preferable. The results of placing implants of larger diameter warrant the extra time and effort. It is important, however, to ascertain whether the root diameter is capable of accommodating the larger-sized implants without fracture or a lateral perforation.

Perform the procedure in the following order: Nos. 45, 50, 55, 60, 70, 80, 90, and 100 reamers should be introduced, each to the same rubber-stoppered 35-mm length (Fig. 17-3, *A*). Rotation must be slow, with no pressure placed on the contra-angle. If the reamer binds, stop the engine, detach the reamer by opening the latch, and back the reamer out by hand. Use the next smaller diameter, again with copious quantities of ir-rigant, and perform the enlargement slowly and with deliber-ation. A safe alternative is using hand reamers that are also available in a wide variety of lengths and diameters from the same manufacturers (Fig. 17-3, *B*). This is far more arduous but much more conservative, since the handheld reamers rarely fracture. None of these intraosseous instruments may be used dry. Frequent pauses for irrigation with the anesthetic syringe offer the greatest levels of assurance of sparing thermal trauma to the bone.

When the proper length and diameter odontoosteotomy has been achieved (35 mm), seek the presence of bone perfo-rations by using a No. 40 hand reamer as a probe. Ensure that neither the opposing nor any lateral cortical plate has been pierced. If the probe should pass out into soft tissues, take a radiograph to recheck the length from apex to cortex so that a shorter length can be selected. Dry and seal the canal and dress it with a dry formocresol dressing. The implant procedure may not be completed until a subse-quent check demonstrates an acceptable environment for doing so.

When the canal and bone are ready to receive an implant, select a stabilizer of the proper diameter. Using a fine diamond disc, score it lightly at a point 15 mm from its apical end. Score it more deeply 35 mm from the apical end so that only a sliver of metal remains. The small amount left should offer just enough strength and rigidity to permit the manipulation and rotation of the implant, application of cement, and seating of the implant (Fig. 17-4).

Shave 1 mm of metal from the apical end so that the im-plant does not rotate in the bone, but rather seats firmly in the apical area, thereby offering a sound bacteriostatic seal.

When the implant is seated, the 35-mm line must be level with the incisal edge. Sponge the implant with saline, place it in the bead sterilizer for 10 seconds, and store it in a sterile medicine-glass of saline. Extra-coarse absorbent points (J & J) should be used to dry the canal. They must be cut exactly 0.5 mm short of the apex (at 19.5 mm). If the points are even slightly overextended, a blood-free tip will never be forth-coming (Fig. 17-5). When the canal is absolutely dry, remove the stabilizer from the saline, dry it in the bead sterilizer, and coat it with a layer of carboxylate cement (e.g., Durelon) from the first line (14 mm from the apex) to the second one (34 mm) (the intracanal portion) (Fig. 17-6). Grasp the implant firmly with a needle holder or pliers, remove the final (and now dry) absorbent point from the canal, and seat the implant using gentle but firm rotation as well as thrust. Stop it at the 34-mm line (Fig. 17-7).

After the extruded cement has hardened completely, twist

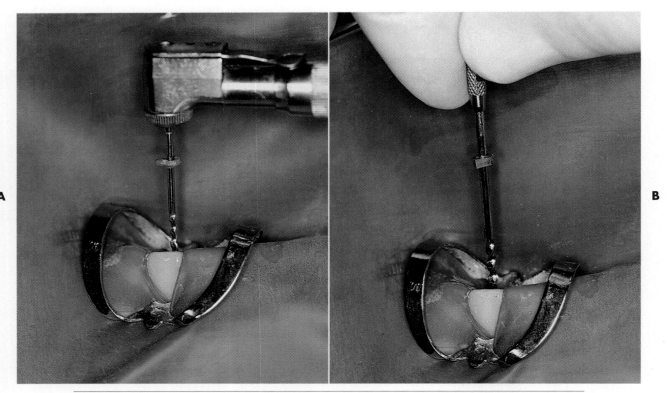

Fig. 17-3 A, Prepare the odontoosteotomy using an ultra–low-speed saline-cooled handpiece with a No. 40 twist drill-reamer to the calibrated length. **B,** Enlarge the canal-bone preparation to at least a size 90 using either engine-driven or hand reamers.

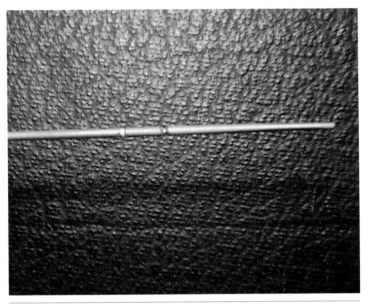

Fig. 17-4 The approximately sized endodontic implant is tried in to verify its accommodation to the full length, and the implant is scored at the tooth's incisal edge and apical end after its removal and drying. A total of 1 mm is removed from the implant's apical tip.

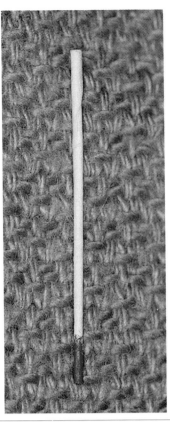

Fig. 17-5 When the canal preparation is completed, there may be the slightest sign of blood on the tip of the inserted paper point. If so, refit a point that is slightly shorter. A totally dry point is mandated before implant cementation.

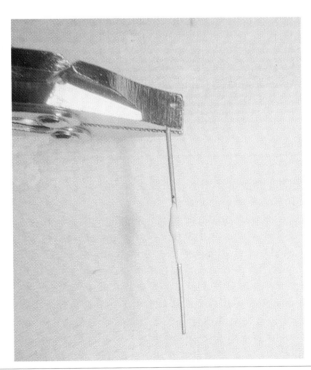

Fig. 17-6 After the canal has been irrigated and dried again, coat the implant with cement between the scores for the entire length of the canal.

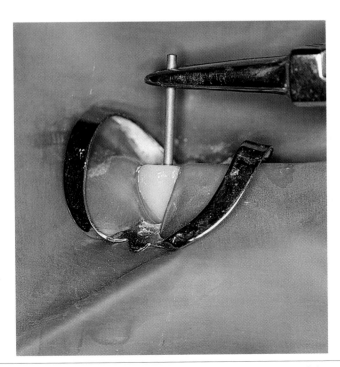

Fig. 17-7 Each implant should be thrust to its full length, and the cement should be allowed to harden.

the protruding end of the implant sharply. It will come away at the deeply scored incisal line. Smooth it level with the lingual surface of the tooth using a pear-shaped diamond drill. Conventional prosthodontic restorations may then be undertaken (Fig. 17-8).

If a classic post-and-core type of restoration is required, the implant has to be scored deeply at 24 mm rather than 34 mm (leaving 10 mm, or one half of the unfilled canal, available). The coronal 10 mm should not be coated with cement. With a simple twist, the extending portion of the implant may be removed after the apical cement has hardened. Subsequent conventional post-and-core management then is made possible coronal to the implant.

If after cementation of a full length implant, the coronal portion of the tooth requires prosthetic augmentation, the implant should be permitted to protrude. Score this portion with a fine diamond to add retention to it, add two or three TMS minim pins, and complete a standard polymeric composite or glass ionomer buildup. This may be prepared for a crown in the classic manner. Place the crown margins on the natural tooth structure apical to the polymeric reconstruction.

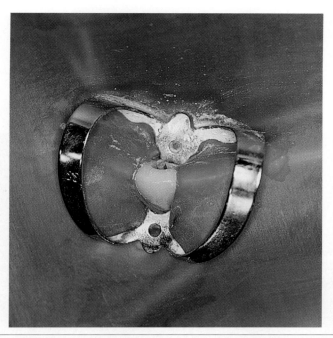

Fig. 17-8   After complete hardening of the cement, twist the protruding end of the implant sharply so that it comes away at the deeply scored incisal line.

Stabilizers for Nonconforming Teeth

Occasionally, an endodontic implant is desirable for a tooth that is procumbent or in some other manner, does not have an axis that when extended beyond the apex, is contained within the bone. Under these circumstances, employing an alternative technique may enable the use of an endodontic stabilizer.

Complete the endodontic therapy in the classic manner, filling to the apex with gutta percha. After satisfactory obtundation, the series of stabilizer odontoosteotomies as described in Part I are performed in an eccentric angulation, keeping the instruments within the subapical bone. Most often, because the

direct extension from the apex would lead to a labial perforation, make the entry through the labial surface. Enter in a direction that carries the drills obliquely into the supporting bone midway between the facial and palatal cortical plates (Fig. 17-9, *A*).

Dry the prepared pathway within the tooth with absorbent points, coat the intradental portion of the implant with carboxylate cement, and seat it firmly. When the cement has set, snap off the implant at the countersunk score mark and cover it with opacifier and a composite polymer (Fig. 17-9, *B*).

Threaded Implants

The preceding sections described the details of the classic tapered, matte-finished variety of endodontic stabilizer. There are also threaded varieties. The techniques used to place them differ slightly from the method formerly described. The first type of implant is threaded along its entire length and may be obtained from Park Dental Research Corporation (Fig. 17-10). To use this type, prepare the host site exactly as described for the smooth implants, and fit the threaded implant using the routine technique. Apply the cement in the same manner as well, and insert the implant by rotating it into place. After the cement hardens, cut the implant at the desired coronal level.

The second type, called the TRI-LOCK endodontic implant, is also available from Park Dental Research (Fig.

17-11). This implant is threaded in two areas: at the apical end, where the implant engages the supporting subapical bone, and at the coronal portion of the tooth, which gains retention within this area. The value of this second design, compared with the all-threaded one, is that a more reliable apical seal can be obtained, since the periapical portion of each implant is matte-finished rather than threaded. To use this design, measure and trim the implant with care so that the bone-threaded portion will be located beyond the apex. After preparing the host site, apply cement only to the intradental portion of the implant and insert it by rotation using finger pressure. (It comes with a large, comfortable key that facilitates digital manipulation.) After the cement has hardened, trim the implant to its appropriate length at the coronal end and restore the tooth in the classic manner.

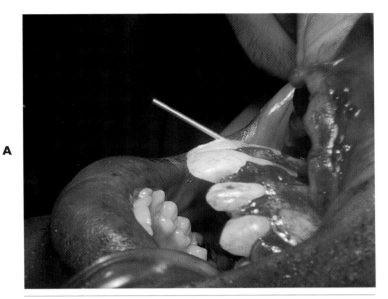

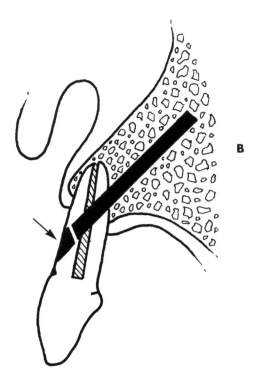

Fig. 17-9 **A,** In cases of unfavorable axial inclinations of teeth that require stabilization, an oblique implant may be placed following an identical technique after conventional endodontic therapy has been completed. **B,** The diagram indicates, in a cross-sectional view, the relationship of the implant to the alveolar bone and its cortical plates and to the endodontically treated root. Before cementing the implant, score it deeply at a level below *(arrow)* the tooth surface. After twisting it off, fill the defect with composite resin.

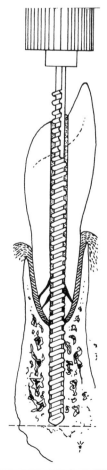

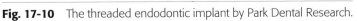

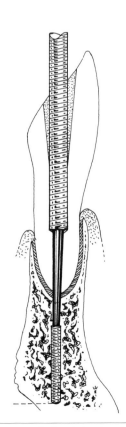

Fig. 17-10 The threaded endodontic implant by Park Dental Research.

Fig. 17-11 The TRI-LOCK endodontic implant by Park Dental Research.

Ceramic-Coated Implants

The Kyocera Company has introduced a single-sized No. 17, tapered, solid aluminum oxide (nonmetallic) endodontic implant, the Bioceram Anchor, that is 40 mm long with a diameter from 1.4 to 1.7 mm (Fig. 17-12). The intradental portion is straight and entirely of the larger diameter. It can be purchased as part of an entire kit containing two diameters of extra-long contra-angle drills, two reamers (A and B), a trial insert (a good idea when using any coated implant system), and some No. 1 measuring rings that serve as disposable depth markers.

Since the system employs the use of only a single-sized endodontic implant, the placement regimen is quite uncomplicated and similar to that described earlier in this chapter. Use drills No. 13 and 17 to enlarge the canal, creating vertical walls. Create the tapered intraosseous component by using hand reamers A and B. On completion, a precise odonto-osteotomy is created. Check its accuracy by placing the try-in. Only after its fit is satisfactory should the implant be cut, prepared, and cemented using glass ionomer or carboxylate cement. The alumina coating presents a promising bone interface and also supplies a good surface for cement adhesion and a reliable apical seal.

Kyocera also offers a No. 21 threaded pin, the Bioceram No. 2 (Fig. 17-13), which is 2.5 mm in diameter and 35 mm long. It should be used for short-rooted teeth that may also require coronal reconstruction. The technique of canal preparation follows conventional methods, and this kit, called the *Bioceram Anchor Pin,* offers four contra-angle spiral drills: No. 13, 17, 19, and 22. The spiral drills, which are gently graduated in diameter, in conjunction with an apicoectomy procedure using a fully elevated flap allow the preparation of the entire tooth and periapical host site. Once this is done, the im-

plant, which must be premeasured, can be affixed with carboxylate cement. For coronal buildups, place a small auxiliary pin (i.e., SMS minim) and allow the anchor pin to protrude for an acceptable length. Teeth treated in this manner may be restored using composites in Ion crowns or similar matrices. Endodontic implant stabilizers offer considerable additional strength, particularly when used in multiples (Fig. 17-14).

After a 6-week postoperative period, "A" splints, ligatures, or other stabilizing devices may be removed. Before removing the fixation, address any significant periodontal deficiencies.

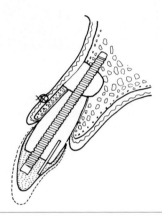

Fig. 17-13   The Bioceram No.2 threaded endodontic Anchor Pin Implant.

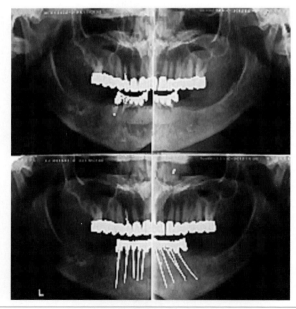

Fig. 17-14   A critically important six-unit mandibular anterior fixed bridge that was virtually lost as a result of trauma was preserved for 17 years using endodontic implant stabilizers.

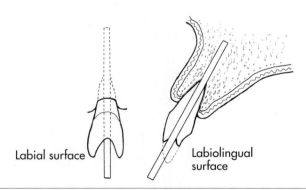

Labial surface   Labiolingual surface

Fig. 17-12   The Bioceram Alumina Anchor by Kyocera.

Suggested Readings

Faban MJ: Endosseous stabilizer implant, *Dent Clin North Am* 24:487-504, 1980.

Fragiskos F et al: A new endodontic stabilizer implant device, *J Prosthet Dent* 65:427-430, 1991.

Frank AL: *The endodontic endosseous implant. Oral implantology,* Springfield, 1970, Charles C. Thomas.

Madison S, Bjorndal AM: Clinical application of endodontic implants, *J Prosthet Dent* 59:603-607, 1988.

Silverbrand H, Rabkin M, Cranin AN: The uses of endodontic implant stabilizers in post-traumatic and periodontal disease, *Oral Surg* 45:920-929, 1978.

18

Transosteal Implant Surgery, Including the Mandibular Staple Bone Plate and Alternatives

ARMAMENTARIUM

Acrylic: self-curing
Burs: rosette egg-shaped, 4-mm diameter
C-clamp drill guide
Diamond drills: Atwood 473 tapered, straight shank
Hall drill
Hemostats: mosquito
Implants: transosteal with internally threaded prosthetic abutments (Fig. 18-1)
Implant kits, proprietary with their complete instrumentation
Pin cutter: orthopedic heavy duty
Retractors: vein and Mathieu
Screws: 7 mm, self-tapping, Vitallium bone
Screwdriver: Vitallium
Twist drills: high-torque, low-speed minidriver (3M) with ⅟₁₆-, ³⁄₃₂-, and ⁷⁄₆₄-inch

CAVEATS

Be careful to keep the bone from being overheated. When placing the drill guide (C-clamp), ensure its stability and position it at exactly at the inframandibular and supramandibular sites at which the implants will enter and exit. Few anatomic problems present with this procedure because virtually no vital structures exist in the proposed operative region. However, awareness of the incisive fossae, oft-present shallow depressions on the mandibular facial surface to the right and left of the midline, and the mental foramina is important. Make the skin incision in a straight line, directly in the first natural skinfold beneath the chin. Cut the bone slowly and keep all drills well cooled and lubricated. If they become dull, change them immediately.

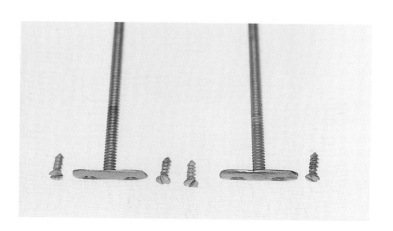

Fig. 18-1 Transosteal implants have threaded abutments ⁷⁄₆₄-inch in diameter, each welded to a cast footplate. The footplate, shaped to fit the inferior border of the mandible, has two countersunk holes that accommodate self-tapping fixation screws.

Single-Unit Transosteal Implant

General anesthesia is preferable for the single-unit transosteal implant procedure, although local anesthesia may be employed. The procedure requires the sterility of an operating room. Prepare the field with povidone-iodine and make a straight skin incision in the first submental natural skinfold (one of Langer's lines) (Figs. 18-2, 18-3). Carry out sharp dissection through the subcuticular tissues, and follow this with blunt dissection of the underlying platysma muscle. Small bleeders are either clamped and tied with a 3-0 plain gut suture or electrocoagulated. Incise the next layer, the periosteum, with a new No. 15 BP blade along the inferior border of the mandible from canine to canine. A new blade ensures that the reflection is clean and the periosteum is protected from being torn. The attachments of the anterior digastric bellies are seen. Elevate them along with the periosteum to expose the inferior cortex (Fig. 18-4). The dissection that was just completed has passed through a number of planes and layers in a rather complex and oblique configuration. The geometry thus created places the skin incision at a considerable distance from the underlying implants. Therefore, even in the case of infection or wound breakdown, dehiscence of the hardware is discouraged.

Next, using a new blade, make a 1-cm incision at each canine area at the crest of the ridge and reflect the mucogingivae to expose the ridge crest at the planned implant exit sites (Fig. 18-5). Place the C-clamp (Fig. 18-6) so that its upper and lower members are located at the exact points of entry and egress planned for the implant. If possible, place the C-clamp

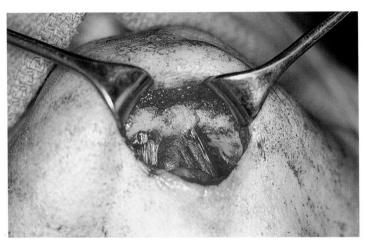

Fig. 18-4 Blunt and sharp dissection is used to expose the inferior border of the mandible. Virtually no vital anatomic structures are present in this area.

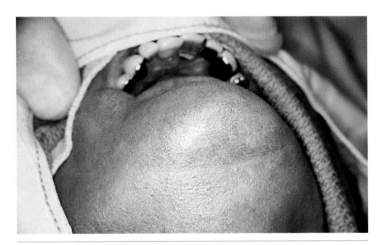

Fig. 18-2 Transosteal implants are placed via a submandibular approach. The procedure, often done under general anesthesia, requires classic skin preparation and draping.

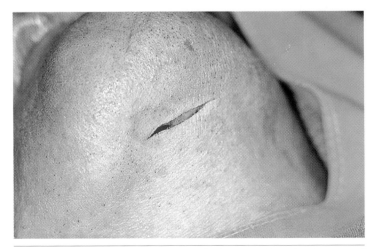

Fig. 18-3 The straight incision through skin is made in the first natural skinfold beneath the chin.

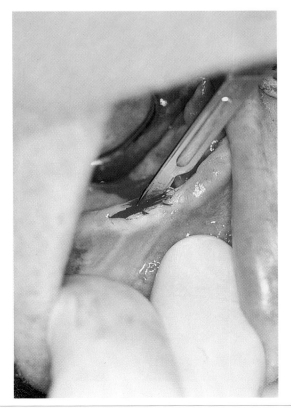

Fig. 18-5 Intraorally, the sites of implant emergence must be exposed by incision and reflection down to the alveolar ridge.

so that the drill is guided to enter the inferior border at a 90-degree angle. This permits the implant footplate to fit snugly against the bone (Figs. 18-7, 18-8).

Tighten the C-clamp and enter the lower guide hole with the smallest-diameter twist drill (³⁄₆₄ inch). It should be sharp and mounted in a 3M air-driven minidriver (Fig. 18-9) with a pistol-grip handle. Start the osteotomy upward toward the alveolar ridge with a steady stream of irrigant directed at the bone entry point. The surgeon should pause and withdraw the drill frequently to keep the internal environment moist

and cool to minimize trauma to the marrow. When the first drill exits through the alveolar ridge and strikes the superior or intraoral member of the C-clamp, stop it instantly. Reverse the drill and keep turning it slowly while withdrawing it. Pass the same drill through the osteotomy by hand to serve as a reamer and debris-remover while copiously irrigating and suctioning the area.

Follow the same principles of low speed drilling applied intermittently with a great deal of irrigation and minimal pressure to enlarge the osteotomy with the ³⁄₆₄-inch drill. Finally, com-

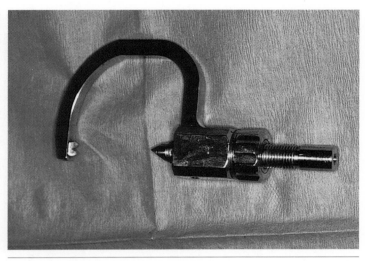

Fig. 18-6 The drill guide, a C-clamp, is designed to be affixed to the mandible in a reliable and stable manner.

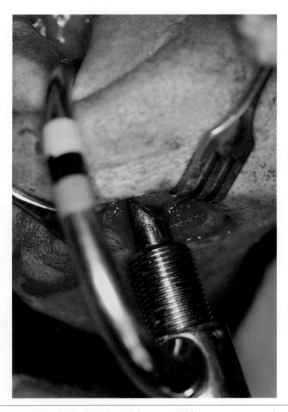

Fig. 18-8 The inferior border of the mandible presents a surface readily receptive to the drill guide's lower member.

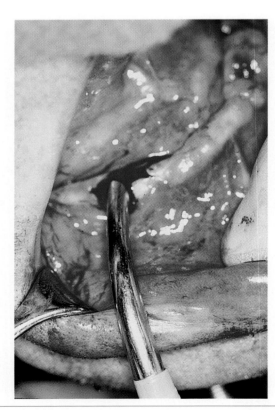

Fig. 18-7 The C-clamp is affixed in its appropriate position and fastened to the inferior and alveolar borders. The intraoral view demonstrates its relationship to the bony ridge.

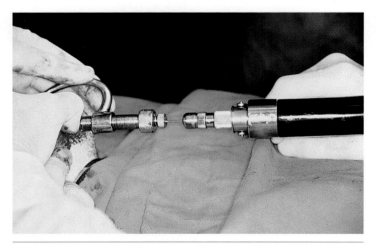

Fig. 18-9 Osteotomies are made using cooled drills in graduated sizes. The power source is an easily controlled air-driven 3M Minidriver.

plete the procedure with the ⁷⁄₆₄-inch drill, creating the proper diameter for placing the transosteal implant (Fig. 18-10).

Ream and irrigate the osteotomy just before seating the implant. If, after it is seated (Figs. 18-11, 18-12), the footplate does not fit intimately against the inferior border (i.e., if the footplate touches at only one end), correction is required. Often, simply rotating the foot-plate 180 degrees may accomplish this. If this does not succeed, note the area that the metal contacted and remove the implant. Contour the bone at the site of contact using a well-irrigated rosette bur so that

the footplate nestles into the cortex. Next, adjust the intra-oral length. Score the protruding portion with the Atwood 473 thin diamond at the desired length, and after removing the implant (which should fit snugly), snip off the excess with an orthopedic pin cutter. Smooth the end with the diamond drill, and reseat the implant. The assistant must hold the footplate firmly against the inferior border with an orangewood stick while a single hole is tapped in the direct center of one of the footplate screw holes using a well-irrigated Atwood tapered drill to the full length of the

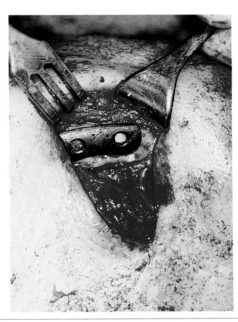

Fig. 18-12 Occasionally, light mallet tapping with an orangewood stick is beneficial in seating the transosteal implant fully.

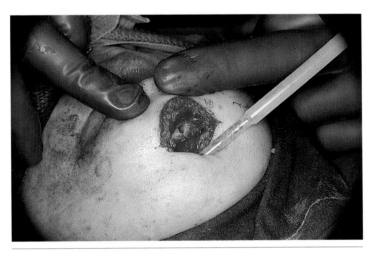

Fig. 18-10 The first osteotomy is made by turning a ³⁄₆₄-inch diameter drill slowly. The low-speed, high-torque Minidriver creates a true, low-trauma intraosseous tract. Each is completed with the use of ⁷⁄₆₄-inch twist drills.

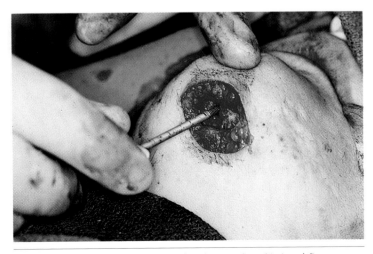

Fig. 18-11 Each implant is found to have a firm frictional fit.

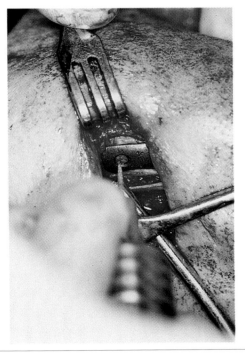

Fig. 18-13 After the satisfactory relationship of the footplate to the inferior border, an Atwood 473 diamond drill is used to pre-tap the holes for footplate fixation.

diamond (Fig. 18-13). Insert a 7-mm self-tapping Vitallium screw and, as it is introduced, make a full turn clockwise and then a half turn counterclockwise. If this is done with care, the screw's progress is slow but predictable. The intraosseous blood serves as a lubricant and prevents binding, which might cause a shearing of the screw head.

The more concentrically the first screw has been placed, the more accurately the footplate fits against the bone. Only after the first screw has been completed should the procedure be repeated for the second one. The second screw is much simpler to place because of the stability offered by the first one. The implant seating is now complete (Fig. 18-14). Additional transosteal implants may be inserted depending on the room available between the mental foramina. Usually, two are used, one at each canine location.

Close the gingivae with a Vicryl continuous horizontal mattress suture (see Chapter 6) (Fig. 18-15). Close the submandibular incision in anatomic layers using 4-0 Biosyn or 3-0 plain, and 5-0 nylon for skin with either an interrupted or a single subcuticular technique (Fig. 18-16). The internally threaded prosthetic abutments may be screwed over the protruding sections intraorally or by using smooth self-curing acrylic balls instead.

These implants may be used for the anchoring of a temporary prosthesis beginning on the day of their placement if this is necessary for patient comfort or cosmesis. Complete healing occurs within 6 weeks (Figs. 18-17 to 18-20).

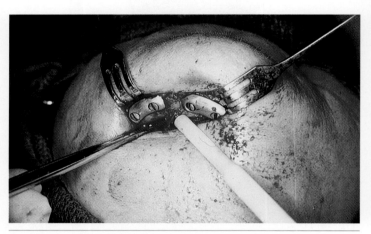

Fig. 18-14 Each self-tapping 7-mm long screw is positioned firmly. This completes the placement of the transosteal implant.

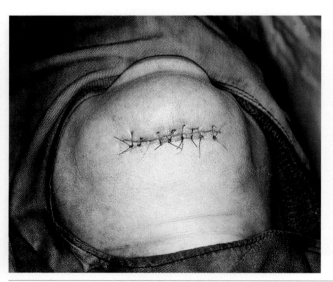

Fig. 18-16 Submandibular closure is performed in anatomic layers. If the digastric muscles are detached, they must be resutured to the bone or implant footplates. Skin may be managed by subcuticular or interrupted sutures.

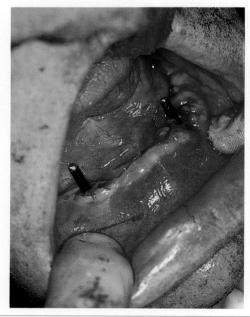

Fig. 18-15 The intraoral closure is made using continuous horizontal mattress or interrupted sutures. The ends of the implants have been polished.

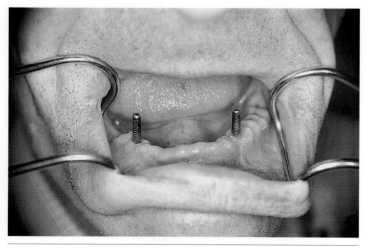

Fig 18-17 Despite the threaded cervices, conscientious hygiene will maintain a healthy, well-keratinized intraoral environment.

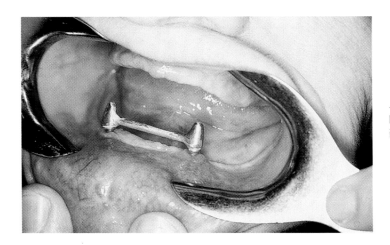

Fig. 18-18   A simple but effective method of using transosteal implants is with the coping bar splint.

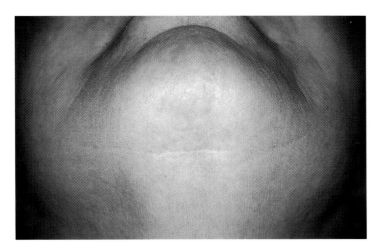

Fig. 18-19   The skin incision heals quickly in a realistic manner because it was made in a natural skinfold.

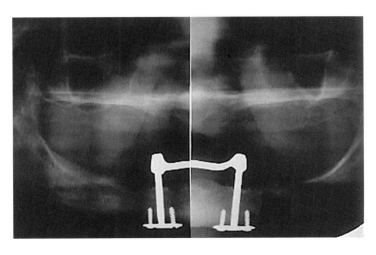

Fig. 18-20   A 5-year postoperative radiograph shows good bone apposition consonant with the clinical appearance.

Mandibular Staple Bone Plate

Place the mandibular staple bone plate in the same region as the transosteal implant and in a similar manner. Since it is a single unit with two abutments, a special drill guide is required.

The following instruments and steps, which make placing the staple different from the single transosteal, should be noted.

Procedure

Make the incision as described for the transosteal implant straight across in the first of Langer's lines in the submandibular skin. Expose the inferior border in a like manner (Fig. 18-21). Expose the anterior alveolar ridge in its entirety

for the application of the drill guide. This guide has the requisite number of holes in it so that the appropriate drill may be used (with stops to govern depth where indicated) to make the proper five or seven osteotomies. Make two of the osteotomies all the way through the alveolar ridge to allow for the exit of the abutments. Although the manufacturer does not recommend this, it is advisable to make saline-cooled, starter osteotomies with smaller-gauge drills (i.e., ⅛ and 3⁄32 inch) before completing them with the 7⁄64-inch drills. At the time of drill-guide application, be sure that all of the parts of the system fall within the anatomic boundaries of the mandible (Fig. 18-22).

When the five or seven osteotomies have been completed using the appropriately stopped twist drills through the tem-

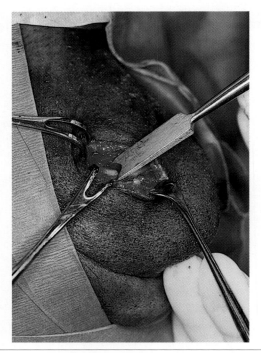

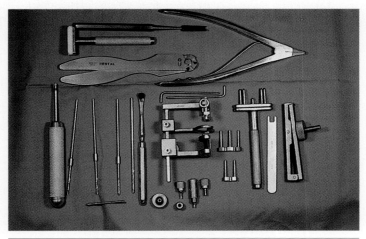

The mandibular staple armamentarium includes a marking guide, tapered twist drills, and an adjustable drill guide, along with a starter and staple extractor.

Fig. 18-21   The inferior border of the mandible is exposed in the same fashion as for the transosteal design. A well-sharpened periosteal elevator facilitates stripping the soft tissue.

plate or drill guide (Figs. 18-23, 18-24), the handheld beveler or a slowly turning rosette bur is used in each osteotomy. The resulting chamfers allow more intimate footplate seating.

Place the selected implant into position (Figs. 18-25 through 18-27), and tap it into place with a mallet using the seating instrument against the footplate (Fig. 18-28). When it rests snugly at the inferior border (Fig. 18-29), place the lock nuts followed by fasteners on each abutment (Fig. 18-30). If adaptation of the implant at the inferior border or alveolar ridge is unacceptable, removal is difficult. It may be attempted using the starter and staple extractor. Wrenches are available for placing of the lock nuts and fasteners. Retention is so good after healing, however, that they may not be necessary (Figs. 18-31, 18-32).

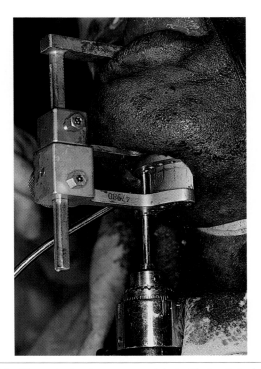

Fig. 18-24 The osteotomies are completed with the ⁷⁄₆₄-inch drills and are beveled slightly either by hand or with a rosette bur to allow intimate setting of the footplate. All of the osteotomies should be inspected for location and integrity.

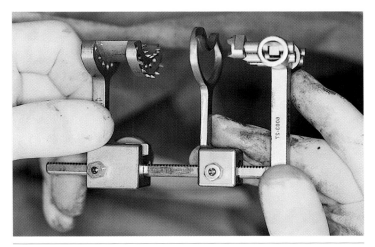

Fig. 18-22 The mandibular staple adjustable drill guide has universal joint bone clamps that make its placement and fixation simple and effective.

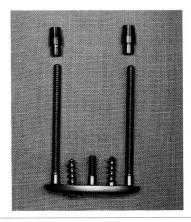

Fig. 18-25 The staple bone plate (Zimmer) will not fit snugly unless bone beveling is performed.

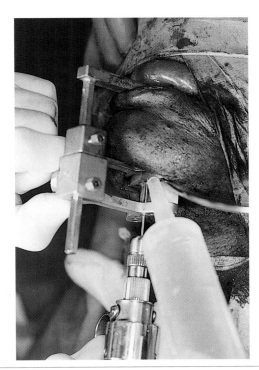

Fig. 18-23 The starter osteotomies are performed with the smaller-gauge drills. For those osteotomies that are not to go all the way through the mandible, self-limiting drills are provided.

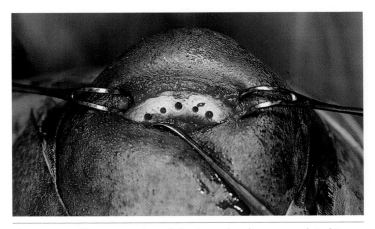

Fig. 18-26 The preparation of the bone has been completed to accept a five-pin mandibular staple bone plate.

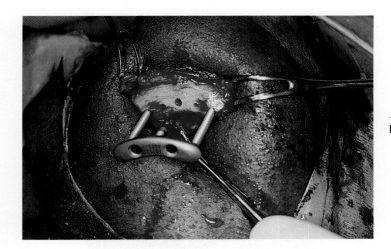

Fig. 18-27 The implant is inserted into the osteotomies.

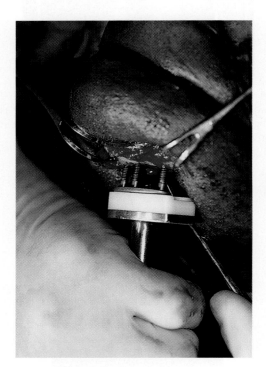

Fig. 18-28 The implant is tapped to place with a mallet by using the plastic-faced seating instrument against the footplate.

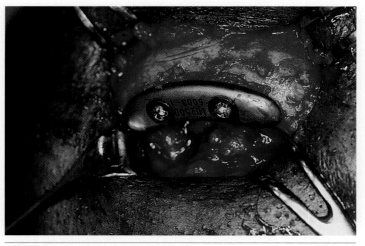

Fig. 18-29 The staple is fully seated, and the second and fourth pins become self-tapping retention screws.

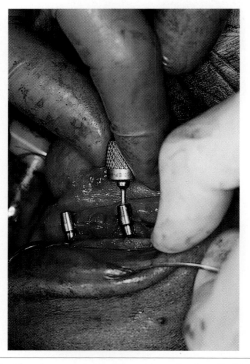

Fig. 18-30 The sleeve nuts are placed by using handheld wrenches.

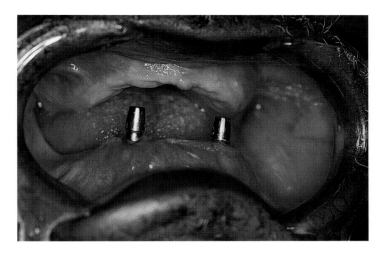

Fig. 18-31 The intraoral tissues are healed completely 2 weeks after surgical placement of the implant.

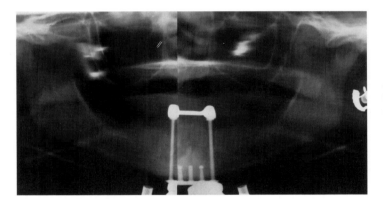

Fig. 18-32 The radiographic appearance of the mandibular staple implant after a coping bar has been placed.

Smooth Staple Implant System (Interphase/Interpore)

The Smooth Staple Implant System is not unlike the Zimmer product described on p. 291. There are a variety of prosthetic options that make it more versatile. In addition, several design features present biologic benefits (Fig. 18-33).

The technique for insertion follows the surgical guidelines as described for the transosteal implant. Submental incision, dissection, and exposure of the inferior mandibular border are exactly the same. The alveolar ridge is denuded in a similar manner. On the bony exposure, clamp a surgical template or guide to the two surfaces to direct the appropriate twist drills from inferior to superior borders.

The implants, which are manufactured of titanium alloy, are available with two (five stations or holes in the footplate) or four (seven stations) abutment designs; the remaining three holes are reserved for shorter, intraosseous fixation screws (of 9-, 12-, and 15-mm lengths). The abutments, which are affixed to the footplate, come in lengths of 21, 29, and 39 mm. The unique benefit offered by these abutments is that they are interiorly threaded, permitting the fabrication of a classically designed fixed-detachable superstructure or mesostructure bar. Another benefit is that they use a smooth transmucosal sleeve

that is screwed down the threaded abutment post to a length that still permits a retentive intraosseous environment and an atraumatic gingival milieu. A unique feature of the Smooth Staple is the flexiguard, which is placed on the permucosal pins to protect the lip and tongue immediately after surgery (Fig. 18-34).

In addition, the internal threading permits the application of titanium alloy top plate or a plastic design that permits casting. This presents a variety of prosthetic options such as the immediate availability of a prefabricated machined titanium top plate mesostructure bar with receptacles that can receive any of the prosthetic components manufactured as coordinating elements (Fig. 18-35). These include Dolder bars, ball fasteners, Dalla Bona attachments, and standard tapered abutments. Laboratory analogs may be obtained for use by the technician.

The single problem in using this system is the need for larger-diameter osteotomies and mucosal openings to accommodate the smooth sleeve. This creates difficulties for the knife-edged ridge and also introduces additional engineering components. The prosthetic versatility of the system, however, presents significant compensation.

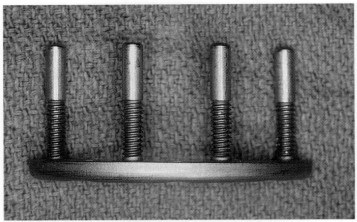

Fig. 18-33 A variation of the staple is the Smooth Staple Implant. This implant has smooth transosseous posts that are internally threaded.

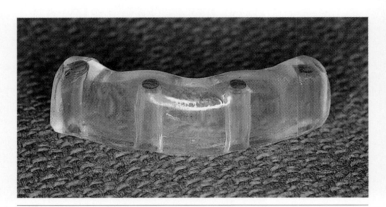

Fig. 18-34 The flexiguard is placed over the transosseous posts at the time of surgery to protect the lip and tongue.

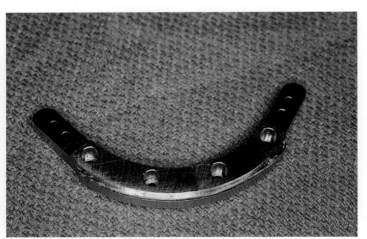

Fig. 18-35 When using the smooth staple in a fixed detachable application, use the prefabricated, machined top plate. This preformed casting eliminates the need for custom impression procedures and fabrications.

TMI (Bosker Transmandibular Reconstruction System)

The TMI system, similar in design and insertion technique, is constructed of an 18K gold alloy and consists of a curved base-plate and fixation screws of various lengths to be used for mandibles of various superoinferior dimensions. A single midline bicortical screw and four additional lateral cortical screws, each of which extends from the inferior border plate well into bone, are included with the kit. Interposed between each bicortical screw are four threaded abutments, each of which serves as a transmandibular bicortical permucosa abutment (Fig. 18-36). The prosthetic techniques involve the use of a superstructure (mesostructure) bar and an overdenture, which is supported with Hader-like clips for attachment. As an option, a fixed prosthesis may be used.

The surgical procedure follows the general techniques of the other products described in this chapter.

As a dividend, the manufacturer presents advice describing a method to improve the submental cosmetics by making an

elliptic incision slightly longer than the base-plate and removing fat and skin. When performing this procedure, divide the platysma muscle, detach the anterior belly of the digastric and the geniohyoid insertions, and incise and reflect the periosteum up to and including the residual ridge. The mental neurovascular bundles are included in this exposure. If the ridge is sharp, use a pear-shaped bur for osteoplasty.

Exercise great care as the quadratus labii inferioris muscles are elevated, since the mental foramina are found directly beneath these attachments.

Apply the base-plate to the inferior border and use it as a surgical template. Align its holes over the bone, placing it with the center hole at the symphysis. Use a stoppered bur after marking the midline with a No. 2 round starter hole using the curved drill guide. This hole should not penetrate the residual ridge.

Employ a bone tap to thread the initial osteotomy. Place

cortical screws, available in four lengths (7 to 16 mm), in the available five locations after repeating the tapping technique used for the midline hole. Use these screws to affix the curved template.

Attach a curved drill guide and tighten it from the inferior border template to the residual ridge at sites from which the transosteal abutments are to emerge. Cut the four key abutment osteotomies with the drill, follow with taps, and place four transosteal abutments of equal lengths through their respective holes until they touch the superior plate passing through keratinized gingiva. Allow six threads to protrude inferiorly. Remove the template, then advance the abutments until they are flush with the inferior border, and affix the baseplate with the same screws that had been used for the template.

Back the threaded abutments into the base-plate's threaded receptacles. Turn them until they become level with the base-plate's inferior surface and then fasten each firmly with an abutment lock screw. Intraorally, fastener nuts placed on the protruding abutments engage the polished per gingival cuffs. Close the wound anatomically in layers.

Initiate the prosthetic steps on the tenth postoperative day. Superstructure bars are an integral part of the procedure and are available in egg-shaped and U-shaped profiles.

Make an impression after transfer copings have been placed on the four abutments. Attach laboratory analogs to them and pour a cast in stone. The laboratory fabricates a bar with soldered abutments, which is placed for verification of passivity. If satisfactory, fasten the bar to the implant complex with lock nuts.

Classic prosthetic techniques complete the procedure. Affix the final denture, which is designed to be totally implant bar–borne, with clips.

The manufacturer states that bone regeneration occurs during the first postinsertion year and that because of a "tented periosteum," bone induction may be noted (Fig. 18-37). Prosthetic tehcniques required to complete these procedures are described in Chapter 26.

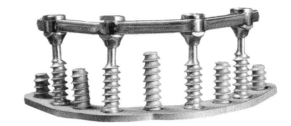

Fig. 18-36　The TMI staple with its innovative abutments and bar offers a number of prosthetic options

(Photo courtesy TMI, Inc.)

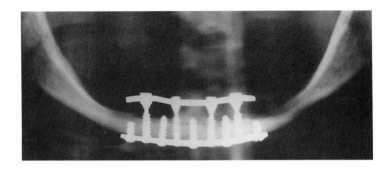

Fig. 18-37　The radiographic results after integration appear to offer support and strength to this atrophied mandible.

Suggested Readings

Bosker H, Van Dijk L: The transmandibular implant: a 12 year follow-up study, *J Oral Maxillofac Surg* 47:442-450, 1989.

Chin DC: Staple implant through bone graft at inferior border of mandible, *Oral Surg Oral Med Oral Path* 56:477-479, 1983.

Cranin AN et al: The transosteal implant: a 17-year review and report, *J Prosthet Dent* 55:709-718, 1986.

Heffez L: A technical note on placement of the mandibular staple bone plate, *J Oral Maxillofac Surg* 43:225-226, 1985.

Helfrick JF et al: Mandibular staple bone plate: long-term evaluation of 250 cases, *J Am Dent Assoc* 104: 318-320, 1982.

Knapp JG, Small IA: Fixed mandibular complete denture prostheses supported by mandibular staple bone plate implant, *J Prosthet Dent* 63:73-76, 1990.

Maxson B et al: Multicenter follow-up study of the transmandibular implant, *J Oral Maxillofac Surg* 47:785-789, 1989.

Powers M et al: The transmandibular implant: a 2-year prospective study, *J Oral Maxillofac Surg* 47:679-683, 1989.

Small IA: Survey of experiences with the mandibular staple bone plate, *J Oral Surg* 36:604-607, 1978.

Small IA: The mandibular staple bone plate: its use and role in prosthetic surgery, *J Head Neck Path* 4:111-116, 1985.295

19

Crête Mince and Other MiniImplant Surgery and Prosthodontics

CAVEATS

As with all endosteal implant procedures, exercise care not to impair vital structures. Using infiltration anesthesia in the mandible helps guide drilling when approaching the mandibular canal, since the patient is able to report lip tingling. Slow drilling to keep intraosseous temperatures low, chilled saline irrigants, carefully planned implant placement, accurately directed drills, maintenance of the integrity of cortical plates, and use of a gentle, pressure-free, well-irrigated sharp instrument offer optimal prognosis. Use the instruments with vertical (not arclike) application, and allow them to find and follow their own paths. The implants themselves are self-tapping. It is mandatory to plan carefully and to fabricate a fixed prosthesis with hollowed pontics designed to serve as their own surgical templates. Small incisions that are cruciform in design (to prevent forced implantation of epithelial cells into the bone) are recommended. Such cells may later proliferate and be responsible for epithelial invagination and failure.

Crête Mince Implants

Crête Mince translates from the French as "thin ridge" (Fig. 19-1). Crête Mince implants were designed and introduced by Michel Chérchève and have been referred to as *C-M* or *M-C* implants. Because of their thinness, they lack strength and cannot be depended on to serve as free-end saddle abutments. However, their versatility and resilience when used in multiples, particularly in pier or interabutment regions, makes them an extremely valuable adjunct to the armamentarium of the eclectic implantologist.

When using Crête Mince implants, place them in medullary bone between cortical plates. Ridge thickness can be as thin as 2.5 mm. Implant lengths are as long as 20 mm, but they may be cut shorter. Attempt to create bicortical osteotomies to gain maximum strength and longevity from these devices.

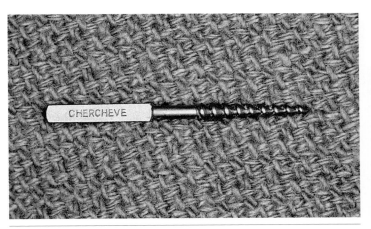

Fig. 19-1 The Michel Chérchève Crête Mince (M-C or C-M) thin ridge implant is now being produced in titanium by Bauer-Chérchève of Germany and by Michel Garard of Megève, France. Although these implants are self-tapping, a No.4 starter bur should be used through the cortex, followed by a series of special twist drills supplied by the manufacturers. Implants of varying lengths are available.

Surgical and Prosthodontic Techniques

The most successful application for C-M implants is in the anterior maxilla or mandible, where a long edentulous span such as from premolar to premolar may be found. Construct fixed bridge prostheses on posterior implants or molars and when available, premolars. In instances requiring superior esthetics, use a unit-built bridge design. This involves the construction of individual cast gold pontics, which are stabilized by internal C-M implants after being connected. Complete each with an individually made telescoped porcelain jacket crown. Using this technique, pin and abut the anterior and formerly unsupported portion of a long bridge to the underlying bone with these multiple threaded pins. The pins serve as reliable anterior pier abutments when used in this fashion. Observation, care, and troubleshooting are consonant with the rules governing other root form implants (Fig. 19-2). In the anterior region, the laboratory should construct an appropriate number of pontics of the classic unit-built design, each well centered over the bony ridge. Each should be hollow from incisal edge to ridge lap with a 2.5-mm diameter accommodation. This is sufficient to accept a C-M implant head. The laboratory should restore each pontic in the complex with a separate porcelain jacket made to telescope over it.

First, place the completed bridge into position. If all standard prosthetic criteria (crown margins, occlusion, and cosmetics) have been met satisfactorily, the bridge should be maintained in position. Each hollow pontic serves as the actual surgical template governing the placement and direction of its implant.

After administering local anesthesia, tattoo each ridge lap through the center of its pontic with an indelible pencil-tipped endodontic explorer. Remove the bridge and make cruciform incisions with a No. 11 blade, using the tattoos to establish their centers. Replace the bridge and perform the osteotomies

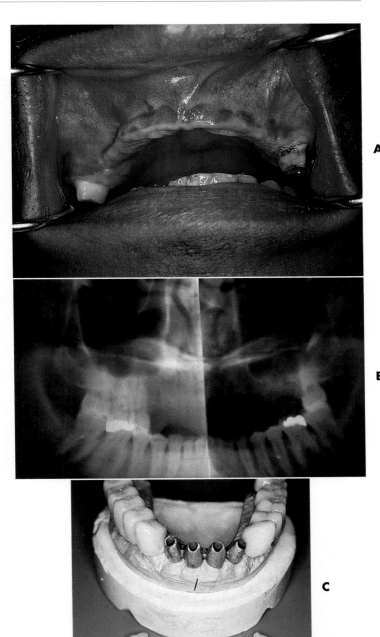

Fig. 19-2 A, A significant traumatic incident caused this long edentulous span. Ridge width was affected materially, but over 15 mm of height remained. **B,** The length of the edentulous spans discouraged any approach involving traditional fixed prostheses. **C,** A fixed maxillary prosthesis was fabricated with six separate anterior porcelain crowns. In this view, four of the six have been removed, revealing the hollow pontic design.
Continued

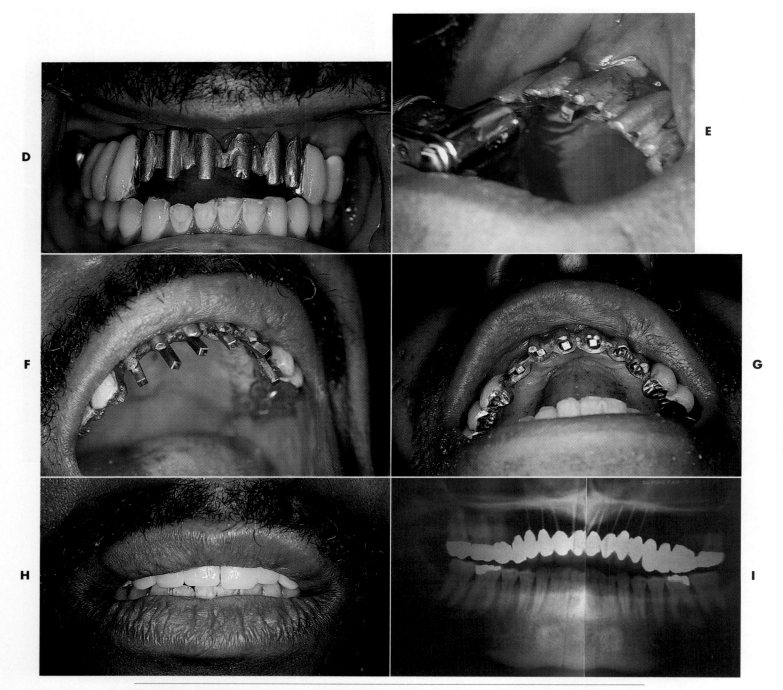

Fig. 19-2, cont'd   D, On the day of surgery, the fixed prosthesis is placed, and local anesthesia is administered. **E,** Each pontic is used as a surgical template, and the twist drills, in graduated sizes and under saline coolant, are used to make the osteotomies. They must be made directly in the center of each pontic so that when the self-tapping C-M implants are introduced, their abutments will be accommodated without trauma within the pontic walls. **F,** All implants have been placed concentrically. **G,** Each implant is shortened so that it will fall within the confines of its assigned pontic and allow complete seating of the individual porcelain crowns. **H,** After abutment scoring, the bridge is cemented using composite resin to lock the pontics to the implants. The jackets are cemented separately to complete the reconstruction. **I,** A panoramic x-ray demonstrates the prosthesis in position, with the implants maintaining integrity anteriorly.

using the pontics as a template to guide the direction and depth of the drills (Fig. 19-3).

Place a No. 1 round XXL bur into the high-speed handpiece and make a penetration only through the cortex. Make a change to the ultra–low-speed system and use copious external saline coolant. Use the 20 mm C-M twist drill next to create an osteotomy to the exact length of the implant and in the direction that the implant should take. Back the drill out slowly by reversing the motor. Irrigate the osteotomy and place the implant into the opening (Fig. 19-4). The handheld ratchet wrench fits over the square head of the implant. Rotate its handle so that it drives (taps) the C-M clockwise into place (Figs. 19-5, 19-6). These implants bite the bone effectively, come to a readily noted stop when fully seated, and create firm seating for themselves. No suturing is required.

Each square implant extension should be lying within its matching pontic's circumference. Remove the bridge and score the heads of the implants with a diamond drill to create undercuts using the high-speed handpiece (Fig. 19-7). Now prepare and cement the bridge using a composite or glass ionomer cement. Place a perforated rubber dam apron around the implants to discourage cement from entering the periimplant spaces (Fig. 19-8). Trim the cement from the open incisal edges of the pontics to restore them to their original contours (Fig. 19-9). Take a postoperative radiograph to confirm implant length and angulation as well as the presence of ectopic cement (Fig. 19-10). Slit and remove the rubber dam apron and after careful isolation of the abutment teeth and implants, place the separate porcelain crowns using properly shaded zinc oxyphosphate cement.

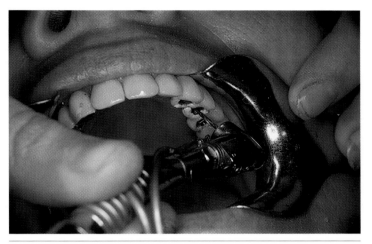

Fig. 19-3 The bridge, which requires stabilization, is supplied by the technician with hollow pontics. The pontics serve as surgical templates for the placement of the implants. Using a low-speed, well-irrigated contra-angle, the twist drill enters one of the pontics and as guided by the pilot hole, pierces the bone to a preplanned depth. An intraoperative radiograph should be taken at this juncture to determine the appropriate angulation and depth.

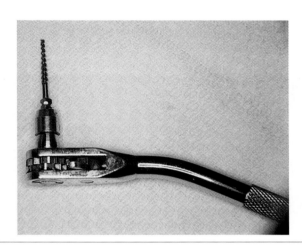

Fig. 19-5 C-M implants may be placed by wheel wrench or ratchet.

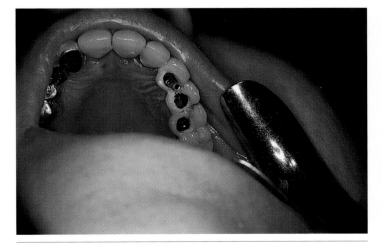

Fig. 19-4 After each osteotomy is completed by using increasingly larger twist drills, the implant is placed by hand. It should occupy the center of the pontic.

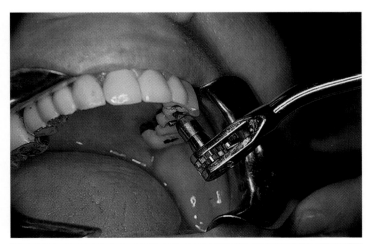

Fig. 19-6 Using a handheld wheel or, for harder bone, a ratchet wrench, drive each implant to its full depth as allowed by the presence of the pontic.

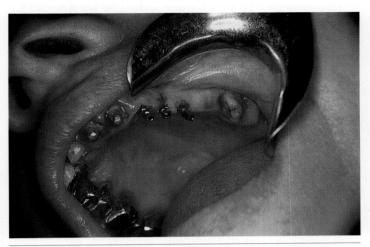

Fig. 19-7 After seating of all of the implants, remove the bridge permitting the final seating of each implant to its full-scored depth. After all of the C-M implants have been seated using the pontic complex as a template, removal and reseating of the bridge may be done with ease. Suturing is not required. Score each implant abutment for cement retention using a fine, water-cooled diamond.

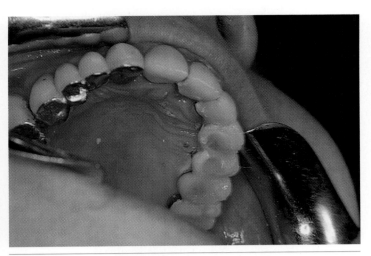

Fig. 19-9 Complete the restoration by removing the dam and placing and polishing occlusal sealers around each implant.

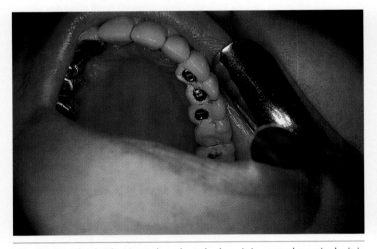

Fig. 19-8 The bridge is replaced, and when it is seated passively, it is cemented with a composite material to the natural abutments. A rubber dam apron is placed over the implants to discourage cement intrusion.

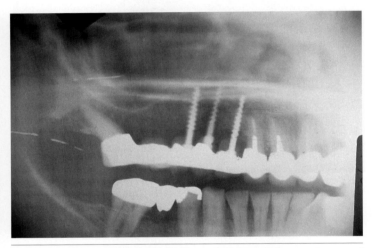

Fig. 19-10 The postoperative radiograph indicates the significance of these implants in supporting what would otherwise be an untenable fixed prosthesis.

Mini Transitional Implants

In a manner similar to that used with Crête Mince implants and with a coordinated simple set of drills, even smaller implants called *mini transitional implants (MTIs)* may be used either for auxiliary, long-term support in conjunction with conventional root form designs. They may also be used solely as interim devices, placed to retain temporary prostheses. Two products currently in use are the Sendax and the Dentatus designs; they are constructed respectively of titanium alloy and CP titanium (Fig. 19-11).

Techniques of placement are straightforward, generally without the requirement of an incision. However, safe practice encourages one. They follow the methods described for the Crête Mince implant and are accompanied by plastic transfer copings that permit the fabrication of fixed acrylic or cast metal prostheses (Fig. 19-12).

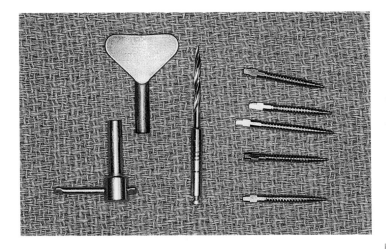

Fig. 19-11   The Dentatus MTI custom consists of a single bone drill, the threaded implants of varying total lengths and two key wrenches for manual insertion.

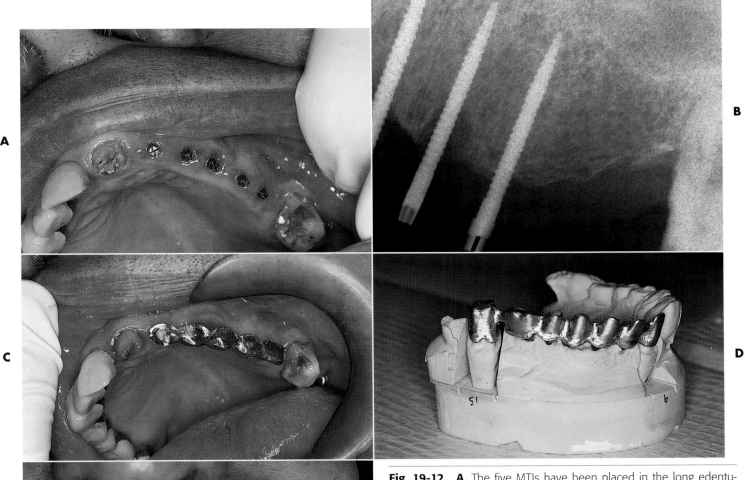

Fig. 19-12 **A,** The five MTIs have been placed in the long edentulous area between the central incisor and the second molar. During the period of postalveoloplasty healing, these implants may be put into function immediately after insertion. They may be used for patients who cannot afford conventional implant reconstruction. **B,** This periapical view demonstrates the position of the most posteriorly placed mini implants in relation to the ridge and maxillary sinus. Good bony integration is evident. **C,** After transferring the position of the mini-implants using plastic transfer housings (available from the manufacturer) nonprecious copings covering the implants are tried in for accuracy of fit. **D,** After a pickup impression of the copings (see Fig. 19-12, C), castings are made from the natural tooth abutments that were soldered to the implant copings. **E,** The completed interim prosthesis is in place; it is fabricated with an Artglass porcelain composite veneer. The material is baked to the surfaces of the nonprecious alloy.

Mini Subperiosteal Button Implants with Intraoral Bar Welding

Drs. Gustav Dahl and Ronald Cullen developed a small, collar button–shaped subperiosteal implant that has been altered in shape by the Park Dental Research Corporation (Fig. 19-13). Insert its 3-mm-diameter, fenestrated base into appropriately sized subperiosteal pockets by means of 3-mm-long full-thickness incisions made at 3-cm intervals parallel with and at the crest of the edentulous mandibular or maxillary ridge. Facially and lingually elevate the periosteum, and insert the flat, slightly carved base of each implant beneath the flaps (Figs. 19-14, *A* through *C*). Complete the procedure with a single pursestring Polysorb suture tied firmly around the protruding abutment. After 6 to 10 implants have been placed strategically, use the Hruska intraoral spot welder to bond half-round titanium bar segments to the abutments (Fig. 19-14, *D*). Make no effort to bend a single curved bar to a shape that can accommodate the implants passively because minor torquing exists even in the hands of the most skilled practitioner. Rather, cut and shape individual bar segments from implant to implant (Figs. 19-14, *E, F*). After completion of the assembly, seat an aggressively routed-out full denture with assurance that it does not contact the implant bar complex. Achieve retention with the use of generous quantities of denture adhesive. Follow with 6 weeks of observation, gentle irrigation, and denture adjustment. If, at that time, the complex is firm, the denture can be adapted to the bar with custom clips or with the addition of a laboratory-processed soft lining (Fig. 19-14, *G*). In some cases, maxillary dentures can be altered by resection of the palatal acrylic, creating a more comfortable horseshoe design.

Suggested Reading

Cranin AN: The Michel Chérchève thin-ridge implant. *Oral Implantology*, Springfield, 1970, Charles C. Thomas, p. 141.

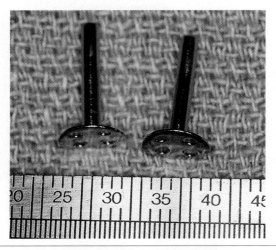

Fig. 19-13 These Park Dental Research titanium mini subperiosteal implants demonstrate their long permucosal extensions (which can be cut to length as needed) and their fenestrated curved bases. These implants, designed at Brookdale, were adapted from the devices introduced by Drs. Dahl and Cullen. Their curved bases can be bent to fit the underlying alveolar ridge.

Fig. 19-14 **A,** The preoperative appearance of the maxilla for which the mini subperiosteal technique is to be used. The patient demonstrates an atrophic ridge that was unsuitable to retain a conventional prosthesis. **B,** After delineating sites for implant placement using a Thompson's marking stick (transferred from the tissue surface of the patient's prosthesis), 1-cm long, full-thickness incisions are made at the crest of the ridge. The mucoperiosteum is elevated buccally and lingually with a periodontal knife in order to accommodate the mini subperiosteal bases. **C,** Each mini subperiosteal implant is inserted by first placing it under the palatal flap and then raising the buccal flap under which the buccal portion of the base is situated. **D,** The Hruska titanium welder consists of a large console attached to an intraoral, handheld clamp and welder. Because of the unique nature of this apparatus, welding titanium to titanium does not generate heat. **E,** A single titanium bar is being welded to two mini subperiosteal implants. Subsequent to this, a bar is welded between the next two implants until all the segments are joined. **F,** The completed bar complex demonstrates all implants joined with individual titanium bar segments in a full arc. The use of a diamond bur allows sharp edges and extensions to be trimmed and smoothed. **G,** Postoperatively, the denture is relined over the implants to ensure that occlusal forces are not transferred to the implants. After a 6- to 8-week healing period, the denture is relined with a semipermanent soft lining material that allows an imprecise but reliable fit around the bar.

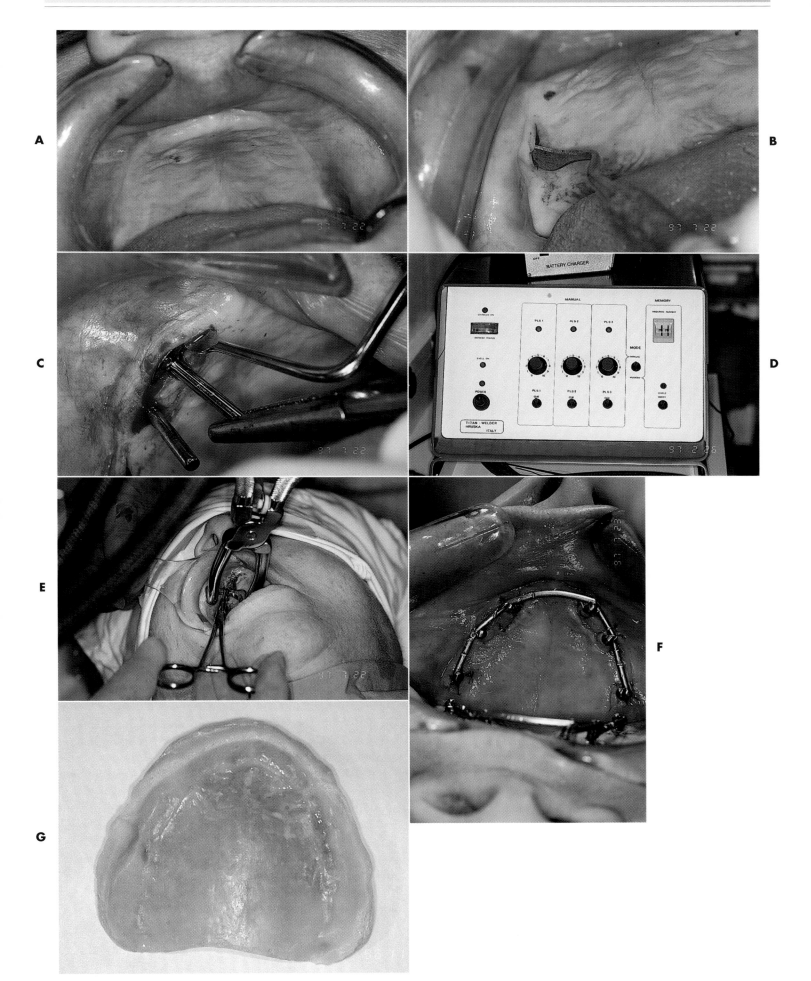

Implant Prosthodontics:

Introduction to Chapters 20, 21, 22, 23, 24, 25, 26, and 27

There is nothing unique involved in the art and science of implant prosthodontics. The novice becomes confused at the entry level when he or she is introduced to the plethora of abutments and attachments made by each company multiplied by the variations and nomenclature that each contributes to the cumulative marketplace.

Added to this prosthetic Tower of Babel are methods of abutment attachment to external and internal hexagonal implant designs using threaded techniques, as well as several variants.

Essentially each company produces restorative systems that are similar to one another. Abutments, after all, must be attached to implants. They will have angulations and shapes required to fill anatomic and esthetic requirements. Patients will request fixed prostheses; dentists will select the option of removable overdentures. Decisions must be made on a basis of occlusal forces, numbers and dimensions of implants, patient compliance, economics, esthetics, and functional requirements.

The following seven chapters will guide restorative dentists and implantologists through each of the available options, problems and their solutions, and the principles of implant occlusion. Since implantology is prosthodontically navigated, the reader should refer to Chapter 5, since the location, design, and number of implants will be selected on a basis of the final prosthetics preferred by consensus after consultation between patient and practitioner.

Once this decision has been made, a classical and unswerving series of orderly procedures must be completed.

This section begins with descriptions of the fabrication of a clear acrylic device, which may go on to serve as a radiographic guide, surgical template, implant locator, and interim prosthesis.

Since implantologists are responsible for maintaining patient comfort, dignity, and self-respect, there must be assurance that, at no time during the entire therapeutic period, will he or she be permitted to function without a prosthesis.

Interim prosthesis are not difficult to prepare, and if designed correctly, can be altered at each phase to continue serving until the final restoration is delivered. Innovative dentistry requires thought, skill, experience, and the guidance offered in the following chapters.

Possibly the most complicated segment of this instructional manual is the section describing abutments. In order to deliver this information and the techniques that follow in a clear and comprehensible fashion, a generic system has been established from which information about individual company's products and techniques can be extrapolated. This includes single tooth restorations, mesostructure bars, overdentures, and fixed prostheses and fixed detachable prostheses, both hybrid and anatomic.

Occlusal principles unique to implant-borne prostheses are included.

Potential problems will be enumerated, and each will be addressed in a manner that will facilitate a solution.

Armamentarium

Standard prosthodontic equipment and supplies
Transfer copings
Implant analogs
Hex drivers
Wrenches
Laboratory anatomic abutments
Plastic copings
A selection of attachments: O-rings, Zest, Zag, ERA, Harder, Dolder

Caveats

Listen to the patient with care. Make final decisions on a basis of good communication; mutual understanding of needs; and a clear, careful, and graphic description of the planned procedures and anticipated results.

There should be no doubt about the patient's expectations. If this is not clarified before the inception of care, the most satisfactory result will be disappointing.

Despite the fact that the doctor's philosophies play a significant role in treatment planning, temper the final prosthetic decision within reason by the expectations of the patient.

When plans are changed or problems arise, frank discussions and disclosures offer the best strategies to maintain high levels of ongoing cooperation.

Do not permit patient enthusiasm to cloud sound diagnostic and evaluative methods. Health status, quality and quantity of bone, operator skills, oral hygiene, and economics are the vital elements that create an admixture of satisfaction and success.

20

Preliminary Prosthodontics: Fabricating a Template

*A*fter the patient has agreed with the treatment plan, the implantologist must comply by performing a series of carefully planned steps.

Fully Edentulous

If the jaw being treated is fully edentulous, whatever the ultimate prosthetic design, supply the patient with a preliminary complete denture. It is also necessary to institute occlusal corrections to the opposing jaw. This may involve balancing the natural dentition, adding crowns or onlays, or completely habilitating the faulty opposing dentition. If for any reason this is not a practical solution, use processed acrylic occlusal onlays as an interim solution. The goal of the restoration should be that the implant-supported jaw be presented with an ideal occlusal relationship.

On the establishment of a satisfactory occlusal height and plane, initiate procedures for the fabrication of an opposing full denture for the operative jaw.

Impression making and record taking may follow classic techniques. Do not complete the denture until the patient registers approval of her or his appearance.

At the time of insertion, a corrected occlusal plane should appose the denture. This may involve increasing the vertical dimension and correcting centric occlusion. The trial period that follows is an essential interval of study that should present assurance that the patient has become acclimated to and comfortable with the changes. If the patient complains of unrelenting facial or temporomandibular joint (TMJ) pain or aching, premature occlusal contact during chewing, or problems with deglutition that are not ameliorated by time, then make accommodations by increasing the interocclusal dimensions and shortening the teeth.

After achieving a satisfactory result, the denture serves as an indispensable guide. It has been designed to govern implant emergence profiles and abutment locations and lengths.

Finalize the treatment plan at this juncture. The choices available are selected on the basis of available bone and its quality; the patient's capabilities, aspirations, and finances; and the operator's skills and prejudices.

The resulting prosthesis may be an overdenture totally supported by the tissue and retained by an O-ring or ball attachments. It may use two implants, three or more implants (with a fixed cemented or fixed-detachable mesostructure bar that may be partly or fully implant supported), or five or more implants (buttressing an anatomic fixed bridge or a bar-borne hybrid fixed prosthesis) (Fig. 20-1). In all events, make the completed support mechanism (abutments, attachments, bars) to fit within the confines of the newly completed denture. If this idealization cannot be satisfied, the final appliance is too large, thereby creating possibly insoluble esthetic and functional problems.

The denture therefore serves significant roles in the processes of planning, management, and fabrication of the complex restorative operation.

If the patient is wearing a denture that satisfies tooth and flange positions, it may be replicated to serve this function. On the other hand, if the existing prosthesis is unacceptable, a new one that presents correct functional and esthetic characteristics is required.

Make an acceptable denture by following the classic steps of prosthesis fabrication.

Make impressions with the use of stock trays with modeling compound or alginate. Also make a counter impression of the opposing arch. Make a record base on the cast of the edentulous arch, followed by a face-bow recording, which is used to mount the maxillary cast. Correct the record base to proper vertical dimension and centric relationship, select and set the denture teeth, and fit the trial denture. Confirm centric and vertical records and obtain approval of esthetics from the patient. This trial denture does not necessarily need processing, but in most cases, it should be completed because it has value as an interim prosthesis.

Replicate the trial denture for use as a surgical template in the following manner:

Fill the lower half of a denture-duplicating flask with alginate and press the denture, tissue side down, into it. Immerse it to half its height. After the alginate has set, trim the excess flask with a Bard Parker No. 10 blade and lubricate lightly. Fill the other half of the duplicator with alginate, spreading it over the occlusal surface of the denture with a moistened finger. Close the duplicator, allow the alginate to set, and open the duplicator to permit removal of the denture. Fill the impression of the denture with cold-cure acrylic using the powder-liquid technique. After filling the impression, close the duplicator again and place it in a pressure pot for complete curing.

After 30 minutes at 300° F, open the duplicator, remove the template, and trim the excess flask with flame-shaped acrylic burs.

In order to permit the template to serve as a device to guide implant positioning, leave the facial surfaces of the teeth intact. The incisal and occlusal surfaces are removed to allow access to the underlying potential host sites. The labial surfaces serve as the most important parameter in governing implant position. Leave a band of lingual or palatal acrylic intact.

This grants rigidity to the template so that it does not bend or fracture. Cut the access opening at least 5 mm beyond the anticipated most distal implant positions to permit flexibility and alteration of planned locations intraoperatively. Implant locations should be idealized just lingual to the cingulum areas of the anterior teeth. This subsequently places the abutments, bars, or both, in the thickest portion of the planned denture. Placement of implants too far lingually places the abutments or bars within the thinnest portion of the denture, which might then undergo premature stress fracture. Be sure to consider the vertical height during implant positioning for overdentures. Consider the heights of the abutments or other attachments, the height of the bar, the height of a superimposed metal casting (if used) the height of the male or female attachments to be placed into the denture acrylic, and the thickness of the denture acrylic. Add these numbers, and the result reveals the total height available for final construction. This number actually represents the vertical distance from the tops of the implants to the incisal edges of the teeth in the surgical template. There should be a minimum of 15 mm available. If this not the case, a variety of shorter abutments may be employed to satisfy the overage (see Chapter 22).

The second function that the denture fulfills is that of a CT radiographic guide (Fig. 20-2). In order to activate this duty, the denture has to be replicated in clear acrylic (Fig. 20-3, *A* through *C*). This may be completed easily by a member of the office staff using a Lang duplicating flask filled with alginate (Fig. 20-3, *D* through *F*). The final clear acrylic reproduction has many valuable uses. In order to enforce its dimensional stability, seat it on its model, place it in a pressure pot, and further cure it by the addition of hot water for 30 minutes (Figs. 20-4 through 20-6).

This multipurpose device fulfills its first critical function if presurgical CT scanning is prescribed. Chapter 4 describes in detail the techniques used for imbedding radiopaque media

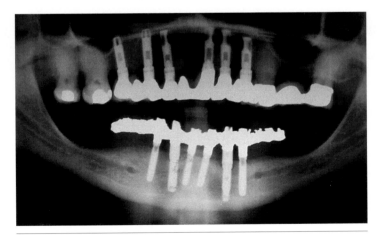

Fig. 20-1 This panoramic radiograph demonstrates a mixed tooth- and implant-supported fixed, cementable, porcelain-fused-to-metal prosthesis in the maxilla and an implant-supported fixed-detachable hybrid mandibular prosthesis.

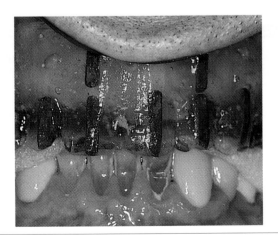

Fig. 20-2 A radiographic template is tried in the mouth to check fit and comfort. By disoccluding the template in the anterior, 3 mm of cold-cure acrylic can be added to allow the jaw to be in a resting position. Petroleum jelly is placed on the opposing dentition to ensure that the cold-cure acrylic adheres to the template only. The radiographic markers in this template are composed of amalgam and acrylic in a 1:3 ratio.

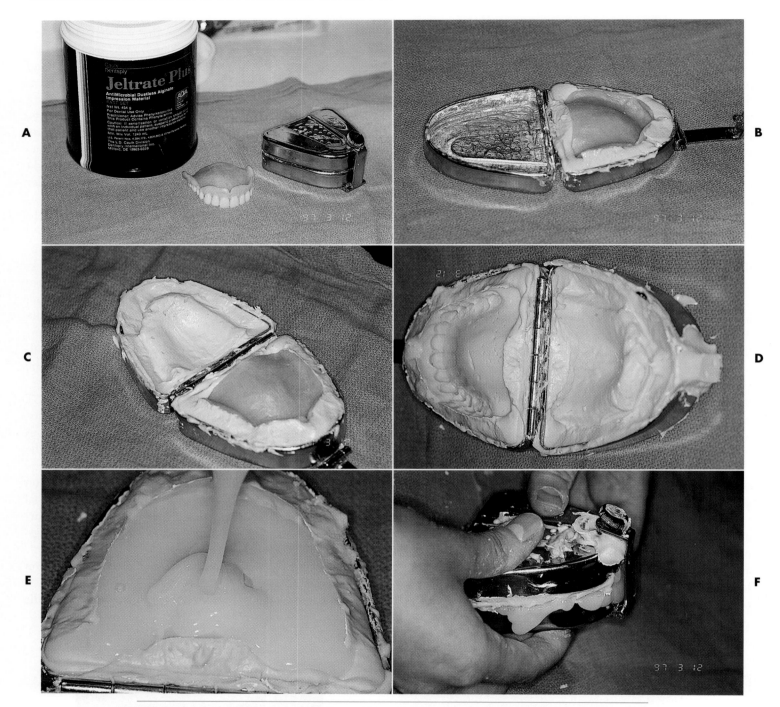

Fig. 20-3 **A,** The Long denture duplicator. The patient's dentures (or acceptable wax try-in) are required to fabricate a duplicate denture. **B,** First, seat the denture into alginate in one half of the denture duplicator. Allow the alginate to set. Subsequent to its setting, place alginate in the other half of the duplicator, and fully close it. **C,** After the alginate is set, separate the two halves, revealing an accurate reproduction of the internal surface of the denture. The fact that alginate does not stick to set alginate allows the two halves to separate easily. **D,** Remove the denture from the set alginate. The reproduced tissue and external surfaces are clearly identified. **E,** Overfill clear, cold-cure acrylic into the concave reproduction of the external side of the denture. **F,** Fully close the duplicator and lock it into position. Excess acrylic must be seen escaping to ensure that no voids are present in the template.

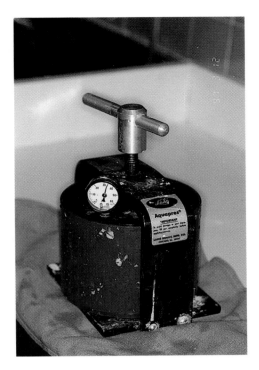

Fig. 20-4   Fill the pressure pot with hot water and place the Lang duplicator in at 30 psi for 30 minutes to allow complete setting of the acrylic.

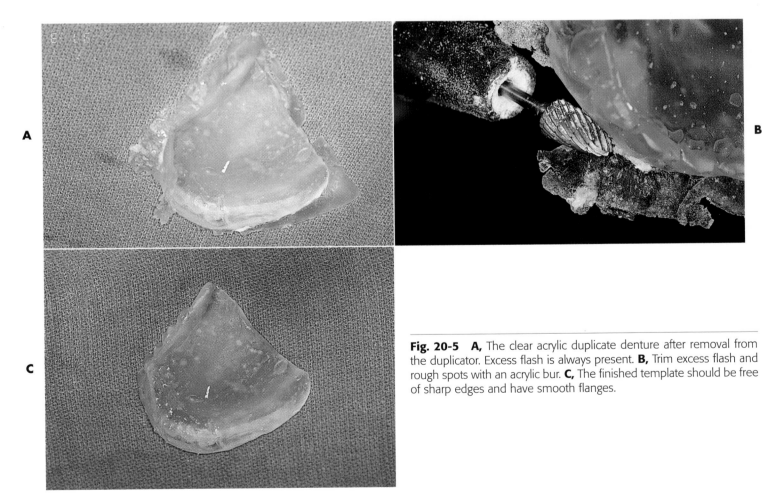

Fig. 20-5   A, The clear acrylic duplicate denture after removal from the duplicator. Excess flash is always present. **B,** Trim excess flash and rough spots with an acrylic bur. **C,** The finished template should be free of sharp edges and have smooth flanges.

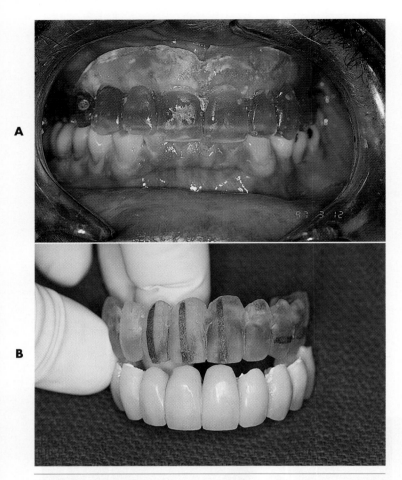

Fig. 20-6 A, The template is tried into the mouth to ensure comfort and proper occlusion. Final adjustments are often required at this step. **B,** A temporary fixed prosthesis may be duplicated in a Lang duplicator to form a surgical template and CT scan template.

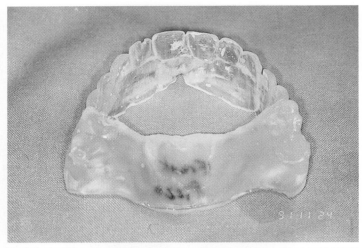

Fig. 20-7 Relieve the template to allow access for surgical placement of implants.

into premeasured grooves that are essential in verifying the locations and dimensions of host sites intraoperatively (Fig. 20-2).

In addition, adding a 3-mm occlusal run to the appliance provides jaw stabilization and comfort in the resting position.

After the appliance had been used for CT scanning, recruit it as a surgical template. An additional alteration is required. Cut away the occlusal, incisal edge and lingual acrylic of all potential implant host sites (Fig. 20-7). This permits surgical access to the bone while the template occupies its anatomic position. The radiopaque markers allow the surgeon to transfer image findings and dimensions directly to the bony host sites (see Chapter 4).

Suturing completes the first stage of implant surgery. The original denture now continues its essential role as a stent and wound protector while providing the patient with continuing cosmetic and functional benefits. It requires alteration and relining to satisfy this need.

In the second stage of surgery, employ the clear replica to localize the buried implants, especially if it was marked with amalgam-filled bur locator holes in the first stage.

After the healing collars or abutments have been attached, the original denture can be again adapted to serve. After stripping the soft lining, rearm it to fit over the permucosal protrusions or transepithelial abutments (TEAs), where it may function through completion of the reconstruction.

As an alternative, trim it back to its dentoalveolar components by grinding away the palate and flanges and use it with cement or even abutment fixation screws as a transitional prostheses. The significance and versatility of this appliance and its clones cannot be overemphasized.

Surgical templates are necessary to accurately and predictably place and position implants. Two different designs of surgical templates are recommended for partially edentulous areas. The first style replicates the provisional denture restoration and is made on the corrected replicated cast. The second style uses an Omnivac template but relies on adjacent teeth and soft tissues for support and positioning. Use the surgical template that replicates the provisional prosthesis rather than an Omnivac when the number of planned implants exceeds two (Fig. 20-8).

Use the Omnivac surgical template, which is simpler to prepare, when there are adjacent teeth that are not being restored. The Omnivac template relies on these fixed structures for support and positioning. Fabricate this type of surgical template by adding wax or denture teeth to the planned operative sites on a stone cast. Trim it below the height of contour of the adjacent teeth, and it will fit snugly and still be removable without difficulty. At the planned implant sites, cut occlusal holes in the Omnivac material. The buccal facings are the most important guides in implant positioning, and they should be preserved. These simple devices are readily sterilized, and they may be retained for use in the second stage of surgery for identification of implant sites. Refer to Chapter 22 for abutment selection after implant exposure.

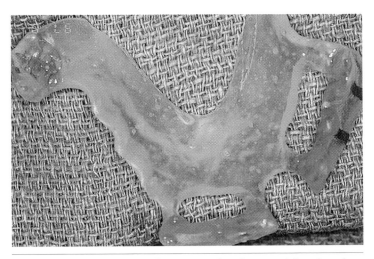

Fig. 20-8 This is an example of a template for a partially edentulous patient. In this case, the template was fabricated from an acceptable acrylic partial denture in a manner described for complete templates. An alternative to this procedure is to fabricate a template based on a suitable wax-up as described in Chapter 4.

Suggested Readings

Binon PP: Provisional fixed restorations supported by osseointegrated implants in partially edentulous patients, *J Oral Maxillofac Implant* 2:173-178, 1988.

Desjardins RP: Prosthesis design for osseointegrated implants in the edentulous maxilla, *Int J Oral Maxillofac Implants* 7:311-320, 1992.

Johns RB, Jemt T et al: A multicenter study of overdentures supported by a Brånemark implants, *Int J Oral Maxillofac Implants* 7:513-522, 1992.

Kallus T et al: Clinical evaluation of angulated abutments for the Brånemark system: a pilot study, *J Oral Maxillofac Implant* 5:39-46, 1990.

Lewis S et al: The "UCLA" abutment, *J Oral Maxillofac Implant*, 3:184-189, 1988.

Lundquist S, Carlsson GE: Maxillary fixed prosthesis on osseointegrated dental implants, *J Prosthet Dent* 50:262-270, 1983.

Misch CE: Density of bone: effect on treatment plans, surgical approach, healing and progressive bone loading, *Int J Oral Maxillofac Implants* 6:23-31, 1990.

Seal DG: Integral implant system prosthodontic considerations, Calcitek, Inc., 1988.

van Steenberge et al: The applicability of osseointegrated oral implants in the rehabilitation of partial edentulism: a prospective multicenter study on 558 fixtures, *Int J Oral Maxillofac Implants* 3:272-281, 1990.

Zobler MN: Reconstruction of the edentulous maxillary arch by using prosthodontic implants, *J Prosthet Dent* 60:474-478, 1988.

21
Provisional Prostheses

There are two stages in the cascade of therapeutic events during which the patient requires a provisional or interim prosthesis. The first is during the integration period after first-stage surgery. The second is after healing collar and abutment placement.

There are several significant factors to consider. Acceptable and believable esthetics are mandated at every stage in oral reconstruction. In addition, sound prosthetic principles must be observed. Well-balanced occlusion and correct centric and vertical dimension are required as well as built-in protection to implant areas during the healing period. If natural teeth are to be used as part of the final restoration, use them for a temporary fixed prosthesis, thereby sparing the gingival tissues overlying the implants. If an opportunity to construct a fixed prosthesis fails to present itself, the necessity arises to construct a tissue-borne removable prosthesis that is broad-based enough to distribute forces evenly. Sound measures incorporate soft relining material (Coe Soft, Viscogel, PermaSoft) that is frequently changed, careful examination of the tissues overlying the operative sites to detect early signs of pressure, and in maxillae, full palatal coverage, despite the fact that this feature does not meet with the approval of many patients.

Totally Edentulous Interim Prostheses

First Stage

The patient usually presents with a complete denture that has been used for the jaw requiring treatment. Chapter 20 describes the machinations required to prepare a new denture and a replicated clear template, which, in their several roles and commutations, serve as a radiographic indicator for CT scans, a surgical template, and as an interim prosthesis. Make these protheses with unfailing attentiveness to classic prosthetic principles. Vertical dimension, centric occlusion, incisal length, free-way space, tooth position and angulation, and patient-approved cosmetics must be satisfied. Except for retention, the final implant-borne prosthesis can never be better than the initial one because the latter's characteristics govern implant locations and emergence angles.

After implant surgery has been completed and hemostasis has been ensured, aggressively ream out the area of the tissue-borne surface of the denture, which approximates the implant sites, with a large round acrylic bur. Manage the flange linings as well as the ridge crest in this fashion so that when seating the denture postoperatively there is no rocking or instability. The relief of acrylic must take into consideration the possible added bulk of bone by expansion techniques or grafting materials, the protrusion of healing screw heads (especially for external hex implants), the increased dimension caused by a bulky suture line (i.e., mattress closures), and edema. The use of the duplicate clear diagnostic plastic base-plate can be used by grinding it until no surgical site mucosal blanching is noted, is of benefit for this critical step. The correction experience then is simplified while replicating the grinding in the interim denture.

After sufficient overcorrection has been made to allow for a several-millimeter thickness of soft lining material, dry, line, and seat the denture and close the patient's mouth into centric position. Perform gentle muscle molding, trim the excess soft material with a No. 11 BP blade in a scalpel handle, and round the borders carefully with sharp sheers to eliminate irritating irregularities.

Occlusal relationships must be precisely the same as they were before these alterations were made.

If vascular oozing continues, facilitate hemostasis by the addition of a 50-50 mix of the powders of denture adhesive and ferric chloride, sprinkled onto the moistened lining with a salt shaker reserved for this use. Additional retention accompanies the rapid coagulation.

Postoperative visits should be in 3-day intervals until wound stability is ensured. After this, visits are made at reasonable intervals for relining and ongoing occlusal adjustments.

Second Stage

The denture is a versatile appliance and lends itself to simple and innovative change as dictated by the patient's prosthetic needs.

Bring its progenitor, the surgical template (which should have been retained) to the host area. With the assistance of the radiopaque markers and carefully made mapping notes,

each implant, although not visible through the mucosa, may be located. (See Chapter 9, Uncovering, p. 187).

After placing healing collars or abutments turn to the acrylic routing burs, this time to make deeper, but more discreet, modifications designed to accommodate the transepithelial abutments (TEAs) in a trauma-sparing environment.

Touching the dried occlusal surfaces of the abutments or collars with pressure indicator paste (PIP) and placing the denture against them now relieved of its soft lining, reveals the exact locations that are in contact (Fig. 21-1). Concentration on the elimination of these areas leads to a prosthesis that is totally relieved of directing pressure to the implants. Again, place a soft lining of choice. Complete definitive prosthetic measures while this removable interim denture continues to serve in its classically versatile manner.

At second-stage surgery, the dentist and patient may find it desirable to substitute a fixed interim prosthesis for the removable one. Base this decision on the same principles that govern the design of fixed prostheses presented in Chapter 24. The following section gives advice on preparing such devices and may be followed with essentially no modifications.

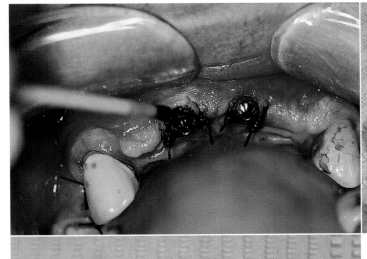
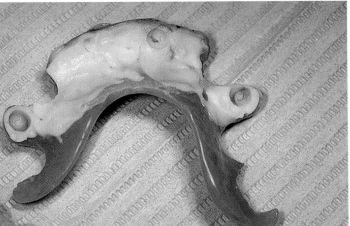
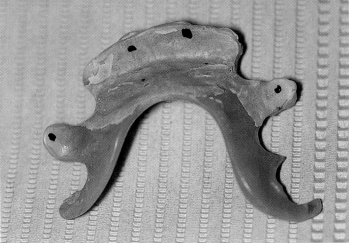

Fig. 21-1 **A,** The first step in adapting a transitional denture to accommodate newly placed healing collars is to outline the collars with a Thompson's marking stick or indelible pencil. **B,** After seating and removing the denture, transfer the markings outlining each implant to its tissue-borne surface. **C,** After the denture base material is reamed aggressively at the sites of the markings, reline it with Coe Comfort or TruSoft.

Partially Edentulous Interim Prostheses

Implant-borne restorations range from single tooth (see Chapter 23), to more sophisticated, complex implant/tooth designs. The provisional prostheses may be removable or fixed, but in all instances it must be kept respectful of the recently submerged implants.

If there is an urgent need for a fixed provisional prosthesis, even in cases in which few or no potential abutments are available, the doctor may plan to add some strategically placed implants at the time of first-stage surgery in addition to those inserted for therapeutic use. Regions such as the tuberosities, pterygoid plates, or interimplant spaces may be suitable for regular or mini implant placement (see Chapters 9 and 19). Although no significant expectations should be held for their long-range prognosis, some mini implants succeed in their ascent to osseointegration and may be kept for incorporation into the final prosthesis. Those that do not require removal because of mobility or bone loss or are not required for final superstructure stabilization because of location or angulation can be shaved level to the gingivae. Periodic radiographic and clinical observation of these interim implants is important because continuing periimplant disease, if present, can affect adjacent teeth and implants. In such cases, immediate removal and repair (see Chapter 24) are indicated.

Single Tooth Implant Restorations

First Stage

The patient may have recently lost an incisor (or another esthetically critical tooth) secondary to trauma. Gingival tissues and bone may be intact or virtually so. In such cases, supply a temporary prosthesis immediately. The following are surgical alternatives:

- Fill the socket with graft material (e.g., tricalcium phosphate [TCP]) and achieve primary coverage by undermining or, if vestibular integrity is inviolable, the use of Alloderm or Regenitex, which may serve as epithelial substitutes.
- Immediately place an implant into the recently vacated alveolus, following the guidelines presented in Chapter 9.
- Allow the injury to heal without treatment. A viable clot serves as the precursor to uncomplicated healing. Sometime before the completion of Σ, Roberts' 20-week bone healing sequence, an implant should be placed or the sanctity of the labial cortical plate will be threatened.

In any event, provide a non–tissue-borne prosthesis to the patient.

A simple alternative is available by bonding an esthetically acceptable acrylic denture tooth to the adjacent proximal enamel surfaces. If occlusal forces appear threatening, an easily fabricated, all-acrylic Maryland-type bridge may be prepared chairside; strengthened, if necessary, with steel mesh or wire; and bonded to the lingual and proximal surfaces of the abutting teeth.

Small, claspless partial dentures (flippers) are discouraged because they permit pressure to be directed to underlying edentulous sites. Postoperative examinations should offer assurance that there is continued stability of the temporary tooth and freedom from ridge lap pressure.

At each stage of treatment from gingivoplasty to grafting and implant placement, the prosthesis may be removed, freshened, and seated again with new cement.

Second Stage

At the time of second-stage surgery, if abutment placement or a contoured healing collar has been used, use of an ion crown will facilitate temporization. Line the crown with a composite and place it with a noneugenol cement (Fig. 21-2).

Partially Edentulous, Multiple Implant Restorations

First Stage

FIXED PROVISIONAL PROSTHESES   After existing pathology has been eliminated by periodontoplasty and endodontic therapy, certain teeth slated for extraction may be retained temporarily, prepared for crowns, and used as abutments for office- or laboratory-processed acrylic Artglass or nonprecious metal fixed bridges. Following this philosophy, teeth that are to be used as abutments for the final prosthesis may be managed in the same fashion. At each visit, remove such bridges, and after the planned therapy has been completed (endodontics, periodontal surgery), replace them with temporary cement. After implants have been placed, carefully manage ridge laps to spare the host sites from injury.

If the condemned teeth are of such poor quality that they cannot be maintained on an interim basis, insert mini implants into nonstrategic areas of the ridge to serve as partial or complete support mechanisms for temporary bridges (see Chapter 19).

Impression and record making for these implant foundations follow classic patterns, with try-ins, occlusal- and tissue-level adjustments, and insertion. Although metal and Artglass provide the most esthetic results, laboratory-processed acrylic bridges present the advantages of adaptability, chairside repair and alteration, ease of construction, ease of adjustment, minimal cost, and simplicity of convertibility after the abutments have been placed.

Fixed provisional restoration is preferable to removable and may be used when fixed abutment support is available. Teeth, implants, or both may supply this support. The teeth that may require extraction can be kept to support the provisional restoration. If implants are used as abutments for provisional prostheses, they may be mature or placed recently for interim support. Although the prognoses for such implants is not as positive as for those that are conventionally placed, many of them survive and contribute to the long-term foundation of the final restorations. There are two designs for fixed provisional restorations. Full-coverage-style bridges of an acrylic or composite with abutment preparations and support from nonprecious metals are one choice.

Strategic implants must be selected. These may have poor prognoses. The requirements for their selection are that they be nonacutely infected and that they cause no pain.

Make diagnostic casts of the operative jaw and mount them against a counter model. If a change in the position of the max-

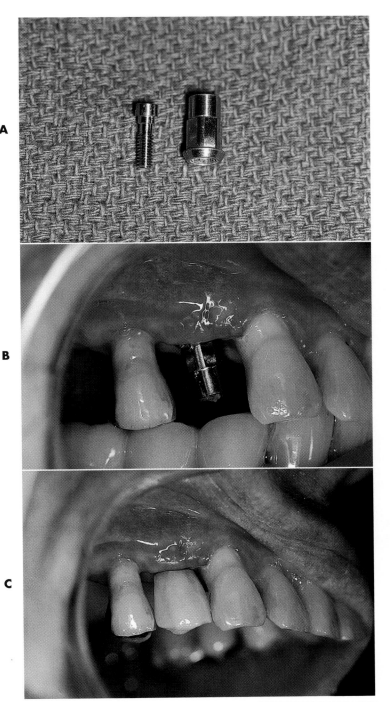

Fig. 21-2 **A,** A hexed temporary cylinder from Implant Innovations uses a central retaining screw. **B,** The temporary cylinder is tightened into place by hand. **C,** An acrylic provisional crown may be relined over the temporary cylinder and then cemented to place, or the provisional may be luted to the temporary cylinder to form a screw-retained provisional restoration.

illary teeth is planned for the provisional restoration, use a face-bow transfer to mount the maxillary cast.

Make changes in tooth position, orientation, shape, or number in wax on the working cast. Replicate this in stone by flasking in alginate. Make a silicone labiomucosal index of the teeth to be provisionalized. This index should include adjacent teeth and gingival tissues. Then prepare all teeth on the diagnostic cast. These preparations should be less than 1 mm in depth. Replicate the altered cast in the form of a refractory model. The laboratory adds wax to the replicated model that should wrap around the lingual surfaces of all of the teeth and extend halfway through the embrasures. There should be no wax on the buccal or occlusal surfaces. Continue the wax over the edentulous areas to accommodate for future implant abutments. Cast the frame in a nonprecious metal and coat its inner aspect with a tooth-colored opacifier to prevent the final acrylic or composite from appearing gray. Place the opaque metal frame on the prepared cast and cover it with the silicone index. Flow wax into the index, creating the planned restoration. Flask, boil out, and use acrylic of the proper shade to replace the lost wax. After curing, deflask, trim, and polish the restoration.

Insert this provisional restoration after preparing the planned abutments in the patient's mouth in the same manner as for normal crowns and then fit and reline the provisional restoration with self-curing acrylic. If the entire arch is being provisionalized, preserve the patient's vertical dimension and maintain or modify it appropriately (Fig. 21-3). Use temporary noneugenol cement (Trial) to cement the provisional prosthesis. It should permit easy removal but maintain its retention in a trouble-free manner. Check the prosthesis for cement integrity monthly and remove it every third month for prophylaxis. Fluoridation is of benefit at these visits as well as the use of a dentifrice at home.

COMPOSITE RETAINED FIXED PROVISIONAL BRIDGE The second choice is the Maryland bridge made either of composite material or of base metal and acrylic. The composite retained fixed bridge is of particular benefit when teeth adjacent to the edentulous area planned for implants are not going to be restored and there is lingual enamel available that does not come into contact with the opposing dentition in centric occlusion or any excursive movements. Fit these lingual surfaces with Maryland-like wings that serve as retentive devices for provisional fixed restorations. Make and mount diagnostic casts of the maxilla and mandible and use wax to incorporate planned changes. Make a stone cast replica of the wax-up and wax the metal framework without preparation or alteration of the natural teeth. Place it on the lingual surfaces of the teeth planned as abutments and extend it halfway into the embrasure spaces, wrapping it around the lingual surfaces of one to three teeth on either side of the edentulous area. The number of adjacent teeth required for abutment support depends on the size of the edentulous span. An edentulous space of two or more teeth should use at least two or more adjacent abutment teeth. The metal frame should cover as much lingual enamel as possible, but it should not interfere with centric supporting stops or excursive movements of the opposing dentition. The thickness of the winged frame should be greater than 1 mm. Cast it in a nonprecious metal, make a silicone index of the teeth to be extracted and the adjacent teeth, and remove the condemned teeth from the cast. Seat the metal frame on the cast, place the silicone index over it, flow wax into the index, and attach it to the cast metal frame. Flask, boil out, and process with appropriately shaded acrylic. After trimming and polishing, cut two to three half round bur holes through the lingual metal wings that seat on the abutment teeth. The metal need not be etched. Make occlusal and esthetic adjustments. Polish the abutment teeth with pumice, then acid-etch them in three spots, and seat the bridge with firm pressure, allowing self-curing composite resin to extrude through the holes in the metal wings. The patient closes his or her teeth in centric occlusion and allows the composite to cure completely. Trim the excess composite resin leaving a button of protruding material at the site of each hole in the metal wings. These buttons retain the fixed bridge mechanically. Bridges made in this fashion may be removed by cutting off the composite buttons (Fig. 21-4).

REMOVABLE PROVISIONAL PROSTHESES Although removable provisional prostheses are simpler to make, require much less preparation of teeth, and circumvent the need for placing mini implants, they present the potential problems of transmitting harmful forces to grafted or implanted sites.

In addition, such prostheses are not appealing to patients; they are bulky and often troublesome prostheses. To fabricate such a device, cast Bonwill clasps with deep and effective occlusal rests. Full palatal or retromolar pad coverage offers effective support, and all saddles require thick soft liners that must be changed with frequency.

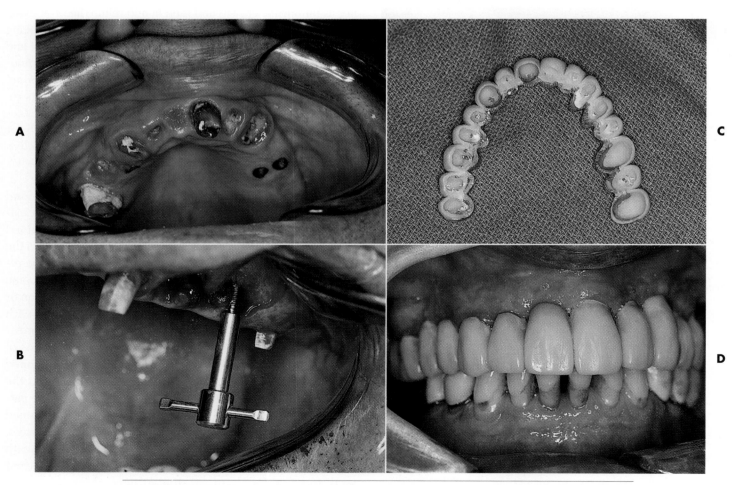

Fig. 21-3 **A,** Teeth that are to be extracted but are not acutely infected or painful may be useful for provisional abutment support. **B,** Mini transitional implants are useful when inadequate teeth are present to support the provisional restoration. **C,** The fixed provisional restoration can be maintained for long periods of time if cast metal reinforcement is processed with the acrylic. **D,** The provisional restoration is relined with autopolymerizing acrylic.

Abutments can be teeth that are to removed, those which are incorporated into the final prosthesis, or other unsullied teeth that may require restorations in order to permit the placement of deep rest seats and clasps.

Second Stage

FIXED PROVISIONAL PROSTHESES   On the occasion of implant exposure for the placement of healing collars or abutments, the all-acrylic prosthesis serves the most protean role. Cut, section, reline, or retrofit it to the TEAs by using PIP to transfer their locations, followed by hollow grinding and then by an autopolymerized resin (Fig. 21-5). At this juncture, the implants can contribute to the prosthesis support mechanism but to an extent not yet quantifiable. By using acrylic as a medium of construction because of its relative softness and compliance, the earliest stage of *progressive loading* is introduced.

PROGRESSIVE LOADING   As weeks elapse during which final prosthetic manipulations are being completed, extract the condemned teeth. Take them out one or two at a time, first from

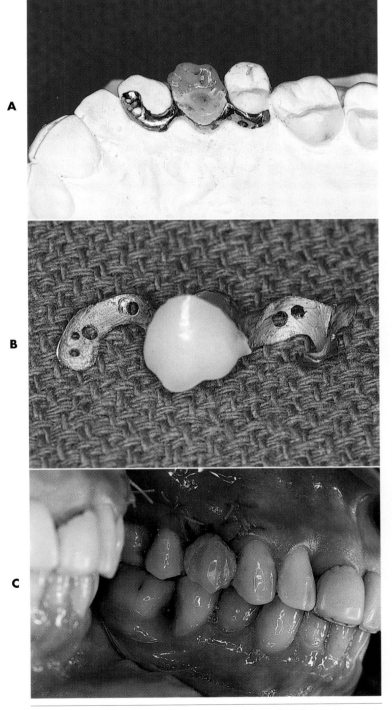

Fig. 21-4 **A,** The cast metal frame should not interfere with centric occlusal stops. **B,** Cut two to three holes through the metal wings to allow composite resin to extrude through them. **C,** Relieve the pontic to eliminate any pressure on the underlying soft tissue.

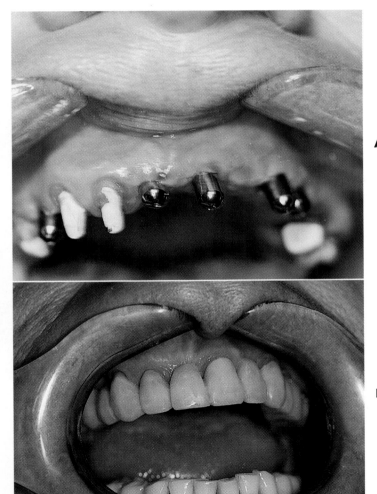

Fig. 21-5 **A,** After placement of gingival healing cuffs, use an indelible pencil to outline the location of each. **B,** The existing fixed temporary acrylic prosthesis is hollowed to conform to the newly placed cuffs and may be placed with temporary cement (e.g., Nogenol).

the areas offering the most peripheral support and subsequently from locations that contribute less buttressing. With each extraction and reaccommodation of the prosthesis, there should be an accompanying analysis and adjustment of the occlusion. These steps amplify the concept of progressive loading, which comes to an end with the delivery of the final prosthesis. If it contains acrylic teeth, the successive occlusal burden is accepted in a subtle way. If porcelain is the occlusal material of choice, the loading is intensified abruptly. In order to buffer this latter step, supply a soft occlusal guard or, more radically, change the acrylic teeth to a composite resin such as Isosit or Artglass, which offers a graduated step before the final insertion of porcelain. During these machinations, control and correct the occlusion and remove the prostheses for purposes of hygiene. Although many variables govern the process of progressive loading (sizes and numbers of implants, density of bone, gnathodynamometry, patient compliance, bruxism, etc.), a salutary result can be achieved by following the regimen described.

Evaluate implants, both traditional and provisional (or mini implants), that had been placed as supports for the prosthesis after the first stage of surgery and that were designed to serve only during the period of osseointegration, after their original function is no longer required.

If they have become integrated, show low Periotest scores, or demonstrate good bone support without significant saucerization, they may be left buried with a sealing screw. Their contribution in this role (as "sleepers") is a contribution to ridge maintenance and availability for use as additives in later times if problems should arise requiring a need for additional abutment support.

If bone loss or fibrous encapsulation mandate implant removals, extricate the implants with minimal trauma, resect the enclosed invaginated epithelium, connective tissue, or granulomata with sharp curettes and a scalpel with a No. 12 BP blade, and fill the osseous defect with demineralized freeze-dried bone (DFDB) particles. Closure should be primary or, if inadequate mucosa is a problem, with Alloderm or Regenetex sutured peripherally to the surrounding gingivae.

As an alternative to cement, attach temporary fixed prostheses to abutments with fixation screws. For this to be effective, the abutment must be well aligned, which may require the use of angled abutments. After the abutments have been put into position, place a temporary cylinder onto each abutment. The fixed acrylic bridge is hollow-ground at the site of each abutment and relined with autopolymerizing acrylic over the cylinders. After making an occlusal hole in each to allow access to the retention screw, affix the prosthesis with the use of several appropriately placed screws (Figs. 21-6, 21-7).

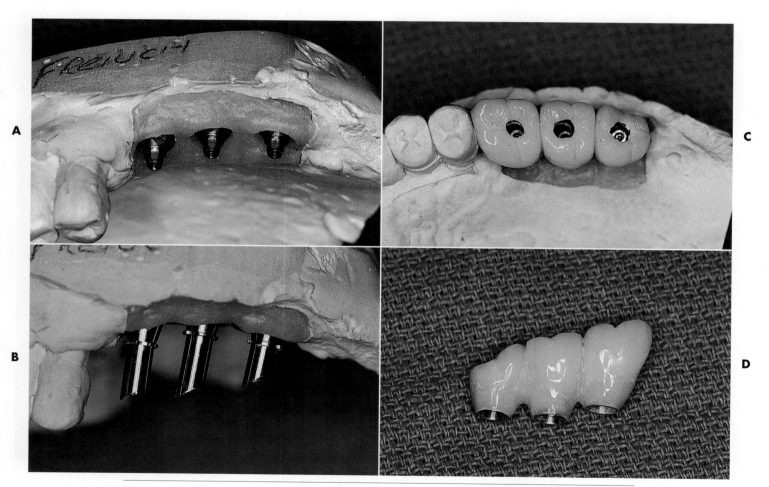

Fig. 21-6 **A,** Conical (Implant Innovations) abutments are on the master cast. **B,** Place temporary cylinders on to the abutments to form a screw-retained provisional restoration. **C** and **D,** Process the temporary cylinders into the acrylic provisional splint with autopolymerizing acrylic resin.

REMOVABLE PROVISIONAL PROSTHESES   On exposure of the implant infrastructures, abutments or healing collars are placed into them with screws. Mark the removable denture, which should not be made containing metal supports in its saddles, with PIP transfers, and ream generously to accommodate the TEAs. Reline these receptacles and the surrounding saddles with Viscogel or another soft material. The full palatal or retromolar pad coverage should remain with hard acrylic linings to offer continued support to the system. Regular and periodic adjustment of these prostheses is advocated during the various stages of superstructure fabrication.

The patient may elect conversion to interim fixed prostheses at this juncture. In such a situation, undertake a classic fixed prosthetic protocol, leading to the fabrication of a cementable or screw-retained acrylic or composite appliance.

As an alternative, the interim denture may be reshaped as a fixed prosthesis by removing palatal and flange extensions, and fitted over the internally threaded abutments. Holes made in corresponding locations will permit entry of fixation screws,

thereby fastening the converted prostheses to the underlying implant support mechanism.

Simple removal and replacement are important factors that govern the design and method of the attachment of interim prostheses because of the numerous occasions at which they must be detached and reset.

Suggested Readings

Adell R et al: A 15-year study of osseointegrated implants in the treatment of the edentulous jaw, *Int J Oral Surg* 10:387-416, 1981.

Axinn S, Boucher LJ: Use of a stabilized record base in osseointegration, *J Prosthet Dent* 59:637-638, 1988.

Balshi TJ: Resolving aesthetic complications with osseointegration using a double casting prosthesis, *Quintessence Int* 17:281-287, 1986.

Balshi TJ, Garver DG: Osseointegration: The efficacy of the transitional denture, JOMI on CD-ROM, *Quintessence* 1(2):113-118, 1986.

English C: An overview of implant hardware, *J Am Dent Assoc* 121:360, 1990.

Ericsson I et al: A clinical evaluation of fixed bridge restorations supported by the combination of teeth and osseointegrated titanium implants, *J Clin Periodontol* 13:307-312, 1986.

Gelfand HB, Ten-Cate AR, Freedman E: The keratinization potential of crevicular epithelium, *J Periodont Res* 48:140, 1977.

Gould TRI, Brunette DM, Westbury L: The attachment mechanism of epithelial cells to titanium in vitro, *J Periodont Res* 16:611, 1981.

Henry PJ: An alternative method for the production of accurate casts and occlusal records in osseointegrated implant rehabilitation, *J Prosthet Dent* 58:694-697, 1987.

Henry PJ: Occlusal considerations in the osseointegrated prosthesis, *Acad Res Dent,* Feb. 1989.

Jemt T: Modified single and short-span restorations supported by osseointegrated fixtures in the partially edentulous jaw, *J Prosthet Dent* 55:243-247, 1986.

Krekeler G, Schilli W, Diemer J: Should the exit of the artificial abutment tooth be positioned in the region of the attached gingiva? *Int J Oral Surg* 14:504-508, 1985.

Lewis S, Parel S, Faulkner R: Provisional implant—supported-fixed restorations, JOMI on CD-ROM, Quintessence, 10(3):319-325, 1994.

Lewis S et al: Single tooth implant-supported restorations, *Int J Oral Maxillofac Implant* 3:25-30, 1988.

Lewis S et al: The restoration of improperly inclined osseointegrated implants, *J Oral Maxillofac Implant* 4:147-151, 1989.

Lewis S et al: The "UCLA" abutment, *Int J Oral Maxillofac Implant* 3: 183-189, 1988.

Misch CE: Single tooth implants: difficult, yet overused, *Dent Today* 2: 46-51, 1992.

Moscovitch MS, Sebastian S: The use of a provisional restoration in implant dentistry: a clinical report, JOMI on CD-ROM, *Quintessence* 11(3):395-399, 1996.

Orhnell L et al: Single-tooth rehabilitation using osseointegration. A modified surgical and prosthodontic approach, *Quintessence Int* 19: 871-876, 1988.

Parel SM et al: Gingival augmentation for osseointegrated implant prosthesis, *J Prosthet Dent* 56:208-211, 1986.

Perri G et al: Single tooth implant, *J Calif Dent Assoc* 17:30-33, 1989.

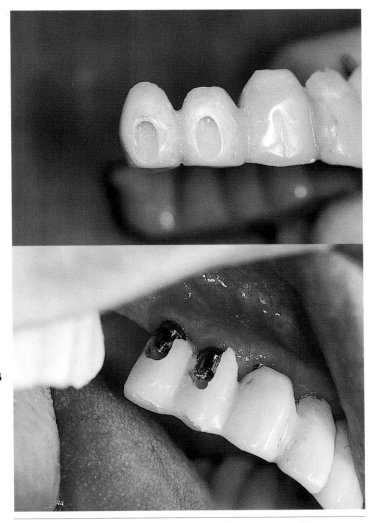

Fig. 21-7   A, By preparing an anatomically correct acrylic temporary fixed-detachable prosthesis, the flawed angulation of the implants can be ascertained by noting their directions of emergence. **B,** Although the screws that appear through the buccal surfaces of the prosthesis can be masked with acrylic, a more satisfactory result is achieved by substituting angled abutments.

22

Root Form Implant Prosthodontics: Abutments

*A*fter completing second-stage surgery and removing the healing collars, start the final restoration. In order to affix a final prosthesis to the implants, abutments must be used as intermediate devices. In the majority of implant systems (two surgical stages), abutments are the components that extend through the gingival tissues overlying the implants. For implants placed in a single stage such as the ITI, Paragon or Park, position the abutments, when attached, above the exposed gingival cuffs (see Chapters 10 and 11).

Abutments may consist of one (Fig. 22-1), two (Fig. 22-2), or three constituents, which may be separate or unified: the base, which fits into the antirotational component of the implant; the head, which protrudes permucosally and serves as the prosthetic retainer; and the retaining screw, which affixes them to the implant. Abutments can be obtained from the manufacturer in machined form or can be custom-cast by a laboratory using manufactured gold or plastic components. Several recently introduced variations include ceramic and other wide esthetic abutments. Tables 22-1 and 22-2 list the specific characteristics of each company's spectrum of available abutments for screw-retained and cementable crowns and copings. In this atlas, implant abutments are referred to as *transepithelial abutments* (TEAs).

There are many options that govern the selection of abutments. Prosthesis design plays a major role in determining the types of abutments to be used.

Whenever esthetically permissible, place the margins of final restorations 2 mm above the gingival tissues. This allows easier access for oral hygiene efforts and minimizes the possi-

bilities of gingival inflammation, which may lead to implant pericervical saucerization. In such areas, select a TEA, which will place the planned crown margin at an optimal location. Determine this location by placing a plastic periodontal probe along the gingival margin adjacent to the healing collar and down to the cervix or by using the collar itself as a guide. By adding 2 mm to that measurement, establish the proper collar height (Fig 22-3). This can be done by the laboratory techni-

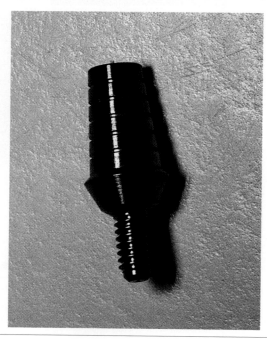

Fig. 22-1   A one-piece abutment may be used to support a cement-retained prosthesis.

Table 22-1   Abutment Options for Cement-Retained Prostheses

NAME	STRAIGHT	ANGLED	CUSTOM-CAST	ESTHETIC	OTHER
Ace Surgical	*	*	*	*a	
Astra	*		*		
Bicon	*	*	*		
BioHorizons	*	*	*		*d
Duo-Dent	*		*		
Imtec	*		*		
Innova	*	*	*	*a	
Lifecore	*	*	*		
Nobel Biocare	*	*	*	*c	*e
Paragon	*	*	*	*a	
Park Dental	*	*	*		
Sargon	*	*	*		
Steri-Oss	*	*	*	*a, *b	
Straumann/ITI	*	*			
Sulzer Calcitek	*	*	*	*a	
3i	*	*	*	*a	

*a: Wide emergence profile.
*b: Tooth-shaped bioesthetic abutments.
*c: CeraOne: ceramic core allows for fabrication of custom-fitted ceramic crown.
*d: Prepable titanium inverse cone, allows for up to 20-degree angulation.
*e: CerAdapt ceramic abutment.

Table 22-2   Abutment Options for Screw-Retained Prostheses

NAME	FLAT TOP	TAPERED	TAPERED ANGLED	DIRECT GOLD
Ace Surgical	*	*		*
Astra		*	*	
Bicon				
BioHorizons	*			*
Duo-Dent				*
Imtec				*
Innova	*			*
Lifecore	*	*		*
Nobel Biocare	*	*	*	*
Paragon	*	*	*	*
Park Dental		*		*
Sargon				*
Steri-Oss	*	*		*
Straumann/ITI		*		
Sulzer Calcitek		*		*
3i	*	*	*	*

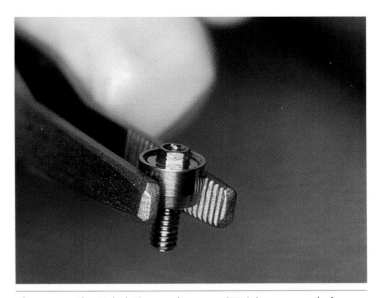

Fig. 22-2 The Nobel Biocare abutment (TEA) is composed of a center screw and an outer housing that fits over the external hex of the implant.

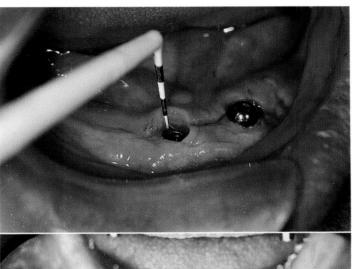

A

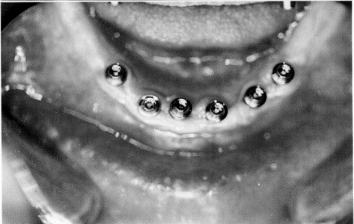

B

Fig. 22-3 **A,** After removing the gingival healing cuff, use a plastic periodontal probe to measure the tissue height, which will determine the selection of a TEA. The TEAs can accommodate a variety of gingival thicknesses. **B,** After measurements indicate soft tissue thicknesses, screw abutments into the implants that have 2 mm of additional height.

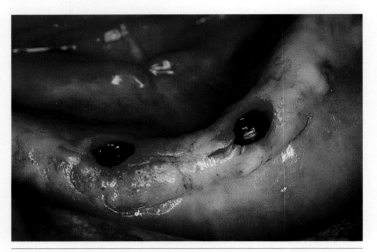

Fig. 22-4 These implants have cervices at the tissue level and may require custom-cast abutments for esthetic restoration.

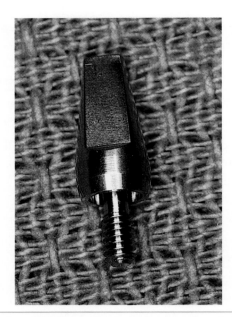

Fig. 22-5 The straight abutment is made with a threaded post.

cian or the practitioner. See Chapter 24 for the steps required to accomplish implant transfer to a cast.

If the location of an implant requires that margins be placed subgingivally, as in cases of esthetic demand or if the patient desires placement to be below the gum margin, make collar heights commensurately shorter.

In some cases, the cervix of an implant is already level with the gingival tissues or possibly slightly below them (Fig. 22-4), and no space has been left for a collar. In such instances, make an esthetic restoration by fabricating a crown directly to the head of the implant. This is commonly done by the use of a manufactured gold or polymeric coping described later in this

chapter. Another alternative, which allows cementation of the prosthesis, is to insert the abutment with a torque wrench and prepare the implant/abutment combination intraorally with a tapered diamond bur and copious irrigation, which creates a subgingival margin. Some systems do not have an abutment or attachment designed to satisfy every requirement of the clinician. There is a wide variety of abutments made with compatible internal thread patterns (Fig. 22-5) and matching antirotational bases available from several manufacturers. The abutments of different companies (i.e., 3i or Impac) therefore may be substituted if they supply a required angulation, dimension, or emergence profile.

Cement versus Screw Retention of Abutment-borne Prostheses

Cement Retention

There is significant controversy in the implant literature regarding cement-retained versus screw-retained prostheses. Screw-retention proponents cite retrievability as its major advantage.

Advantages

Cement retention, however, offers many benefits, including the following:
Cemented, fixed restorations tend to loosen less often than those affixed by screws.
Superstructures are more passive because of the space created for the cement.
Occlusal surfaces remain intact because there are no screw holes, which allows better axial loading of the supporting implants.

Esthetics are improved because the occlusal surfaces are not marred by screw heads or the patches used to cover them.
Fewer occlusal porcelain fractures occur because of occlusal surface integrity.
If cement washes out, it is easily corrected by replenishment.
Chairside fabrication techniques are virtually the same as for conventional fixed prosthetic construction.
Manipulation in posterior regions is easier with cement than with screws and screwdriver management.
Cementation is an ordinary and familiar function in prosthodontics.
Screw retention is more expensive as a result of additional components and increased numbers of clinical and laboratory procedures.
Inventories of small screw parts are more complex and costly.
Loosening of fixation screws leads to mobility of implant components, which may cause related problems such as soft

tissue hypertrophy or ingrowth, loose or fractured screws in abutments, fractured porcelain, and disintegration of implant host sites.

Disadvantages

Cement retention presents some potential shortcomings as well:

Abutments sometimes must be prepared intraorally.
Gingival retraction may be needed, which increases chair time and requires the use of local anesthetics.
When permanent cements are used, evaluation and maintenance of the implant/abutment complex is difficult.
Loosening of some components in permanently cemented bridges creates major problems when removing the entire prosthesis becomes necessary.
Temporary cements, when used, may wash out prematurely. This causes improper loading, prosthesis dislodgment, foul taste as a result of food impaction, and the proliferation of endotoxin-forming organisms.

Screw Retention

Screw-retained prostheses offer benefits that deserve serious consideration. The primary advantage is greater prosthetic flexibility. Although cementation is used primarily for conventionally designed crown and bridge prostheses (whether single tooth or full arch), they lose efficacy if there is insufficient height. In such instances, screw retention permits the use of abutments that are short, or of low profile. In addition, screws provide reliable security when mesostructure bars (see Chapter 26) of limited vertical dimension are made quite close to the mucosa and offer reliable support to hybrid prostheses, which must be removed for hygiene (see Chapter 24) (Fig. 22-6).

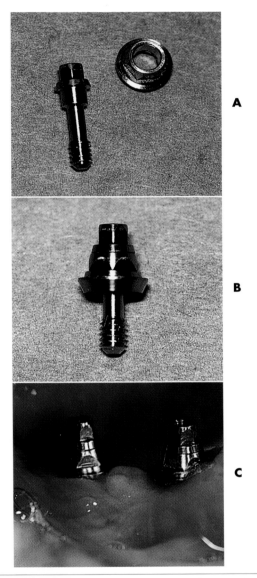

Fig. 22-6 **A,** The Nobel Biocare system supplies the practitioner with the EsthetiCone abutment. It consists of a threaded central screw and a cone component that is made available in three heights. This is designed to satisfy the esthetic requirements in a variety of clinical situations. **B,** EsthetiCone components are shown when coupled. **C,** The selection of the proper EsthetiCone brings the cervical margin of the abutment to a point level with or just below the free gingival margin.

Attachment of Abutments to their Implants

Most current systems mandate the attachment of abutments to implants by use of retaining screws, which pass through the abutment and into the implant's threaded internal receptacle.

Abutments for Flat-surfaced Implants

Abutment/implant interfaces vary depending on whether antirotational devices are included. Implants that do not have an-

tirotational elements are flat surfaced and usually demand the attachment of one-piece abutments (Fig. 22-7). Traditionally, these implants are used only when multiple units are to be splinted by connecting their overlying crowns or bars, which generally are cement retained, thereby preventing abutment malrotation. The use of flat-surfaced implants, however, should not be used for single-tooth restorations because the lack of an antirotational feature results in persistent abutment and prosthesis loosening.

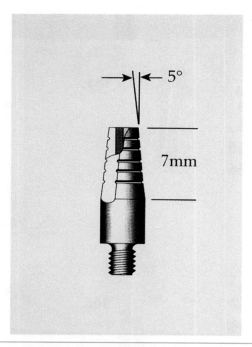

Fig. 22-7 A one-piece abutment has the screw and outer housing in one machined piece. An independent screw is required to retain a restoration into the top of this TEA.

Table 22-3 Methods of Antirotational Connection Between Implants and Abutments

NAME	EXTERNAL HEX	INTERNAL HEX	SPLINE	MORSE TAPER
Ace Surgical	*			
Astra				*
Bicon				*
BioHorizons	*			
Duo-Dent	*			
Imtec	*			
Innova	*			
Lifecore	*			
Nobel Biocare	*			
Paragon	*	*		
Park Dental	*		*(internal)	
Sargon	*			
Steri-Oss	*			
Straumann/ITI				*
Sulzer Calcitek	*		*(external)	
3i	*			

Abutments for Implants with Antirotational Features

Antirotational Features of Various Implant Systems

Antirotational features on implants inhibit unwanted movement of their overlying abutments. Antirotational components in current use include the external hex, the internal hex, the spline type interface, the Park star, and the Morse taper. Table 22-3 presents the distribution of these features in the various implant systems currently available.

THE EXTERNAL HEX   The external hex (Fig. 22-8) is the most widely available antirotational component found in implants. This design offers a great variety of restorative options due to the interchangeability of abutments among manufacturers. For example, the hexagonal geometry found atop the 3.8 mm Steri-Oss implant is compatible with the abutments available for Nobel Biocare implants, including the ceramic Cer-Adapt design.

THE INTERNAL HEX   The internal hex (Fig. 22-9) is available only in implants belonging to the Paragon system. This geometry offers several advantages. It provides a more precise implant to-abutment interface and allows easier intraoral abutment connection. In addition, there is less abutment movement once it is seated and fastened. Because of its meticulous fit, the internal hex has fewer screw-loosening problems. The internal hex permits implant cover screws to be seated level with the top of their implants at stage one surgery in contrast to the external hex designs, which are forced to incorporate cover screws that seat above the level of the implant. Therefore, in-

ternal hex implants permit simpler suturing and greater assurances of primary closure. In addition, because there is no protrusion above the bone, there are fewer opportunities for injury to the implant or its overlying tissues from prostheses.

THE SPLINE ATTACHMENT AND VARIATIONS   Splines are fin-to-groove antirotational configurations with a long and successful history in engineering. The designers of the Calcitek implant chose this strategy, thereby creating an extremely effective external source of antirotation. Each of the six external components, which are called *tines,* protrude 1 mm from the implant and are matched to a female embedded in the abutment base. Using this system, angled abutments from 15 to 25 degrees have rotational opportunities at 60-degree intervals, thereby permitting six different angles. After final positioning, a torque wrench set at 30 N/cm is used for fixation (Fig. 22-10).

For those who prefer the benefits of internal antirotational devices (see Chapter 23, Single Tooth Implants, p. 341), Jack Wimmer of Park Dental Research has designed an abutment-keyed-to-implant complex that offers protruding extensions from the abutment base, which fit precisely into six females placed in the implant top. Six rotational directions are made available in the Startech when there is a need for an angled abutment (Fig. 22-11).

THE MORSE-TAPER (COLD-WELD) ATTACHMENT   Bicon (formerly Stryker) makes a finned implant fitted with a 5-degree, tapered-wall, one-piece abutment post (Fig. 22-12). It provides almost unremovable stability in both straight and angled designs by firm tapping. 3i and other manufacturers make two-

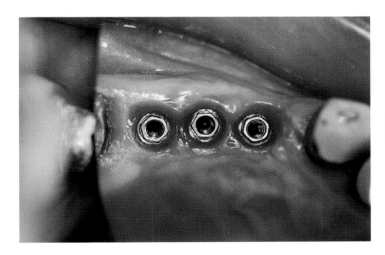

Fig. 22-8 Abutments that require antirotation must engage the external hex found on the top of these implants.

A B

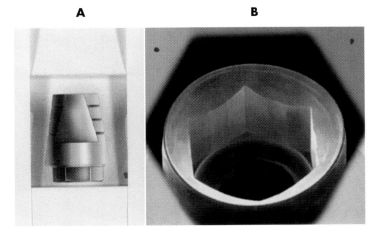

Fig. 22-9 A, Abutments for internal hex implants seat into the hexagonal depression **(B)** of the implant as opposed to external hex abutments, which seat onto the implants.

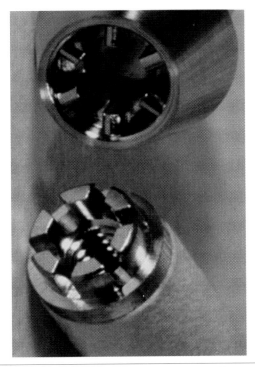

Fig. 22-10 Sulzer-Calcitek's spline is a fin-to-groove design, which creates a successful extracoronal antirotational relationship.

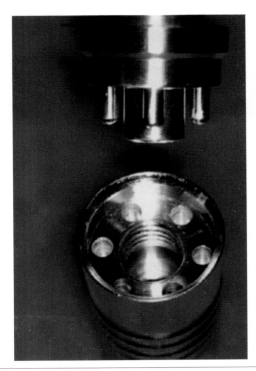

Fig. 22-11 Park Dental Research has designed an internal antirotational modification. The abutment has protruding extensions, which slide into females placed into the implant's top surface.

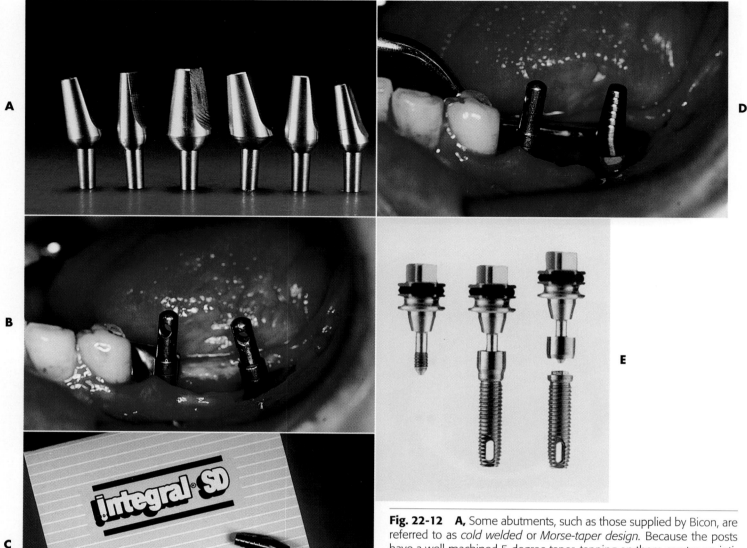

Fig. 22-12 **A,** Some abutments, such as those supplied by Bicon, are referred to as *cold welded* or *Morse-taper design.* Because the posts have a well-machined 5-degree taper, tapping on them creates an intimate relationship with the implant, which resists rotation and even removal. **B,** Submergible (two-stage) implants may be placed in nonparallel posture as seen by the two trial-seating devices. **C,** Angled abutments are available in 15- and 25-degree inclinations. **D,** Alignment is ensured with use of correctly angled abutments, which must be placed into the implant before seating. **E,** This antirotational abutment (Paragon) is made in similar fashion to those of other manufacturers (3i, Lifecore). The internal Morse-taper abutment produces a cold-weld, which is resistant to rotation.

piece Morse-taper abutments available. These are also straight or angled and have the benefit of an infinite selection of angulations by appropriately positioning the abutment within the implant (which has an 8-degree internal taper) and activating the cold-weld feature by torquing down the fixation screw with 35 N/cm of force. Further information on Morse-taper abutments can be found later in this chapter.

Abutments that Engage the Antirotational Component

The antirotational features used for abutment stabilization are commonly available in two pieces, which demands that the abutment be seated on the implant, thereby engaging the an-

tirotational component. Once this is achieved, use a retaining screw to tighten the abutment to the implant (Fig. 22-13).

To ensure that the abutment is securely fastened to the implant and after radiographic verification, tighten the retaining screw with a torque wrench (Table 22-4) in order to secure the implant with a firmness not possible with finger force alone. Torque values typically will vary from 10 to 45 N/cm. Refer to the manufacturer's instructions for guidance. Another critical factor that requires consideration when a retaining screw is fastened is the phenomenon of thread stretch. This is caused by relaxation of the screw metal after it has been tightened. To ensure continuing screw tightness, retorque the screw subsequently with the proper force for up to four additional procedures over a 1-week period. Two-piece designs permit abutments, which engage the

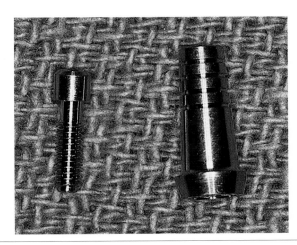

Fig. 22-13 A central retaining screw is used to fix this Steri-Oss abutment to the implant after the abutment engages the external hex on the implant.

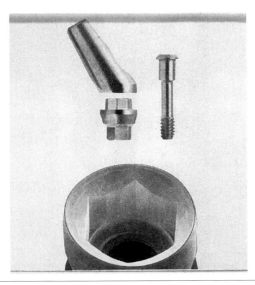

Fig. 22-14 This angled abutment system, made by Paragon, is presented with three components. The collar, with its hexagonal base, is seated into the implant. The external hex protruding from the collar is octagonal and offers any one of three angled abutments (15-, 20-, 25-degree) and eight potential positions. The entire system therefore offers 24 possible combinations of angle and direction.

Table 22-4	Torque Wrenches	
NAME	**METHOD**	**TORQUE VALUES N-CM**
Ace Surgical	Hand torque wrench	10,20,30
BioHorizons	Hand torque wrench	20,30
Imtec	Hand torque wrench	20
Innova	Hand torque wrench	20,30
Lifecore	Hand torque wrench	10,20,30
Nobel Biocare	Electric console/handpiece	10,20,32,45
Paragon	Hand torque wrench	20,30
Park Dental	Rachet	10-170
Steri-Oss	Hand torque wrench	15,35
Sulzer Calcitek	Hand torque wrench	20,30
Vident	Hand-operated contra-angle	10,20
3i	Hand-operated contra-angle	10,20,32

Torque: a force acting through a moment arm. It can be expressed in units of Newton-centimeters, or foot-pounds.

antirotational components of their implants to be fabricated in either straight or angled designs from 10 to 30 degrees. Angled abutments may be placed in any one of six positions overlying the hexagon or spline, thereby granting 60-degree rotational variations to help achieve parallelism or to alter emergence profiles. Also available are three-piece designs, which consist of an angled abutment, an interposed collar (each with its own antirotational component), and a fixation screw. The cervical element allows up to eight angulations, which adds to the versatility of the reconstruction when necessary. By using abutments of 15, 20, and 25 degrees, for example, 24 different choices are made available. However, the added device increases costs, makes manipulation more difficult, and imposes an additional potential site of failure (Fig. 22-14).

Custom Abutments

Custom-cast abutments (UCLA design, Impac) are made when precise angulations are required for proper prosthetic positioning. UCLA abutments are fabricated on models obtained from implant transfer impressions. Plastic patterns or manufactured gold collars engage the implant hexagonal antirotational component and are augmented with wax or acrylic. The resulting casting offers an abutment of flawless size and angulation. The plastic patterns that engage the hex and that require casting offer a less precise implant-to-abutment interface than the cast-to-gold cylinders currently available (Fig. 22-15, A-G).

Abutments that Bypass the Antirotational Component

The option of bypassing the antirotational component of the implant is available by the selection of one-piece abutments similar to those used on flat-surfaced implants. Since these abutments do not engage the antirotational hexagons of their implants because they have hollow housings in their bases, they may be used only for multiple-splinted superstructures (overdentures; hybrid fixed-detachable prostheses; and multiple-tooth, porcelain-fused-to-metal crowns) (Figs. 22-16, 22-17, and 22-18).

Abutments for Implants with the Morse-taper Interface

Implants designed with Morse-taper interfaces engage their abutments by using a five-degree angulated, friction-fit internal wall into which an abutment with a rounded male exten-

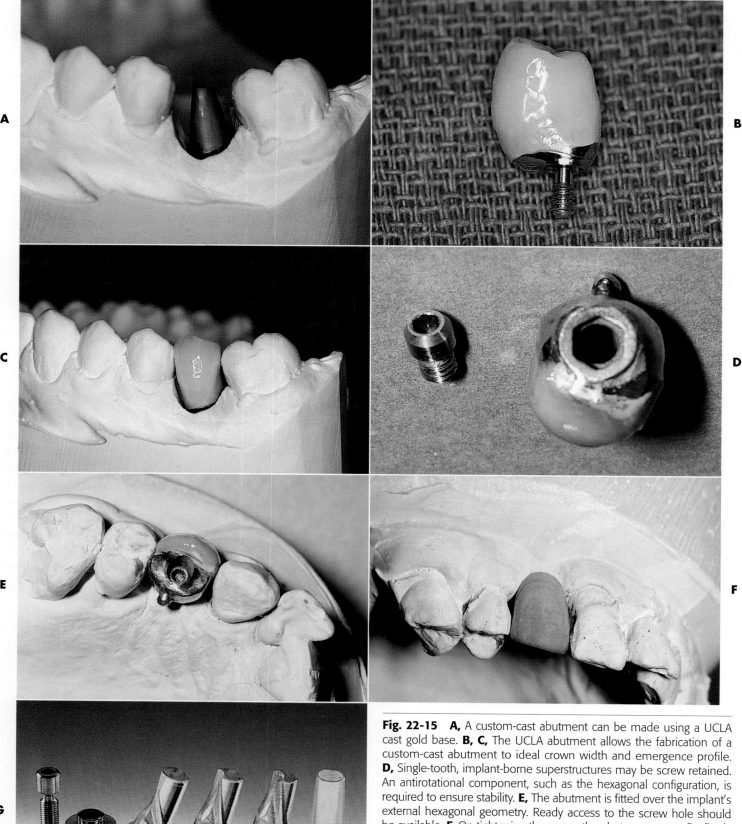

Fig. 22-15 A, A custom-cast abutment can be made using a UCLA cast gold base. **B, C,** The UCLA abutment allows the fabrication of a custom-cast abutment to ideal crown width and emergence profile. **D,** Single-tooth, implant-borne superstructures may be screw retained. An antirotational component, such as the hexagonal configuration, is required to ensure stability. **E,** The abutment is fitted over the implant's external hexagonal geometry. Ready access to the screw hole should be available. **F,** On tightening the screw, the abutment crown fits firmly in position without the necessity of wings or rests on adjacent teeth. **G,** The Impac IPA–Infinite Position Abutment—is available with a high noble metal base suitable for a variety of implants, to which a plastic head may be fitted at virtually any direction. Angles are from 0 to 20 degrees and after determining the desired position and angulation, it may be cast in gold to the base. These abutments are screw retained.

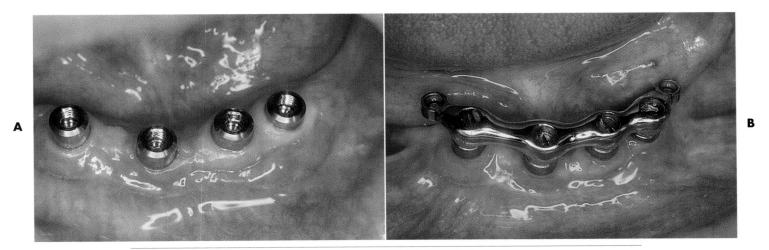

Fig. 22-16   After placement of TEAs, coping bar splints, made following the directions in Chapter 26, are placed as a fixed-detachable system using distally cantilevered ERA attachments.

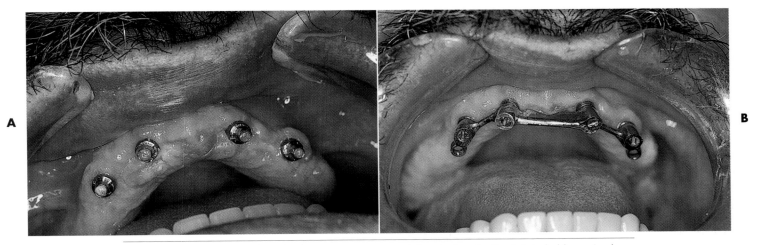

Fig. 22-17   Maxillary root form implants can serve as retaining devices for fixed-detachable coping bars.

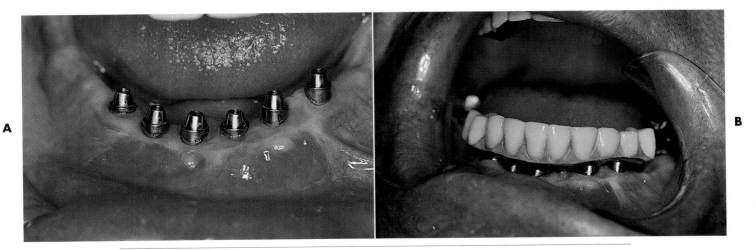

Fig. 22-18   **A,** The Sustain system was used for this mandibular rehabilitation. **B,** These six implants permitted the construction of a fixed-detachable, hybrid high-water, full-arch splint with two bilateral cantilevered pontics (see Chapter 25).

sion is placed (Fig. 22-12, *E*). Fixation in some implant designs is further achieved by tightening a central screw. Manufacturers of these designs state that the abutments achieve antirotational properties due to the cold-weld phenomenon that occurs after placing and torquing the abutment. 3i manufactures an 8-degree Morse taper abutment for its Osteotite hybrid design implant, which permits standard crown and bridge fabrication procedures.

An alternative design using the Morse taper is the screwless, press-fit abutment (Bicon Implant System). These abutments are of the one-piece variety and are tapped directly into position, thus creating a cold-weld interface (Fig. 22-12, *A*). When positioning angled abutments, use extreme caution before tapping them into place, because this system may seriously discourage abutment removal for angulation or other adjustments.

Abutment Designs

Abutments that Require Crown or Coping Cementation

Cemented prostheses may be selected in all-traditional porcelain, fused-to-metal applications ranging from single-tooth replacement to full-arch restoration (see Chapter 23). Cemented mesostructure bars are also used as alternatives to screw-retained overdenture bars (see Chapter 26). However, the screw-retained bar is more frequently used because of its necessary low profile mandated by the additional height required for the overdenture. Do not use cementation for fixation of hybrid acrylic/metal prostheses (see Chapter 25), because they need to be removed for hygienic purposes. Abutments for cementable prostheses offer classical fixed-bridge tapers and gingival or subgingival finishing lines, and after they are screwed to their supporting implants, the cemented superstructures are prosthetically managed in the classical fixed prosthodontic mode. When natural teeth and implants are to be used as abutments for cemented prostheses, make cast gold copings and cement them to protect each natural tooth. Make these copings parallel to the implant abutments to create insertion paths for long-span fixed prostheses. When completed, these prostheses function conveniently with temporary cement, which permits removability without the complex, costly, and time-consuming problems caused by screw fixation. There is some question, however, related to the natural tooth root intrusion phenomenon that has been reported when temporary cement is used. For practitioners who suspect that this may occur, permanent cementation of the bridges is suggested.

Abutments for Cement Retention

Straight Abutment

Straight abutments are indicated for replacing single teeth and for larger prostheses up to full arch, implant-borne reconstructions. They may be used, however, only when their emergence profiles are or can be made parallel. For single tooth habilitation, choose abutments that engage a requisite antirotational component of the implant. In applications in which multiple splinted or joined components are planned, use less costly implants without antirotational components.

Straight abutments, if not quite parallel to one another, can be prepared to proper contours by one of two methods.

The first is direct preparation in the mouth after the abutment is firmly seated by torque wrench. Use copious irrigation and a diamond bur to ensure that minimal heat is transmitted from the abutment to the implant and its host site bone.

The second and preferable option in preparing a straight abutment is to make an implant transfer impression. To do this, place a transfer coping on each implant and make either an open or closed tray impression (see Chapter 23). Place implant analogs into the copings, pour a stone cast, and select and place the final abutments on the implant analogs (Fig. 22-19). The resulting articulated model allows direct bench preparation of the abutments with respect to size, shape, inclination, and parallelism. Another benefit of using this technique is the saving of valuable chair time.

Straight Abutment Variants

Traditional straight abutments are obtainable with one or two components. Those with two parts engage the antirotational component present in implants (internal or external hex, spline). One-piece designs, if they bypass the antirotational component, should only be used in multiple implant reconstructions. One-piece designs are also used for Morse taper connections and can be used for single or multiple implant reconstructions.

Additional straight abutments include emergence profile designs, which have broad bases of varying heights and widths depending on gingival depth and diameters of adjacent teeth (Fig. 22-20). They are intended to deliver an improved emergence profile, which grants a higher level of esthetics to the completed prosthesis or crown. This option is especially useful in single tooth replacements of maxillary centrals and for molars being restored on single implants.

Steri-Oss produces a system of abutments that are designed to simulate the shape of teeth. These Bio-Esthetic abutments are selected at the time of implant placement. This is possible only if the surgeon has acquired a costly array of abutments. The chosen abutments are retained and upon second-stage surgery, placed immediately to contribute to gingival contour.

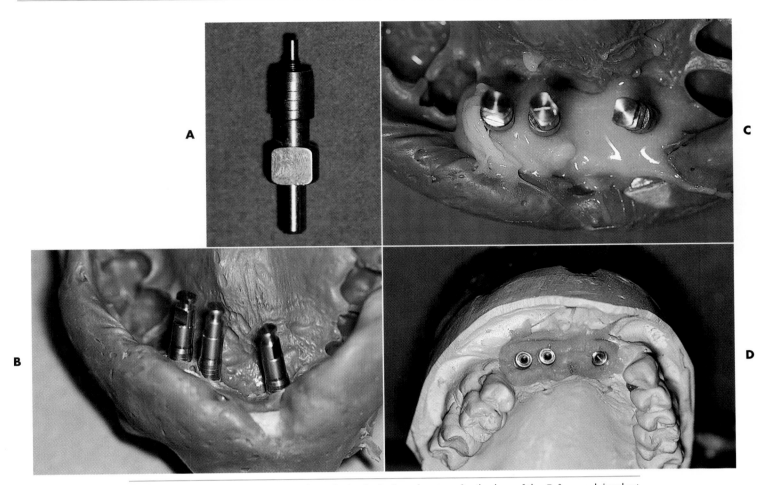

Fig. 22-19   A, This Implant Innovations device is designed to transfer the hex of the Brånemark implant to the working cast. **B,** Pick up the hex transfer copings in an Impregum impression and over each, place a hex-bearing implant analog. **C,** Place TruSoft polymeric material at the base of the analog complex to a depth simulating the natural gingivae. This will exteriorize the analogs and permit easy placement and removal of prosthetic components. **D,** The poured "soft tissue" model has a compliant and readily manageable zone of TruSoft surrounding the implant analogs. The prosthesis may be completed, through each phase, using an articulated cast prepared as is this one.

Angled Abutments

Abutments are available from implant manufacturers in angulations from 10 to 30 degrees. One-piece designs (those without screws) are only available for those with the Morse taper, which are tapped into position (Bicon) (see Fig. 22-12, A), or for implants without an antirotational component (see Fig. 22-12, B, C, D). Most manufactured abutments are available in the two-piece design (Figs. 22-21, 22-22). Such configurations permit the abutments to be seated on their implants and then tightened using the center screw. These abutments must engage the antirotational component of the implant before torquing (see Chapter 23). Three-part abutments are those with separate bases which, on their deep surfaces, engage the antirotational component that supplies an external hex, which allows six possible angulations in which the abutment component may be placed on their superficial surfaces, an additional antirotational component is found that supplies an external hex, which allows six additional possible angulations in which the abutment component may be placed. Despite the many

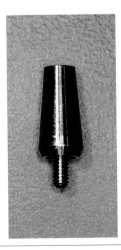

Fig. 22-20   This natural profile abutment from ImplaMed comes in varying widths for different tooth sizes.

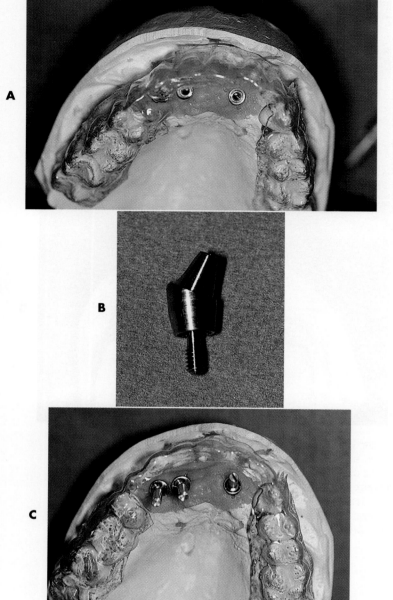

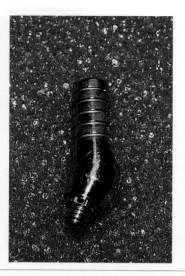

Fig. 22-22   Calcitek makes both 15- and 25-degree angled abutments. Each is supplied with an offset screw that will secure the abutment at the proper angle in any one of eight positions. The Omniloc is manufactured with an octagonal design. An additional 24 positions can be realized by using their Universal abutment in conjunction with their angled head, for a total of 32 selections.

Angled Abutment Variants

Angled abutments can be obtained with a variety of base widths and heights, which contribute to esthetics by improving emergence profiles and allowing placement of abutment margins subgingivally (Fig. 22-24).

In addition, custom-cast abutments can be made by the laboratory technician using plastic patterns to which wax or acrylic can be added (Fig. 22-25). The advantage of these abutments is that they can be tailor-made precisely to the situation at hand so that directions and dimensions not available from standard designs are producible. As previously discussed, the implant-abutment interface can be fabricated from either plastic burn-out patterns or cast to machined gold components. The latter choice offer a more precise implant-abutment interface. Disadvantages of these designs include the fact that they are costly and that the individually made components are subjected to casting inaccuracies (Fig. 22-26). Of particular concern is the antirotational component casting (in two-piece abutments) or the screw (in one-piece abutments), which consistently require exquisite fitting and adjustment modifications.

Paragon offers 15- and 25-degree angled abutments with straight or parallel cuff lengths that are from 1 to 5 mm. This permits the elimination of a separate collar component and, as such, contributes to simplicity (Fig. 22-27).

Nobel Biocare offers an array of esthetic abutments for crown cementation only. The CeraOne system provides a ceramic cap to which a porcelain crown is baked. The cap engages the underlying titanium abutment and upon completion can be cemented (Fig. 22-28). The CerAdapt system allows the practitioner to use an all-ceramic abutment. This abut-

Fig. 22-21   **A,** Of these three Nobel Biocare implants, the right lateral and canine demonstrate that their angulations will project straight abutments through the labial surfaces of those teeth in the template. This would create an unacceptable situation, since the fixation screws would appear labially in the final restorations. **B,** Nobel Biocare offers a 30-degree angled abutment to solve the problems of poor angles of emergence. **C,** With 30-degree angled abutments, the problem of superlabial pronation has been solved.

additional positions available with this design, it is often difficult to manipulate intraorally, and its multiple small parts portend increased possibilities of component loosening.

Manufactured angled abutments can be further modified chairside or in the laboratory as described for straight abutments (Fig. 22-23).

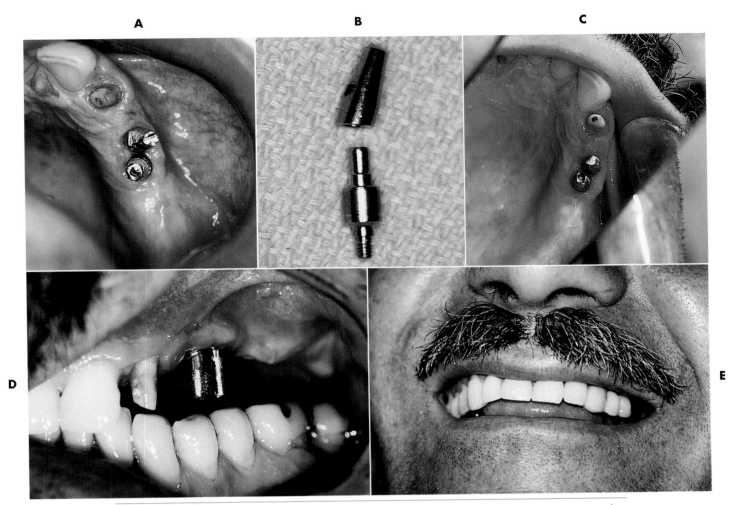

Fig. 22-23 **A,** Two Integral implants, although osseointegrated, are of significantly divergent angles. **B,** The O-butment Company supplies an Integral-compatible screw-in base, which, after placement, allows for a 15-degree angled head to be spun into a position of parallelism. When this requirement is satisfied, the head is cemented. The angled abutments solve the problem of nonparallelism, as may be seen from occlusal (**C**) and lateral (**D**) views. **E,** The completion of this prosthesis is not only esthetic, but is facilitated technically by the achievement of conforming abutment angulations.

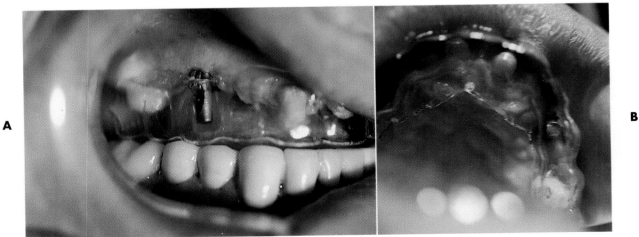

Fig. 22-24 A satisfactory technique for achieving the correct angulation of an abutment is to use the clear prosthetic template as a guide. This should be evaluated both laterally and occlusally to ascertain accuracy in all directions.

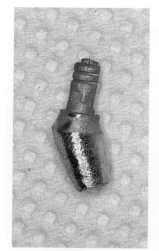

Fig. 22-25 Abutments can be custom-cast for any implant system, either threaded or not, and may be angulated precisely to satisfy the requirements of any situation.

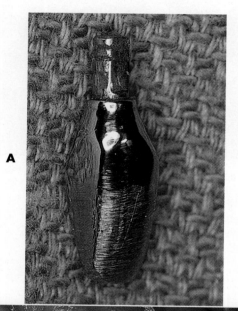

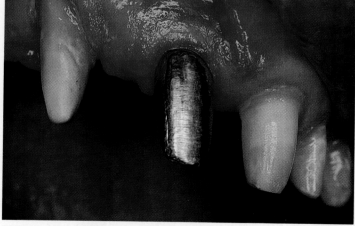

Fig. 22-26 **A,** This permucosal abutment was custom-cast. It was designed to be cemented into the implant body, has a highly polished cervix, and a matte-finished abutment, all in a single unit. **B,** After cementation, the custom abutment is seen to be parallel to adjacent teeth and is prepared to receive a conventional ceramo-metal crown, which is made in the classic manner.

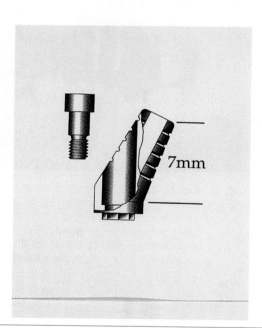

Fig. 22-27 This angled abutment with a collar as a single unit is available in angles of 15 and 25 degrees with cuff lengths varying from 1 to 5 mm in height. This design simplifies the operation of angled abutment seating.

ment provides a high level of esthetics but may sacrifice long-term strength when compared with metal base abutments (Fig. 22-29).

Abutments that Require Screws for Crown or Coping Retention

Screw-retained prostheses can be utilized for affixing any implant modality from traditional porcelain-fused-to-metal replacements (single tooth or full arch), to mesostructure bars for overdentures and for fixed-detachable hybrid designs. Though costly and more complex, this method of fixation offers great versatility, particularly in cases of limited available height.

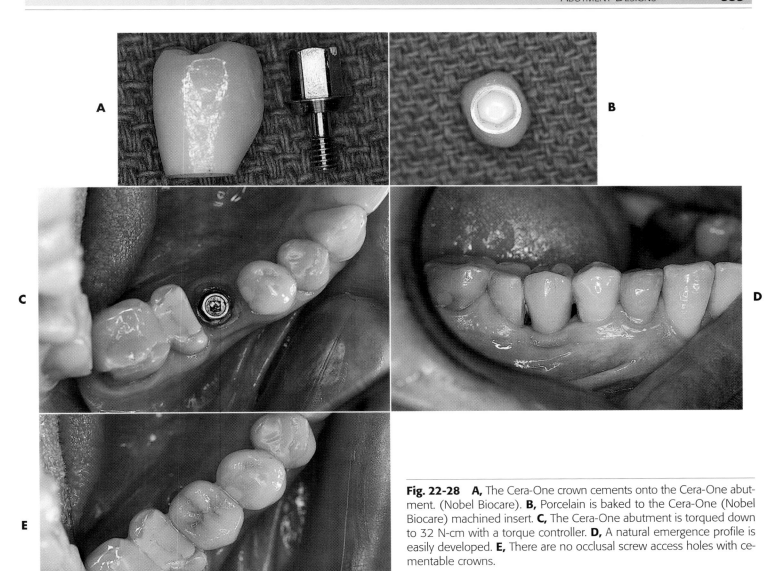

Fig. 22-28   A, The Cera-One crown cements onto the Cera-One abutment. (Nobel Biocare). **B,** Porcelain is baked to the Cera-One (Nobel Biocare) machined insert. **C,** The Cera-One abutment is torqued down to 32 N-cm with a torque controller. **D,** A natural emergence profile is easily developed. **E,** There are no occlusal screw access holes with cementable crowns.

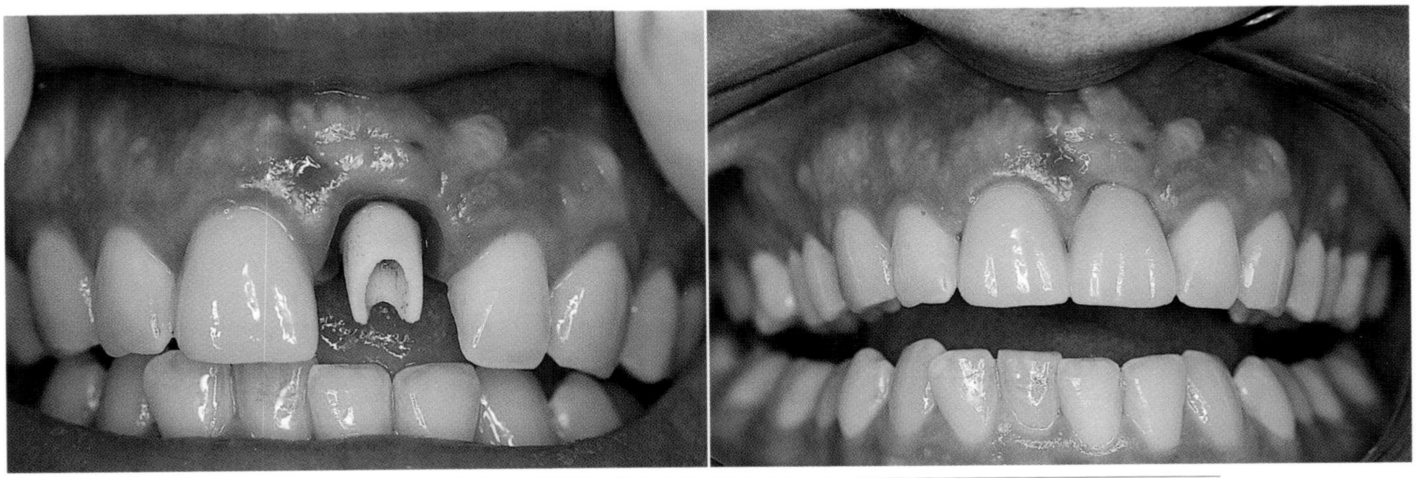

Fig. 22-29   A, The Ceradent All Ceramic abutment is prepared with a diamond bur. **B,** An All Ceramic crown is cemented over the Ceradent abutment (Nobel Biocare) for ideal esthetics.

Abutment Types

Flat-topped Abutments

Flat-topped abutments are similar to the original Brånemark-style abutments used to support bars for overdentures or fixed-detachable hybrid prostheses. They do not engage the antirotational components of the implants. They can be used, therefore as well, with implants lacking antirotational components. However, these abutments must be used in multiple implant reconstructions because of this deficiency. These abutments are available in a variety of lengths, and their selection is based on the height of the gingival tissue (see Fig. 22-27).

The benefit of this design is its simplicity. The disadvantage is that it does not have a means to resist counterrotational forces and thus is unsuitable for single-tooth replacement. Because of its straight emergence profile, it often provides an unesthetic result in porcelain-fused-to-metal applications, particularly in the anterior maxilla.

Tapered Shouldered Abutments

Tapered shouldered abutments are used in a variety of situations from bars to overdentures and hybrid overdentures to single-tooth replacements.

Because of their tapered top designs, resistance to lateral forces is enhanced, and a lower profile abutment collar is possible. The latter allows the clinician to place the margins of the abutment subgingivally, which can encourage the most esthetic restorative results. These abutments typically bypass the implant antirotational component and thus must be used in multiple tooth situations. When compared with the flat-topped abutment, less room is permitted for the divergence of implants. Typically, a tapered shoulder is angled at 9 to 15 degrees, thus allowing a divergence between implants of between 18 and 30 degrees (Fig. 22-30).

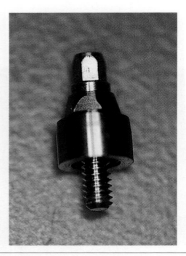

Fig. 22-30 This Implant Innovations conical abutment engages an external hex and offers considerable levels of flexibility in regard to superstructure design and emergence profile.

Tapered Shouldered Variants

Variations of this design include those with an array of shoulder widths and heights to permit more esthetic restorations by subgingival placement and more naturally appearing graduated emergence profiles. Angled, tapered-shouldered abutments are also available and allow the correction of wide divergencies of implant angulations and more significantly, offer opportunities otherwise unavailable, which permit retaining screws to exit through occlusal surfaces.

Another alternative to this design is the addition of an antirotational component to the tapered top of the abutment. This feature allows the application of single-tooth reconstruction. These designs must engage the antirotational component of the implant and therefore must consist of two parts. An exception to this is the one-piece Octabutment from Straumann, which prohibits rotation by its cold-weld Morse taper (Figs. 22-31). Gold copings that key to the antirotational components are available for most systems and can be shaped by waxing to them and casting the combination. Impac makes two gold/platinum abutments, which may be used for a wide variety of implants with both external and internal hex designs. They are available in tapered and bulb-shaped configurations for screw retention or cementation. These POQ abutments permit direct porcelain firing, which can be extended subgingivally.

Direct Gold Copings

The use of copings permits the implantologist to bypass the abutment entirely. They consist of two parts: coping and screw. Porcelain is baked directly to the coping, resulting in a crown, which attaches directly to the implant body. The coping is designed to engage the antirotational component of the implant. Direct gold copings are fabricated from UCLA-type plastic burn-out patterns, which may or may not be used with a cast-to-gold cylinder. This type of abutment is used for single tooth restorations that do not require any alterations or adjustments of angulation, thus allowing the screw to exit through the occlusal surfaces of posterior teeth and at the cingula of anterior teeth (Fig. 22-32). Due to the angulation at which most anterior implants are placed, this design has limited use in such applications. This abutment is particularly useful in situations that have limited interocclusal space, those with minimal soft tissue thickness, and those that require the placement of subgingival margins. This abutment is also useful in the fabrication of bars used for overdentures or fixed-detachable prostheses. In cases where there is minimal interocclusal clearance, prohibiting the use of either flat or tapered shoulder abutments, the solution is to create a bar that is cast directly to the implant heads by the use of plastic burn-out patterns or cast-to-gold cylinders (see Chapter 25).

Abutments for Overdentures

These abutments are used only in cases of soft tissue-borne, non-bar supported overdentures maintained directly by a minimal number of (two or three) implants used in the mandible. These may apply to bar overdentures as well, if the attachments are soldered to or cast as part of the bars (i.e., ERA or O-ring components incorporated into mesostructure bars). Spheroflex ball abutments made by Preat key into metal-based females processed into overdentures. These abutments are made available for use with natural teeth in the form of endodontic posts.

These abutments are typically available from implant manufacturers and most often consist of a male component, which is screwed directly into the implant head and a female component, which is processed into the denture. New entries into the field include the Lifecore O-ring, Della Bona, and three-sized snap abutment products. Paragon's one stage implant also offers a ball screw for overdenture retention. Exceptions to the conventional design are the Zest/ZAAG and ERA systems, which use male components in the denture, while the abutment serves as the female. The males pivot up to 10 degrees and may be changed in less than 1 minute. These abutments are available in either one- or two-piece configurations, are angled at 15 and 25 degrees when necessary, and come in various lengths (3.0, 4.0, 5.0 mm), allowing supragingival abutment placement. Attachment of the devices is facilitated by use of simple armamentaria (see Table 5-2 for a list of attachments commonly used for these applications and Chapter 26 for insertion instructions). When considering the use of these anterior-based systems, ensure that the attachments will allow rotation of the denture posteriorly to avoid overloading the implants (Fig. 22-33).

Immediate Impression Implants

Steri-Oss and others have introduced implants with attached abutments, designed for immediate postinsertion impression making. These extension pins are shaped to be seated into an

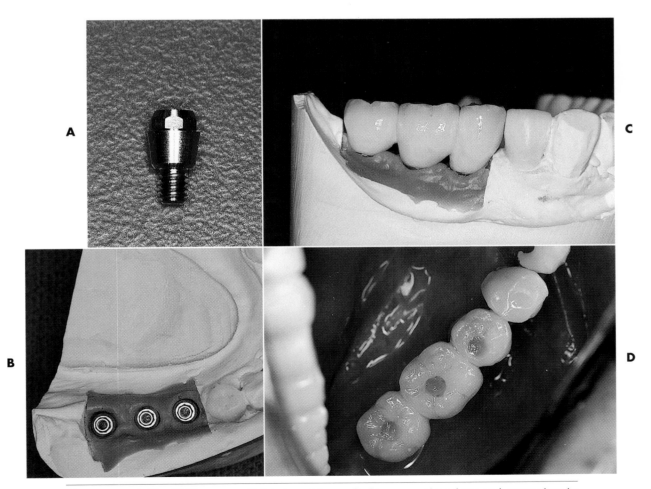

Fig. 22-31   A, The ITI/Straumann Octabutment is supplied in a one-piece form and screws into its matching ITI one-stage implant. **B,** The soft tissue cast allows easy access to the Octabutment analog. **C,** Ideal tooth contours can be made emanating from the Octabutment. **D,** Occlusal screw access holes must be closed with composite resin.

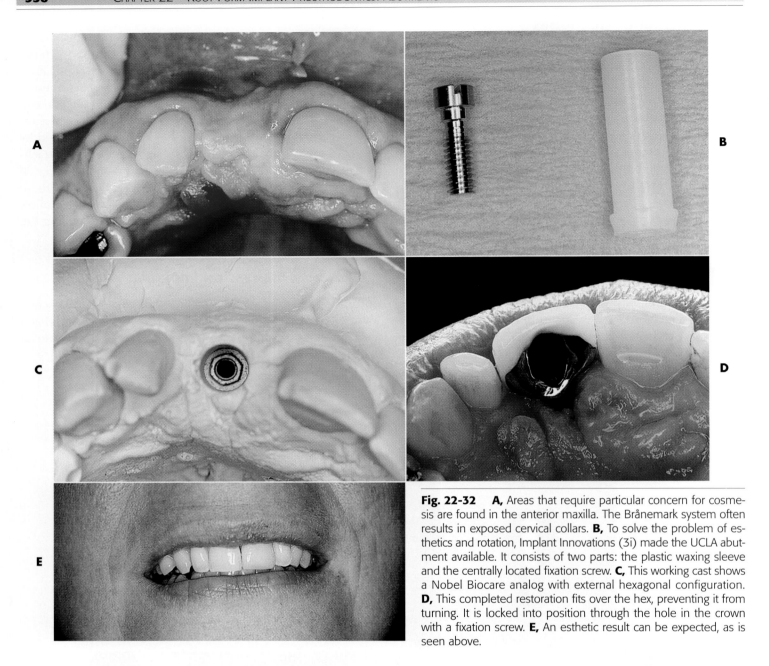

Fig. 22-32   **A,** Areas that require particular concern for cosmesis are found in the anterior maxilla. The Brånemark system often results in exposed cervical collars. **B,** To solve the problem of esthetics and rotation, Implant Innovations (3i) made the UCLA abutment available. It consists of two parts: the plastic waxing sleeve and the centrally located fixation screw. **C,** This working cast shows a Nobel Biocare analog with external hexagonal configuration. **D,** This completed restoration fits over the hex, preventing it from turning. It is locked into position through the hole in the crown with a fixation screw. **E,** An esthetic result can be expected, as is seen above.

Fig. 22-33   Abutments need not be splinted in osseointegrated reconstruction, as may be seen with these four "trailer-hitch" designs used for O-ring fixation of an overdenture.

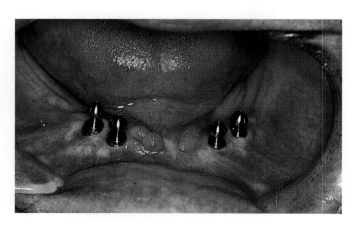

elastomeric impression material onto which implant analogs are fitted. The resulting model permits very early provisional restorations (ideally to be made in the laboratory) inserted on the day of abutment placement and influences well-controlled and predictable soft-tissue healing (Fig. 22-34).

One-Stage, Two-piece Implants

Following the philosophies of the TPS screw (Straumann, Park), and the ITI implant, a number of manufacturers are making a two-piece implant for immediate exposure after insertion. Paragon (Fig. 22-35) presents a threaded implant of the hybrid

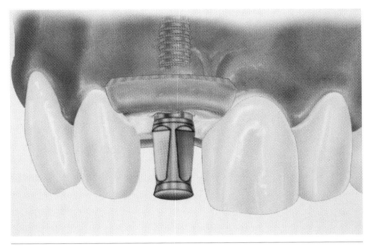

Fig. 22-34 This Steri-Oss system permits the impression pin to be picked up by an elastomer at the first-stage implant insertion visit. Early placement of interim prostheses are thereby facilitated (see p. 341).

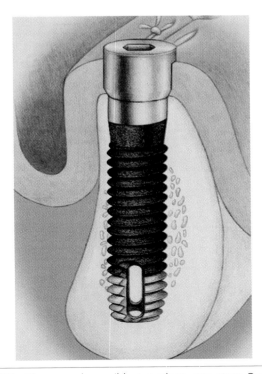

Fig. 22-35 The nonsubmergible two-piece, one-stage Paragon implant, similar designs of which are made available by many manufacturers, instructs the clinician to affix the cap screw or an esthetic abutment to the implant body with a screw, before suturing.

variety (different apical-to-cervical textures) to which a capscrew is attached just before suturing. The capscrew or an esthetic abutment (to influence gingival contouring) is left in position for the entire period of osseointegration. The benefits of using one-piece implant designs (see Chapter 11) include:
- Second-stage surgery is eliminated.
- The seam between the abutment and the implant is suragingival.
- Osseointegration accompanies healing with the same prognosis as is offered by two-stage implant design.

Suggested Readings

Assif D et al: Comparative accuracy of implant impression procedures, *Int J Periodontol Rest Dent* 12:113-121, 1992.

Bahat O: Osseointegrated implants the maxillary tuberosity: report on 45 consecutive patients, *Int J Oral Maxillofac Implants* 7:459-467, 1992.

Balshi TJ: Resolving asesthetic complications with osseointegration using a double casting prosthesis, *Quint Int* 17:281-287, 1986.

Balshi TJ et al: Three-year evaluation of Branemark implants connected to angulated abutments, JOMI on CD-ROM *Quintessence* 12(1):52-58, 1997.

Binon PP: Provisional fixed restorations supported by osseointegrated implants in partially edentulous patients, *J Oral Maxillofac Implants* 2:173-178, 1987.

Carr AB: A comparison of impression techniques for a five-implant mandibular model, *J Oral Maxillofac Implants* 6:448-455, 1991.

Clinical procedure for single tooth abutment, *Nobelpharma AB*, 1988:5.

Cox J, Zarb G: Alternative prosthodontic superstructure designs, *Swed Dent J* (Suppl) 28:71-75, 1985.

Desjardins RP: Prosthesis design for osseointegrated implants in the edentulous maxilla, *Int J Oral Maxillofac Implants* 7:311-320, 1992.

Diaz-Arnold AM et al: Prosthodontic rehabilitation of the partially edentulous trauma patient by using osseointegrated implants, *J Prosthet Dent* 60:354-357, 1988.

Finger IM, Guerra LR: Integral implant-prosthodontic considerations, *Dent Clin North Am* 33:793-819, 1989.

Gelfand HB, Ten Cate AR, Freedman E: The keratinization potential of crevicular epithelium: In vitro, *J Periodont Res* 48:140, 1977.

Gould TRI, Brunette DM Westbury L: The attachment mechanism of epithelial cells to titanium in vitro, *J Periodont Res* 16:611, 1981.

Henry P: Occlusal considerations in the osseointegrated prosthesis, *Academy of Restorative Dentistry*, February 1989.

Jemt T: Modified single and short-span restorations supported by osseointegrated fixtures in the partially endentulous jaw, *J Prosthet Dent* 55:243-247, 1986.

Johns RB, Jemt T et al: A multicenter study of overdentures supported by Brånemark implants, *Int J Oral Maxillofac Implants* 7:513-522, 1992.

Kallus T et al: Clinical evaluation of angulated abutments for the Brånemark system: a pilot study, *J Oral Maxillofac Implant* 5:39-46, 1990.

Kinsel RP: Universal abutments for implant prosthodontics: a case report, JOMI on CD-ROM *Quintessence* 9(3):361-366, 1994.

Krekeler G, Schilli W, Diemer J: Should the exit of the artificial abutment tooth be positioned in the region of the attached gingiva? *Int J Oral Surg*, 1985, 14:504-508.

Lekholm U, Jemt T: Principles for single tooth replacement. In Albrektsson T, Zarb G, editors: The Brånemark osseointegrated implants, Chicago, 1989, *Quintessence*.

Lewis S: An esthetic titanium abutment: report of a technique, *J Oral Maxillofac Implant* 6:195-201, 1991.

Lewis S et al: The restoration of improperly inclined osseointegrated implants, *J Oral Maxillofac Implant* 4:147-151, 1989.

Lewis S et al: Single tooth implant supported restorations, *Int J Oral Maxillofac Implant* 3:25-30, 1988.

Lewis S et al: The "UCLA" abutment, *J Oral Maxillofac Implant* 3:184-189, 1988.

Loos L: A fixed prosthodontic technique for mandibular osseointegrated titanium implants, *J Prosthet Dent* 55:232-242, 1984.

Lunquist S, Carlsson GE: Maxillary fixed prosthesis on osseointegrated dental implants, *J Prosthet Dent* 50:262-270, 1983.

Misch CE: Single tooth implants: difficult, yet overused, *Dent Today* 2:46-51, 1992.

Nelson DR, Von Goten AS: Prosthodontic management of the hydroxy-apatite–augmented ridge, *Gen Dent* 315-319, 1988.

Orhnell L et al: Single tooth rehabilitation using osseointegration. A modified surgical and prosthodontic approach, *Quintessence* 19:871-876, 1988.

Perri G et al: Single tooth implant, *J Calif Dent Assn* 17:30-33, 1989.

Preiskel HW, Tsolka P: The DIA Anatomic Abutment System and Telescopic Prosthesis: a clinical report, *JOMI on CD-ROM Quintessence* 12(5):628-633, 1997.

Rangert BR, Sullivan RM, Jemt TM: Load factor control for implants in the posterior partially edentulous segment, *JOMI on CD-ROM Quintessence* 12(3):360-370, 1997.

Rasmussen EJ: Alternative prosthodontic technique for tissue-integrated prostheses, *J Prosthet Dent* 57:198-204, 1987.

Seal DG: Integral implant system prosthodontic considerations, *Calcitek Inc.*, 1988.

Spector MR, Donovan TE, Nicholls JI: An evaluation of impression techniques for osseointegrated implants, *J Prosthet Dent* 63:444-447, 1990.

Strid KG: Radiographic results. In Bränemark P-I, Zarb GA, Albrektsson T, editors: *Tissue integrated prosthesis: osseointegration in clinical dentistry*. Chicago 1995, *Quintessence* pp 187-198.

van Steenberge et al: The applicability of osseointegrated oral implants in the rehabilitation of partial edentulism: a prospective multicenter study on 558 fixtures, *Int J Oral Maxillofac Implant* 3:272-281, 1990.

Zobler MN: Reconstruction of the edentulous maxillary arch by using prosthodontic implants, *J Prost Dent* 60:474-478, 1988.

23

Root Form Implant Prosthodontics: Single Tooth Implant Restorations

*P**atients should always** be informed of all treatment options for replacing missing single teeth. The following are indications to consider when using an implant-supported crown to replace a single missing tooth.

The teeth adjacent to the edentulous span may be minimally restored or unrestored. There may be recent restorations placed in or on them that are satisfactory and as such, using these teeth as abutments for a fixed prosthesis would be unnecessarily invasive. On the other hand, the adjacent teeth may be compromised with poor prognoses but might not require immediate removal. If there is bone loss or active disease nearby, however, the surgeon must be convinced that the planned host site will not be compromised.

Provisional Restorations

The single tooth edentulous area will require a provisional restoration in order to maintain esthetics and function and to prevent movement of adjacent or opposing teeth during the period of osseointegration (see Chapter 21). The provisional restoration may be a removable partial denture (flipper) or a fixed prosthesis. The latter requires that a pontic be supported by adjacent teeth. This should be done only when the teeth require significant restoration. In such instances, a pontic may be cantilevered from one adjacent tooth with a full coverage acrylic/composite restoration or supported bilaterally. However, when such peripheral care is required, reconsider the need for an implant. Discourage removable appliances because their tissue-borne saddles may cause ischemia or in some other manner injure the implant host site.

Composite Retained Provisional Restorations

As an alternative, use teeth adjacent to an edentulous anterior area to support a composite retained bridge (Maryland-type bridge) (see Chapter 21, p. 314).

Surgical Templates

Surgical templates are required for the placement of all implants, including the single tooth designs. The simplest and most effective type of template for limited surgical sites is the Omnivac style (see Chapter 20).

Impressions at Stage One Surgery: Implant Placement

When conventional, two-stage implants are placed, the surgeon may elect to make an impression of the implant after it has been seated. This permits the fabrication of a master cast with an implant analog in position. Provisional or even final restorations can be fabricated on this master cast and will be available for insertion at the time of exposing the implant (stage two). Such a maneuver will allow the soft tissues to heal in an ideal contour as influenced by the restoration. In addition, treatment time is shortened. Steri-Oss provides a design that facilitates this procedure.

After implant insertion, seat an impression coping that is accommodated by the hexagonal (or other) antirotational characteristic (Fig. 23-1, A).

The coping, which will be either of the tapered or the square/locking design, will have a center screw, which is to be turned clockwise until it engages the implant. Before full tightening, turn the coping until it drops into a nonrotational mode by nestling over the hex. Then completely tighten the center screw (Fig. 23-1, B). Using a paralleling technique, take a radiograph to verify complete seating of the impression coping.

A polyether or similar semirigid impression material should be used in a standard stock tray. If a square/locking impression coping is chosen, an open style impression tray is mandated. Tapered copings, on the other hand, can be accommodated by conventional trays.

Open trays require that a window directly over the copings. To do this, modify a stock tray. When the tray is seated, the center retaining screw of the coping must protrude through the opening. Heat a square of pink base-plate wax and place it over the opening. Seal it with sticky wax, thereby closing the tray over the coping (Fig. 23-1, C). Seat the tray into the patient's mouth while the wax is still warm. This allows the center retaining screw to leave an indentation in it. After the proper adhesive is used, make an elastomeric impression using a syringe followed by seating of the tray.

When the impression material has set, peel back the pink base-plate wax. Turn the center screw, which is visible, counterclockwise until it becomes completely disengaged from the

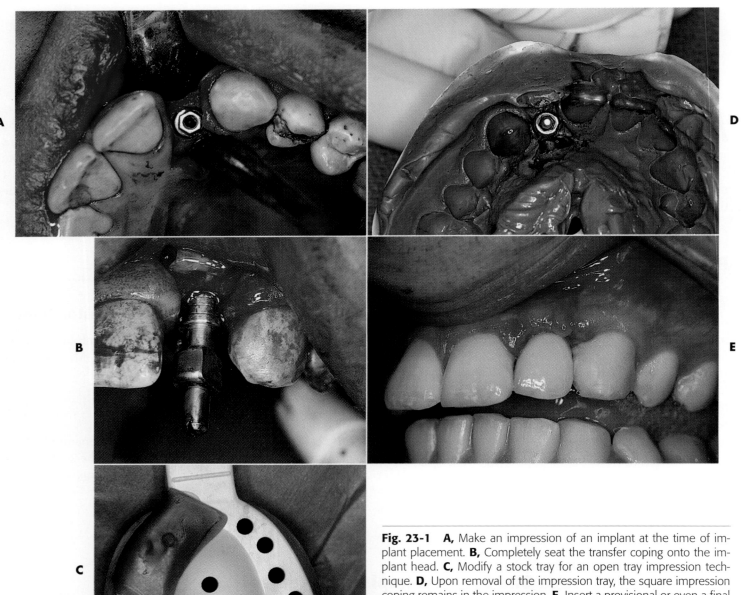

Fig. 23-1   **A,** Make an impression of an implant at the time of implant placement. **B,** Completely seat the transfer coping onto the implant head. **C,** Modify a stock tray for an open tray impression technique. **D,** Upon removal of the impression tray, the square impression coping remains in the impression. **E,** Insert a provisional or even a final restoration at the time of second stage surgery.

implant. The impression tray now may be removed. The coping will come away with the impression. Secure an appropriately selected implant analog to the square locking impression coping within the impression material and pour a stone cast.

The nonlocking/tapered impression coping will remain attached to the implant upon removal of the impression tray (Fig. 23-1, *D*). It is removed from the impression, and a properly matching implant analog is attached to it. Reseat the coping with analog in the impression. To avoid errors in orientation, accurately place these tapered copings, which have flat sides or similar identifying characteristics, so that the implant analog in its model will occupy a position exactly replicating

the posture of the dental implant that has just been placed surgically. Pour a stone cast.

Place the healing screw into the implant and tighten it. Do not allow the implant to rotate. If it does, it has not been placed to its full depth and such movement will require a new impression. Suturing can now be completed.

The master cast made from either of these impressions will permit the selection and completion of an abutment and allow a provisional or final restoration to be made to ideal tooth contours during the integration period. The abutment and restoration may be inserted at stage two surgery with the expectation that the soft tissues will heal to their outlines (Fig. 23-1, *E*).

Abutments

There are two types of abutments (see Chapter 22). They may be designed to receive screw- or cement-retained restorations. Abutments must always be detachable from these implants. Most abutments are screw-retained. A few other designs are fastened by a Morse taper design (or cold weld). These do not require antirotational devices or cementing media and often are retrievable).

Select the type of abutment before implantation, because it may affect implant positioning. Screw-retained crowns may

be fitted to prefabricated abutments, which are screwed into the implant. These abutments are supplied with copings to which the complete crowns are cast. Center screws pass through these crowns and engage them to the abutments.

"UCLA" type crowns also may be made screw-retained. These constructions, described in Chapter 22, seat on the implant and are cast abutment-to-crown as a single entity. The unit is affixed to the implant by the use of a center screw (Fig. 23-2).

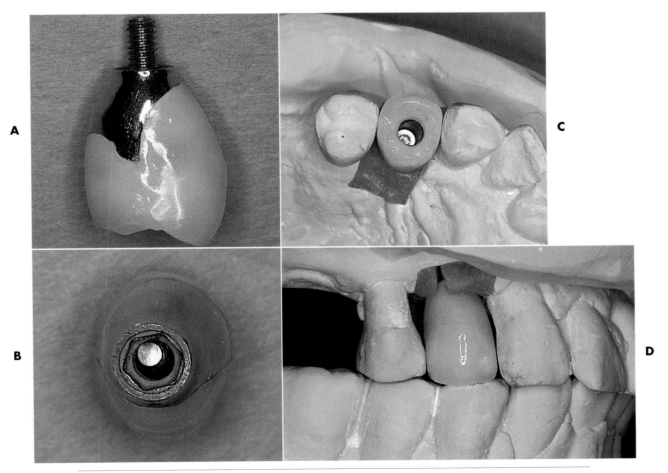

Fig. 23-2 A, B, A one-piece abutment and crown (using an externally hexed UCLA abutment) is designed with an emergence profile that flows from the implant head. **C,** Place the implant in the appropriate prosthetic position to allow the fabrication of a screw-retained one-piece UCLA abutment and crown. **D,** Shape and characterize the restoration to match the adjacent teeth.

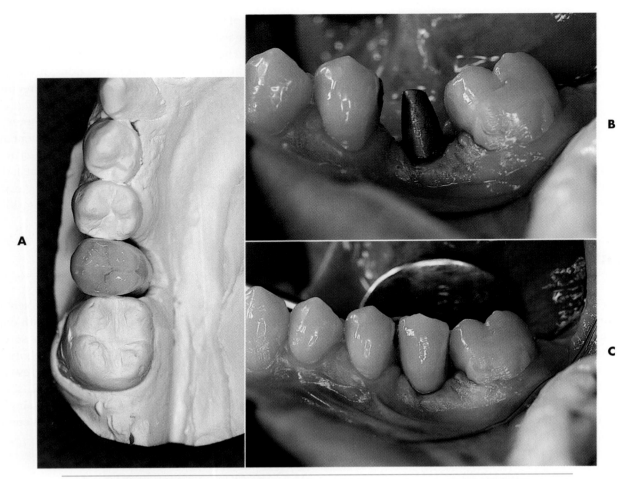

Fig. 23-3   A, The cementable crown eliminates the unsightly occlusal screw access hole. **B,** Abutments for cementable crowns may be prefabricated or custom-made using an UCLA abutment as its base. **C,** The cementable crown is cemented with a light, temporary cement.

Cement-retained restorations fit over abutments that are screw retained to their implants. These abutments are available in prefabricated form or may be custom cast. Many prefabricated abutments are supplied with machined copings that fit precisely over them. When these copings are picked up with an impression, the laboratory will be able to wax and cast a crown to it. When positioning or emergence profile demands a custom coping, make it by fitting a machined coping to the implant. The laboratory can transform the impression transfer into an abutment casting that it fabricated from a wax-up.

Select or make all abutments so that their crown shoulders will seat no more than 1 mm below the free gingival margin (Fig. 23-3). This allows for effective removal of cement and facilitates oral hygiene procedures.

All components chosen by the restorative dentist must be designed for use with single tooth restorations. These must be characterized by antirotational features such as hex configurations in or on the implants and matched by the abutments.

Impression Techniques

As noted in preceding paragraphs, there essentially are two impression techniques. The first uses the square impression coping, which locks into the impression material and is removed with the tray. The second involves a tapered coping, which remains in place after the impression tray has been removed. The technique of impression making varies slightly, depending on which coping design has been chosen. After the healing abutment and the temporary restoration have been removed from the implant, place the impression coping upon it. As described previously, after properly engaging the coping to the hex, tighten the center screw firmly. Verify seating by a radiograph.

Depending on whether the square or tapered abutment is used, select an open or closed tray. Make the open tray from a stock selection merely by cutting a fenestration through its top at a place directly opposite the implant coping. Seal this opening using pink base-plate wax secured by a periphery of sticky wax.

Next, seat the tray. Allow the protruding coping to mark its presence in the soft pink wax.

Use Impregum or another form polyether as an impression material. Accuracy will be fostered by using a syringe before seating the tray. After an interval of 7 minutes to allow for stable setting of the elastomer, peel away the pink wax and expose the fixation screw. Counterclockwise turning will remove the screw, thereby disengaging the square coping.

Remove the impression at this time, and the coping will come away with it. After the removal of the impression, screw an implant analog to the coping and pour a model. The laboratory can then proceed with the fabrication or selection of the abutment and crown.

The tapered coping will remain on the implant after removal of the impression tray. It will have to be unscrewed and seated in the Impregum. Accurate seating is facilitated by keying the flat side of the coping into its matching impression. This second technique, although similar, (i.e., a regular closed tray is used) is not as accurate in transferring the components from mouth to model.

Soft Tissue Model

Make a soft tissue model if the impression coping is found to be seated below the free gingival margin.

To do this, inject a soft tissue material in a syringe (e.g., Gi mask, Vestogum Espe) around the portion of the coping that protrudes out of the impression. Cover the coping and at least 2 mm of the implant analog with the soft tissue material. After

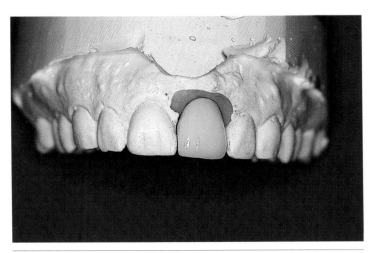

Fig. 23-4 The soft tissue model made with Vestogum allows access to contour the cervical and subgingival portions of the restoration regardless of the existing gingival anatomy.

the soft tissue material sets, trim it evenly with a sharp knife and pour stone into the impression to form a cast. Since the gingival tissues on the cast will be soft, their resiliency allows for accurate subgingival shoulder adaptation (Fig. 23-4). If an abutment is selected and inserted before making the final impression, the impression techniques and creation of the master cast remain the same. Select an impression coping for use on the chosen abutment. The choice of impression techniques remains the same.

Provisional Restorations Used During Prosthesis Fabrication

The provisional restoration fabricated for service during implant healing may be used during the restorative phase of treatment as well. However, if no provisional restoration was used during the implant healing phase, a provisional fixed restoration to the implant may be desirable to mold the soft tissues. Design this interim restoration as the final restoration is planned to look. It may be cemented or screw-retained and made on the stone cast or directly in the patient's mouth. To anchor it, use the final abutment.

Crown Design

Design the crown to have an emergence profile consonant with the outline and cement-to-enamel junctions of the adjacent teeth. Screw-retained crowns should have machined copings as their bases to retain them to their abutments, or directly to the implant (as for a UCLA-type crown). Make screw access holes through the cingulum areas for anterior teeth and through the central fossae for posterior teeth.

Cementable crowns should have abutments with a 6-degree taper for support. Abutments should be as long as possible for better retention of crowns. For anterior teeth, shape abutments toward the projected incisal edges of the crowns for posterior teeth. Design them to project toward the central fossae.

Block out adjacent embrasure areas as much as practicable to inhibit food impaction. Modification of adjacent teeth surfaces that form contact areas with the implant crown is required. Flattening of these surfaces will allow broader contacts and prevent excessive embrasure spaces. This will still permit good levels of oral hygiene. Metal in crowns must be of the precious variety. All components mating with the implant should be premachined. Porcelain, composite materials, or acrylic may be applied to the metal substructure.

Abutment Insertion

After removing the healing abutment/provisional restoration, rinse the implant interior with saline or chlorhexidine in a syringe.

Insert the abutment and tighten the center screw clockwise. Correct orientation of the abutment may be recorded from the master cast before the screw is completely tightened. Rotate the abutment until it drops into place. When it is completely seated, tighten the center screw. Verify the seating by radiography (Fig. 23-5). Once proper seating is confirmed, torque down the abutment to its appropriate preload level as suggested by the manufacturer. Take appropriate antitorque measures by stabilizing the abutment with a cone socket pliers or a manufacturer-designed antitorque device.

Crown Insertion

After seating the crown, adjust the mesial and distal contact points. If a cementable crown fails to seat completely, and the contact points have been relieved, apply manual pressure to seat it with a cotton-wood bite stick. Seat screw-retained crowns by slowly tightening the center screw clockwise. If pressure is encountered, which may be seen as blanching of the gingival tissue, halt tightening until the blanching dissipates (over 2 to 5 minutes). If necessary, proceed with tightening slowly until complete seating is achieved. A measurable torque driver is recommended to apply torque to all screws. All screws should be of a hex or other internal engaging design for easy screwdriver use. If a cementable crown has been used, a light temporary cement should be applied that will permit it to be removed about once a year. Judgment and experience will contribute to the selection and change of thin cement, when necessary. A radiograph confirms the complete seating of such crowns.

Consider fabrication of a removable cosmetic gingival prosthesis in the following situations:

1. The final result demonstrates a crown that is longer than its neighbor in a patient with a high lip line.
2. The emergence profile of the implant at the abutment junction presents overly narrow contours not soluble by a custom-cast abutment or a therapeutically contoured crown.
3. The distance from the contact point to the alveolar crest is greater than 5 mm, so that a natural, realistic papilla may not materialize.

This procedure is accomplished by replicating the completed case using an accurate elastomeric impression material (a polyether is recommended). Send this to the laboratory along with a close-up, noncolor-distorted photograph of the area. The sophisticated technician will survey the cast, establish a path of insertion for the prosthesis, and fabricate it of cured pink resilient Gingivamoll available from the Preat Corporation. Leave slight undercuts, which will permit positive retention, but still allow removal. After making a try-in to assess fit, contour, color, retention, and ease of manipulation by the patient, and after corrections are completed by the restorative dentist, it is returned to the laboratory for completion. The prescription should offer advice about the basic shape and shade deficiencies, if any. The photograph will emphasize additional characteristics by pointing out things such as blanching, pigmentation, gingival notching, melanosis, and other salient characteristics of the adjacent natural gingivae (Fig. 23-6).

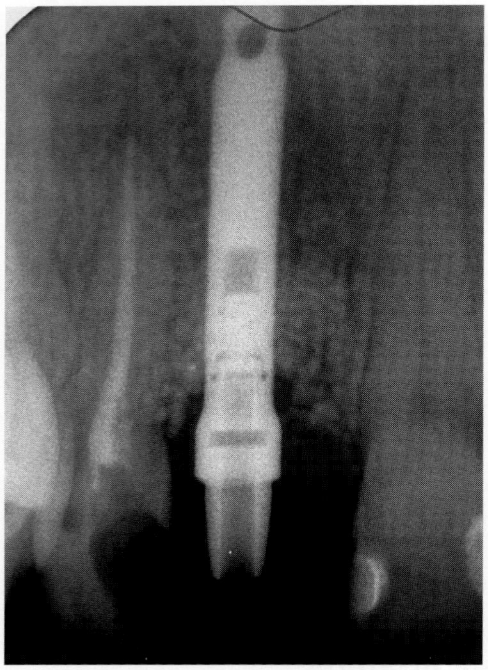

Fig. 23-5 The radiograph must parallel the implant and abutment to be perpendicular to the implant/abutment interface. In this manner, complete seating of components is confirmed.

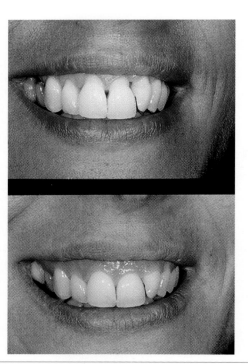

Fig. 23-6 Soft cosmetic gingival prostheses (Gingivamoll) serve very effectively as masks to cover unattractive embrasures. In addition to being of benefit for single tooth restorations, they may be adapted for use with "high-water" full arch splints (see Chapter 24, p. 359).

Make several prostheses at the same time in case of loss, breakage, or color change. Keep each in a hydrated environment when not in use. Remove the intraoral prosthesis daily for cleaning and the institution of proper oral hygiene maneuvers.

Occlusion

After satisfactory placement of the restoration, adjust occlusion for light centric contact (see Chapter 27). Eliminate excursive contacts by using adjacent teeth for guidance. Light protrusive contact is acceptable for anterior teeth.

Polish, reinsert the crown, and screw it in place using the manufacturer's recommended torque level. Place a cotton pellet on top of the screw to protect it. Place an easily removable soft, light-cured material (e.g., Fermit) on top of the cotton pellet, filling the screw access chamber to within 4 mm of the top of the chamber. Etch the metal and place a primer and a bonding agent. Place a light-cured composite material, filling the screw access hole. Finish it in contiguity with the adjacent occlusal restorative material. Recheck the occlusion and polish the composite polymer.

Suggested Readings

Bahat O: Osseointegrated implants: report on 45 consecutive patients, *Int J Oral Maxillofac Implant* 7:459-467, 1992.

Carr AB: A comparison of impression techniques for a five-implant mandibular model, *J Oral Maxillofac Implant* 6:448-455, 1991.

Desjardins RP: Prosthesis design for osseointegrated implants in the endentulous maxilla. *Int J Oral Maxillofac Implants* 7:311-320, 1992.

Finger IM, Guerra LR: Integral implant-prosthodontic considerations, *Dent Clin North Am* 33:793-819, 1989.

John RB, Jemt T et al: A multicenter study of overdentures supported by Brånemark implants, *Int J Oral Maxillofac Implant* 7:513-522, 1992.

Katona TR, Goodacre CJ, Brown DT, Roberts E. Force-movement systems on single maxillary anterior implants: effects of incisal guidance, fixture orientation, and loss of bone support, JOMI on CD-ROM (1997 © Quintessence Pub. Co.), 1993 Vol. 8 No. 5 (512-522).

Lewis S: An esthetic titanium abutment: report of a technique, *J Oral Maxillofac Implant* 6:195-201, 1991.

Ohrnell LO et al: Single-tooth rehabilitation using osseointegration. A modified surgical and prosthodontic approach, *Quintessence Int* 19:871-876, 1988.

Rasmussen EJ: Alternative prosthodontic technique for tissue-integrated prostheses, *J Prosthet Dent* 57:198-204, 1987.

Strid KG: Radiographic results. In Brånemark P-I, Zarb G, Albrektsson T, editors: Tissue-integrated prosthesis, Chicago, 1995, Quintessence, pp. 187-198.

van Steenberge et al: The applicability of osseointegrated oral implants in the rehabilitation of partial edentulism: a prospective multicenter study on 558 fixtures. *Int J Oral Maxillofac Implants* 3:272-281, 1990.

24

Implant Prosthodontics: Fixed and Fixed-Detachable Prosthesis Design and Fabrication

*S*everal *options exist* for the patient who requests a fixed prosthesis. The appliance may be made so that it cannot be removed (cemented), or it can be fabricated so that the clinician (but not the patient) can remove it by backing off its fixation screws. The term that describes this type of prosthesis is *fixed-detachable*.

Prosthesis Support Requirements

In the mandible, for full-arch fixed or fixed-detachable prostheses using root form implants, the implantologist should observe some general guidelines. If usable bone is available only between the mental foramina, insert a minimum of five properly spaced root form implants.

In maxillae, a full-arch fixed prosthesis requires a minimum of six root form implants because of the decreased density of the bone. Once again, space the implants properly.

Always keep in mind that implant length plays a significant role in determining the amount of allowable cantilever extension. Implants 18 to 20 mm long offer much greater resistance to failure than those 8 or 10 mm long. Therefore, permit maximum distal extension only with the longer implants (i.e., 15 mm in mandibles).

Insert submergible blade implants in place of root forms if anatomic conditions dictate their use. In a few instances, their abutments have attachments compatible with root forms of the same manufacturer.

Single-stage implants are one-piece devices that protrude through the gingival tissue. Abutments may be attached to them. The heads of the implant project into the oral cavity im-

mediately on insertion. Such implants include blades and root forms (e.g., Kyocera single crystal sapphires, ITI threaded designs), as well as subperiosteal implants. In general, use these implants as distal or pier abutments for fixed (cementable) bridges rather than for the detachable types. (The ITI design may be used for detachable designs.) Along with adjacent natural teeth, employ them for coping bar overdentures as well.

The best design for the restoration is often one in which the superstructure occupies a position high above the tissues to permit easy access for oral hygiene ("high-water" design), or it may rest directly on or even below the gingiva for a more esthetic result. The patient's compliance and willingness to allow this design is often not forthcoming because of speech, saliva, and food-lodging problems. The ultimate benefits that accrue to such acceptance, however, make the effort a worthy one. Make special considerations for oral hygiene when planning a prosthesis of the latter type (see Chapter 29, Maintenance and Hygiene, p. 446). The patient's manual dexterity plays an important role in the levels of home care performance; be sure to consider this factor when selecting superstructure type and design.

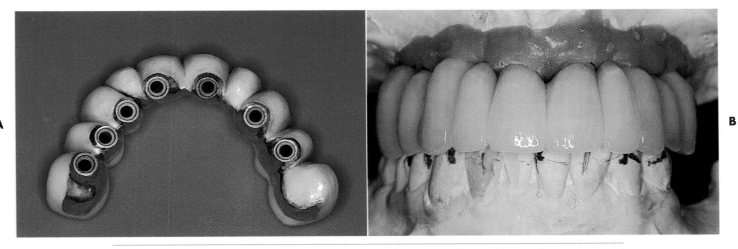

Fig. 24-1 **A,** The UCLA design, one-piece abutment and crown may be used for multiple units of fixed screw-retained bridgework. **B,** The UCLA abutment allows the greatest room for developing an esthetic emergence profile.

Use UCLA and similar custom-cast abutments when reorientation reangulation or esthetic demands require that no metallic implant, collar, or transepithelial abutment (TEA) material be seen at the gingival margin. For example, less than 1 mm of gingival tissue overlying the implant may exist, and on uncovering the implant, the standard TEA (1 mm or more in height) places the margin of the restoration supragingivally. In such cases, attach a specially designed abutment to the implant, solving the cosmetic problem (Fig. 24-1).

Preparatory Phases

Staging

Submergible (Two-stage) Implants

Abutments (TEAs) for submergible implants are designed to be attached after integration has taken place. Allow implants to integrate following surgery for 4 to 6 months, depending on location. If desirable, existing or new removable or fixed prostheses are used during this period, opt for a design that spares the operative sites from contact. If this is not feasible, then relieve the ridge laps over the implant sites and reline them with a soft material. Chapter 20 presents the details of temporization. Once the integration period has been completed, each implant is ready to receive its TEA. Chapter 22 offers advice as to the proper selection and methods of attachment of abutments.

Restoration of Single-stage Implants

Single-stage implants (implant heads that are allowed to protrude from the time of insertion) succeed best if they are permitted to remain in a trauma-free environment for an initial 12-week healing period. If the surgeon places them in a position that requires coverage for esthetic reasons, the permucosal restoration should be relieved so the implant heals free of trauma. For implants requiring stabilization, accomplish this using a temporary splint, which should have been fabricated before surgery. On removal of the splint, undertake classic single tooth restorative procedures. There are several single-stage systems (i.e., ITI), which can be placed into immediate function.

Provisional Prostheses

After the TEAs are in place, they will require a temporary prosthesis. Such a restoration protects the abutment heads, provides the patient with a more stable interim prosthesis, and adds comfort. It also establishes esthetics, tooth form, and occlusal stability. The temporary prosthesis is sometimes referred to as a *provisional prosthesis.* For detailed instruction on the selection, conversion, and fabrication of these interim prostheses, see Chapter 20.

Temporary Removable Prostheses

If the patient is wearing a complete denture, modify it at the same appointment when inserting the abutments. Transfer the positions of the abutments to the tissue-borne surface of the prosthesis using an indelible pencil. Relieve these areas with an acrylic bur to create space for each abutment. When the denture seats completely over the abutments, reline it with a temporary soft relining material (e.g., Coe-Soft). The denture is now secure, stable, and comfortable.

Conversion Prostheses

Other interim prosthesis options are available. One logical approach is to create a fixed-detachable temporary prosthesis from a denture. Transfer the positions of the abutments to the denture, using PIP or Thompson's sticks, and drill holes completely through the acrylic base at each site. This permits the denture to be seated passively over the abutments. Attach plastic waxing sleeves or temporary metal copings provided by the manufacturer to each abutment by their fixation screws. If using plastic waxing sleeves, score and roughen them with a bur to create mechanical retention, because acrylic does not bond to them. Block out all areas adjacent to the metal TEAs with periphery wax before seating the fenestrated denture. Paint pink self-curing, hard relining acrylic around each plastic waxing sleeve or notched metal coping, ensuring reliable adhesion. Following the setting of the acrylic, remove the fixation screws from each abutment, remove the denture and luted sleeves, and complete final curing in a pressure pot. Use the denture to reconfirm passive seating. Trim excess acrylic from the undersurface to leave space around each abutment for proper oral hygiene. Cut away all flanges to the crest of the ridge, creating a convex, highly polished undersurface. Reduce the posterior saddles of the denture distally so that no more than 15 mm of denture extends beyond the distal portion of the most posterior abutment. Flanges and soft tissue ridge lap contact are important in these areas for additional support. This technique has converted the denture into a temporary fixed-detachable prosthesis. The screws and denture have to be removed from the patient's mouth each time there is a prosthetic visit.

Provisional Fixed Prostheses

If planning simple fixed prostheses, make a temporary acrylic bridge on natural and implant abutments in the classic manner and cement it into place with a soft, noneugenol cement (e.g., Trial).

Impression Making

Fixed-cementable Prostheses

Single-stage Implants

In single-stage implants, such as blade, subperiosteal, and Kyocera root form implants the abutments are attached. Obtain a working or master cast to fabricate a final prosthesis. Acquire this cast and its dies by making an impression of the abutments using any comfortable technique. First employ alginate in a stock tray. Pour a cast and prepare a custom resin impression tray. Use any conventional technique with judicious application of gingival retraction cord around teeth and, if needed, around implants. Elastomeric impression materials are recommended. Pour all dies in epoxy resin for strength (Fig. 24-2, 24-3).

Two-stage Implants

MORSE-TAPER (COLD-WELD) ABUTMENTS   Traditional root form implants and single-stage implants such as ITI and Screw-Vent (which, although considered single stage, have attachable abutments) represent this group. If a system with nonscrew attached abutments is being used, such as Bicon, insert them so that a classic impression procedure may be undertaken.

THREADED ABUTMENTS: ONE-PIECE (WITHOUT COLLARS)   In order to produce a working cast for this rarely used type of abutment, screw them (which have one flattened side) into their implants. Check their alignment and relationships of fit clinically and with bitewing x-rays, and, if necessary, correct the alignment with cooled diamond stones.

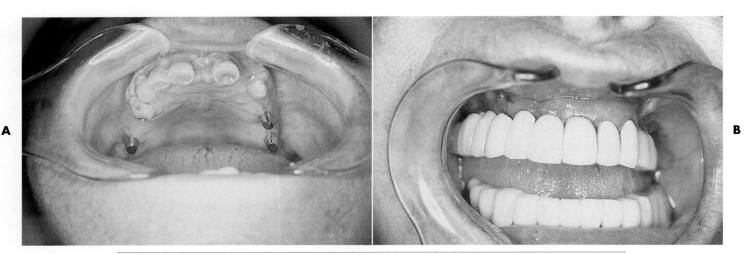

A   B

Fig. 24-2   A, A fixed prosthesis is sometimes desirable for the restoration of a universal subperiosteal implant combined with natural abutments. **B,** This composite veneered gold coping bridge serves both functionally and esthetically as a final prosthesis. If temporary cement is used, supply the natural teeth with gold copings.

If the alignment of the TEAs is acceptable after their initial placement, score each of them with a ¼-inch round bur at the gingival margins. This level is important to record in areas of esthetic concern. Then number the TEAs with the same bur, return them to the mouth, pack retraction cord, and make an impression in the conventional manner.

The scoring instructs the laboratory at which point to end the restorations, or, as an alternative, the laboratory can shorten the margins and return the abutments for a new master impression. One of these strategies is necessary because there are no shoulders or finishing lines to indicate where the crowns must terminate. The laboratory should pour the impression in epoxy resin and then proceed with fabrication of the superstructure (Fig. 24-4).

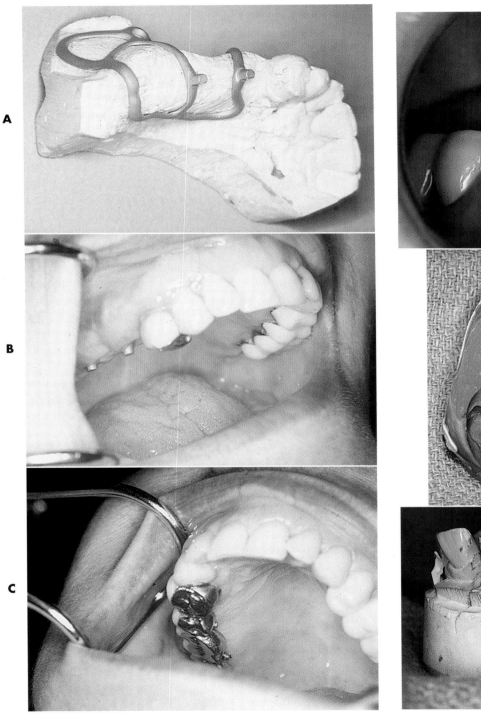

Fig. 24-3 **A** and **B,** Interocclusal distances do not permit the creation of full-sized abutments for this subperiosteal implant. **C,** Retention of the fixed prosthesis was achieved with the use of lingually placed headless Howmedica screws, which, when tightened, nestled into female recesses placed on the implant abutments.

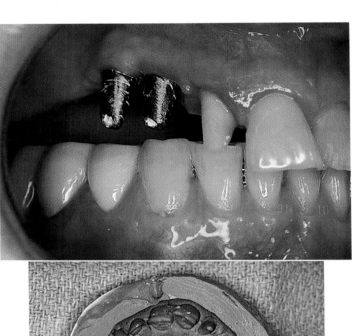

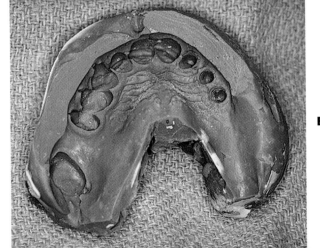

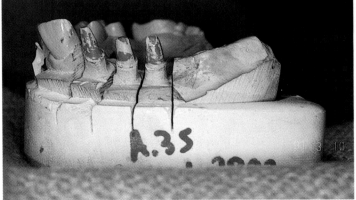

Fig. 24-4 **A,** Cemented or threaded abutments may be designed for fixed retainers to be attached with hard cement. **B,** A polyether (Impregum) impression is made using the classic technique for fixed prostheses. **C,** A master cast is made on which the final prosthesis may be fabricated.

If location, angulation, or emergence profile present problems, solutions are best achieved on a master cast rather than directly in the mouth. To accomplish this, obtain a transfer of the relationship of the implants to their surrounding tissues and teeth. Transfer copings may be used. There is one flat side on the tapered copings to ensure that they seat accurately into the impression. After tightening the abutments securely to the implants and making radiographic confirmation of complete seating, screw the appropriately selected transfer copings to the abutments. As an alternative, make direct impressions of the implants. This requires the acquisition and placement of abutment analogs for each implant. Make impressions with either a closed or open-top tray, depending on the design of the transfer device. The techniques for doing this are as follows: (Fig. 24-5).

After the removal of the impression, unscrew the copings or abutments from the implants and seat them into it. Their flat sides ensure accurate placement. Attach an implant analog (nonprecious replicas of the implants are available from each manufacturer) to each TEA that is accurately lodged in the impression and produce a final master cast. Use the analog appropriate for the specifically chosen TEA. For example, if the TEA serves as an abutment for a cementable fixed bridge, the analog represents the implant only. With this type, place the TEA into the analog in the master cast to permit fabrication of the bridge. However, if the TEA is for use in creating a fixed-detachable restoration, then make the impression with a transfer coping on the TEA. Leave the TEA in the patient's mouth following the impression while removing the transfer coping. Then insert the transfer coping into the impression. Attach an analog representing the TEA and implant to the transfer coping and pour the impression in die-stone. The heads of these analogs serve as the TEAs and are used as such by the laboratory.

After separation, a master cast has been created with each implant placed precisely as it exists in the mouth. Articulate it to the counter model with an appropriate interocclusal record using wax or polyether. If the abutments are poorly aligned, select angled types and insert them into the analogs following information available in Chapter 22. If angulation correction cannot be satisfied using manufactured abutments, the laboratory can make custom castings. If the prosthesis involves both natural teeth and implants, choose one of the following options:

1. Cover natural teeth after preparation with cemented copings; follow with a full arch of porcelain-fused-to-metal crowns, thereby splinting the teeth and implant abutments together. Such splints may be attached safely using temporary cement (Fig. 24-6).
2. Place interlocks between natural teeth and implants and use permanent cement for the natural tooth segments (Fig. 24-7). Make a trial fitting at each step. Passive seating of the metal substructure is imperative.

Fixed-Detachable, Unit Type (Anatomic) Fixed Prostheses

Many patients request fixed-detachable restorations, which more closely resemble the appearance of natural teeth and do not give the artificial appearance of the high-water hybrid design with its pink acrylic base. This is a particularly significant factor for patients who have high lip lines.

If the implants are located in acceptable anatomic positions, the laboratory provides a restoration designed as with individual crowns, each over its own TEA and with classically designed pontics representing any teeth missing between them. This technique requires that the laboratory be supplied with the preprosthetic index, articulated casts, waxing sleeves, and fixation screws. If the implants have been placed in proper positions and correctly angulated and spaced, the prosthesis may be screwed down directly. The result is far more realistic but less easily cleaned than the hybrid. Development of a proper emergence profile is essential. To do this, place each implant 3 mm below the level of the cementoenamel junctions of the adjacent teeth that are part of the planned final restoration. Make individual castings for the implant abutments and attach pontics to them in appropriate segments. Take impressions for assembly only after satisfactory individual seatings. The particular implant system in use determines the positions of the crown margins. Complete the crowns at the gingival levels or extend the castings slightly below them. In cases of thin gingivae, choose TEAs that have commensurately narrow cervical zones. If permitting the margins to be supragingival does not create an esthetic problem, it certainly facilitates oral hygiene measures and contributes to the health of the investing tissues. Design the pontics with modified ridge laps to make hygienic measures easier to perform.

Although it is possible to make fixed-detachable superstructures with single-stage implants, and even with subperiosteal and transosteal implants, the surgeon usually employs the classic, two-stage submergible type for the fabrication of these versatile prostheses. When using submergible implants, impression techniques may vary. An open tray or closed tray technique may be used.

Closed Tray Technique

The closed tray technique requires a custom impression tray. Make an alginate impression with the healing collars in position. After pouring, the implant locations are evident on the cast. Block out each healing collar on the cast with a tube of hard wax 5 mm in diameter and 15 mm in height. Aluminum shells or annealed copper bands function well as matrices. Use petroleum jelly to lubricate the tubes and mold a self-curing resin tray over them. The wax spacer provides the tray sufficient relief to permit room for impression posts that must be placed into the TEAs.

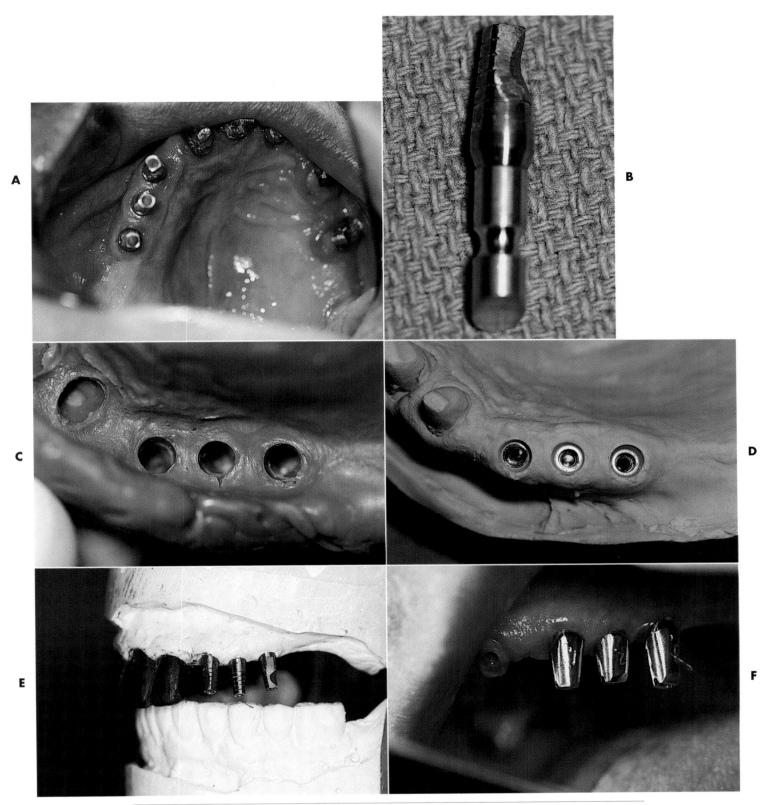

Fig. 24-5 **A,** Three maxillary Integral implants have become integrated, permitting placement of threaded abutments. Because of malalignment, they are to be used only for transferring locations and angulations of the implants. **B,** Flattening one surface of its coronal morphology modifies each coping. This ensures positive seating in the pickup impression. Attach a prosthetic implant analog to this altered coping. **C,** Make a polyether impression by picking up the three modified abutments. **D,** Pour the master cast with each analog accurately placed to represent its anatomic location. **E,** After the casts are articulated and the abutments screwed into place in the analogs, the malalignment of the implant bodies is demonstrated. **F,** The lack of parallelism is so significant that proper relationships are achieved only by the use of newly constructed custom-cast abutments.

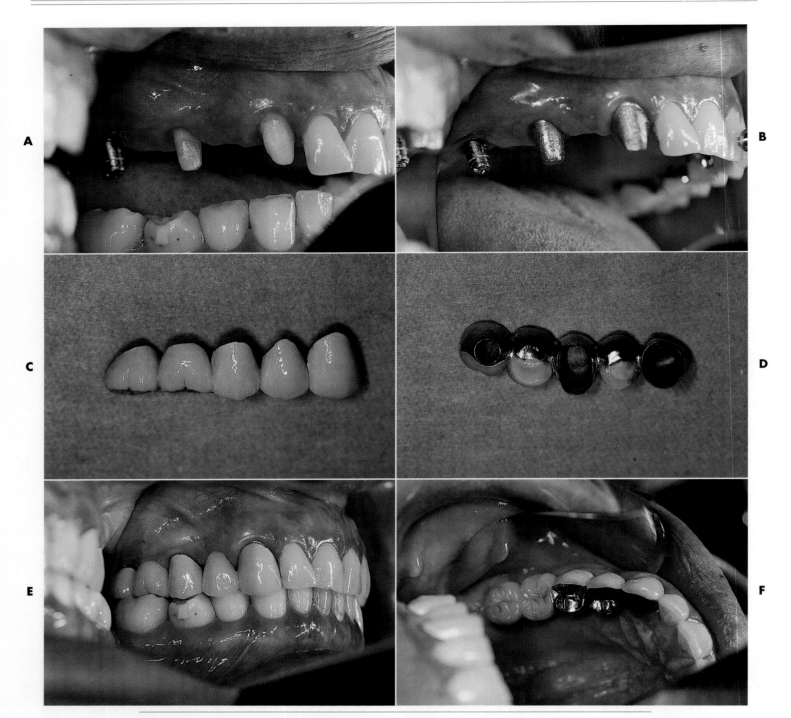

Fig. 24-6   A, A fixed implant abutment is placed in parallel configuration with two anterior natural abutments. **B,** Each tooth is protected with a cemented gold coping. **C,** The protected natural abutments enable the practitioner to make a one-piece casting without fear of caries if temporary cement failure occurs. **D,** The design permits the prosthesis to be easily cleaned. **E,** Temporary cement is used for this five-unit fixed prosthesis without fear of the onslaught of caries. **F,** For an occlusal view, the buccolingual tables are designed to deliver forces with minimal trauma to the supporting abutments. This prosthesis is ceramo-metal; subsequent adjustments, repairs, and prophylaxes are facilitated by its retrievability as a result of using temporary cement.

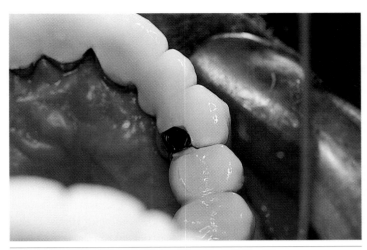

Fig. 24-7 If gold copings are undesirable because of dimensional restrictions, make interlocks between natural and implant abutments so that permanent cement may be used to protect the natural teeth.

Remove the intraoral healing collars (no local anesthesia is needed) and replace them with TEAs. Insert an impression post or coping into the threaded receptacle of each TEA.

Make the final impression using a rigid elastic polyether impression material (Impregum) to ensure that the impression posts or copings remain firmly placed in their correct positions. Examine each impression post for the presence of a thin slot or a small depression on its head (used for screwing them into place). Block out this slot or depression with wax before making the impression because recording it interferes with the accurate reseating of the posts or copings into the impression. After removing the impression, unscrew the posts or copings from their TEAs and attach them to the implant analogs supplied by the manufacturer (Fig. 24-8). Place these combined units into the impression, box and pour them in a hard dental stone like Velmix. The laboratory uses the resulting cast to complete construction of the prosthesis. If subgingival margins are required, soft tissue models are required. Insert a soft tissue material, such as GI mesh around each abutment analog in the final impression before pouring with stone.

Open Tray Technique

This impression technique uses square impression posts around which elastomeric materials lock, making it impossible to remove the impression before backing off the retaining screws. To allow this maneuver, these systems require a specially constructed impression tray that must be supplied with a window on its occlusal surface. To fabricate such a tray, make a study model with the TEAs in position in the implants. Erect a chimney of wax 15 mm in height to surround them. Next, soften and press one layer of pink base-plate wax over the abutments and adjacent edentulous ridges to serve as relief for the fabrication of a tray. Place resin over the wax in all areas except over the chimney. After curing and trimming the tray, access to the TEAs is available from above. Attach the

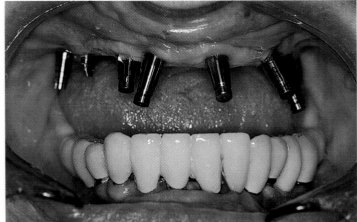
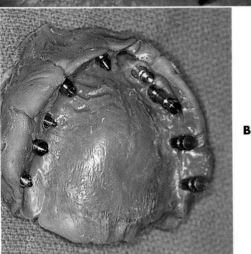

Fig. 24-8 A, Seat tapered impression copings on the implant abutments. **B,** Insert the tapered impression copings with the appropriate analog immediately after removing of the impression from the patient's mouth.

square impression posts to the TEAs using specially supplied long screws. Tie dental floss in figure-8 patterns joining the impression posts, and paint Duralay or GC Pattern resin incrementally over the floss, thus forming a solid matrix. Ensure that the custom tray, when tried in, is not encumbered by the splinted complex. Place a piece of softened base-plate wax over the open window and press until the heads of the impression posts make indentations into it. Remove the tray and seal the wax roof to the housing using sticky wax. The indentations in the wax made by the impression posts are excised through its full thickness. Replace the tray, and ensure that the top of the screwed impression posts can be seen through the holes just made.

Make the final impression using a standard elastomeric technique. Express impression material from a syringe around all of the TEAs before seating the tray, which is filled with the same material. The tray, if seated accurately, demonstrates impression material extruding through the holes just cut in the wax. After setting, excise the extruded impression material with a scalpel using a No. 11 BP blade, revealing each of the long screw heads. Back out these screws, allowing removal of the impression. Retain the square posts in the impression. Attach the appropriate implant analogs, and pour the model in die-stone material.

A working model now has been produced that permits the construction of a fixed-detachable prosthesis (Fig. 24-9, *A-C*).

Interocclusal Record Making

The recording of the correct maxillomandibular position is critical for the establishment of the proper occlusion and design of a prosthesis. Standard record-making techniques may be used for all but fixed-detachable bridges. For the latter, obtaining the highest level of accuracy requires an alternative technique.

Make a record base on the master cast by relieving it using a single layer of base-plate wax, which should be placed around each of the implant sites. The implant analogs and abutments should be visible through the wax. It is not necessary to use every implant in order to stabilize the base; alternate ones do this, as long as tripodal stabilization is achieved. Place a fixation screw into each of three disparate implant abutments of choice and lubricate the cast with a thin layer of petroleum jelly. Make a self-curing resin record base over the base-plate wax and incorporate the fixation screws into it. Bases produced in this manner should not have any tissue contact except on the edentulous saddles and, when screwed into position, is rigid and stable. Place the wax bite blocks used as recording media on the base just before its insertion. Leave the screw holes so that the base may be removed. Register the maxillomandibular position in the usual manner, take a face-bow transfer, and mount the cast on a semiadjustable articulator, as described in Chapter 4. This prepares the case for the laboratory phases.

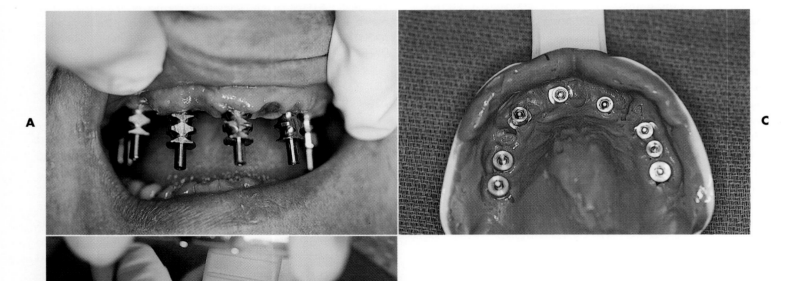

Fig. 24-9   **A,** Place Implamed square implant impression copings directly onto the implant heads. **B,** The center retaining screws for the square impression copings are seen in the pink wax on the open impression tray. **C,** After unscrewing them, remove the square impression copings with the impression.

Superstructure Fabrication

Casting Materials

A precious alloy with a low level of in-solution ionic activity (such as palladium, platinum, or gold alloys) is preferred for the fabrication of all implant-borne castings. Never use nonprecious metals. Try-in all castings to ensure passive seating. If there is any doubt about the passivity of the fit, section the casting and take a relationship for soldering. Cast metal frameworks from precious metals. Evaluate all bare interface joints clinically, and, if they are not easily visible, evaluate them radiographically. When passive seating is satisfactory, use porcelain, acrylic, or composite material to finish the prostheses (Fig. 24-9, *D, E*). Consideration of the occlusal materials in the opposing arch provides guidance in the selection of the veneering substances.

Veneering Materials

Veneering materials may be porcelain, acrylic, or composite resins. Porcelain is a material used extensively in restorative procedures because it is esthetic and maintains its shape and color with reliability. However, porcelain is hard, brittle, and resistant to repair. The larger an implant prosthesis is, the less acceptable porcelain is as a veneering material. It has never been shown, however, that porcelain is more destructive to the supporting tissues as a result of its hardness, and therefore it is not contraindicated for this reason.

Do not use the acrylic resins on occlusal surfaces because of their low levels of resistance to abrasion. The singular advantage of the resins is that they are easily and readily repaired and that this can be done with prostheses that are fixed in position. Fixed-detachable prosthesis repairs pose much less of a problem, regardless of the material from which they are made.

Recent improvements in the qualities of composite resins have made them strong and quite resistant to abrasion. They are stable in color and readily repairable either in situ or on the bench. Composites such as Isosit are the most versatile and popular of the veneering materials for implant-borne fixed superstructures.

As the number of splinted teeth increases, so does the likelihood that a restoration does not seat passively. Give attention to the design of the framework. Minimize the number of units splinted after evaluating the benefits of clinical splinting. At the try-in visit, a porcelain-metal bridge may not seat fully if the prosthesis is designed to fit below the gingival margins. Ask the patient to bite gently but firmly on a cottonwood bitestick for 5 full minutes. If blanching of the soft tissue is noted, these tissues are preventing the full seating of the restoration. If after 5 minutes the blanching persists, make mesial and distal crevicular releasing incisions on either side of the blanched gingivae to allow them to receive the crown margins passively. If there is no blanching and the restoration does not seat, reexamine the frame-to-abutment relationships. The baking of porcelain sometimes causes the substrate to warp or distort. Check this by reseating the restoration on the verified analog cast.

Follow this strategy for cementable and screw-retained restorations. With the latter, after using the bite stick, employ continued gentle incremental screw tightening for 5 minutes until accomplishing complete seating. Surgical release of the tissues also may be required. Topical or local anesthesia may be required when seating prostheses. When in doubt about complete seating, take radiographs. Evaluate the restoration for shade, shape, overall esthetics, emergence profile, embrasure design, ability to be cleaned, and occlusion (Fig. 24-9, *F-I*). Light centric occlusion is desirable with balanced excursive contacts. If the restoration is going to be actively used for excursive function, then canine guidance is desirable in lateral movements, and anterior guidance is required in protrusive movements. Follow the instructions presented in Chapter 23 for closure of screw access holes.

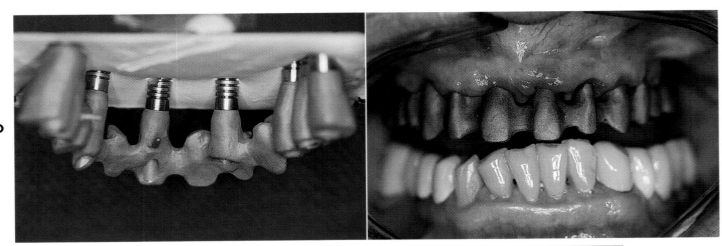

D   **E**

Fig. 24-9, cont'd   D and **E,** After laboratory assembly, the metal casting must seat with complete passivity.   *Continued*

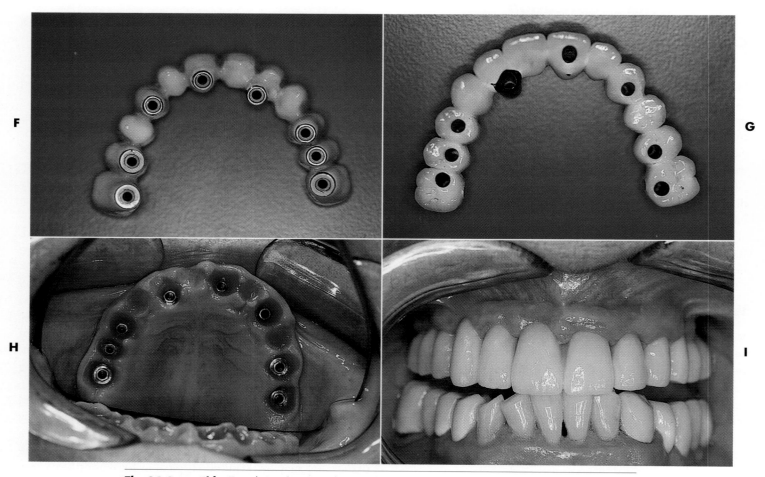

Fig. 24-9, cont'd **F** and **G,** After porcelain application, recheck the restoration for passive seating. **H,** Debride the implant interiors carefully. **I,** Seat the prosthesis and again check for passivity by affixing only one screw at a time.

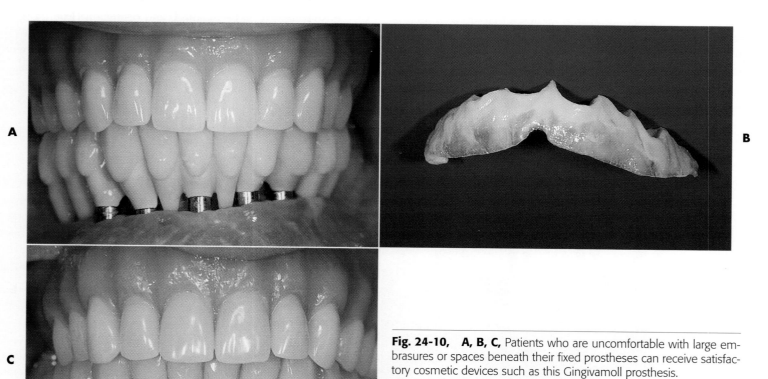

Fig. 24-10, **A, B, C,** Patients who are uncomfortable with large embrasures or spaces beneath their fixed prostheses can receive satisfactory cosmetic devices such as this Gingivamoll prosthesis.

(Courtesy of Preat Corporation, San Mateo, Calif.)

A measurable torque driver is recommended for applying torque to all screws. All screws should be of a hex or other internal engaging design for ease of use with screw hex, Allen wrench, or nut drivers.

Make a fixed bridge design to simulate natural teeth as they emerge from the soft tissue. Begin development of emergence through the soft tissues by abutment selection and restoration style. If implants are positioned very far lingually, such situations may not be possible. If implants are not placed below the level of the cementoenamel junction (CEJ) of adjacent teeth, it is not possible to accomplish esthetic restorations without the addition of ridge lap acrylic additives. This mandates frequent hygiene visits and more meticulous home care. Large embrasure areas are desirable and are more easily cleaned, but patients tend to accumulate food in these areas and object to them. These embrasures may be closed and completely obliterated, but they may not compress the soft tissues. They must permit the patient to pass floss and a Proxybrush beneath the ridge laps and adjacent to the abutments and are a poor but often necessary choice. As an adjunct, which will allow the embrasures to remain open, a Preat Gingivamoll soft prosthesis can be given to the patient for cosmetic use. The patient must remove this frequently at home for oral hygiene (Fig. 24-10).

Cantilevering

When using at least five evenly distributed root form implants of 15-mm length each in the anterior mandible, the maximum allowable extension is 15 mm cantilevered from the distal implant on either side. For the maxillae, cantilevering is discouraged, and it is absolutely contraindicated with blade implants.

Fixed-detachable Superstructures

A fixed-detachable prosthesis can be designed in two basic forms. The first is the traditional "high-water" hybrid design introduced by the Brånemark group. The second is the unit type or anatomic fixed bridge prosthesis made possible only if the implants are placed accurately in natural tooth positions at the time of surgery. The latter technique is successful only if the prosthetic workup was impeccable and the placement of implants governed carefully by using a surgical template (see Chapter 4).

"High-water" or Hybrid Design

This method allows more flexibility in cases in which implants have been placed at irregular intervals or at nonconforming angles. The techniques for design fabrication are described in Chapter 25.

Insertion of the Prosthesis

After the completion and insertion of the finished prosthesis, check all occlusal contacts and make the necessary corrections. Review oral hygiene procedures and ensure that the patient is able to maintain a high level of cleanliness (see Chapter 29).

Covering Screw Holes in a Fixed-detachable Bridge

At the time of initial insertion of the bridge, do not cover the screw openings with a polymeric composite or cement. If it has to be removed for adjustments, the presence of the masking material adds a considerable amount of chair time. Once the clinician and patient are satisfied with the prosthesis and the patient's ability to maintain a satisfactory level of oral hygiene has been demonstrated, affix the crowns with screws, tighten them to the manufacturer's recommended levels with a torque wrench, and cover the screw access openings with self-curing or light-cured composite resin. Place the resin in the opening only after the screw slots have been blocked out with temporary stopping, cotton, Cavit, gutta percha, or Fermit (Fig. 24-11). This prevents damaging the screw slot

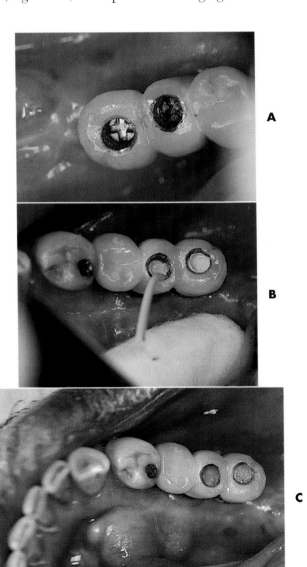

Fig. 24-11   A, Screw access holes must be easy to reach with a straight or offset screwdriver. **B,** After screw fixation is achieved, use gutta percha plugs to cover their heads. **C,** Final restorations with esthetic, smooth, readily removable screw covers are achieved with a light-cured composite material of a slightly different shade so that it may be easily detected.

while drilling out the composite at future times when retrieval is required. Implaseal, a nonhardening grout, serves as a hygienic sealant when placed beneath crowns before screw fixation. Sometimes, screws loosen repeatedly. This annoying event can be discouraged by the use of Implaseal or Cekabond. These sealing materials are nonirritating, and they discourage the screws from backing out spontaneously without creating difficulties at times of removal. On each occasion of removal, the sealant, which pulls away easily from the screw threads, must be renewed.

Cementation

The final cementable fixed prosthesis can be inserted with a soft, temporary cement initially and maintained in this fashion indefinitely if this is the choice of the clinician and patient. Temporarily cemented prostheses must be removed regularly, particularly when natural teeth are involved, to check for cement washout. Whenever possible, protect all natural teeth with individual telescopic gold copings, which are to be placed with a permanent cement. After a trial period of 2 to 4 weeks, cement the prosthesis permanently in the conventional manner.

Suggested Readings

Adell R et al: A 15-year study of osseointegrated implants in the treatment of the edentulous jaw, *Int J Oral Surg* 10:387-416, 1981.

Assif D et al: Comparative accuracy of implant impression procedures, *Int J Periodontol Rest Dent* 12:113-121, 1992.

Augthun M, Conrads G: Microbial findings of deep peri-implant bone defects, *Int J Oral Maxillofac Implant* 12:106-112, 1997.

Axinn S, Boucher LJ: Use of a stabilized record base in osseointegration, *J Prosthet Dent* 59:637-638, 1988.

Becker W et al: Clinical and microbiologic findings that may contribute to dental implant failure, *Int J Oral Maxillofac Implant* 5:31-38, 1990.

Bergendal B, Palmqvist S: Laser-welded titanium frameworks for fixed prostheses supported by Osseointegrated implants: a 2-year multicenter study report, JOMI on CD-ROM *Quintessence* 10(2):199-205, 1995.

Beumer J, Lewis SG: The Brånemark implant system: clinical and laboratory procedures, *Ishiyaku EuroAmerica*, St. Louis, 1989.

Blitzer A, Lawson W, Friedman W, editors: *Surgery of the paranasal sinuses*, Philadelphia, 1985, WB Saunders.

Briner WW et al: Effect of chlorhexidine gluconate mouth rinse on plaque bacteria, *J Periodont Res* 16(suppl):44-52, 1986.

Caplanis N et al: Effect of allogeneic, freeze-dried, demineralized bone matrix on guided bone regeneration in supra-alveolar peri-implant defects in dogs, *Int J Oral Maxillofac Implant* 12:634-642, 1997.

Carr AB, Brunski JB, Hurley E: Effects of fabrication, finishing, and polishing procedures on Preload in prostheses using conventional 'gold' and plastic cylinders, JOMI on CD-ROM, *Quintessence* 11(5):589-598, 1996.

Casewell WC, Clark AE: Dental implant prosthodontics, Philadelphia, 1991, Lippincott.

Castelli W: Vascular architecture of the human adult mandible, *J Dent Res* 42:786-792, 1963.

Cox J, Zarb G: Alternative prosthodontic superstructure designs, *Swed Dent J* (Suppl)28:71-75, 1985.

Craig RG: A review of properties of rubber impression materials, *Mich Dent Assoc J* 59:254, 1977.

Cranin AN: The Anchor oral endosteal implant, *J Biomed Mater Res* 235(suppl 4):1973.

Dawson PE: Evaluation, diagnosis, and treatment of occlusal problems, ed 2, St Louis, 1989, Mosby.

Dharmar S: Locating the mandibular canal in panoramic radiographs, *Int J Oral Maxillofac Implant* 12:113-117, 1997.

Diaz-Arnold AM et al: Prosthodontic rehabilitation of the partially edentulous trauma patient by using osseointegrated implants, *J Prosthet Dent* 60:354-357, 1988.

Eriksson I et al: A clinical evaluation of fixed bridge restorations supported by the combination of teeth and osseointegrated titanium implants, *J Clin Periodontal* 13:307-312, 1986.

Eriksson RA, Albrektsson T: Temperature threshold levels for heat-induced bone tissue injury, *J Prosthet Dent* 50:101, 1983.

Gallagher DM, Epker BN: Infection following intraoral surgical correction of dentofacial deformities: a review of 140 consecutive cases, *J Oral Surg* 38:117-120, 1980.

Grazer G, Myers M, Tranpour B: Resolving esthetic and phonetic problems associated with maxillary implant supported prostheses: A clinical report, *J Prosthet Dent* 62:376-378, 1989.

Grondahl K, Lekholm U: The predictive value of radiographic diagnosis of implant instability, *Int J Oral Maxillofac Implant* 12:59-64, 1997.

Henry PJ: An alternative method for the production of accurate casts and occlusal records in osseointegrated implant rehabilitation, *J Prosthet Dent* 58: 694-697, 1987.

Hulterstrom M, Nilsson U: Cobalt-chromium as a framework material in implant-supported fixed prostheses: a preliminary report, JOMI on CD-ROM *Quintessence* 6(4):475-480, 1991.

Hulterstrom M, Nilsson U: Cobalt-chromium as a framework material in implant-supported fixed prostheses: a 3-year follow-up report, JOMI on CD-ROM *Quintessence* 9(4):449-454, 1994.

Humphries RM, Yamen P, Bloem TJ: The accuracy of implant master casts constructed from transfer impressions, *J Oral Maxillofac Implants* 5:331-336, 1990.

Hurzeler M et al: Treatment of peri-implantitis using guided bone regeneration and bone grafts, albone or in combination, in beagle dogs. II. Histologic findings, *Int J Oral Maxillofac Implant* 12:168-175, 1997.

Jemt T, Linden B, Lekholm U: Failures and complications in 127 consecutively placed fixed partial prostheses supported by Brånemark implants: from prosthetic treatment to first annual checkup, *Int J Oral Maxillofac Implant* 7:40-45, 1992.

Jemt T: Modified single and short-span restorations supported by osseointegrated fixtures in the partially edentulous jaw, *J Prosthet Dent* 55:243-247, 1986.

Jensen S et al: Tissue reaction and material characteristics of four bone substitutes, *Int J Oral Maxillofac Implant* 11:55-67, 1996.

Judy WK: Multiple uses of resorbable tri-calcium phosphate, *New York Dent J* 53:1983.

Kan J et al: Mandibular fracture after endosseous implant placement in conjunction with inferior alveolar nerve transposition: a patient treatment report, *Int J Oral Maxillofac Implant* 12:655-660, 1997.

Kan J et al: Endosseous implant placement in conjunction with inferior alveolar nerve transposition: an evaluation of neurosensory disturbance, *Int J Oral Maxillofac Implant* 12:463-471, 1997.

Knudson RC et al: Implant transfer coping verification jig, *J Prosthet Dent* 61:601-602, 1989.

Laney WR, Gibelisco JA: *Diagnosis and treatment in prosthodontics*, Philadelphia, 1983, Lea & Febiger, p. 169.

Lang B, Mossie H, Razzoog M: *International workshop: biocompatibility, toxicity and hypersensitivity to alloy systems used in dentistry*, Ann Arbor, Mich., University of Michigan Press.

Leghissa G, Botticelli A: Resistance to bacterial aggression involving exposed nonresorbable membranes in the oral cavity, *Int J Oral Maxillofac Implants*, 11(2):210-215, 1996.

Loos L: A fixed prosthodontic technique for mandibular osseointegrated titanium implants, *J Prosthet Dent* 55:232-242, 1984.

Mason M et al: Mandibular fracture through endosseous cylinder implants, *J Oral Maxillofac Surg* 48:311-317, 1990.

Misch CE, Crawford EA: Predictable mandibular nerve location—a clinical zone of safety, *Int J Oral Implant* 7:37-44, 1990.

Misch CE: Blade vent implant: still viable, *Dent Today* 8(9):34, 42, 1989.

Misch CE: Direct bone impression—material and techniques, *International Congress of Oral Implant,* 1st Subperiosteal Symposium, San Diego, October, 1981.

Misch CE: *Protect the prosthesis (manual).* Misch Implant Institute, 1990.

Mombelli A et al: The microbiota associated with successful or failing osseointegrated titanium implants, *Oral Microbiol Immunol* 2:145, 1987.

Mordenfeld A, Andersson L, Bergstrom B: Hemorrhage in the floor of the mouth during implant placement in the edentulous mandible: a case report, *Int J Oral Maxillofac Implant* 12:558-561, 1997.

Nelson DR, Von Gonten AS: Prosthodontic management of the hydoxyapatite-augmented ridge, *Gen Dent* July-August: 315-319, 1988.

O'Roark WL: Improving implant survival rates by using a new method of at risk analysis, *Int J Oral Implant* 8:31-57, 1991.

Palmqvist S et al: Marginal bone levels around maxillary implants supporting overdentures or fixed prostheses: a comparative study using detailed narrow-beam radiographs, *Int J Oral Maxillofac Implants* 11(2):223-227, 1996.

Parel SM et al: Gingival augmentation for osseointegrated implant prosthesis, *J Prosthet Dent* 56:208-211, 1986.

Pertri WH: Osteogenic activity of antibiotic-supplemented bone allografts in the guinea pig, *J Oral Maxillofac Surg* 42:631-636, 1984.

Phillips KM et al: The accuracy of three implant impression Techniques: a three-dimensional analysis, JOMI on CD-ROM *Quintessence* 9(5):533-540, 1995.

Rejda BV, Peelen JCJ, Grot K: Tri-calcium phosphate as a bone substitute, *Bioengineering* 1:93, 1977.

Rosenquist B: A comparison of various methods of soft tissue management following the immediate placement of implants into extraction sockets, *Int J Oral Maxillofac Implant* 12:43-51, 1997.

Sager RD, Thies RM: Implant-retained precision two-stage single tooth replacement, *J Oral Implantol* 17:166-171, 1991.

Salcetti J et al: The clinical, microbial, and host response characteristics of failing implant, *Int J Oral Maxillofac Implant* 12:32-42, 1997.

Salinas TJ et al: Spark erosion implant-supported overdentures: clinical and laboratory techniques, *Implant Dent* 1:246-251, 1992.

Scher EL: The use of osseointegrated implants in long-span fixed partial prosthesis: a case report, *J Oral Maxillofac Implants* 6:351-355, 1991.

Schnitman PA et al: Immediate fixed interim prostheses supported by two-stage threaded implants: methodology and results, *J Oral Implantol* 16-95-103, 1990.

Schnell RJ, Phillips RW: Dimensional stability of rubber base impressions and certain other factors affecting accuracy, *J Am Dent Assoc* 57:39, 1958.

Simion M et al: Treatment of dehiscences and fenestrations around dental implants using resorbable and nonresorbable membranes associated with bone autografts: a comparative clinical study, *Int J Oral Maxillofac Implant* 12:159-168, 1997.

Spector MR, Donovan TE, Nicholls JI: An evaluation of impression techniques for osseointegrated implants, *J Prosthet Dent* 63:444-447, 1990.

Stefani LA: The care and maintenance of the dental implant patient, *J Dent Hygiene* 10:447-466, 1988.

Symposium on Retrieval and Analysis of Surgical Implants and Biomaterials, *Society for Biomaterials,* Snowbird, Utah, 1988.

Takeshita F et al: Histologic study of failed hollow implants, *Int J Oral Maxillofac Implant* 11(2):245-254, 1996.

Taylor TD: Fixed implant rehabilitation for the edentulous maxilla, *J Oral Maxillofac Implant* 329-337, 1991.

Teixeira E et al: Correlation between mucosal inflammation and marginal bone loss around hydroxyapatite-coated implants: a 3-year cross-sectional study, *Int J Oral Maxillofac Implant* 12:74-81, 1997.

Thomson-Neal D et al: A SEM evaluation of various prophylactic modalities on different implants, *Int J Perio Rest Dent* 4;1989.

Tolman DE, Keller EE: Management of mandibular fractures in patients with endosseous implants, *Int J Oral Maxillofac Implants* 6:427-436, 1991.

Tulasne JF: Implant treatment of missing posterior dentition. In Zarb G, Albrektsson T, editors: *The Brånemark implant,* Chicago, 1989, Quintessence.

van Steenberge et al: The applicability of osseointegrated oral implants in the rehabilitation of partial edentulism: a prospective multicenter study on 558 fixtures, *Int J Oral Maxillofac Implant* 3:272-281, 1990.

Viscido A: Submerged function predictive endosteal blade implants, *J Oral Implant* 15:195-209, 1974.

Walton JN, Gardner FM, Agar JR: A survey of crown and fixed partial denture fixtures: length of service and reasons for replacement, *J Prosthet Dent* 56(4):416-421, 1986.

Weinmann JP: Biological factors influencing implant denture success, *J Implant Dent* 2:12-15, 1956.

Weiss CM: A comparative analysis of fibro-osteal and osteal integration and other variables that affect long-term bone maintenance around dental implants, *J Oral Implant* 13:467-487, 1987.

Wolinsky LE, Camargo PM, Erard JC: A study of in vitro attachment of *Streptococcus sanguis* and *Actinomyces viscosus* to saliva-treated titanium, *Int J Oral Maxillofac Implant* 4:27-31, 1989.

Zablotsky M. Meffert RM, Caudill R et al: Histological and clinical comparisons of guided tissue regeneration on dehisced hydroxylapatite-coated and titanium endosseous implant surfaces: a pilot study, *Int J Oral Maxillofac Implant* 6:295-303, 1991.

25

Implant Prosthodontics: Hybrid Bridge Fixed-Detachable Prosthesis Design and Fabrication

Fully Edentulous Arch

*T*he *hybrid bridge* is a fixed bridge made of denture teeth processed to a cast metal barlike framework. The prosthesis must be screw retained, and it is usually used in arches that are completely edentulous. Its prognosis is best when the opposing arch is complete denture or another hybrid bridge. Mandibular prostheses require a minimum of five implants; maxillary hybrid bridges require six or preferably, more. The greater the number of maxillary root form implants placed (even up to 12), the better the prognosis. The hybrid bridge is a less costly bridge to make, and it is less demanding technically to fabricate than fixed or fixed-detachable prostheses. It is a useful bridge for patients who have significant loss of alveolar dimension, whose teeth would appear unrealistically long were a conventional construction technique used. The most valuable of the benefits attributed to the hybrid is that it can serve well both functionally and cosmetically when implant emergence angles prohibit classic techniques of construction.

Provisional Restoration

The completely edentulous jaw may be restored with one of two types of provisional prostheses before and during implant treatment. The provisional restorations may be complete removable dentures or provisional fixed bridges made subsequent to the second stage of surgery. Chapter 21, Interim Prostheses, (p. 317) describes in detail the manner in which any of the designs selected for patient comfort can be fabricated.

Surgical Template

A surgical template is necessary to accurately and predictably place and position implants. The surgical template for a hy-brid bridge should demonstrate what the final prosthesis looks like, including buccal position, incisal edge position, overall height, and cingulum and occlusal areas of the teeth. If the patient is wearing a denture in which tooth positions are to be replicated, use this denture as a guide for construction of the surgical template. If planning altered tooth positioning, construct a trial denture that demonstrates the new dental alignment and use it for template duplication. Chapter 20 gives techniques for fabricating these invaluable devices.

Abutment Selection

After exposing the implants and removing healing collars, choose the abutments. Use shouldered, standard, or conical variety abutments for hybrid bridges (see p. 336, Chapter 22). The abutments act as platforms on which the hybrid bridge framework seats. Select abutments of a height that will place their interfaces with the hybrid cast framework at the level of the soft tissue. This allows the prosthesis to be adapted to the soft tissues, thereby blocking out all spaces. It discourages food from becoming lodged beneath the framework, and neither saliva nor air can escape from beneath the ridge lap. The soft tissue beneath the hybrid frame is sufficiently compliant to allow a Proxybrush to perform successful ablutions. Abutments may be fitted directly in the patient's mouth or from the master cast after impressions are completed. After firmly placing the abutments using a recommended torque wrench, make impressions using the square or tapered coping techniques as described in Chapter 24 (Fig. 25-1, *A-K*).

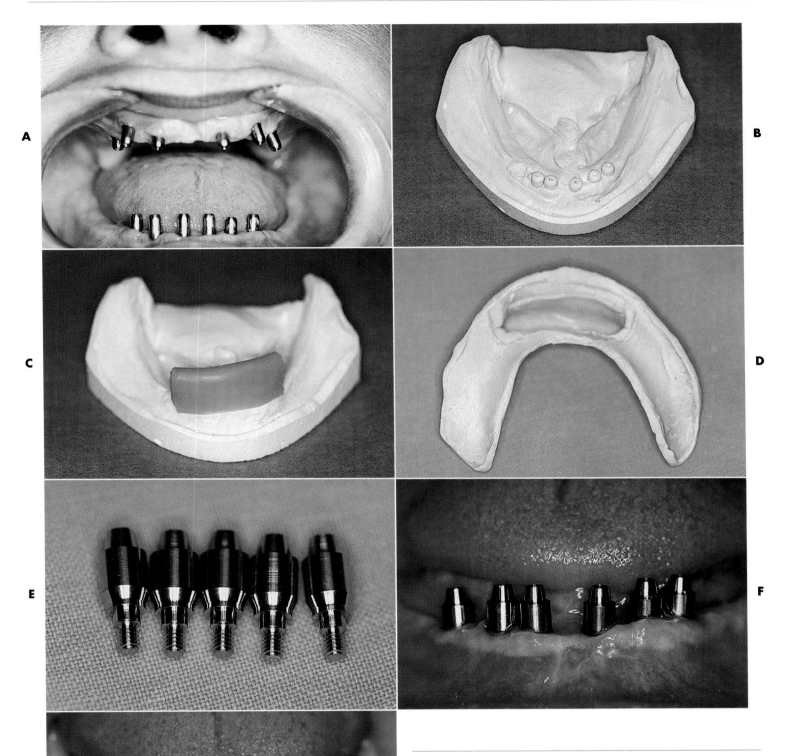

Fig. 25-1   A, Six Integral implants have become integrated in the parasymphyseal area. Healing collars are in position for 2 weeks. **B,** Make a stone cast from an alginate impression of the six healing cuffs. **C,** Use base-plate wax to block out the entire healing cuff zone to a width of 5 mm and a height of 15 mm. **D,** Make an autopolymerizing or Triad tray that is designed to accommodate the boxed area. **E,** Select nonfluted abutments to be threaded into the implants. These abutments are designed to receive fixed-detachable restorations. **F,** Screw the abutments into position. Radiographs must verify proper seating. **G,** Screw transfer copings into the threaded receptacles of the abutments.

Continued

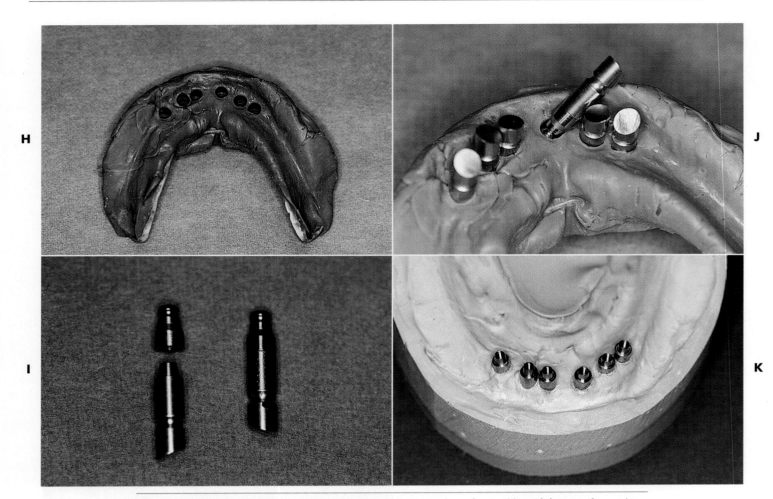

Fig. 25-1, cont'd **H,** Make an Impregum impression to register the position of the transfer copings. **I,** Supply each transfer coping with a prosthetic abutment analog (left). They are connected by a threaded relationship (right). **J,** Fit each transfer coping-abutment analog complex into the Impregum impression, as may be seen by the positioning of the right central incisor. **K,** Pour a master cast in stone. The prosthetic abutment analogs are replicated in their true anatomic positions.

Prosthetic Technique

Complete the final casts by using analogs on which the final hybrid bar is fabricated. Follow the guidelines presented in Chapter 21 to convert temporization from a relined overdenture to an interim fixed prosthesis.

Screw-retained provisionals may use temporary cylinders of the type that seat directly on the implant head or on top of a final abutment. Make a hole completely through the provisional restoration to allow the chimney of the abutment cylinder to pass through it or at least to be seen through it. This allows access to the retaining screw. Process the cylinder to the provisional restoration with self-curing acrylic directly in the patient's mouth. Exercise care when luting the cylinders. Small paintbrush acrylic slurry increments prevent filling of the screw access holes. Additionally, place a cotton pellet into each screw access hole to protect the screw heads from becoming covered. Wax is an unsuitable blocking agent because it dissolves as the monomer contacts it. After tacking the cylinders into position, allow 10 minutes to elapse for the acrylic to set. Removing the temporary before chemical stabilization causes shrinkage, which will hamper accuracy.

Once the master cast has been trimmed, make a verification jig. Make the verification tip by luting together cylinders or transfer copings placed in the master cast. GC Pattern may be used to lute them together. Then try in the luted assembly on top of the implant abutments. Insert and tighten only one screw. Then examine all the abutment coping interfaces for complete passive seating. If any joint is open, cut the assembly with a thin disc. Then seat the coping with its retaining screws and lute the assembly together again. Modify the master cast by repositioning the analog, or attach a series of analogs to the assembly and place them in die-stone to create a solder index. When it fits passively, fabricate the final hybrid bar on the master cast (Fig. 25-1, *L-O*).

Mount the maxillary cast to a semiadjustable articulator with the face-bow record, and mount the mandibular cast to the maxillary cast using the centric oriented record base. Set the appropriate teeth on the record base. Complete a try-in next. Verify the centric relation, vertical dimension, and overall esthetic appearance (Fig. 25-1, *P-R*).

Once the tooth try-in is complete, fabricate the metal framework to support the restoration. The laboratory makes a silicone index of the tooth position and its relationship to the master cast (Fig. 25-1, *S*). Wax the frame in relationship to

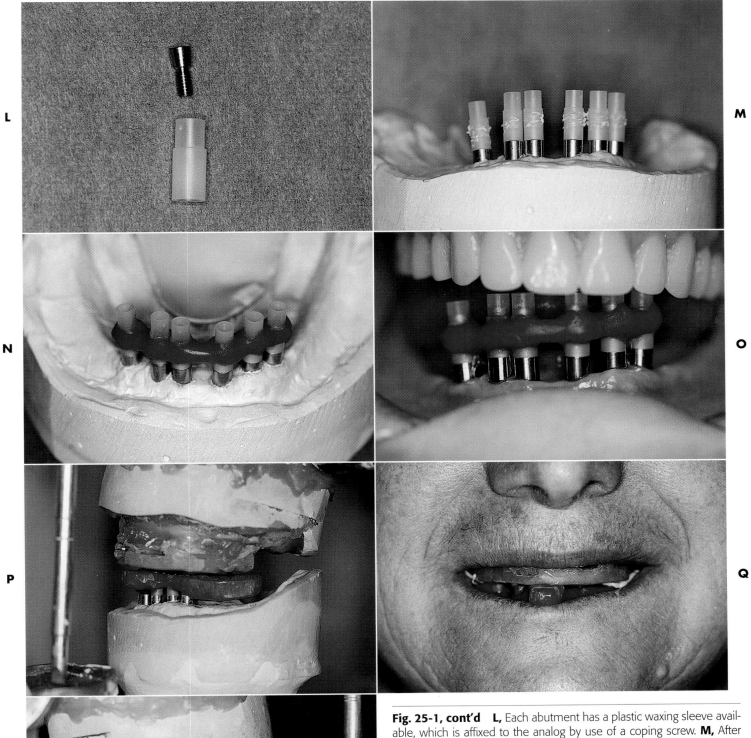

Fig. 25-1, cont'd   L, Each abutment has a plastic waxing sleeve available, which is affixed to the analog by use of a coping screw. **M,** After abrading the surfaces of the sleeves, screw each into position on the cast.   **N,** Fabricate a verification jig using GC Pattern or Duralay resin, which bonds mechanically to the abraded sleeve surfaces. This is used to stabilize the sleeves during the refitting maneuver over the actual implants in the patient's mouth. **O,** By placing a single distal fixation screw, the entire complex should fit intimately and accurately into place without torquing or lifting. **P,** Replace the verification jig and abutment assembly on the master cast and make a wax rim to fit over the GC Pattern resin. **Q,** Using the rim, register vertical and centric recordings. **R,** Affix the casts to a semiadjustable articulator, and wax teeth with respect to incisal length, midline, labial position and inclination.

Continued

tooth position. The framework is designed to support denture teeth that are processed to it and to include female receptacles through which fixation screws are placed and activated. To fabricate this, fit gold copings to each flat or tapered abutment analog and incorporate them into a waxed outline of the bar. Make a precious metal (platinum, palladium, or gold) casting with retention loops placed for acrylic attachment. After receiving a high polish, affirm the following requirements: The metal frame should come down to touch the alveolar ridge adjacent to the implants and may extend posteriorly in the mandible 15 mm distally from the most posterior implant abutment. In maxillae, avoid cantilevers.

Metal Framework Try-in

Seat the metal framework into position over the abutments and insert and tighten one screw of the most distal abut-

ment on one side with a torque driver. Evaluate all abutment-framework interfacial relationships clinically, and if they are not easily visible, evaluate them radiographically. The framework should be seated on all abutments. Loosen the screw and tighten a second screw on the other end of the frame. The same satisfactory criteria must be satisfied. Now insert and tighten all of the screws to finalize the assessments of accurate fit. Then remove the framework and replace protective caps onto the abutments. If the framework does not seat passively (one or more interfaces show gaps), section and reconnect it until satisfactory.

After the metal framework is acceptable, return it to the laboratory for setting of the denture teeth and final wax-up. Try-in the hybrid bar with teeth into the patient's mouth and confirm the centric relation, vertical dimension, and esthetics. The final laboratory task is processing the denture teeth with acrylic to the metal frame (Fig. 25-1, *T-W*).

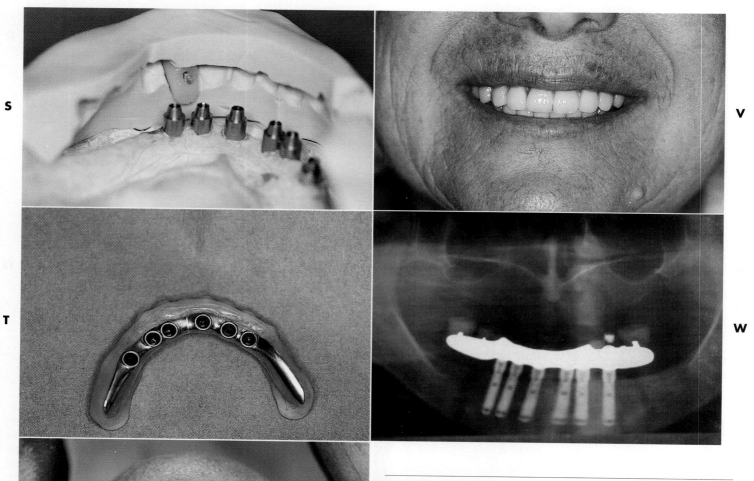

Fig. 25-1, cont'd **S,** Make a silicone impression of the trial bridge on the master cast. Remove each tooth from the wax-up and seat each into the silicone index. This serves to guide the location of the waxed superstructure in relationship to the teeth that are borne by it. **T,** The surface of the completed prosthesis is designed for access and ability to be cleaned easily. **U,** Location of the fixation screws creates an esthetic and functional result. **V** and **W,** The hybrid superstructure, both clinically and radiographically, reveals an esthetic prosthesis that has become an integral component of the patient's masticatory apparatus.

Insertion

At the last clinical visit, torque the abutments down to the manufacturer's recommended levels and insert the completed prosthesis over the abutments. Insert and tighten all the screws. Evaluate the tissue contact. It is considered satisfactory if there is no visible space between the prosthesis and the alveolar ridge, but floss can be passed beneath it (Figs. 25-2, 25-3).

Occlusion

Evaluate the occlusion after fixation of the hybrid. There should be even contact on all of the teeth in centric relation. Develop a mutually guided occlusion in lateral excursive movements, placing the canine and incisors on the working side into function. There should be anterior guidance in protrusive movements.

Now remove the prosthesis, and after polishing, reinsert it with all screws placed to their manufacturer's suggested levels using a torque controller. The screw access holes may be covered with a cotton pellet and temporary sealing material such as Fermit. Take final radiographs, panoramic and periapical, at the time of completion to document the condition of the implants and adjacent bone as well as the seating of all components. This film also acts as a baseline for future comparisons.

Make an appointment with the patient for examination in 1 month. Reevaluate the prosthesis relative to esthetics, occlusion, and the patient's ability to maintain good oral hygiene. Once satisfied with all of these aspects, close the screw access holes definitively with composite material. After placement of a cotton pellet over the screw, light process Fermit to protect it. Leave 4 mm of the coronal access chamber clear. Etch the metal and place a primer and bonding agent followed by light-cured composite, which can be blended with the occlusal restorative material. Recheck the occlusion and finally, polish the composite.

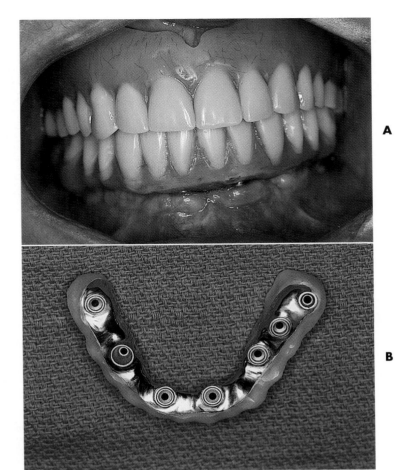

Fig. 25-2   A, B, The cast metal hybrid framework may be designed to touch the gingival tissues as long as it can be hygienically cleaned.

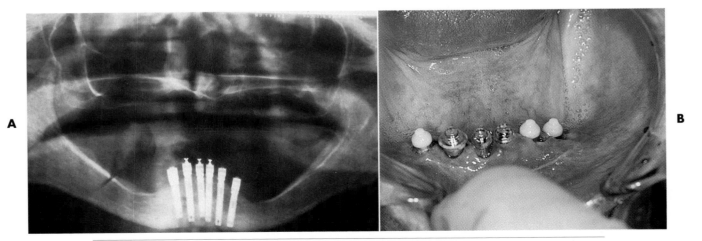

Fig. 25-3   A, A radiograph of six parasymphyseal well-integrated Brånemark implants. Each has its TEA screwed into place. **B,** Clinical view of Brånemark implants with attached TEAs. Three have healing caps covering them. These caps offer a smooth, plaque-free surface during the period of prosthesis construction.

Continued

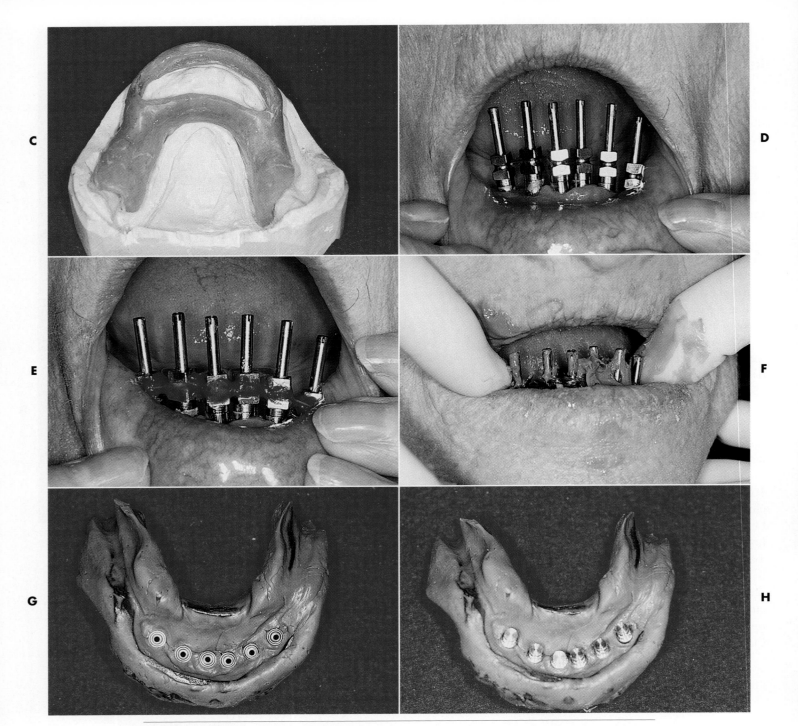

Fig. 25-3, cont'd **C,** Impression making begins with the fabrication of a well-extended autopolymerized tray. The fenestration permits access to the implant sites. **D,** Screw square transfer copings to the TEAs (after healing cap removal) using long threaded guide pins. **E,** A figure-8 continuous floss lattice is covered with GC Pattern or red Duralay, thus assembling the six-abutment complex. **F,** When the tray is seated, the guide pins protrude through the chimney fenestration. Following this, press a piece of softened base-plate wax over the pins, thus sealing the tray and creating a method of gaining compression of the impression material around the implants. When these steps are completed, remove the tray and use polyether (Impregum) to record the final impression. Some of the material escapes from around the guide pin access holes. **G,** After the polyether has set, unscrew the protruding pins, permitting removal of the impression tray with the transfer copings, bound with acrylic and floss retained within the impression material. **H,** Attach a brass abutment analog to each transfer coping. **I,** Pour the master cast, thus relating the abutment analogs to one another and to the other anatomic structures with accuracy. **J,** Place the final gold copings supplied by Nobel Biocare on the analogs. Lute them with GC Pattern resin and, on their removal in a single unit, try them into the mouth for purposes of verification of accuracy of the cast. **K,** Efforts at achieving accuracy are sometimes unsuccessful. In this instance, it is obvious that the gold copings on the patient's right side have not gone to position. **L,** Remove the assemblage and use a disc to section it at the point of suspected error. **M,** The two parts are seated successfully, as is evident from the precise marginal relationships of all of the gold copings. Strategically placed guide pins hold the segments securely into position while new GC Pattern material is used to relute the parts. **N,** Process three well-located gold copings into a final record base. By so doing, the base-plate will be affixed firmly in place so that accurate vertical and centric relationships will be achieved. **O,** Employ classic prosthodontic techniques that include assessments of anatomic distances and relationships. **P,** Make centric and vertical dimension recordings.

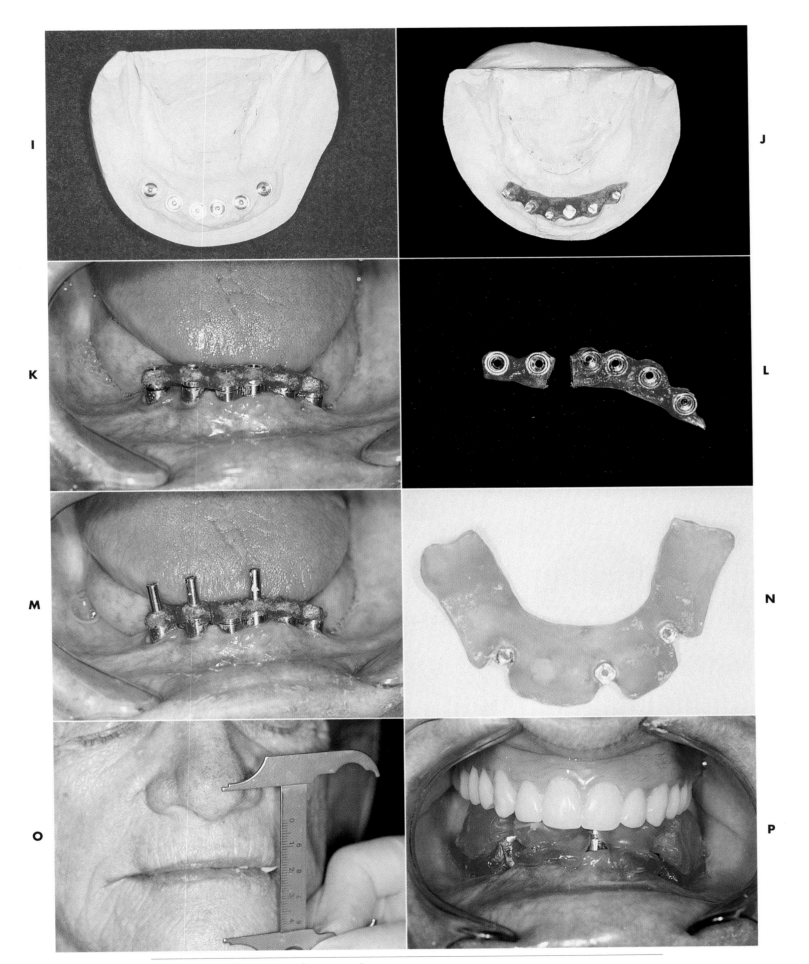

Fig. 25-3, cont'd For legend see opposite page.

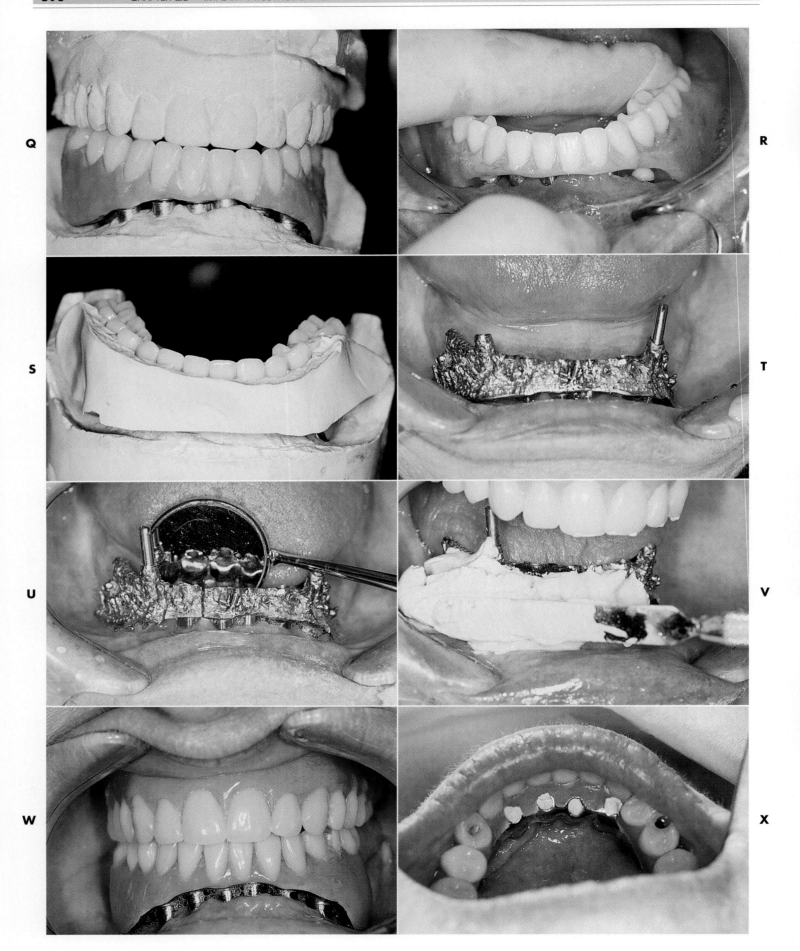

Fig. 25-3, cont'd **Q,** Select the teeth and set them into wax using a semiadjustable articulator. **R,** Give the patient the opportunity to evaluate the esthetic aspects of the prosthesis at the same visit during which the practitioner assesses function. **S,** Use polyvinylsiloxane putty to make an impression of the labial surfaces of the teeth and denture base. Following its removal, unscrew the denture base, set the teeth into the putty, and place the gold copings into position on the abutment analogs. Wax a bar incorporating the copings and the putty impression, with teeth in place, using it to determine the shape and size of the bar. **T,** After the bar is cast, place it over the implants and retain it with a single screw, which permits a test for total passivity during seating. **U,** In cases of inaccurate seating, cut the bar and use a plastic index for reassembly. **V,** A plaster index is an effective method of making a solder index. **W,** Aggressively trim away the labial flange to permit convenient measures of hygiene and ease of observation. **X,** From the occlusolingual view, the fixation screws are well concealed, easy to clean, and accessible for removal and replacement. Temporary stopping may be used to cover the screws during the early trial visits.

Partially Edentulous Arch

The responsibility of the fixed-detachable hybrid lends benefits for the restoration of partially edentulous sites as well as for the fully edentulous jaw. Hybrids and adaptations have the capabilities of solving problems of implant placement, location, angulation, and emergence profile, which, when using conventional fixed or fixed-detachable techniques, might render the implants useless. Any number of missing teeth beyond one can be replaced using the hybrid design.

The principles governing presurgical planning, fabrication of temporary prostheses, and surgical templates have been described clearly in Chapters 5 and 20. Implant placement must be optimally performed, using as large a number as practicable. The decision to use the hybrid often can be made by careful analyses at the treatment planning stage (Fig. 25-4).

The technique for bar fabrication follows the methods described for the fully edentulous arch in every detail. In approaching the partially edentulous arch, the presence of natural teeth facilitates record making, which offers guidance as to centric relationship, vertical dimension, free-way space, and tooth alignment.

After exposing the implants and allowing the gingival contours to mature, screw the final flat or tapered abutments to place using a wrench set to the recommended torque. Affix abutment transfer copings of the square or tapered variety with secondary screws, again with appropriately applied force, and make an elastomeric impression. Confirm the accuracy of coping positions in the impression by inspection, attach abutment analogs, and pour the cast in stone.

Make a semianatomic articulator face-bow mounting. Verify the accuracy of the articulator relationship by analyzing dental wear facets or by using tooth-mounted wax rims on base-plates.

Wax and cast the prosthesis in a precious alloy following the descriptive paragraphs given in the first part of this chapter.

Validate accuracy of ridge lap relationships and implant interfaces by inspection and alternating individual placement of fixation screws. Perform sectioning if an inaccuracy, such as rocking, is detected. Lute the segments with GC Pattern and solder for reconnection.

After the bar fits properly, wax the teeth to it, correct gingival contours, and place and screw the prosthesis into position. The design of partial hybrid dentures permits successful daily hygiene measures by the patient and periodic removal by the implantologist for maintenance and repair.

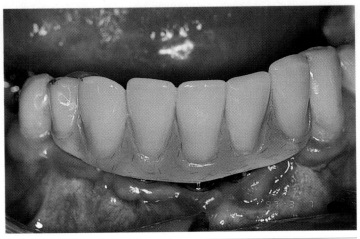

Fig. 25-4 The hybrid bridge can be a functional, low-cost fixed prosthesis for a partially edentulous arch.

Electronic Discharge Machining or Spark Erosion

Electronic discharge machining (EDM) or spark erosion uses milling and electrical technology to create hybrid-type overdentures that seat with precision on mesostructure bars that are attached by screw retention to implants. Such prostheses are designed for pure implant support and may serve the roles of replacing all or several missing teeth. They offer excellent mechanical retention and a flange-free construction, facilitating oral hygiene measures. The accuracy of the machined fit between the two-degree tapered bar and its matching female is within 10 mμ. Despite its initial cost and the demands of prosthetic skill, the spark erosion hybrid prosthesis offers the benefits of simple placement and removal, stable, firm retention, and the elimination of screws for fixation.

Fabrication of this system requires the completion of a primary cast mesostructure bar, machined facially and lingually, whose sides converge with a two-degree taper (Fig. 25-5, A). These bars, made by the spark erosion technique, are shaped and machined without heat and are designed to be attached to a number of well-placed implants by screw fixation. Because of the special demands placed on this retention system, the number of implants should be the same as are ordinarily placed for fixed prosthesis support.

Make impressions for bar fabrication following the steps presented in the paragraphs of this chapter for hybrid bar construction.

When boxing the impression, allow sufficient labial room for the placement of a facial index, which should be made from the interim denture. Its position determines the height and location of the machined bar.

The bar must satisfy the accepted levels of flawless fit; if it does not, the classic corrective measures of verification are required (see Chapter 24). Once fitted, screw the bar firmly atop the supporting implant abutments.

Design the denture/hybrid superstructure with the assistance of the index and cast in a high–platinum content precious metal. Its transfer to the master cast with the primary

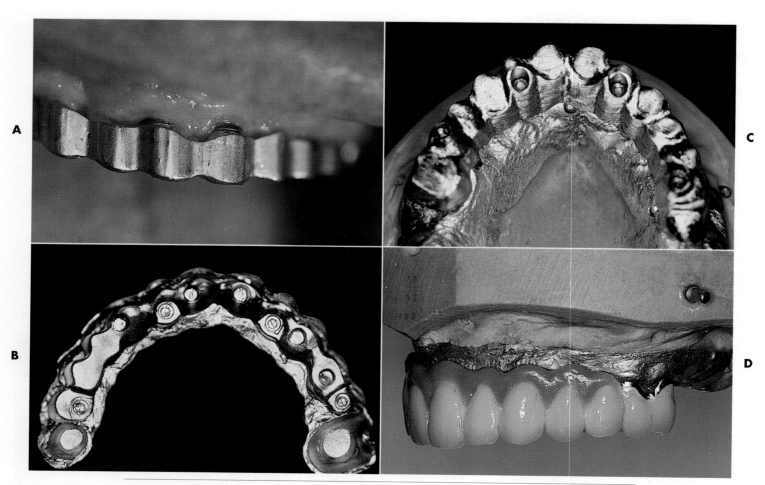

Fig. 25-5 **A,** Electron discharge machining or spark erosion techniques were used to mill this mesostructure bar shown attached to implants with fixation screws. **B,** The armature or skeleton to which the porcelain is baked and the denture teeth are processed, is milled intimately to fit by a precise frictional relationship to the mesostructure bar. **C,** The external surface of this structure is prepared to receive the processed prosthesis. **D,** The completed spark erosion fabricated mesostructure bar, with a totally porcelain baked superstructure may be maintained by a frictional relationship or if additional retention is desired, by the use of strategically related latches, such as Ceka-like attachments.

(Courtesy Dr. Aram Sirakian).

bar positioned on the implant/coping analogs confirms the accuracy of casting. Then, using a reverse polarity ionization technique, complete the electronic erosion of the secondary bar (Fig. 25-5, *B, C*). Achieve secondary retention with two or more Ceka-like attachments, or simple swivel latches, to derive primary retention from the precise relationship of the bar and a number of strategically placed vertical fins.

After final precision milling, set and process the denture teeth, hybrid fashion, to the secondary bar or as an alternative, bake it with teeth and gingiva from porcelain (Fig. 25-5, *D*). Adjust it intraorally, and give the patient training in regard to removal and insertion techniques as well as oral hygiene strategies. This is an extremely satisfactory alternative method for affixing hybrid prostheses to their supporting implants.

Suggested Readings

Ampil JP et al: Use of magnets for staple mandibular implants, *J Prosthet Dent* 55:367-369, 1986.

Bahat O: Osseointegrated implants and maxillary tuberosity: report on 45 consecutive patients, *Int J Oral Maxillofac Implants* 7:459-467, 1992.

Batenburg R, Reintsema H, van Oort R: Use of the final denture base for the intermaxillary registration in an implant-supported overdenture, JOMI on CD-ROM, *Quintessence* 8(2):205-207, 1993.

Bodine RL et al: The subperiosteal implant denture program at the University of Southern California. II. Prosthodontic preparations for oral surgery, *J Oral Implantol* 7:11-32, 1977.

Brewer AD, Morrow RM: *Overdentures*, ed 2, St Louis, 1980, Mosby.

Davidson TJ, Ruff S: A prosthodontic technique for the ramus endosseous frame implant, *J Prosthet Dent* 47:535-538, 1982.

Davis D, Rogers J, Packer M: The extent of maintenance required by implant-retained mandibular overdentures: a 3-year report, *Int J Oral Maxillofac Implant* 11(6):767-774, 1996.

Desjardins RP: Prosthesis design for osseointegrated implants in the edentulous maxilla, *Int J Oral Maxillofac Implant* 7:311-320, 1992.

Engquist B et al: A retrospective multicenter evaluation of osseointegrated implants supporting overdentures, JOMI on CD-ROM, *Quintessence* 1(2):113-118, 1997.

Galandi ME et al: Evaluation of two bar systems for denture retention under simulated loading conditions, *Z Zahnarztl Implantol* 5:33-37, 1989.

Gillings BR: Magnetic denture retention systems, *Int Dent J* 34:184-197, 1984.

Goll GE, Smith DE: Technique for fabrication of the mandibular denture over the staple bone implant using a permanent heat-cured base, *J Prosthet Dent* 53:820-824, 1985.

Guerra LR et al: Modifications of the superstructure for the staple implant, *J Prosthet Dent* 52:858-861, 1984.

Hadeed GJ, Pipko DJ: Non-vertical loaded minimal stress attachment with the mandibular staple bone plate, *J Prosthet Dent* 53:824-827, 1985.

Hallman W et al: A comparative study of the effects of metallic, nonmetallic, and sonic instrumentation on titanium abutment surfaces, *Int J Oral Maxillofac Implant* 11:96-100, 1996.

Humphris GM et al: The psychological impact of implant-retained mandibular prostheses: a cross-sectional study, JOMI on CD-ROM, *Quintessence* 10(4):437-443, 1995.

Jemt T, Book K, Karlsson S: Occlusal force and mandibular movements in patients with removable overdentures and fixed prostheses supported by implants in the maxilla, *Int J Oral Maxillofac Implant* 8:301-308, 1993.

Johns RB, Jemt T et al: A multicenter study of overdentures supported by Branemark implants, *Int J Oral Maxillofac Implant* 7:513-522, 1992.

Loos LG: A fixed prosthodontic technique for mandibular osseointegrated titanium implants, *J Prosthet Dent* 55:232-242, 1986.

Maxon BB et al: Prosthodontic considerations for the transmandibular implant, *J Prosthet Dent* 63:554-558, 1990.

Mericske-Stern R: Clinical evaluation of overdenture restorations supported by osseointegrated titanium implants: a retrospective study, JOMI on CD-ROM, *Quintessence* 5(4):375-383, 1990.

Mericske-Stern R: Oral tactile sensibility recorded in overdenture wearers with implants or natural roots: a comparative study. Part II, JOMI on CD-ROM, *Quintessence* 9(1):63-70, 1994.

Mericske-Stern R et al: In vivo measurements of maximal occlusal force and minimal pressure threshold on overdentures supported by implants or natural roots: a comparative study. Part I, JOMI on CD-ROM, *Quintessence* 8(6):641-649, 1997.

Mericske-Stern R et al: Three-dimensional force measurements on mandibular implants supporting overdentures, JOMI on CD-ROM, *Quintessence* 7(2):185-194, 1992.

Meyer JB, Kotwal KR: Clinical evaluation of ramus frame and staple bone implants, *J Prosthet Dent* 55:87-92, 1986.

Naert I et al: Overdenture supported by osseointegrated fixtures for the edentulous mandible: a 2.5-year report, *J Oral Maxillofac Implant* 3:191-195, 1988.

Palmqvist S, Sondell K, Swartz B: Implant-supported maxillary overdentures: outcome in planned and emergency cases, JOMI on CD-ROM, *Quintessence* 9(2):184-190, 1997.

Parel SM: Implants and overdentures: the osseointegrated approach with conventional and compromised applications, *J Oral Maxillofac Implant* 1:93-99, 1986.

Petropoulos VC, Smith W, Kousvelari E: Comparison of retention and release periods for implant overdenture attachments, JOMI on CD-ROM, *Quintessence* 12(2):176-185, 1997.

Quirynen M et al: The influence of titanium abutment surface roughness on plaque accumulation and gingivitis: short-term observations, *Int J Oral Maxillofac Implants* 11(2):169-178, 1996.

Salinas TJ et al: Spark erosion implant–supported overdentures: clinical and laboratory techniques, *Implant Dent* 1:246-251, 1992.

Sirila HS et al: Technique for converting an existing complete denture to a tissue-integrated prosthesis, *J Prosthet Dent* 59:464-466, 1988.

Smedberg J-I et al: A new design for a hybrid prosthesis supported by osseointegrated implants: Part II: Preliminary clinical aspects, JOMI on CD-ROM, *Quintessence* 6(2):154-159, 1997.

Spiekermann H, Jansen VK, Richter EJ: A 10-year follow-up study of IMZ and TPS implants in the edentulous mandible using bar-retained overdentures, *Int J Oral Maxillofac Implant* 10:231, 1995.

Stefani LA: The care and maintenance of the dental implant patient, *J Dent Hygiene* 10:447-466, 1988.

Van Steenberge et al: The applicability of osseointegrated oral implants in the rehabilitation of partial edentulism: a prospective multicenter study on 558 fixtures, *Int J Oral Maxillofac Implant* 3:272-281, 1990.

Versteegh P et al: Clinical evaluation of mandibular overdentures supported by multiple-bar fabrication: a follow-up study of two implant systems, JOMI on CD-ROM, *Quintessence* 10(5):595-602, 1995.

Vigolo P, Millstein PL: Evaluation of master cast techniques for multiple abutment implant prostheses, JOMI on CD-ROM, *Quintessence* 8(4):439-445, 1997.

Wismeyer D, van Waas M, Vermeeren J: Overdentures supported by ITI implants: a 6.5-year evaluation of patient satisfaction and prosthetic aftercare, JOMI on CD-ROM, *Quintessence* 10(6):744-749, 1997.

Zarb GA, Janson T: Laboratory procedures and protocol. Tissue-integrated prostheses. In Branemark P-I, Zarb GA, Albrektsson T, editors: *Osseointegration in clinical dentistry*, Chicago, 1985, Quintessence.

26

Implant Prosthodontics: Overdentures and Their Mesostructure Bars

*O*verdentures are the recommended prostheses for many types of implant systems and are relatively economical and easy to use. In order to have a successful result with overdentures, both esthetically and functionally, and for complete subperiosteal, ramus frame, transosteal, or root form implants, proper positioning of a mesostructure bar is essential. If the bar is in an inappropriate location (e.g., impinging on the tongue space or placed too far labially, creating an unesthetic or dysfunctional situation), a surgically acceptable implant may not be restorable. In addition, if inadequate vertical dimension has been left for construction of the overdenture, successful use of the implant may be impossible.

The preoperative procedure of making a surgical template as described in Chapters 4 and 20 should serve as a guide in placing a bar or implants designed to hold a bar in the most optimal positions. The template can be used at the time of surgery to guide the placement of transosteal, blade, and root

form or ramus frame implants, at least within the limits of the available bone. It may also be used after implant integration to guide bar placement. Such a template may also cause the surgeon to abandon the procedure entirely because prosthetic restoration may be impossible.

If planning a complete subperiosteal casting, place the clear surgical template over the bone model (although its fit is only approximate) to govern bar placement by the laboratory. At the time of the first-stage surgery (if the computer-assisted design–computer-assisted manufacture [CAD-CAM] or stereolithographic method has not been chosen), take an impression of the opposing arch and a wax or Optosil putty interocclusal recording with the bone exposed at the correct vertical dimension and centric relationship (Fig. 26-1). This permits the accurate mounting of the bone model and the proper placement of the abutments (Fig. 26-2). CAD-CAM technology creates a more significant problem because even the most

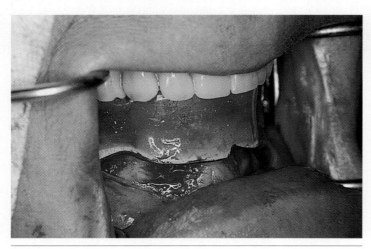

Fig. 26-1 A centric and vertical dimension recording may be taken with a wax rim to establish a relationship between the bony mandible and the fixed anatomic structures of the maxillae.

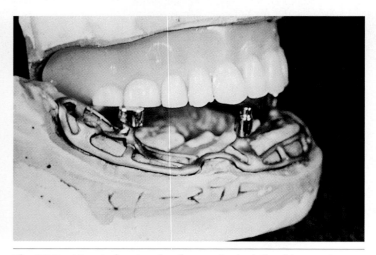

Fig. 26-2 Mounted casts using the acquired relationship permit accurate placement of abutments or a Brookdale bar.

splendidly executed cast is returned without its relationship to the opposing jaw. The CAD-CAM section in Chapter 14 gives a solution to this problem. Following the tube-and-stylus technique described ensures accurate bar or abutment placement.

Chapter 5 explains bar attachment designs. If making the bar separately from the implants, make it of the fixed-detachable or the cemented variety and fabricate it in accordance with the techniques outlined in Chapters 24 and 25. Of course, a bar may also be a part of the implant infrastructure casting, as with ramus frame and subperiosteal designs.

Full Subperiosteal Implants

The prosthetic technique of choice for the complete subperiosteal implant is an overdenture. Full-arch fixed splints have been used, but they are not the recommended treatment primarily because of hygiene considerations.

If centric relationship and vertical dimension records were taken at the first stage of bone surgery, the laboratory can articulate the bone impression model with reliability. Once it is articulated, the information needed to fabricate the implant is available, and an interim or temporary denture may be made for the patient (Fig. 26-3). The surgeon may insert this at the time of surgery and use it during the period of healing (Fig. 26-4). The temporary denture usually consists of anterior teeth and posterior bite blocks. The laboratory can make a temporary denture with a CAD-CAM model as well, if the tube-and-stylus method is followed. However, if a 1-day, two-stage procedure is being followed, it is virtually impossible for the laboratory to have time to fabricate a temporary overdenture. In such cases, the patient's existing denture may be modified to fit over the implant. After aggressive reaming, use a soft liner material such as Coe Comfort, Viscogel, or Softone. It is important that there be no soft tissue contact anywhere beneath the denture base. The denture should be completely implant borne. This is also true for the final superstructure restoration. Tissue contact or pressure could lead to dehiscence of the implant infrastructure. After readapting the denture to the Brookdale bar, dismiss the patient and allow 6 weeks for healing before fabricating the final prosthesis.

The impression procedure requires taking precautions not to lock material under the bar or to force material beneath the tissues surrounding the implant cervices. Block out the area under the bar with a soft (e.g., periphery) wax or blockout ma-

terial and, following this, make an impression with an alginate material in a stock tray (Figs. 26-5, 26-6). Pour the impression with die-stone and use the cast to fabricate a custom tray (Fig. 26-7). Use this tray to record the final impression with an elastomer such as Impregum, once again being sure to block out the areas under the bar (Fig. 26-8). Make the final cast of an epoxy material using the centrifuge technique to obtain accuracy, density, and strength (Fig. 26-9). This method ensures a detailed duplication of the bar and its retention devices such as O-rings, trailer hitches, or Zest anchors.

Next, make an acrylic, heat-cured, final denture base for

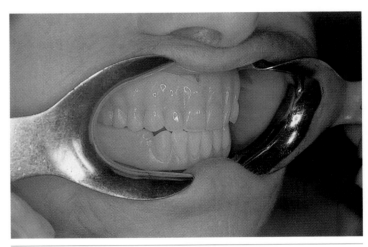

Fig. 26-4 A temporary overdenture may be worn over a newly placed subperiosteal implant throughout the postoperative period and until the patient is supplied with the final prosthesis. It must be totally implant-borne.

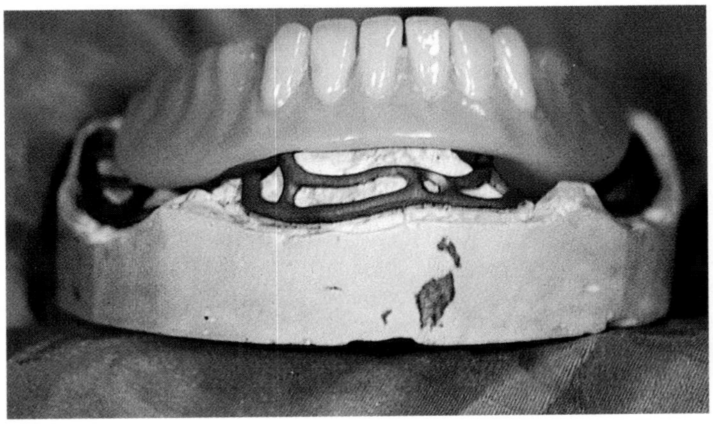

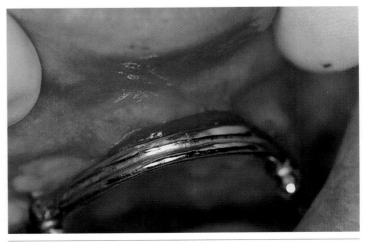

Fig. 26-5 Blocking out undercuts beneath the bar with periphery wax facilitates impression making.

Fig. 26-3 Accurate mounting permits the fabrication of a temporary (six anterior teeth and posterior bite block) overdenture, which may be inserted immediately after implant placement.

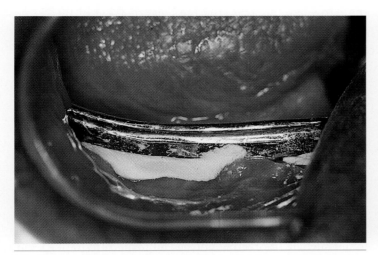

Fig. 26-6   Ultradent block-out material is effective and lends itself to this application with ease before making a final impression.

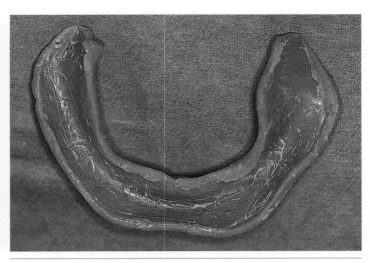

Fig. 26-7   Custom trays may be made of acrylic, Triad, or shellac.

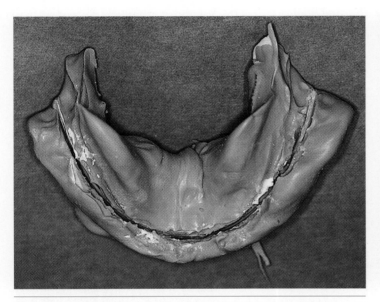

Fig. 26-8   Impressions must be taken only after bar and other structural undercuts are blocked out. Polyethers or polyvinylsiloxanes may be used for these impressions.

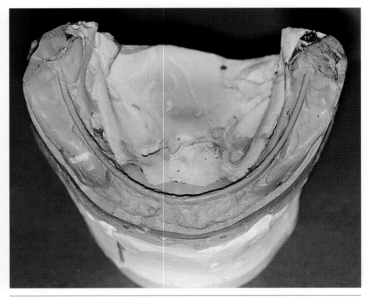

Fig. 26-9   The laboratory should be instructed to make casts of epoxy material. This withstands the machinations to which the laboratory subjects it.

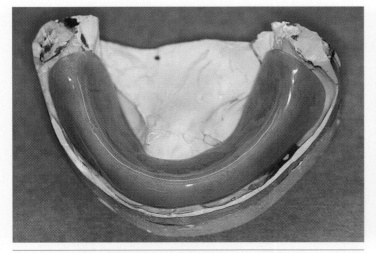

Fig. 26-10   A heat-cured polymethylmethacrylate final denture base offers the most accurate method of acquiring records.

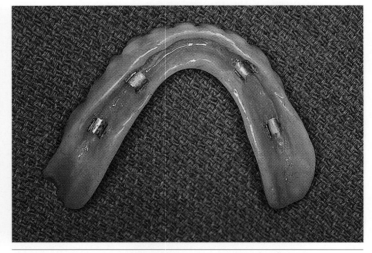

Fig. 26-11   Place the retentive devices planned for the superstructure in the base before recording prosthetic registrations. This grants the stability required for recording accurate relationships.

the establishment of maxillomandibular records (Fig. 26-10). If retentive devices are being used as means of attachment, the laboratory should incorporate them into the base so that its final position permits the making of accurate records (Figs. 26-11, 26-12). After deeming the trial setup as satisfactory, use this base as the final one onto which to process the teeth (Figs. 26-13 to 26-15).

Use zero-degree acrylic denture teeth to minimize oblique and lateral forces that are transmitted to the implant (Figs. 26-16, 26-17).

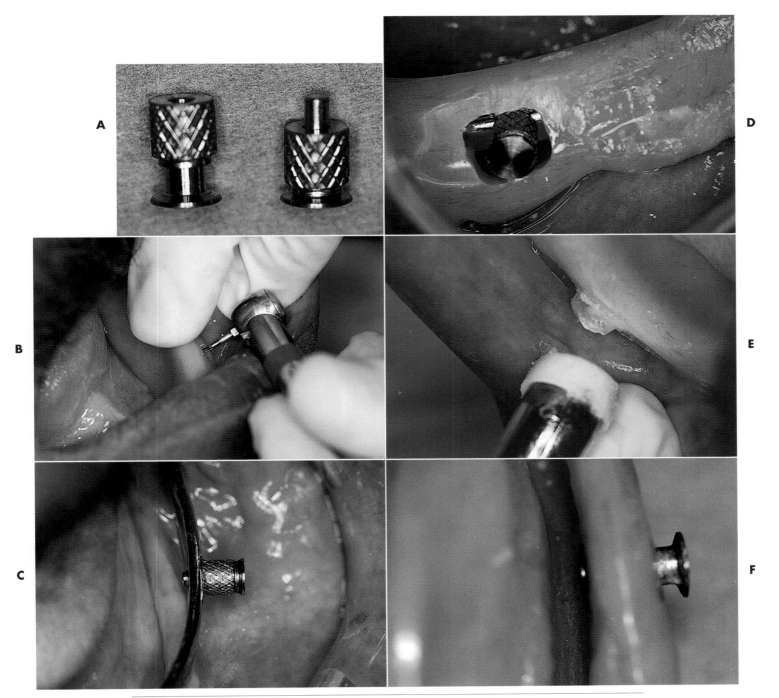

Fig. 26-12   A, One successful retentive device is the Lew attachment (Park DRC). This photograph shows a pair of them in opened (released) and closed (fixed) positions. The protruding pin gains retention by fitting into a groove made in the mesostructure bar. **B,** When the mesostructure bar has not been designed with a retentive groove or notch, such a receptacle can be cut into it by using a diamond or fissure bur. **C,** The relationship of the Lew attachment to the fenestration cut for it in the Brookdale bar. **D,** Open the overdenture buccal flange to reveal the attachment site. Into this, process the Lew attachment. **E,** Use light-cured composite to tack the attachment to the denture. **F,** A profile view of the flange, with the attachment in open position fully processed into it. When the patient presses the button after complete seating of the denture, the pin locks it into place and the head becomes flush with the flange.

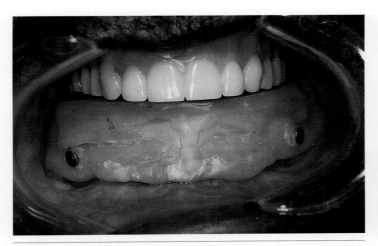

Fig. 26-13   Initiate the final denture construction technique by record making with a wax rim that has been mounted on the stabilized base. The base is retained by Lew attachments.

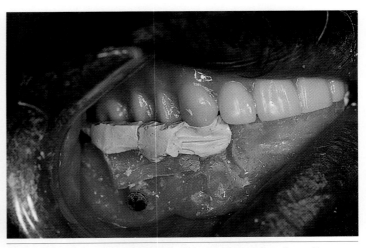

Fig. 26-14   Register centric and vertical relationships after adjustment of the rim by using a rapid ZOE impression paste (Opotow or Bosworth's Superbite).

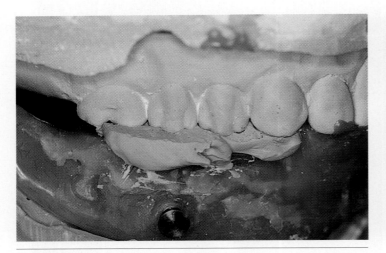

Fig. 26-15   Transfer the base-plates to a semiadjustable articulator. Face-bow mounting contributes to accuracy.

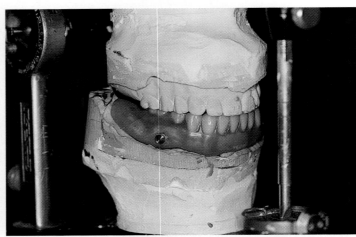

Fig. 26-16   The initial try-in has the teeth set into wax on the final, attachment-supplied denture base.

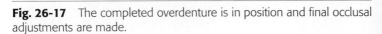

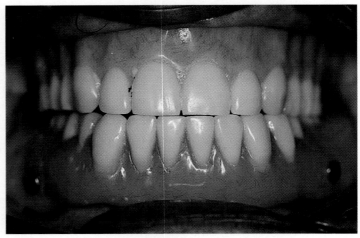

Fig. 26-17   The completed overdenture is in position and final occlusal adjustments are made.

Universal Subperiosteal Implants

The universal or bilateral subperiosteal implant is a full arch casting placed in the presence of natural teeth, which its peripheral struts circumvent. The usual reconstructive technique is an overdenture with cast gold copings placed on the natural teeth (Figs. 26-18 to 26-20).

Make telescopic copings on the natural teeth after the tissues have healed. If these copings are placed beforehand, gingival recession takes place at their margins. If a single-cast gold coping splint is cemented for the natural teeth, then employ standard impression techniques for the fabrication of the overdenture. The basis for the anchorage of natural teeth and subperiosteal implant abutments is dissimilar, so one-piece coping bar splint is not advisable. Individual gold copings protect the natural teeth from caries and facilitate hygiene procedures.

The overdenture fabrication method follows the techniques previously described in this chapter. When the over-

denture has been completed, there are two options if clips are to be used:

- The laboratory may process the clips into the denture base on an epoxy model. Since the most accurate method for record making is to use stabilized bases, laboratory-processed custom clips processed into such bases yield more accurate results.
- The clips may be cold-cured into position directly in the mouth at the time of denture insertion (Fig. 26-21, *A, B*) in the following manner:
  1. Cut a window through the lingual or palatal flange of the denture over the areas of the planned clips (Fig. 26-21, *C*). These windows must allow the denture to seat passively without interferences and permit the visualization of the bar resting beneath it (Fig. 26-21, *D*).
  2. Remove the denture. Place the attachments (clips with retention wings) on the implant bar, block out all undercuts beneath the bar so that the denture cannot become locked to it, and paint a small amount of pink cold-cure denture base acrylic onto the retention wings (Fig. 26-21, *E, F*).
  3. Reseat the denture over the attachments on the bar immediately, and allow the acrylic to polymerize.
  4. When the luting becomes firm, remove the denture with its clips and fill in the remaining spaces between the attachments and denture with additional acrylic (Fig. 26-21, *G*).
  5. Fill in the operative fenestrations in the lingual or palatal flanges with pink polymer, replace the denture, and ask the patient to close into centric relationship. Hold the entire assembly in place until the acrylic sets (Fig. 26-21, *H*). If the denture becomes locked under the bar, reopen the lingual windows and remove the acrylic that has fastened it into place with a bur. Then remove the denture, reblock the undercuts with wax, and repeat these procedures, doing as much of it as possible with the denture out of the mouth.

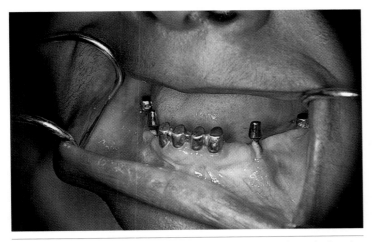

Fig. 26-18 Manage a universal subperiosteal implant by splinting the patient's remaining four mandibular incisors with gold copings.

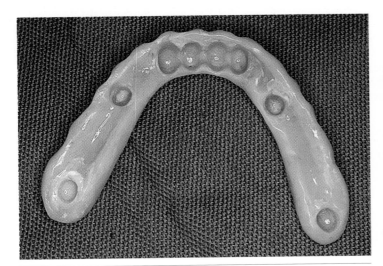

Fig. 26-19 Reline the overdenture, which may be used with or without a bar, depending on retention requirements, when necessary.

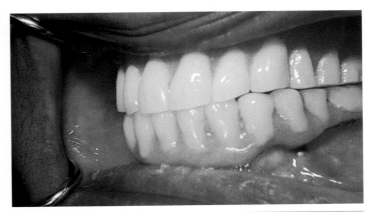

Fig. 26-20 The completed overdenture satisfies the needs of function and esthetics.

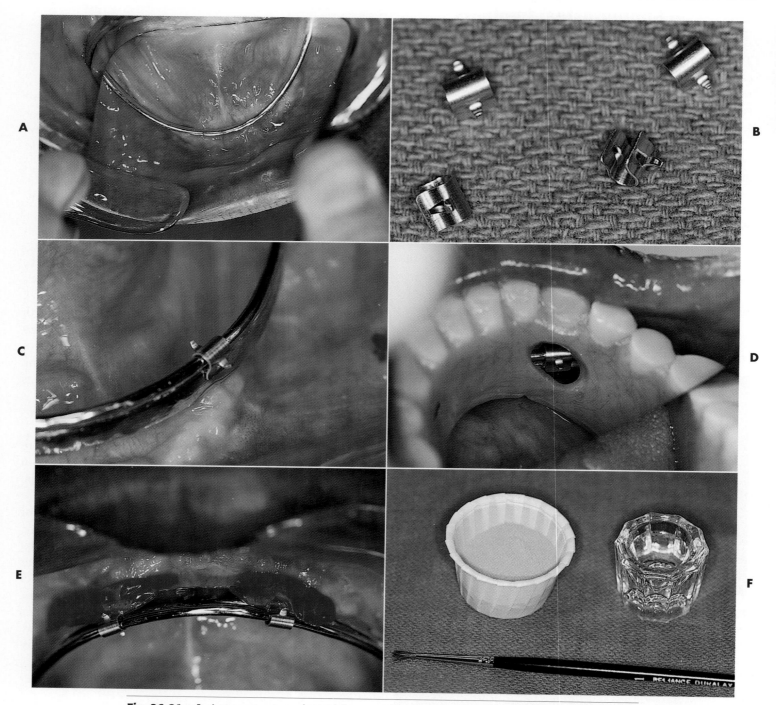

Fig. 26-21 **A,** A mesostructure planned for reception of Hader clips. **B,** Precious metal Hader clips, each of which is supplied with retention wings. **C,** Place clips in selected strategic numbers and locations on the bar. Retention wings should be readily accessible. **D,** Cut windows through the lingual flange of the overdenture at each clip site. The denture is seated, offering clear access to each device. **E,** The area beneath each clip is blocked with wax. **F,** Use a strong, quick-setting, autopolymerizing resin such as GC Pattern for processing the clips to the denture.

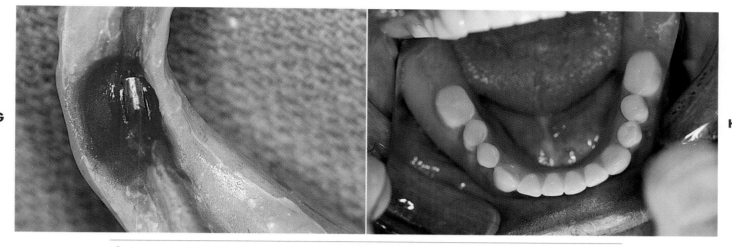

Fig. 26-21, cont'd   G, After processing, the stark contrast of the repair material to the denture acrylic makes correction, retrieval, and change of clips a simple task. **H,** Final finishing should include masking the bright red with pink denture material in areas where esthetics dictate such change.

A "sloppy" or imprecise fit overdenture may also be completed clinically. The denture must seat passively, without contacting the underlying bar. Do not block out undercuts beneath the bar or elsewhere. Place pink, cold-cure denture reline acrylic (e.g., Durabase) into the dried denture. Lubricate the bar with a thin layer of petroleum jelly (Vaseline). Seat the denture over the bar and ask the patient to close into centric position. After the initial set (approximately 1 minute), lift the denture, place it under cold running water briefly to dissipate the heat, and then reseat it. Repeat this process of removal and replacement of the denture every 15 seconds until the acrylic comes to a final set. At this time, it has developed considerable retention, but it still permits removal with some effort. Complete the procedure by trimming excess acrylic and polishing the peripheral areas (Fig. 26-22).

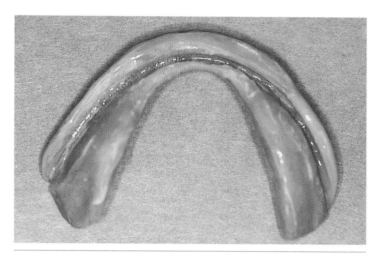

Fig. 26-22   The "sloppy" fit overdenture is managed by chairside reline procedures. Care must be exercised to prevent the denture from becoming locked beneath the bar during the application of hard self-curing resin.

Ramus Frame Implants

The ramus frame implant has, as an integral part of it, a bar to retain an overdenture. The bar, which is rectangular, does not offer the option of permitting attachments to be incorporated into it. The denture may be retained by custom-made clips or by "sloppy fit." Zero-degree teeth are recommended with ramus frame implants and the occlusion should be adjusted, as described for the subperiosteal implant.

Transosteal Implants

As with all types of implants, do a careful preprosthetic workup before placement of transosteal implants to establish their planned labiolingual positions. The staple implant, a special type of transosteal implant, may be limited somewhat in the positioning of its abutments. Single transosteal implants, on the other hand, may be inserted in positions at which they are of the most prosthetic value, particularly if a proper surgical template, as described in Chapter 9, was used during insertion.

The preferred method for the restoration of transosteal implants is with overdentures. The abutments are connected with a bar (Figs. 26-23, 26-24). There are many attachments from which to choose (e.g., O-rings, clips, magnets, "ball" attachments, Zest anchors, or "sloppy" fit).

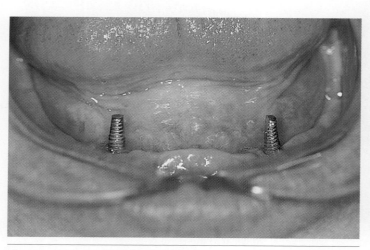

Fig. 26-23   Internally threaded, chrome alloy abutments are available for transosteal implants.

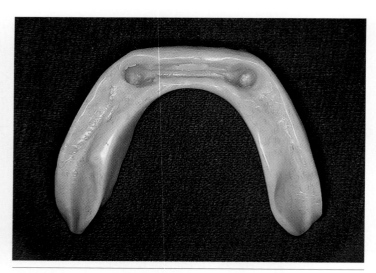

Fig. 26-25   The overdenture, which is both bar- and tissue-supported, must demonstrate good peripheral extension and accurate fit.

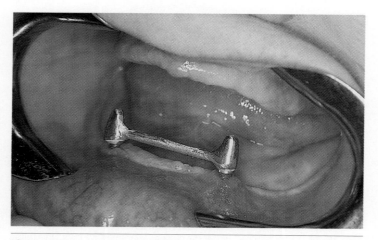

Fig. 26-24   Routine prosthodontic techniques supply the patient with a precious metal coping-bar splint.

When fabricating a soft tissue–borne denture that is to be bar retained, make an accurate impression of the soft tissues as well as the bar (Fig. 26-25). Fabricate a custom tray, allowing sufficient internal height for the implant and transfer copings. Manufacturers supply transfer copings for the fabrication of the master or working cast. After placing them over the implant abutments, make a wax relief. This permits the tray to be seated passively. Border mold the tray to record all landmarks as for a conventional denture, and make the impression using a standard technique with a stiff polyether material such as Polygel or the polyvinylsiloxane, Reprosil. When removing the impression, pour a die-stone model. Then fabricate the mesostructure bar and final overdenture on the master model. (If the final restoration is to approximate the soft tissue, then fabricate a soft tissue model with Vestogum, as described in Chapter 20.)

The construction of the denture should follow acceptable prosthetic techniques and guidelines.

Root Form Implants

The overdenture is a good prosthetic option for patients who seek prosthesis stability and retention but do not mind that the prosthesis is removable. It is required for patients who do not have sufficient bone and soft tissue and require the benefits of bulk offered by such designs. In addition, the economics affected by placing minimal numbers of implants demand the trauma-sparing behavior delivered by overdentures. Essentially, the overdenture is the fundamental prosthesis, the linchpin, of implant-borne reconstruction. There are several types of overdentures, and each has its purpose and requirements. If individual attachments are affixed to these implants, the attachments offer retention for the denture, but the hard and soft tissues supply all of the support. Although retentive,

there is slight movement of the denture on the soft tissues. When using a bar to splint implants, the overdenture derives retention from attachments adapted to the bar and support from the bar and implants as well as from the soft and hard tissues. As greater numbers of implants are added and bar length increases, an increasing amount of support comes from the bar and implants. The result is greater stability of the prosthesis. Unlike mandibles, which may have as few as two implants for overdenture support, maxillary overdentures require a minimum of four implants splinted with a bar to serve as support mechanisms.

The projected designs of the final prostheses govern the number of root forms placed. Solid, secure overdenture prostheses require at least four implants in the mandible and five in the maxilla. If the aim is to obtain moderate retention with the use of a tissue-borne overdenture that offers the benefits of stress-breaking or if economics is a factor, a good result may be achieved with two implants. Make the bar connecting them as a straight segment so that the internal clips or attachments fitted to it permit the saddles to rotate against the resilient bearing tissues covering the posterior ridges. If the bar is curved or the attachments poorly aligned, the saddles are not stress-broken and excessive stresses are transferred to the implants.

The abutments for overdentures may contain housings for fixation screws; in such cases, the bar can be screwed into them just as if it were a fixed-detachable prosthesis. Alternately, these coping bars may be cemented.

The choices for abutments and their retentive devices are the same as those for all fixed-detachable devices, and the options for the use and correction of misaligned or angled implants are also the same as those described in Chapter 22 (Abutments, p. 333) and Chapter 28 (Diagnosis and Treatment of Complications, p. 404).

Provisional Restorations

The provisional restoration used during implant treatment often is a complete denture. Although laboratory-processed temporary prostheses are an option, Chapter 21 describes the various designs and techniques available for temporization.

Surgical Templates

Surgical templates are designed to guide implant location, angulation, and placement and must conform to all functional esthetic requirements. See Chapters 4 and 20 for design and fabrication instructions.

Final Prosthesis Fabrication

After the implants have been uncovered and the soft tissues have healed, initiate fabrication of the final prosthesis.

For a stable and retentive overdenture, a mesostructure bar may incorporate any of the attachments, which are described in Table 5-1. In cases in which five or six implants have been used, cantilever the bar past the last implant on either side. The length of the extensions depends on the number and length of the implants. In cases of six implants of 13-mm length or greater, the cantilevered bars may extend 15 mm in the mandible, but this practice should be eschewed in maxillae. Fewer or shorter implants allow use of commensurately shorter extensions. If the record base used was screw-retained, the reliability of this technique permits the laboratory to incorporate the attachments directly into the denture at the time of processing. If the base was not stabilized with screws, the attachments usually have to be processed into the denture while stabilizing it intraorally. Use cold-cured acrylic through lingual operative fenestrations as described in Fig. 21-A-H and the accompanying text. If making rotating or other stress-broken prostheses, make the bar shorter, since the overdenture is to be retained by only two or three implants.

Zero-degree denture teeth are recommended for use in overdentures. If a patient has any remaining natural teeth that are periodontally sound, include them in the bar configuration. If the bar is to be screw retained, there is a prosthetic complexity using natural teeth. If it is to be cemented, its removal becomes difficult or impossible. Additionally, the cement has the potential of washing out from under castings, which may lead to decay of the natural teeth. To avoid such occurrences, place individual gold copings on natural teeth to protect them from caries. Then fit the bar over the copings and implants, thus safely incorporating the natural teeth in the reconstruction.

If a fixed-detachable concept is the desirable approach and the patient has a combination of implants and natural teeth, make impressions of those teeth after their preparations, fabricate copings, and pick them up in a master impression. The laboratory can solder internally threaded sleeves to the coping occlusal surfaces (TSFH, available from Paragon). This permits the natural teeth to join the implants in a classic fixed-detachable system, either for bar or other more realistic types of prostheses (Fig. 26-26).

In situations in which a reconstruction is limited to the use of two implants and as a result of anatomic considerations in the structure of the patient's arch they are too far apart to be connected, it is acceptable to use them as freestanding abutments with attachments for overdentures. The attachments used most frequently in these situations are Zest anchors (Fig. 26-27), ERA attachments, or O-rings (Fig. 26-28). Screw either into the threaded housing of its implant and cold-cure the retentive component into the patient's denture through lingual fenestrations. In these situations, keep the attachments as low to the tissue as possible to avoid unfavorable crown-root ratios.

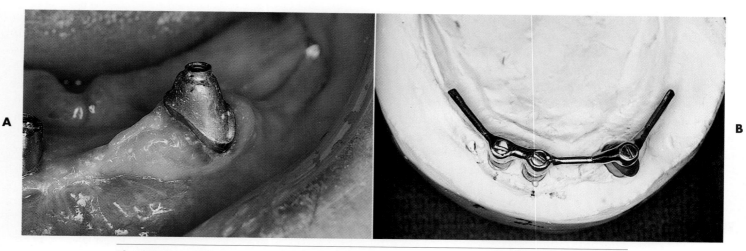

Fig. 26-26   **A,** When it is preferable to use a fixed-detachable coping bar splint in the presence of natural teeth, the internally threaded TSFH (Paragon) attachment can be soldered to the coping. **B,** In such a fashion, the resulting splint can be attached by screws to all supporting abutments, whether natural or implant-borne.

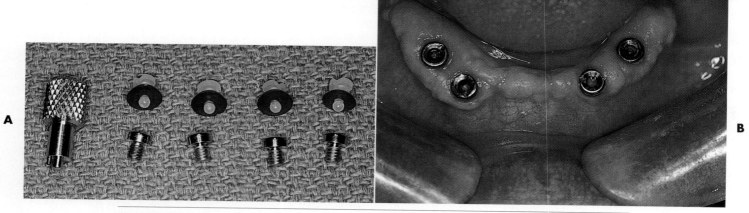

Fig. 26-27   **A,** Zest attachments offer good sources of overdenture support. The attachments are threaded and the instrument on the left serves to insert them into the threaded interiors of osseointegrated implants. Above each attachment is a white plastic retentive device that is to be processed into the overdenture. The washers are used for their stabilizing effects and, after the processing procedure, are discarded. **B,** Four well-integrated implants are shown, each with a Zest female anchor screwed into place.

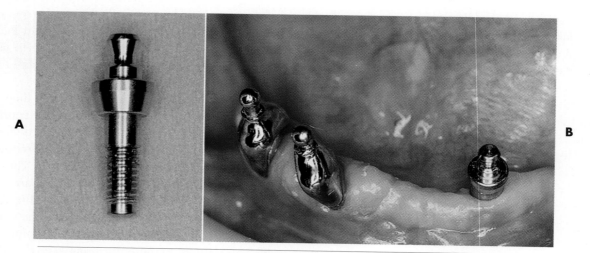

Fig. 26-28   **A,** An O-ring male attachment is placed as it relates to a root form implant. **B,** O-rings, when processed into an overdenture, may seek retention from natural teeth (right mandible) as well as implants (left). There is sufficient resilience in design to permit their use with multiple abutments irrespective of their support mechanisms or imperfect parallelism.

Abutment Selection

Select abutments after the impressions are made so that implant positions may be studied. Remove the healing collars using a counterclockwise motion with a screwdriver compatible with the implant system. Measure the tissue depths using a periodontal probe and replace the healing abutments one implant at a time. If the healing abutments are left out for extended periods of time, the tissue may be drawn over the implant peripheries. The patient then will have pain on reinsertion of the healing abutments. Select abutments 1 mm longer than the tissue depth measurements.

For a bar overdenture, choose a shouldered abutment that accepts a screw-retained bar. For individual attachment-type abutments, make sure the implants are parallel to one another. If they are not, angled abutments that permit parallelism are required. Divergence of the abutments causes divergent paths of removal, which may be responsible for attachment breakage, premature wear of the attachments, or unnecessary stress to the implants.

Impression Making for Overdentures

Fabricate a custom tray. This tray should have full-flange extensions as if it were designed for a conventional denture impression. The tray must be capable of accommodating the implant abutments and impression copings (Fig. 26-29). Insert the custom tray over the abutments and impression copings, and adjust its borders. Manipulation of the tray should not be limited by the presence of the copings (Fig. 26-30). Complete the border molding, and perform final seating of the tray (Fig. 26-31). The impression making section of Chapter 24 describes in detail the principles of this procedure(Fig. 26-32).

On completion of the impression, place protective caps on the abutments, using either square or tapered abutment transfer copings (Fig. 26-33). Relieve the provisional denture and reline it with a soft tissue liner; reseat it and check for proper occlusion.

If individual attachment abutments are planned, use the impression copings as the portions of the attachments that are affixed to the denture base. If adapting this technique, coat the attachments with adhesive and place them on the abutments. Pick them up with the impression into which the individual attachment abutment analogs will then be placed.

Now make a master cast. Bead, box, and pour the final impression in dental stone. A soft tissue model is required if the soft tissues touch the impression copings when making impressions of the implants. Chapter 23 gives instructions on fabrication of soft tissue casts.

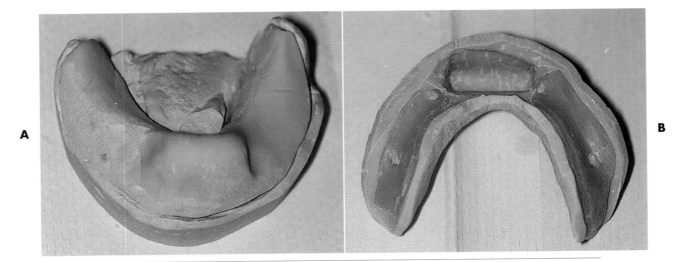

Fig. 26-29 **A,** Coping bar fabrication must begin with the construction of a polymeric custom tray, which has a housing large enough to accommodate abutments and transfer copings. **B,** The tissue-borne side of the tray demonstrates the pink wax relief areas for the ridges as well as the adequacy of the housing.

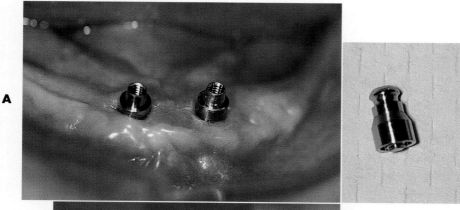

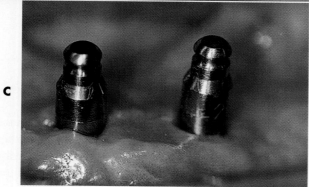

Fig. 26-30 **A,** Screw final titanium abutments into place in root form implants. Each abutment is supplied with internal threading. **B,** Transfer copings are made to be seated by threading into the TEAs. **C,** Screw each transfer coping tightly into its matching abutment.

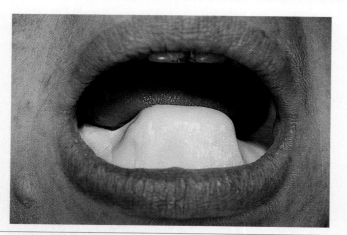

Fig. 26-31 After the tray is seated freely and comfortably over the TEA transfer coping complex, it is border-molded in an acceptable manner.

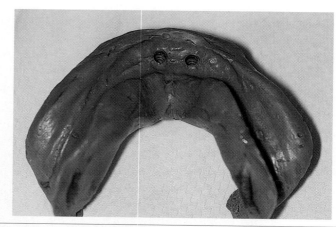

Fig. 26-32 The final impression accurately records all tissues and transfer copings.

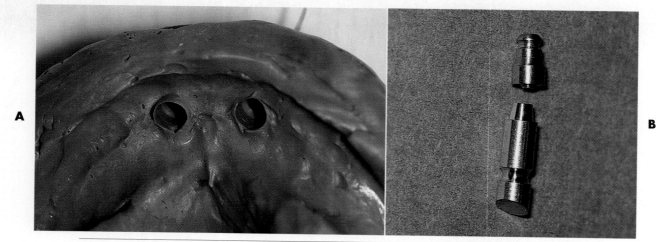

Fig. 26-33 **A,** Important detail is recorded most successfully by use of an impression syringe. **B,** Each transfer coping is removed from its abutment and screwed into a prosthetic implant analog. These mated components are seated into the impression. Pour the cast in yellow stone.

Verification Jig, Vertical Dimension, and Centric Relation

Once the master cast has been trimmed, make a verification jig by placing square/locking impression copings on top of the abutments or implant analogs on the cast. Use a stable acrylic resin (GC Prep) to lute them into a unit.

Use a traditional base-plate, made sufficiently large to accommodate the capped abutments (Fig. 26-34, *A, B*), to record centric relation, vertical dimension, and esthetic contours. Articulator mount it using a face-bow transfer (Fig. 26-34, *C*). Remove the caps from the abutments. Select teeth of an appropriate shade and mold (Fig. 26-34, *D, E*). Place the verification jig on the abutments, and tighten a screw at one end.

Follow the sequence described in Chapter 25, which describes the fabrication and use of the verification jig.

These steps are required only when designing multiple splinted units. On satisfactory seating of the copings, transfer them to a working cast, set appropriate teeth on the record base, and schedule a try-in. After verification of vertical dimension, tooth shade, tooth shape, and the overall esthetic appearance of the overdenture, place a cast metal frame into it. The space accommodation for the abutment and bar creates weak points in the denture that may cause wear or fractures. Make the cast metal frame of a nonprecious metal; it serves

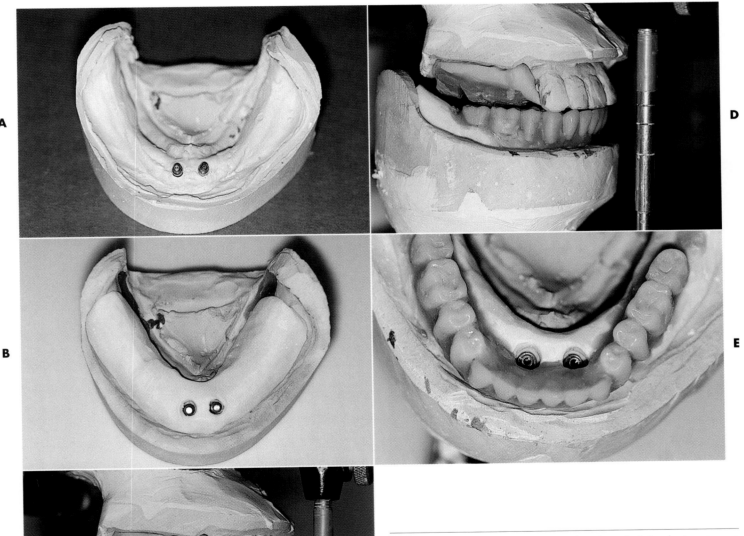

Fig. 26-34 A, Place abutment analogs into their implant mates on the working cast. **B,** Process an accommodating base-plate to the cast. **C,** Lute a wax rim to the base-plate for purposes of recording centric relationship and vertical dimension. **D,** Set teeth in wax to an ideal plane. **E,** The abutments may be visualized from above in their accurate relationship to the denture base.

most successfully if it accommodates the implant abutments, attachments, and bar (Fig. 26-35). Make the metal frame when the record base is prepared. If electing construction of the metal frame after the tryin phase, reset the teeth on the casting and try in the denture before processing.

The laboratory may now also fabricate the bar with attachments. Cast these bars of precious metal. Use machined gold copings for the bar-abutment interface. The machined copings along with their appropriate retaining screws are available from the manufacturer of the abutments. Position the bar on the abutments with an index of the waxed-up denture in position. In this manner the bar and attachments may be positioned relative to the tooth and flange positions. Ideally, place the bar just lingual to the cingulum areas of the anterior teeth. This permits maximum vertical space. The positioning of the attachments depends on their design, how they function, and how the denture uses them. If using two implants with a Hader Bar for attachment, make sure the bar is perpendicular to the posterior alveolar ridges. Use a single clip as the attachment to the bar. In this manner, the clip may rotate around the bar at 90 degrees to the posterior alveolar ridges.

Cantilever bar extensions are not permissible. If ERA attachments are used, place them distal to the most posterior abutment on either side of the bar.

Try in the bar and denture wax-up along with the casting. Reconfirm the denture esthetics, centric relation, and vertical dimension. Fit the bar by removing the protective caps from the abutments and tightening a screw on the side with the most distal abutment. Evaluate all abutment-bar interface joints clinically, and if they are not easily visible, examine them radiographically for reverification. Now insert all other screws and tighten them to ensure flawless seating. Then remove the bar and replace the protective caps on the abutments. Process the denture but not the internal attachments. Instead, make space accommodation for them available.

At the insertion visit, remove the protective caps and insert the bar. Insert the gold screws used to retain the bar with a torque wrench to the manufacturer's advised level.

Adjust the denture base flanges and occlusion using a philosophy that governs the rules for conventional dentures (Fig. 26-36).

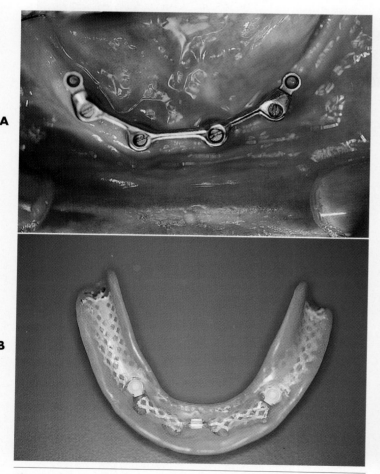

Fig. 26-35 **A, B,** Although the mandible can be restored with two implants, a more reliable fixation is ensured with four implants and a fixed-detachable bar that offers Hader clip and ERA retentive devices to an overdenture that it supported as well in the saddle areas.

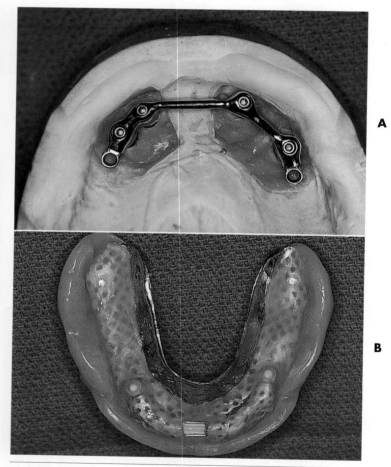

Fig. 26-36 **A** and **B,** Four maxillary implants with a fixed-detachable bar offer a variety of attachments ensuring firm retention without a need for full palatal coverage.

Attachment Connection

Ideally, insert the attachments (Fig. 26-37) after 1 week of denture wearing to allow the new denture to completely settle to its resting position. When inserting the attachments, block out all adjacent undercuts on the abutments and bar 180 degrees to prevent locking of acrylic to the bar (Fig. 26-38). Seat the attachments into or onto the bar in their appropriate positions. The attachments cannot interfere with the complete seating of the denture (Fig. 26-39). Paint self-curing denture repair acrylic onto the attachment and into the appropriate position in the denture. Place the denture and allow the acrylic to set. After removing the denture, evaluate the relationship and stability of each attachment. If too little acrylic had been placed to retain the attachment, it will have remained on the bar, but its indentation is seen in the denture. Additional acrylic is required. Apply in small increments to prevent locking of the denture on the bar. After adding and curing adequate acrylic, remove the excess flash and reevaluate and adjust the occlusion. Polish and insert the denture, giving the patient instructions on its care and use (Fig. 26-40). Although the laboratory can place attachments, the numerous transfers almost always cause inaccuracies. Precision is most readily achieved by direct intraoral assemblage.

Make an appointment to see the patient for additional adjustments 2 weeks after attachment insertion. The attachment may loosen slightly after the first month of use. Some attachments can be retightened. Others should be replaced when they are no longer retentive. The time interval depends on the type of attachment used and the individual using them. Patients are generally told to have the attachments replaced between 6 months and 2 years. Take a final radiograph, panoramic, or periapical at the time of the initial denture insertion visit to document the condition of the implants and adjacent bone as well as the seating of all components. This film also acts as a baseline for future comparisons.

For specific bar designs and detailed description of bar shapes, their modes of anchorage (cemented, fixed-detachable) as well as the versatile and wide variety of attachments, refer to Chapters 5 and 26.

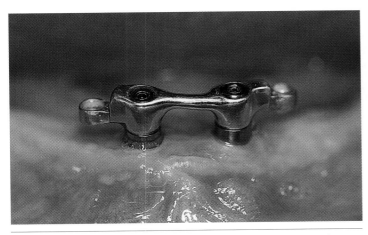

Fig. 26-37 Wax the copings and bar on the working cast and, upon their casting and completion, screw them to position into the abutments.

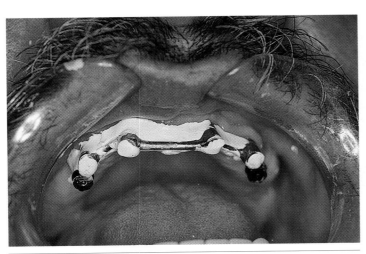

Fig. 26-38 ERA black attachments are placed directly in the patient's mouth, and undercuts are blocked out in preparation for denture relining and pickup of the attachments.

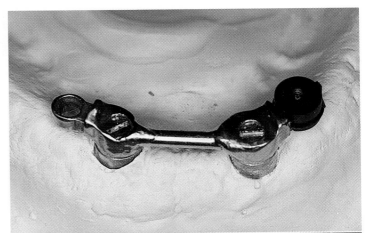

A

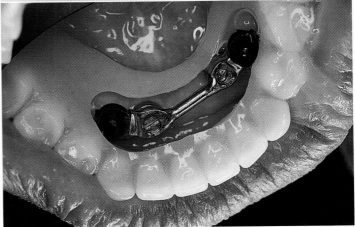

B

Fig. 26-39 **A,** The assembly on a working cast for an ERA attachment overdenture includes the actual coping bar splint that has been seated on the implant analogs. **B,** In order to ensure that adequate clearance is allowed, use the black attachments for this critical step of transferring the male components into the overdenture via a lingually created fenestration.

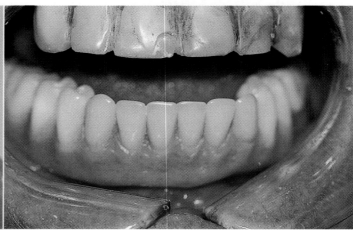

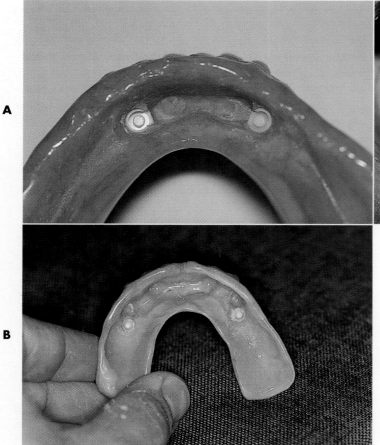

Fig. 26-40 **A,** Affix the attachments, after being placed on the bar, to the denture through lingual window directly in the mouth. **B,** Remove the black processing attachments after completion of the assembly, and use attachments of appropriate retention to replace them. **C,** The ERA retained denture is finished, polished, and inserted.

A Modified Transfer Technique

Marc Kaufman

As an alternative to the classic methods of impression making for overdentures, a modified technique has been used, yielding high levels of accuracy. The standard procedure for the transfer of implant and abutment position to a working cast has been hindered by multiple transfers and record reproductions and the errors induced by these many steps, serving to delay completion of the patient's prosthetic appliances. A transfer technique that uses custom impression trays fabricated from surgical templates permits a single-visit transfer of centric occlusion, vertical dimension, tooth position, and implant or abutment location.

Traditionally, the prosthetic phase begins with the fabrication of a cast by making an alginate impression of the healing abutments. Then the implantologist uses the cast to fabricate a custom tray. This is followed by the making of a final impression using implant transfer copings secured by guidepins. The implant transfer copings are luted together with a polymer to increase the accuracy of the registration. The second phase involves using the master cast to fabricate a record base. The base is required to register interocclusal relationships, a step that is mandated for articulation of the casts. This technique for both partially and totally edentulous patients often requires four or more visits.

The modified technique permits registration of implant location, tooth position, and centric relation to be established in a single visit. It may be used for any type of full-arch reconstruction, and it offers the additional advantage of requiring minimal use of prosthetic components. While this technique may be used for any type of implant-borne reconstruction, the focus of this method is for overdenture construction.

Select appropriate abutments for a bar overdenture prosthesis at the time of second-stage surgery. Estimate tissue heights by means of a millimeter probe before implant uncovering or by tissue depth measurements taken at the time of healing abutment placement. The surgical template used in this technique is a duplicate of the patient's existing provisional denture (Fig. 26-41). The template reproduces the correct tooth position at the established vertical dimension. Use the surgical template to check the angulation, height, and location of each abutment relative to the patient's prosthetic plan. Place transfer copings over each abutment (Fig. 26-42), and modify the surgical template by creating internal clearance so that it may be used as a custom tray. This permits it to be fully seated when the abutments and transfer copings are in place. Shorten the transfer copings, if needed, to permit the patient to close in centric with the template and transfer copings in place (Fig. 26-43). After checking the position of the template for accuracy in vertical dimension and centric occlusion, make the impression by placing a polyether impression material into the modified tray, seating it, and guiding the patient's mandible into centric occlusion (Fig. 26-44). After removing the tray, verify occlusal registrations and seat the transfer copings into their appropriate positions within the impression.

This procedure has related both arches in centric occlu-

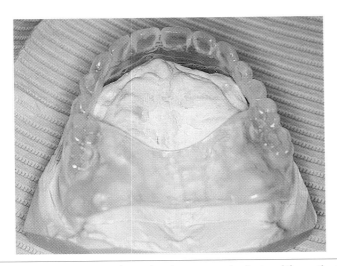

Fig. 26-41 This surgical template is an exact duplicate of the patient's transitional denture.

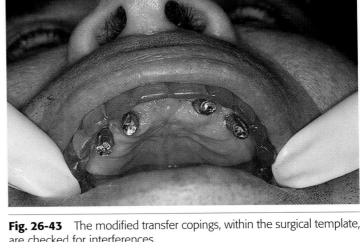

Fig. 26-43 The modified transfer copings, within the surgical template, are checked for interferences.

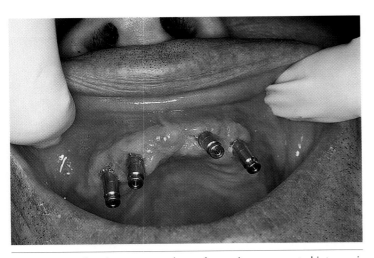

Fig. 26-42 The abutments and transfer copings are seated into position before the final impression is made.

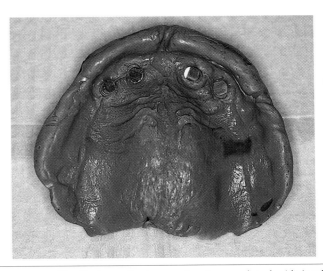

Fig. 26-44 The final transfer impression is completed with implant analogs and transfer copings reseated.

sion and vertical dimension, as well as registering tooth position and abutment location in one step. Send the counter cast and abutment analogs to the laboratory, where the master model will be articulated to it. The laboratory fabricates and returns the custom bar (Fig. 26-45) and waxed overdenture (Fig. 26-46) with the teeth set into position (Fig. 26-47), according to the information obtained from the single impression. If inaccuracies are discovered, section the bar and reconnect it by means of applying a stable polymer as described in Chapter 24. Remove the joined sections in their proper relationship with the use of a polyether impression material in the wax record base. Accomplish this by removing the attachments from the base before picking up the bar and using an impression wash material with the patient closed in centric position.

Address discrepancies in tooth position, as well as problems associated with centric accuracy or lip line contour, by adjusting the wax set-up at chairside. After completing the corrections, reline the trial base with a polyether impression material and pick up the bar to compensate for the changes in

the soft tissue morphology caused by the surgical uncovering procedure. The laboratory pours a new master cast and completes the processing of the case for delivery on the patient's third visit (Fig. 26-48).

This technique can simplify overdenture construction when the supporting implants are only mildly divergent. When implant angulations are greater, however, the modified technique saves great deal of time and effort.

The impression and transfer technique described may be used with any dental implant system for the entire spectrum of prosthetic design. Although this technique saves chair time, it requires the development of additional skills. It is necessary, as well, to establish a relationship with a dental laboratory that is capable of executing the steps necessary to satisfy these procedures. If this technique is performed correctly, its benefits become apparent because of its efficiency and economics of time.

Give the patient techniques for overdenture removal. A proper removal strategy reduces the tendency for attachment wear and breakage as well as minimizing the placement of

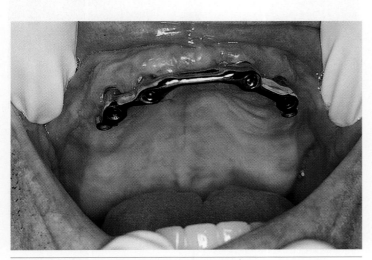

Fig. 26-45 The cast bar is tried-in and checked for accuracy.

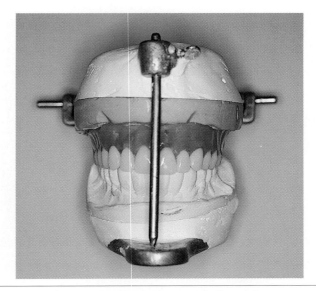

Fig. 26-47 The wax overdenture is set-up before try-in.

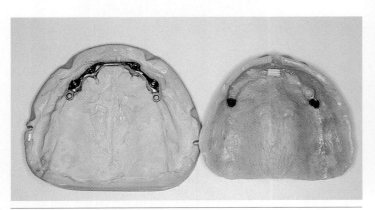

Fig. 26-46 The fabricated bar and wax-up are tried-in with their attachments in place.

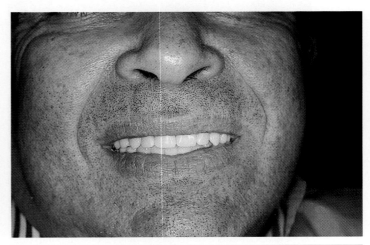

Fig. 26-48 The completed case is inserted on the third visit.

torque on the implants. The patient should be instructed to do the following:

1. Bite his or her teeth together.
2. Place one thumbnail under the overdenture flange in each canine area.
3. Open his or her jaw in a straight downward direction.

Remove the overdenture as it comes away above the thumbs. This technique is not effective if Lew attachments are used because they can be opened most easily when the patient's teeth are closed.

Suggested Readings

Ampil JP et al: Use of magnets for staple mandibular implants, *J Prosthet Dent* 55:367-369, 1986.

Batenburg R, Reintsema H, van Oort R: Use of the final denture base for the intermaxillary registration in an implant-supported overdenture, JOMI on CD-ROM, *Quintessence* 8(2):205-207, 1993.

Bodine RL et al: The subperiosteal implant denture program at the University of Southern California. II. Prosthodontic preparations for oral surgery, *J Oral Implantol* 7:11-32, 1977.

Botta FD: Acute diarrhea, *La Rev du Praticien* 1:113-120, 1995.

Bouma J et al: Psychosocial effects of implant-retained overdentures, JOMI on CD-ROM, *Quintessence* 12(4):515-522, 1997.

Brewer AD, Morrow RM: *Overdentures,* ed 2, St Louis, 1980, Mosby.

Civitelli R, Gonnelli S, Zacchei F et al: Bone turnover in postmenopausal osteoporosis. Effect of calcitonin treatment, *J Clin Invest* 82:1268-1274, 1988.

Consensus Development Conference: Diagnosis, prophylaxis and treatment of osteoporosis, *Am J Med* 94:646-650, 1993.

Cram DL, Roberts HD: Ramus endosseous frame implant for use with patient's dentures, *J Am Dent Assoc* 84:156-162, 1972.

Davidson TJ, Ruff S: A prosthodontic technique for the ramus endosseous frame implant, *J Prosthet Dent* 47:535-538, 1982.

Dawson PE: *Evaluation, diagnosis, and treatment of occlusal problems,* ed 2, St Louis, 1989, Mosby.

Engquist B et al: A retrospective multicenter evaluation of osseointegrated implants supporting overdentures, JOMI on CD-ROM, *Quintessence* 1(2):113-118, 1997.

Falk H et al: Occlusal force patterns in dentitions with mandibular implant-supported fixed cantilever prostheses occluded with complete dentures, *J Oral Maxillofac Implant* 4:55-62, 1989.

Falk H et al: Occlusal interferences and cantilever joint stress in implant-supported prostheses occluding with complete dentures, *J Oral Maxillofac Implant* 5:70-78, 1990.

Galandi ME et al: Evaluation of two bar systems for denture retention under simulated loading conditions, *Z Zahnarztl Implantol* 5:33-37, 1989.

Gerber A: Complete dentures (I). Color Atlas, *Quintessence International* 7:27-32, 1974.

Gerber A: Complete dentures (II). The stability of maxillary dentures during mastication. Color Atlas, *Quintessence International* 8:27-32, 1974.

Gerber A: Complete dentures (III). Better stability for mandibular dentures. Color Atlas, *Quintessence International* 9:31-36, 1974.

Gerber A: Complete dentures (IV). The teamwork of dentures in chewing-function. Color Atlas, *Quintessence International* 10:41-46, 1974.

Gerber A: Complete dentures (V). Functional dynamics determines the type of occlusion. Color Atlas, *Quintessence International* 11:43-47, 1974.

Gerber A: Complete dentures (VI). Mastication (ev-function) centric for fit and tissue comfort. Color Atlas, *Quintessence International* 12:33-38, 1974.

Gershkoff A, Goldberg NI: Further report on the full lower implant dentures, *Dent Dig* 56:11, 1950.

Gillings BR: Magnetic denture retention systems, *Int Dent J* 34:184-197, 1984.

Goldberg NI, Gershkoff A: Fundamentals of the implant denture, *J Prosthet Dent* 2:1-90, 1952.

Goldberg NI, Gershkoff A: Implant lower dentures, *Dent Dig* 5:11, 1952.

Goldberg NI, Gershkoff A: Six-year progress report on full denture implants, *J Implant Dent* 1:13-16, 1954.

Goldberg NI, Gershkoff A: The implant lower denture, *Dent Dig* 55:490-493, 1949.

Goll GE, Smith DE: Technique for fabrication of the mandibular denture over the staple bone implant using a permanent heat-cured base, *J Prosthet Dent* 53:820-824, 1985.

Guerra LR et al: Modifications of the superstructure for the staple implant, *J Prosthet Dent* 52:858-861, 1984.

Hadeed GJ, Pipko DJ: Non-vertical loaded minimal stress attachment with the mandibular staple bone plate, *J Prosthet Dent* 53:824-827, 1985.

Hallman W et al: A comparative study of the effects of metallic, non-metallic, and sonic instrumentation on titanium abutment surfaces, *Int J Oral Maxillofac Implant* 11:96-100, 1996.

Harris ST, Watts NB, Jackson RD et al: Four-year study of intermittent cyclic etiodronate treatment of postmenopausal osteoporosis: three years of blinded therapy followed by one year of open therapy, *Am J Med* 95:557-567, 1993.

Hobo S et al: Osseointegration and occlusal rehabilitation, *Quintessence* (Tokyo), 1990, pp. 323-326.

Humphris GM et al: The psychological impact of implant-retained mandibular prostheses: a cross-sectional study, *JOMI on CD-ROM, Quintessence* 10(4):437-443, 1995.

Jemt T, Book K, Karlsson S: Occlusal force and mandibular movements in patients with removable overdentures and fixed prostheses supported by implants in the maxilla, *Int J Oral Maxillofac Implant* 8:301-308, 1993.

Johns RB, Jemt T et al: A multicenter study of overdentures supported by Branemark implants, *Int J Oral Maxillofac Implant* 7:513-522, 1992.

Lew I: An implant case study of twelve years duration, *J Implant Dent* 8:41-49, 1962.

Lew I: Full upper and lower dentures implant, *Dent Concepts* 4:17, 1952.

Lew I: Case histories and reports: upper and lower implant dentures—fixation with surgical prosthetic splinting, *J Implant Dent* 1:36-38, 1955.

Lew I: Progress report on full implant dentures, *J Prosthet Dent* 3:571, 1953.

Lew I: Implant and denture: a simplified upper technique using immediate prostheses, *Dent Dig* 58:10, 1952.

Linkow LI: The pterygoid extension implant for the totally and partially edentulous maxillae, *Dent Concepts* 12:17-28, 1973.

Loos LG: A fixed prosthodontic technique for mandibular osseointegrated titanium implants, *J Prosthet Dent* 55:232-242, 1986.

Lundgren D et al: The influence of number and distribution of occlusal cantilever contacts on closing and chewing forces in dentitions with implant-supported fixed prosthesis occluding with complete dentures, *J Oral Maxillofac Implant* 4:277-284, 1989.

Martel M: Position paper: occlusal considerations for implant restorations, *Dent Implantol Update*, January 1991, pp. 4-5.

Matson MA, Cohen EP: Acquired cystic kidney disease: occurrence, prevalence, and renal cancers, *Medicine (Baltimore)* 69(4):217-226, 1990.

Maxon BB et al: Prosthodontic considerations for the transmandibular implant, *J Prosthet Dent* 63:554-558, 1990.

Mericske-Stern R: Clinical evaluation of overdenture restorations supported by osseointegrated titanium implants: a retrospective study, *JOMI on CD-ROM, Quintessence* 5(4):375-383, 1990.

Mericske-Stern R: Oral tactile sensibility recorded in overdenture wearers with implants or natural roots: a comparative study. Part II, *JOMI on CD-ROM, Quintessence* 9(1):63-70, 1994.

Mericske-Stern R et al: In vivo measurements of maximal occlusal force and minimal pressure threshold on overdentures supported by implants or natural roots: a comparative study. Part I, *JOMI on CD-ROM, Quintessence* 8(6):641-649, 1997.

Mericske-Stern R et al: Three-dimensional force measurements on mandibular implants supporting overdentures, *JOMI on CD-ROM, Quintessence* 7(2):185-194, 1992.

Meunier PJ: Les osteoporeuses, *La Rev du Praticien* 5:1059-1135, 1995.

Meyer JB, Kotwal KR: Clinical evaluation of ramus frame and staple bone implants, *J Prosthet Dent* 55:87-92, 1986.

Misch CE: Prosthodontic options in implant dentistry, *Int J Oral Implant* 7:17-21, 1991.

Naert I et al: Overdenture supported by osseointegrated fixtures for the edentulous mandible: a 2.5-year report, *J Oral Maxillofac Implant* 3:191-195, 1988.

Palmqvist S, Sondell K, Swartz B: Implant-supported maxillary overdentures: outcome in planned and emergency cases, *JOMI on CD-ROM, Quintessence* 9(2):184-190, 1997.

Parel SM: Implants and overdentures: the osseointegrated approach with conventional and compromised applications, *J Oral Maxillofac Implant* 1:93-99, 1986.

Petropoulos VC, Smith W, Kousvelari E: Comparison of retention and release periods for implant overdenture attachments, *JOMI on CD-ROM, Quintessence* 12(2):176-185, 1997.

Richter EJ: Basic biomechanics of dental implants in prosthetic dentistry, *J Prosthet Dent* 61:602-609, 1989.

Sakaguchi RL, Borgersen SE: Nonlinear contact analysis of preload in dental implant screws, *JOMI on CD-ROM, Quintessence* 10(3):295-302, 1995.

Sirila HS et al: Technique for converting an existing complete denture to a tissue-integrated prosthesis, *J Prosthet Dent* 59:464-466, 1988.

Versteegh P et al: Clinical evaluation of mandibular overdentures supported by multiple-bar fabrication: a follow-up study of two implant systems, *JOMI on CD-ROM, Quintessence* 10(5):595-602, 1995.

WHO Study Group: *Assessment of fracture risk and its application to screening for postmenopausal osteoporosis.* In WHO Technical Report Series 843, Geneva, 1994, World Health Organization, pp. 1-129.

Wismeyer D, van Waas M, Vermeeren J: Overdentures supported by ITI implants: a 6.5-year evaluation of patient satisfaction and prosthetic aftercare, *JOMI on CD-ROM, Quintessence* 10(6):744-749, 1997.

Zarb GA, Janson T: Laboratory procedures and protocol. Tissue-integrated prostheses. In Branemark P-I, Zarb GA, Albrektsson T, editors: *Osseointegration in clinical dentistry*, Chicago, 1985, Quintessence.

27

Principles of Occlusion in Implantology

Ival G. McDermott

cclusal scheme design for implant-supported prostheses is often only briefly discussed in implantology
literature. Yet, as with all phases of prosthodontics,
occlusion is a critical factor in the success or failure of implant-
supported restorations. Tremendous effort has been made
to design complex and intricate implant infrastructures for
these prostheses. It is of equal or greater importance to design restorations that use occlusal forces constructively, not
destructively.

An understanding of implant-supported prosthetic occlusion begins with some basic assumptions drawn from knowledge of natural and prosthetic occlusion.

First, the patient controls the occlusal forces on natural
teeth in response to proprioception. Since natural periodontal
ligament–mediated proprioception does not occur with implants, its protective influence is lost in determining mandibular velocity and displacement. This means occlusal forces on
implant-supported prostheses must be, if anything, more carefully designed and exactly accomplished than tooth-supported
prostheses.

Second, no single occlusal scheme can be used for every
type of restoration. The purpose and mechanism of complete
denture occlusion is different from that of a single crown
restoration. For implant-supported prostheses, the occlusal
scheme must suit the purpose and location of the restoration.

Third, two arches are involved in every occlusion. Whether
the implant-supported prosthesis occludes with natural dentition, tooth- or tissue-supported prostheses, or another
implant-supported prosthesis, is of critical interest, because
each of these prostheses exerts a different range of forces in
both functional and resting movements.

Finally, the natural resorption pattern of edentulous alveolar bone is almost never parallel to the ideal occlusal plane
of the dentition. In determining abutment height and position,
not only adequacy of interarch space but also orientation of

the plane of occlusion must be considered, for it is impossible
to achieve an optimum occlusal scheme with a disrupted or
incorrectly oriented plane of occlusion (Fig. 27-1).

In all phases of prosthetic rehabilitation, design the occlusal scheme to meet the requirements of its oral situation.
When an implant-supported prosthesis replaces a single tooth
in an otherwise intact dental arch, design the occlusion like
that of a tooth-supported single restoration. This is generally
agreed to include lighter-than-normal tripodal centric occlusal
contacts to prevent supereruption of the opposing natural
tooth. Since teeth have a periodontal ligament, they are mi-
croscopically compressible. Take centric stops by having the
patient close hard in centric. It is necessary to compress the
adjacent periodontal ligaments to prevent hyperocclusion of
the implant restoration. The implant-supported prosthetic
crown should follow the guidance of natural teeth in working
relationships, similar to other fixed restorations bounded by
intact natural teeth (Fig. 27-2).

Use canine disclusion in cases in which natural canine
teeth are present and periodontally strong. Where replacing
canine teeth with implant-supported prostheses that occlude
with natural teeth or other implant-supported prostheses,
group function occlusion supported by natural teeth or other
implant-supported prostheses is preferable to avoid loading a
single supporting implant during disclusion. Group function
occlusion provides occlusal contact in centric position and in
working movements but complete disclusion in balancing positions (Fig. 27-3).

By far the most controversial design for implant-supported
prosthetic occlusion is in the totally edentulous mandible
opposing the edentulous maxilla. The osseointegrated, subperiosteal, staple, and other implant types were originally designed to treat patients who use maxillary dentures with little
difficulty but have unfavorable hard- and soft-tissue configurations for retention and stability in the mandibular arch. It is

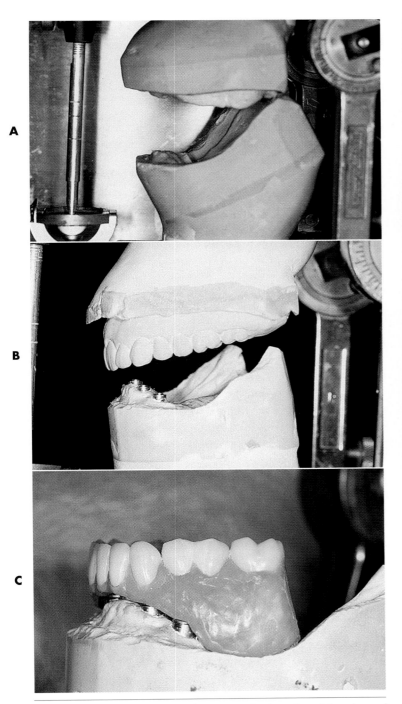

Fig. 27-1 Adequacy of interarch space and orientation of the plane of occlusion must be considered in designing a restoration that provides a balanced occlusal scheme.

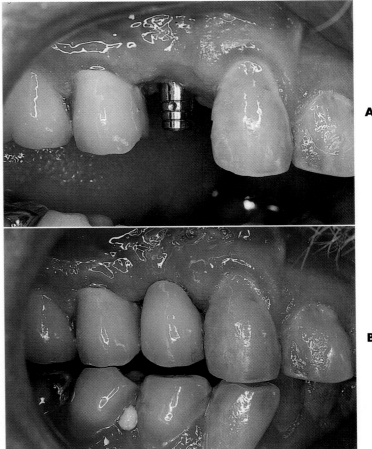

Fig. 27-2 Implant-supported prosthetic crowns bounded by natural teeth should follow their guidance in working relationships, similar to other fixed restorations. The canine guidance found in these arches is maintained after restoration of the implants.

still probably the oral situation most frequently treated with implant dentistry.

A similarity in occlusal scheme requirements exists between the case of maxillary complete denture or mandibular implant-supported prosthesis and the combination of the maxillary complete denture and mandibular distal extension removable partial denture. Both situations provide a maxillary denture that rests on movable and depressible tissue and a mandibular arch with dentition, either natural or artificial, essentially fixed into place.

At first glance, it would seem that the principles of complete dentures apply to implant-supported prosthesis restorations, but the quality of prosthesis support in the two cases is different. In conventional complete denture cases, both dentures are free to move on the tissues, and balanced occlusion (dynamic occlusal contacts throughout the arch) is usually accomplished, at least in part, by denture base movement on resilient tissue. This is especially true of flat plane cases, which have no cuspal inclines to compensate for Christensen's phenomenon (the disclusion of posterior teeth in protrusive position). In dynamic occlusion with complete dentures, each base moves slightly, and compressive force delivered to tissue is relatively low. Tissue proprioception is a limiting factor, because the patient patterns his or her movements to seat, rather than to unseat, his or her mandibular denture.

In the complete denture or implant-supported prosthesis, only the maxillary denture moves in function. Do not rely on soft tissue resiliency and denture movement to assist in balancing dynamic occlusal contacts without excessive compressive and tensile forces under the denture base. Occlusal forces generated against the maxillary denture by the implant-supported prosthesis are of similar magnitude to cantilever

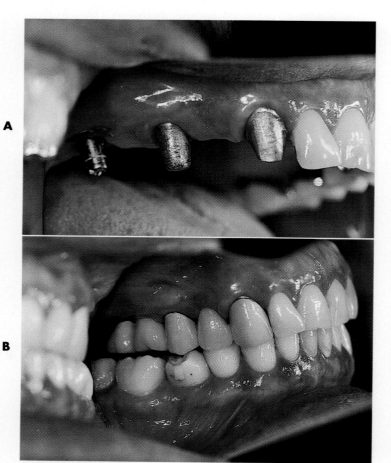

Fig. 27-3 For canine area implant supported crowns, group function occlusion supported by natural teeth or implant-supported prostheses is preferable to canine guidance to avoid loading a single supporting implant during disclusion.

restorations using natural teeth. These forces are many times greater than would be possible with even a well-supported mandibular complete denture, and tissue proprioception of the mandibular denture base is no longer significant. An occlusal scheme that requires movement of the maxillary restoration could predispose the patient to combination syndrome, as has been documented in patients using maxillary denture restorations that provide only anterior tooth contacts in protrusive position.

Clinical signs of this combination syndrome derive from hyperfunction in the anterior area of the arches resulting from Christensen's phenomenon. They include excessive resorption of maxillary anterior alveolar bone, downgrowth of maxillary tuberosities, and a lowering posteriorly of the occlusal plane of the prostheses. The need for an early refining of the maxillary denture signals a rapid degenerative change related to occlusion for this type of restoration.

To avoid initiating this syndrome in patients treated with maxillary complete dentures and mandibular implant-supported prosthesis restorations, an occlusal scheme that is bilaterally balanced during dynamic occlusion is necessary. In 1923, Rudolf Hanau formulated the Hanau Quint as an aid to achieving balanced denture occlusion, and it is quite useful in the complete denture or implant-supported prosthesis situation. It states:

$$< \frac{CG \quad IG \qquad PO \quad CC \quad CH}{\triangle} >$$

where CG is the condylar guidance, IG is the incisal guidance, PO is the plane of occlusion, CC is the compensating curve, and CH is the cusp height.

Simply, this means that factors on the left side of the equation must be offset or balanced by factors on the right. Condylar guidance and incisal guidance are factors that are not within the control of the dentist. Condylar guidance is a function of the anatomy of the temporomandibular articulation. The esthetic position of the anterior teeth, natural or artificial, sets the incisal guide. Factors on the right are within the control of the dentist: orientation of the plane of occlusion of the prosthesis, compensating curve of the plane, and cusp height of the artificial teeth. Making the occlusal plane, the compensating curve, or the cusp height steeper promotes balance by providing more posterior tooth contact during protrusive and lateral movements.

Although the orientation of the plane of occlusion and compensating curve are defined as within the dentist's control, the position of the maxillary tuberosity limits them, especially in patients who had retained natural mandibular anterior teeth before implant placement. Also, the bisection of the retromolar pad is a commonly accepted landmark for orientation of the occlusal plane, and this can limit posterior elevation and use of a steep compensating curve. The factor most easily within the dentist's control is the cusp height of the artificial teeth selected for the prosthesis, and many clinicians, especially those who have considered the potential for combination syndrome, recommend use of cusp or fossa occlusion to provide balance in complete denture or implant-supported prosthesis cases.

Attempts to provide occlusal balance in complete denture or implant-supported prosthesis restorations may cause problems. One problem is the absence of molar occlusal contacts in the shortened arch form usually used for implant-borne cantilever prostheses. It is generally suggested to limit such cantilevers to 15 mm posterior to the posterior implant abutment. This scheme provides occlusal contacts only back to premolars or first molars. Further extension posteriorly will direct unfavorable forces to the implants.

Another issue that could argue against the use of cusp or fossa-balanced occlusion is the introduction of horizontal, non-axial forces on the implants during posterior cusp–guided disclusion. This concern has prompted some clinicians to use either a totally flat plane scheme or the reduction of cusp height to the point that the anterior teeth accomplish disclusion. Most complete denture or implant-supported prosthesis cases are made with implant support that extends only to the canine region, so, in essence, no posterior tooth contacts are directed along the long axes of the implants even in centric closure. The number and location of implants in fully implant-supported fixed prostheses and saddle and flange extensions to use soft tissue support for implant-supported overdentures compensate for this. In either case, the implant-supported prosthesis in the mandibular arch has a far greater potential for destruction of the edentulous maxilla than the maxillary denture has for the implants, whatever their type or configuration.

When only a limited number of implants can be placed, the restoration of choice is often the implant-supported overdenture. Some authors have advocated a round configuration clip bar extending between two implants only, permitting free rotation of the denture vertically under posterior loading and sparing the implants in occlusion. An unwanted side effect of such a design is the potential for mandibular posterior bone loss and eventual anterior tooth occlusion in centric relationship closure, as well as in eccentric movements. If using this design, take care in follow-up visits to evaluate occlusion, reline if necessary, and be ready to change occlusal philosophy if rapid mandibular posterior or maxillary anterior bone resorption occurs.

Creating a Balanced Occlusal Scheme

Many dentists and laboratories have grown used to arranging only flat or semianatomic artificial teeth for contact in centric relationship. A brief review of waxing balanced occlusion may be helpful.

1. Face-bow mount the master casts in centric relationship at the determined vertical dimension of occlusion.
2. Use a semiadjustable articulator, and set the condylar elements and incisal guide table with the use of an interocclusal record made in edge-to-edge protrusive position (Fig. 27-4).
3. Mark the land area of the mandibular cast to show the level of the bisection of the retromolar pads.
4. Trial-insert the maxillary anterior teeth for esthetic position before beginning the full setup. Also trial-insert the mandibular anterior teeth, whose position is in part determined by the implant abutments, and adjust the horizontal and vertical overlap to approximately 2 mm in both dimensions. Ideally, this has been worked out in trial dentures before implant placement and planned with the use of a surgical template to ensure abutment alignment within an acceptable range for esthetic artificial tooth arrangement (Fig. 27-5).
5. Arrange maxillary 30-degree cusp posterior teeth with a plane of occlusion so that the first molar mesiolingual cusp bisects the retromolar pad and a steep compensating curve begins there and rises above the plane 1 to 2 mm (Fig. 27-6).
6. Arrange mandibular 30-degree cusp posterior teeth to provide tight occlusal contacts when viewed from the lingual and buccal aspects (Fig. 27-7).
7. Unlock the condylar elements and move the articulator into protrusive position with the incisors at edge-to-edge relationship to check for cusp tip contacts of all posterior teeth (Fig. 27-8).
8. Move the articulator into right and left working positions to check for cusp-to-fossa contacts in working positions and cusp tip contacts in balancing positions, as viewed from buccal and lingual aspects (Fig. 27-9).
9. Reestablish that the anterior teeth are just out of contact in protrusive and lateral excursions (Fig. 27-10).

Because the semiadjustable articulator has a straight line condylar path, it cannot duplicate mandibular movements with precision. Before trial insertion, arrange teeth as perfectly as possible, but be ready to make another protrusive record, especially when what is seen in the mouth appears different from what is on the articulator. It is better to process the dentures with excessive cuspal contact in lateral and protrusive positions, since this allows for adjustment in a functional grind-in procedure. It is easy to remove excessive cusp height, but it is impossible to add it if the cusp tips fall short of obtaining balance. In that instance, balance has to be obtained by grinding anterior teeth, with the attendant loss of esthetics.

A successful modification of full cusp balance that may offer advantages is the lingualized occlusion scheme. In this scheme, obtain balance by continuous contact of the maxillary lingual cusps with the occlusal table of the mandibular teeth during dynamic occlusion.

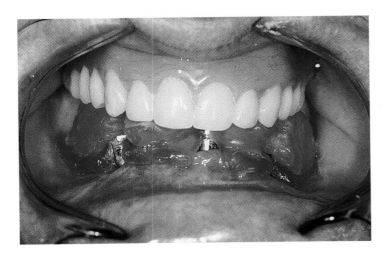

Fig. 27-4 Use a protrusive record to program the semiadjustable articulator condylar elements and incisal guide table. Make this record with wax rims or after the trial insertion of anterior teeth.

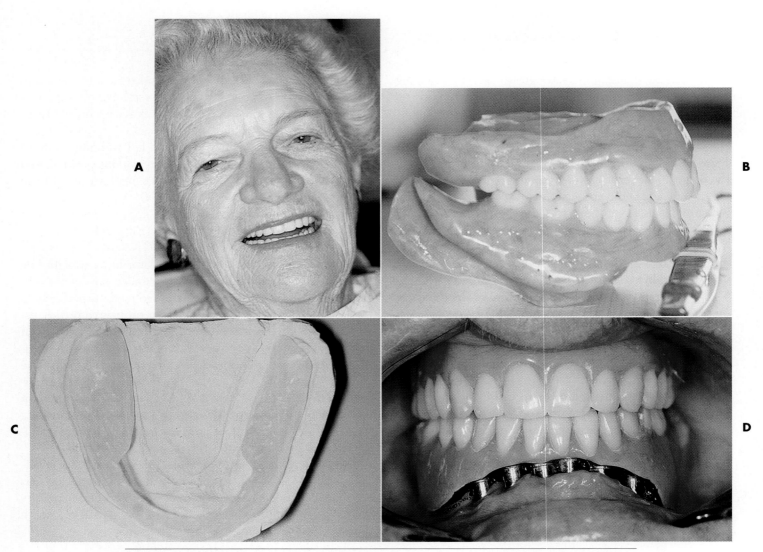

Fig. 27-5   A-D, Perform a trial insertion to evaluate esthetic tooth position before beginning the full set-up. Usually, this duplicates tooth position of dentures made before implant placement. Use of a surgical template can aid in abutment alignment within an acceptable range for esthetic artificial tooth arrangement.

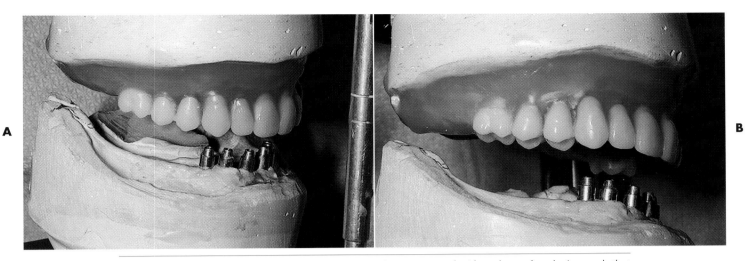

Fig. 27-6   A, Maxillary 30-degree cusp posterior teeth are arranged with a plane of occlusion such that the first molar mesiolingual cusp bisects the retromolar pad and a steep compensating curve begins there and rises above the plane 1 to 2 mm. **B,** They are arranged such that only lingual cusps touch the plane of occlusion.

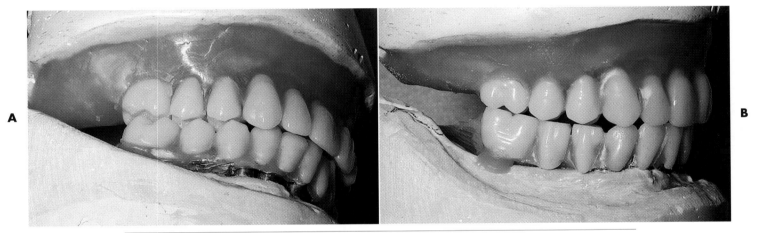

Fig. 27-7   A, Mandibular 30-degree cusp posterior teeth are arranged to provide tight occlusal contacts as viewed from the lingual and buccal aspects. **B,** These flat or semiautomatic posterior teeth are arranged to provide tight occlusal fossa contacts with the maxillary lingual cusps. Buccal cusps should be out of occlusion in centric and eccentric positions.

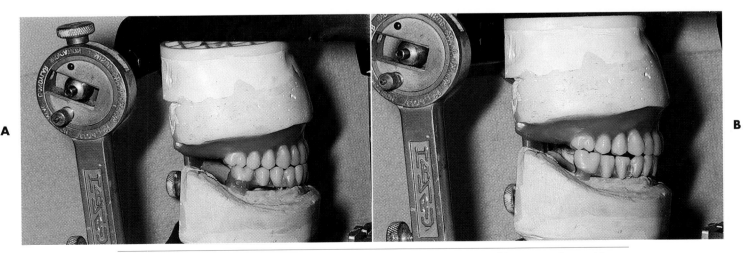

Fig. 27-8   A, Condylar elements may be unlocked and the articulator moved into protrusive position to check for cusp tip contacts on all posterior teeth at the anterior edge-to-edge position. **B,** The maxillary lingual cusp tips of all posterior teeth should contact the mandibular fossae at the edge-to-edge position.

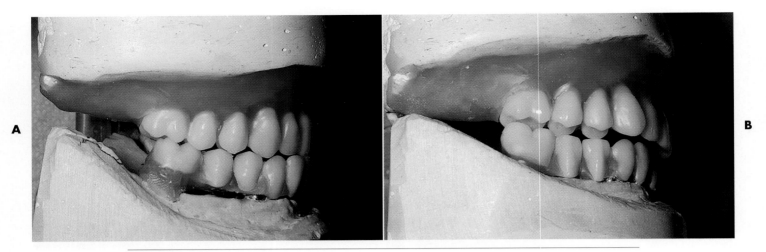

Fig. 27-9 **A,** The articulator may be moved into right and left working positions to check for cusp-to-fossa contacts in working and cusp tip contacts in balancing positions, as viewed from buccal and lingual aspects. **B,** The arrangement should provide cusp-to-fossa contacts in a small range of working and balancing positions.

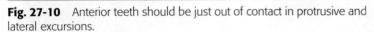

Fig. 27-10 Anterior teeth should be just out of contact in protrusive and lateral excursions.

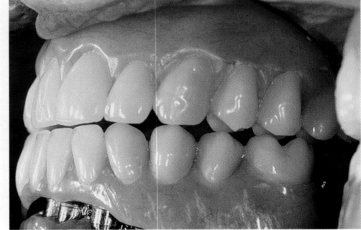

Functional Adjustment for Balanced Occlusion

Clinical remount procedures using an articulator can reestablish coincidence between centric relation closure and maximum intercuspation. A stable, unstrained, intercuspal position is the most important aspect in a cusped occlusion. A laboratory remount of freshly processed dentures before decasting, although advocated by some authors, can cause gross inaccuracies if processing shrinkage has caused the dentures to distort by pulling away from the master casts. It is preferable to decast and finish the prostheses and insert them before any occlusal adjustment. Usually, little distortion occurs in implant-supported prostheses with metal infrastructures. Insert and tighten them into place on their supporting implants before occlusal registration. Disclose tissue-borne opposing "dentures with pressure indicator paste (PIP), and remove interferences to vertical seating without occlusal contact (Fig. 27-11).

Make a new centric relation record to reestablish centric relation occlusion on the articulator (Fig. 27-12). It is inadvisable, however, to attempt to duplicate dynamic occlusion mechanically, so use functional methods such as chew-in techniques, centric-bearing devices, and occlusal indicator waxes instead (Fig. 27-13). To avoid losing balanced contacts, make adjustments in the form of sharpening cusps and deepening or widening fossae. It is preferable to adjust the maxillary denture, as opposed to the mandibular implant-supported prosthesis, to avoid flattening the orientation of the occlusal plane or compensating curve. Occlusion for implant-supported restorations holds a major key to long-term success, not only for the prostheses but also for the remaining oral supporting structures they approximate.

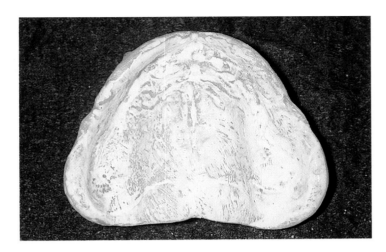

Fig. 27-11 Seat tissue-borne opposing dentures under finger pressure using pressure indicator paste, and eliminate interferences to vertical seating.

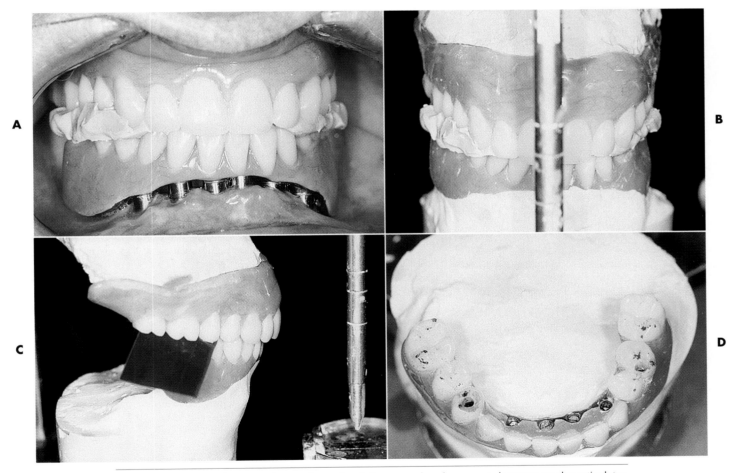

Fig. 27-12 A-D, Make a new intraoral centric relation record and remount dentures on the articulator. Adjust articulating paper markings until uniform contact in centric relation has been established.

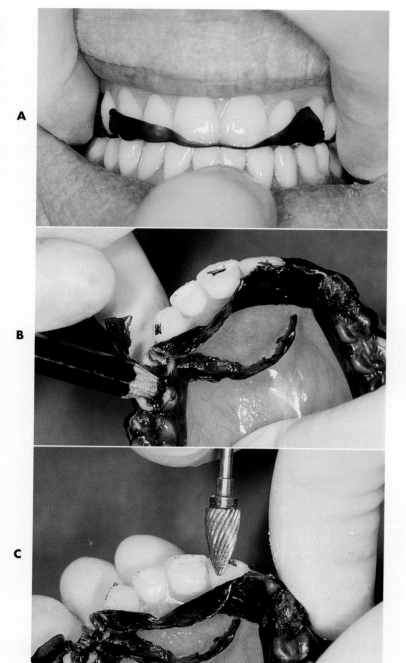

Fig. 27-13 **A-C,** Occlusal indicator wax is useful for marking areas of premature contact in excursive movements of the mandible. Grasp the maxillary denture firmly at the zygomatic buttress areas to avoid denture movement during record making. Uniform contact on posterior tooth fossae and cuspal inclines is desired. Remove contact on anterior teeth (proximal to the canine cusp tip) from maxillary lingual or mandibular incisal surfaces.

Suggested Readings

Ali A et al: Implant rehabilitation of irradiated jaws: a preliminary report, *Int J Oral Maxillofac Implant* 12(4):523-526, 1197.

Asikainen P et al: Osseointegration of dental implants in bone irradiated with 40, 50, or 60 gy doses. An experimental study with beagle dogs, *Clin Oral Implant Res* 9(1):20-25, 1998.

Augthun M, Conrads G: Microbial findings of deep peri-implant bone defects, *Oral Int J Maxillofac Implant* 12:106-112, 1997.

Balshi TJ: Resolving aesthetic complications with osseointegration using a double-casting technique, *Quintessence* 17:281-287, 1986.

Becker W et al: Clinical and microbiologic findings that may contribute to dental implant failure, *Int J Oral Maxillofac Implant* 5:31-38, 1990.

Branemark P-I et al: An experimental and clinical study of osseointegrated implants penetrating the nasal cavity and maxillary sinus, *J Oral Maxillofac Surg* 42:497-505, 1984.

Briner WW et al: Effect of chlorhexidine gluconate mouth rinse on plaque bacteria, *J Periodont Res* 16(suppl):44-52, 1986.

Brogniez V et al: Prosthetic dental rehabilitation on osseointegrated implants placed in irradiated mandibular bone. Apropos of 50 implants in 17 patients treated over a period of 5 years, *Rev Stomatol Chir Maxillofac* 97(5):288-294, 1996.

Brygider RM: Precision attachment-retained gingival veneers for fixed implant prostheses, *J Prosthet Dent* 65:118-122, 1991.

Brygider RM, Bain CA: Custom stent fabrication for free gingival grafts around osseointegrated abutment fixtures, *J Prosthet Dent* 62:320-322, 1989.

Caplanis N et al: Effect of allogenic, freeze-dried, demineralized bone matrix on guided bone regeneration in supra-alveolar peri-implant defects in dogs, *Int J Oral Maxillofac Implant* 12:634-642, 1997.

Carlson B, Carlsson GE: Prosthodontic complications in osseointegrated dental implant treatment, JOMI on CD-ROM, *Quintessence* 9(1):90-94, 1994.

Carr AB, Laney WR: Maximum occlusal force levels in patients with osseointegrated oral implant prostheses and patients with complete dentures, JOMI on CD-ROM, *Quintessence* 2(2):101-108, 1987.

Castelli W: Vascular architecture of the human adult mandible, *J Dent Res* 42:786-792, 1963.

Chiche G et al: Auxiliary substructure for screw-retained prostheses, *Int J Prosthodont* 2:407-412, 1989.

Christiansen RL: Latent infection involving a mandibular implant: a case report, *J Oral Maxillofac Implant* 6:481-484, 1991.

Dahlin C et al: Generation of new bone around titanium implants using a membrane technique: an experimental study in rabbits, *J Oral Maxillofac Implant* 4:19-25, 1989.

Davenport WL et al: Salvage of the mandibular staple bone plate following bone infection, *J Oral Maxillofac Surg* 43:981-986, 1985.

Davies JM, Campbell LA: Fatal air embolism during dental implant surgery: a report of three cases, *Can J Anaesth* 37:112-121, 1990.

Dharmar S: Locating the mandibular canal in panoramic radiographs, *Int J Oral Maxillofac Implant* 12:113-117, 1997.

Eckert SE et al: Endosseous implants in an irradiated tissue bed, *J Prosthet Dent* 76(1):45-59, 1996.

Esser E et al: Dental implants following radical oral cancer surgery and adjuvant radiotherapy, *Int J Oral Maxillofac Implant* 12(4):552-557, 1997.

Falk H, Laurell L, Lundgren D: Occlusal force pattern in dentitions with mandibular implant-supported fixed cantilever prostheses occluded with complete dentures, *J Oral Maxillofac Implant* 4:55-62, 1989.

Falk H, Laurell L, Lundgren D: Occlusal interferences and cantilever joint stress in implant-supported prostheses occluding with complete dentures, *J Oral Maxillofac Implants* 5:70-77, 1990.

Fisch M: Causes of failure with intraosseous implants, *Int Dent J* 33:379-382, 1983.

Franzen L et al: Oral implant rehabilitation of patients with oral malignancies treated with radiotherapy and surgery without adjunctive hyperbaric oxygen, *Int J Oral Maxillofac Implant* 10(2):183-187, 1995.

Gallagher DM, Epker BN: Infection following intraoral surgical correction of dentofacial deformities: a review of 140 consecutive cases, *J Oral Surg* 38:117-120, 1980.

Gammage DD: Clinical management of failing dental implants: four case reports, *J Oral Implantol* 15:124-131, 1989.

Garfield RE: Implant prostheses for convertibility, stress control, esthetics, and hygiene, *J Prosthet Dent* 60:85-93, 1988.

Granstrom G et al: Titanium implants in irradiated tissue: benefits from hyperbaric oxygen, *Int J Oral Maxillofac Implant* 7(1):15-25, 1992.

Grondahl K, Lekholm U: The predictive value of radiographic diagnosis of implant instability, *Int J Oral Maxillofac Implant* 12:59-64, 1997.

Hobo S, Ichida E, Garcia LT: *Osseointegration and occlusal rehabilitation*, Chicago, 1990, Quintessence.

Hurzeler M et al: Treatment of peri-implantitis using guided bone regeneration and bone grafts, alone or in combination, in beagle dogs. Part II. Histologic findings, *Int J Oral Maxillofac Implant* 12:168-175, 1997.

Ibbott CG: In vivo fracture of a basket-type osseointegrating dental implant: a case report, *J Oral Maxillofac Implant* 4:255-256, 1989.

Jensen O, Nock D: Inferior alveolar nerve repositioning in conjunction with placement of osseointegrated implants: a case report, *Oral Surg Oral Med Oral Pathol* 63:263-268, 1987.

Jisander S et al: Dental implant survival in the irradiated jaw: a preliminary report, *Int J Oral Maxillofac Implants* 12(5):643-648, 1997.

Kan J et al: Mandibular fracture after endosseous implant placement in conjunction with inferior alveolar nerve transposition: a patient treatment report, *Int J Oral Maxillofac Implant* 12:655-660, 1997.

Keller EE: Placement of dental implants in the irradiated mandible: a protocol without adjunctive hyperbaric oxygen, *J Oral Maxillofac Implant* 55(9):972-980, 1997.

Keller EE et al: Mandibular endosseous implants and autogeneous bone grafting in irradiated tissue: a 10-year retrospective study, *Int J Oral Maxillofac Implant* 12(6):800-813, 1997.

Laboda G: Life-threatening hemorrhage after placement of an endosseous implant: report of a case, *J Am Dent Assoc* 121:599-600, 1990.

Lambert P, Morris HF, Ochi S et al: Relationship between implant surgical experience and second-stage failures: DICRG interim report no. 2, *Implant Dent* 3:97, 1994.

Laney WR, Gibelisco JA: *Diagnosis and treatment in prosthodontics*, Philadelphia, 1983, Lea & Febiger, p. 169.

Lang B, Mossie H, Razzoog M: *International workshop: biocompatibility, toxicity and hypersensitivity to alloy systems used in dentistry*, Ann Arbor, 1985, University of Michigan Press.

Larsen PE: Placement of dental implants in the irradiated mandible: a protocol involving adjunctive hyperbaric oxygen, *J Oral Maxillofac Surg* 55(9):967-971, 1997.

Leghissa G, Botticelli A: Resistance to bacterial aggression involving exposed nonresorbable membranes in the oral cavity, *Int J Oral Maxillofac Implant* 11(2):210-215, 1996.

Lillard JF: Resolution of a complicated implant case using accepted multimodal guidelines, *J Oral Implantol* 17:146-151, 1991.

Lindquist LW, Rockler B, Carlsson GE: Bone resorption around fixtures in edentulous patients treated with mandibular fixed tissue-integrated prostheses, *J Prosthet Dent* 59:59-63, 1988.

Lundgren D et al: The influence of number and distribution of occlusal cantilever contacts on closing and chewing forces in dentitions with implant-supported fixed prosthesis occluding with complete dentures, *J Oral Maxillofac Implant* 4:277-284, 1989.

Martel M: Position paper: occlusal considerations for implant restorations, *Dent Implantol Update* January 1991; 4-5.

Martin IC et al: Endosseous implants in the irradiated composite radial forearm free flap, *Int J Oral Maxillofac Implant* 21(5):266-270, 1992.

Mason M et al: Mandibular fracture through endosseous cylinder implants, *J Oral Maxillofac Surg* 48:311-317, 1990.

Misch CE: *Protect the prosthesis* (manual). Misch Implant Institute, 1990.

Misch CE, Crawford EA: Predictable mandibular nerve location—a clinical zone of safety, *Int J Oral Implant* 7:37-44, 1990.

Misch CE et al: Postoperative maxillary cyst associated with a maxillary sinus elevation procedure: a case report, *J Oral Implantol* 17:432-437, 1991.

Mombelli A et al: The microbiota associated with successful or failing osseointegrated titanium implants, *Oral Microbiol Immunol* 2:145, 1987.

Mordenfeld A, Andersson L, Bergstrom B: Hemorrhage in the floor of the mouth during implant placement in the edentulous mandible: a case report, *Int J Oral Maxillofac Implant* 12:558-561, 1997.

Niimi A et al: A Japanese multicenter study of osseointegrated implants placed in irradiated tissues: a preliminary report, *Int J Oral Maxillofac Implant* 12(2):259-264, 1997.

Nyman S et al: Bone regeneration adjacent to titanium dental implants using guided tissue regeneration: a report of two cases, *J Oral Maxillofac Implant* 5:9-14, 1990.

O'Roark WL: Improving implant survival rates by using a new method of at-risk analysis, *Int J Oral Implant* 8:31-57, 1991.

Pertri WH: Osteogenic activity of antibiotic-supplemented bone allografts in the guinea pig, *J Oral Maxillofac Surg* 42:631-636, 1984.

Richter EJ: Basic biomechanics of dental implants in prosthetic dentistry, *J Prosthet Dent* 61:602-609, 1989.

Sakaguchi RL, Borgensen SE: Nonlinear contact analysis of preload in dental implant screws, JOMI on CD-ROM, *Quintessence* 10(3):295-302, 1995.

Salcetti J et al: The clinical, microbial, and host response charactistics of the failing implant, *Int J Oral Maxillofac Implant* 12:32-42, 1997.

Schon R et al: Peri-implant tissue reaction in bone irradiated the fifth day after implantation in rabbits: histologic and histomorphometric measurements, *Int J Oral Maxillofac Implants* 11(2):228-238, 1996.

Sclaroff A et al: Immediate mandibular reconstruction and placement of dental implants at the time of ablative surgery, *Oral Surg Oral Med Oral Pathol* 78(6):711-717, 1994.

Simion M et al: Treatment of dehiscences and fenestrations around dental implants using resorbable and nonresorbable membranes associated with bone autografts: a comparative clinical study, *Int J Oral Maxillofac Implant* 12:159-168, 1997.

Stefani LA: The care and maintenance of the dental implant patient, *J Dent Hygiene* 10:447-466, 1988.

Sullivan DY et al: The reverse torque test: a clinical report, *Int J Oral Maxillofac Implant* 11:179-185, 1996.

Symposium on retrieval and analysis of surgical implants and biomaterials, Society for Biomaterials, Snowbird, Utah, 1988.

Takeshita F et al: Histologic study of failed hollow implants, *Int J Oral Maxillofac Implant* 11(2):245-254, 1996.

Taylor TD et al: Osseointegrated implant rehabilitation of the previously irradiated mandible: results of a limited trial at 3 to 7 years, *J Prosthet Dent* 69(1):60-69, 1993.

Teixeira E et al: Correlation between mucosal inflammation and marginal bone loss around hydroxyapatite-coated implants: a 3-year cross-sectional study, *Int J Oral Maxillofac Implant* 12:74-81, 1997.

Thomson-Neal D et al: A SEM evaluation of various prophylactic modalities on different implants, *Int J Perio Rest Dent* 4: 1989.

Tolman DE, Keller EE: Management of mandibular fractures in patients with endosseous implants, *J Oral Maxillofac Implant* 6:427-436, 1991.

Walton JN, Gardner FM, Agar JR: A survey of crown and fixed partial denture fixtures: length of service and reasons for replacement, *J Prosthet Dent* 56(4):416-421, 1986.

Watzinger F et al: Endosteal implants in the irradiated lower jaw, *J Craniomaxillofac Surg* 24(4):237-244, 1996.

Weinmann JP: Biologic factors influencing implant denture success, *J Implant Dent* 2:12-15, 1956.

Weischer T et al: Concept of surgical and implant-supported prostheses in the rehabilitation of patients with oral cancer, *Int J Oral Maxillofac Implant* 11(6):775-781, 1996.

Weiss CM: A comparative analysis of fibro-osteal and osteal integration and other variables that affect long-term bone maintenance around dental implants, *J Oral Implantol* 13:467-487, 1987.

Wolinsky LE, Camargo PM, Erard JC: A study of in vitro attachment of *Streptococcus sanguis* and *Actinomyces viscosus* to saliva-treated titanium, *Int J Oral Maxillofac Implant* 4:27-31, 1989.

Zablotsky M, Meffert RM, Caudill R et al: Histological and clinical comparisons of tissue regeneration on dehisced hydroxylapatite-coated and titanium endosseous implant surfaces: a pilot study, *Int J Oral Maxillofac Implant* 6:295-303, 1991.

Zarb GA, Schmitt A: The longitudinal clinical effectiveness of osseointegrated dental implants: the Toronto Study. Part III. Problems and complications, *J Prosthet Dent* 64:185-194, 1990.

28

Diagnosis and Treatment of Complications

This chapter offers a variety of techniques that may be used if problems arise. The chapter is divided into three major parts:

1. Intraoperative complications
2. Short-term complications (those that occur during the first 6 months after surgery)
3. Long-term complications

CAVEATS

Do not attempt heroic efforts. It is always safer (personally, professionally, and legally) to remove a failing implant or, at the outset, to decide not to insert one. Use good sense and sound clinical judgment tempered with experience in making a decision to perform a salvage operation. At this juncture, it would be useful to review the section on "Surgical Anatomy," p. 55 in Chapter 4 and all of Chapters 6, 7, 8, and 9.

ARMAMENTARIUM

Acrylic, self-curing
Bone files
Burs: 700 L, 701 L, 2 L, 4 L, 6 L friction-grip
Curettes: surgical and periodontal
Electrosurgical unit
Explorer/millimeter probe
Forceps:
  Adson toothed and nontoothed pickup forceps
  Gerald toothed and nontoothed pickup forceps
  Kelly and tonsil (curved) hemostatic forceps
  Rongeur side- and end-cutting
  Wire twisting forceps, heavy duty
Gelfoam, surgical bone wax, Avitene
Handpieces, high- and low-speed, straight and angled, Impactair
Hemostats: mosquito, Kelly
Hypodermic needles, 18-gauge disposable, 1½-inch
Local anesthetic syringes, needles, and solutions
Mallet, nylon-covered
Mirror (front surface)
3½-inch, 18-gauge spinal needle with stylet (for the zygoma)
1½-inch needle (for the mandible)
Needle holders

Nerve hooks
Periosteal elevators
Osteotomes: curved and straight
Pliers:
  College pliers, with plastic tips
  Titanium-tipped cone-socket pliers (2)
Polyethylene (intravenous) tubing
Prep tray for sterilizing the operative site
Retractors: sweetheart (tongue), baby Parker, blunt (Mathieu) rakes, large blunt rakes, Army/Navy, beaver tail (Henahan), McBurney, vein, Leahy
Sable paint brush (0-0)
Scalpel handles (2), Bard Parker No. 3
Scalpel blades Nos. 10, 11, 12, 15
Scissors: Metzenbaum, curved, sharp tissue, and suture
Sponges, 2 × 2-inch, 4 × 4-inch
Suction tips (Yankauer and Frazier), plastic
Sutures, 3-0 black silk, 4-0 dyed Vicryl, 3-0 plain gut, 4-0 chromic gut on tapered and cutting needles
Towel clamps
Wire, monofilament No. 2 stainless steel in 12- to 18-inch lengths
Wire cutters, shears, and nippers

Intraoperative Complications

Endosteal Implants

Oversized Osteotomy

ROOT FORMS   The best way to manage problems is to practice avoidance. Most systems, including Nobel Biocare, 3i, Calcitek, Steri-Oss, and Paragon, offer implants of several diameters. On making the discovery during the placement of a 3.5-mm diameter implant that the endosteal threads have been stripped, place a larger diameter implant (if the ridge is 6 to 7 mm wide) that successfully retaps and grasps the internal environment of the osteotomy. The Nobel Biocare design offers a 4-mm implant to serve as a replacement if the surgeon strips the bone while seating the standard 3.75-mm size. The Steri-Oss series is available in 3.25 mm, 3.8 mm, and larger diameters. An additional advantage is that these implants get wider toward their coronal ends. The Steri-Oss Mini series 3.8-mm-diameter implant does not have a threaded backup size. However, a press-fit 3.8-mm design is available, and it may be used as a substitute for the stripped threaded implant site (Fig. 28-1).

Calcitek makes a 3.25-mm, small-diameter (SD) implant as well as one with a standard 4-mm diameter; both are hydroxyapatite (HA)-coated, press-fit designs. Use the larger size in cases of failure to gain frictional grip of the SD implant.

A helpful hint when placing implants of the Nobel Biocare, Swede-Vent, or 3i type clones in maxillae and in soft mandibles is not to use the counter-sink and bone-tapping or threading instruments. Rather, because of the compliance so often found in maxillary bone, permit the implants to tap themselves into position. These systems are technique sensitive. Do the last two steps, bone tapping and implant seating, with an ultra–low-speed handpiece or by hand. The threads are fine and closely approximated to one another. Using an electric or a nitrogen-powered motor diminishes tactile sensitivity for even the most skilled of surgeons. If the bone lacks sufficient density to stop the rotation by frictional braking, continuing rotation of the bone tap or the implant itself has the potential of stripping the internal bony threads. Therefore, perform the tapping and seating operations with discrimination and care, using a mark on the rotary instrument to dictate the exact moment to reverse the motor direction. One safer approach is to stop the motor at a point four to five rotations from final seating and complete the procedure with the handheld ratchet wrench (Fig. 28-2). Hold the wrench near its working end to neutralize the great leverage offered by its long handle. This leverage, if not governed carefully, may be responsible for stripping the internal bony threads. Make the preliminary efforts of placement by attempting to turn the implant with the wheel only (Fig. 28-3). If, after all of these precautions, the implant does not come to a final and firm stop, remove it and insert the next-larger diameter implant, placing it without the formality of bone-tapping or threading devices. Practice and experience helps flatten the learning curve.

If the osteotomy becomes oversized during the insertion of a press-fit or a threaded implant from a system without an available larger diameter, remove the implant and place some

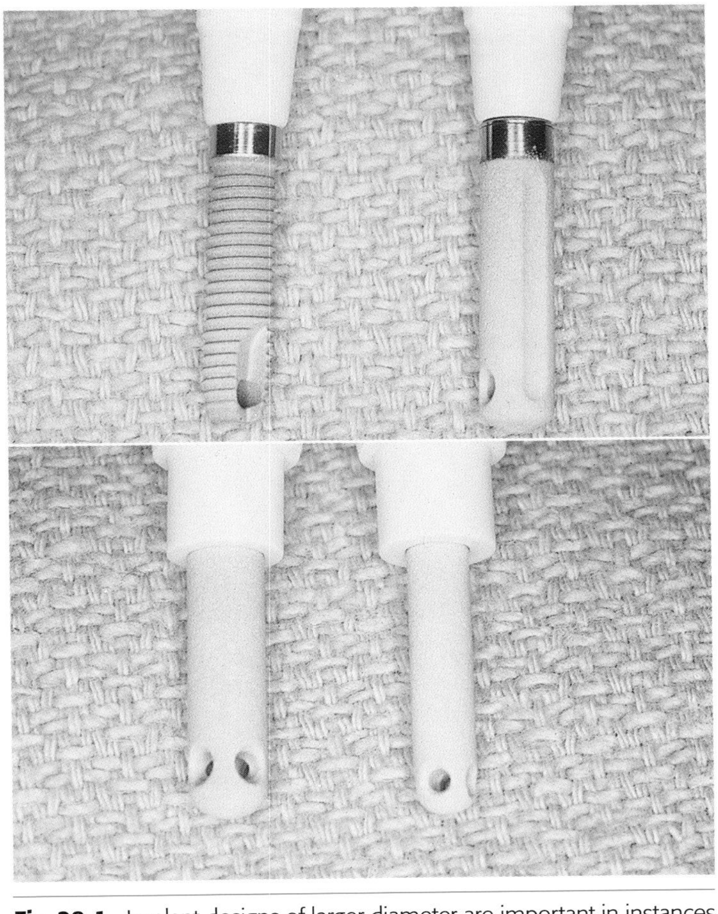

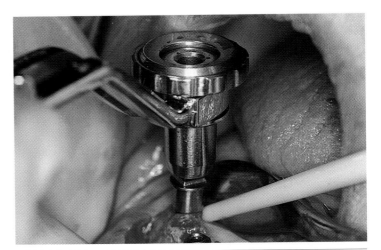

Fig. 28-1   Implant designs of larger diameter are important in instances of oversized osteotomies. If an implant does not fit snugly, a larger design is used. **A,** Steri-Oss: threaded design-supplanted by press-fit. **B,** Calcitek Integral: same design, but a larger diameter implant.

Fig. 28-2   If there is too much resistance to permit threading with the wheel wrench, use the ratchet. The highest level of control is obtained by holding it near its center and supporting with the other counter-torquing hand. As leverage is increased, tactility diminishes.

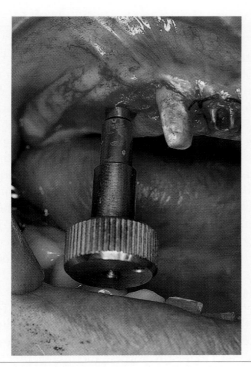

Fig. 28-3 Threaded implant systems supply the clinician with wheel wrenches that are used in less dense bone for discriminate rotation.

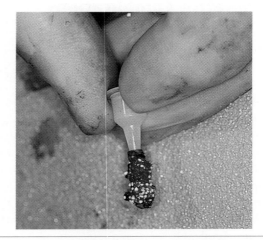

Fig. 28-4 Achieve improved retention for HA-coated, press-fit implants by moistening them in blood and rolling them in 40- to 60-mesh HA. The adherent particles serve to wedge the implant firmly into its host site.

40-mesh, particulate HA graft material against the internal walls of the osteotomy. Roll the implant, moistened in blood or saline, in the particulate slurry until a thin layer of the slurry clings to it. Then reinsert it to achieve a frictional fit. Successful osseointegration can be developed in this manner. A maximum space of 0.5 mm is allowable for the practice of this technique (Fig. 28-4).

BLADE AND PLATE-FORM IMPLANTS The following suggestions are suitable for one-piece and submergible blades. If the osteotomy is larger than the blade infrastructure, trim a second Omni or Ultronics blade (which are supplied in "blank" form) longer or deeper to create a frictional fit within the bone slot (if anatomic structures permit). With all non–HA-coated blades, custom, and catalogue, achieve primary retention by bending the infrastructure into a gently curved "S" pattern. This offers a primary frictional fit by locking the blade into position while the process of osteogenesis is taking place. Bend blades using two titanium-tipped, cone-socket pliers to apply very gentle but firm pressure so that the bends are gradual rather than acute (Fig. 28-5).

In cases of interfacial voids of more than 0.5 mm, using particulate graft material mixed with demineralized freeze-dried bone (DFDB) is strongly recommended as an osteoinductive grout.

Perforations of Cortical Plates: Root Form, Plate-Form, and Blade Implants

When performing osteotomies for the seating of endosteal implants—laminar, grooved, slotted, or cylindrical—it is possible

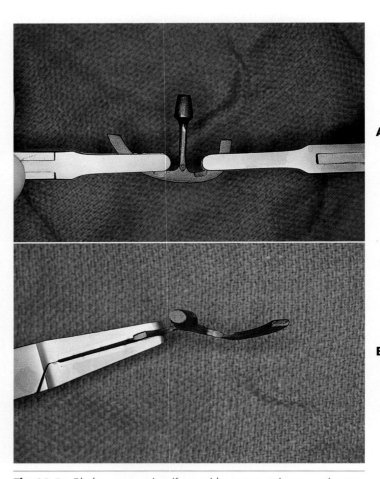

Fig. 28-5 Blade osteotomies, if too wide, may require corrective maneuvers. The use of titanium-tipped, cone-socket pliers to bend gentle irregularities into the infrastructure offers instant retention.

that even if the host site is capacious, misdirection of a drill or the presence of an unexpected anatomic irregularity (e.g., the submandibular fossa beneath the mylohyoid ridge) may cause a perforation, either medially, laterally, or apically (Fig. 28-6). When ridge width is lacking while instituting expansion techniques, fracture may occur with displacement or even loss of

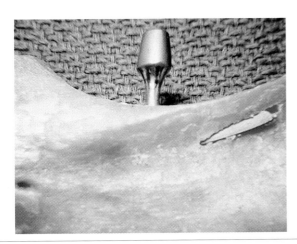

Fig. 28-6 A constant awareness of anatomic characteristics prevents cortical plate perforations. Such events occur with no signal to the surgeon. After completion of osteotomies and before implant placement, make soundings with a blunt probe.

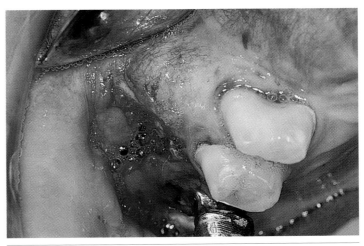

Fig. 28-8 To avoid calamitous maxillary sinus complications, test the osteotomy by asking the patient to exhale gently through the nose while compressing the nares. Bubbling indicates an oroantral communication.

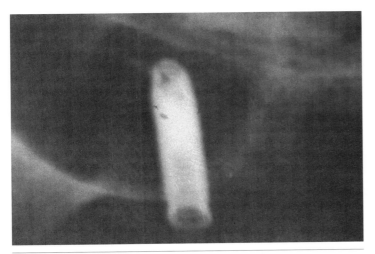

Fig. 28-7 Antral floor perforations should be discouraged. A few millimeters of overextension are allowable because the sinus membrane may be pushed upward and remain intact. Greater penetration mandates instant removal of the implant and primary repair with a pedicle graft.

the cortical segment. If periosteum is attached to the endangered cortical plate, replacing it after implant insertion and suturing presents a good prognosis for healing. If the fragment becomes detached, it can be wedged back into position, but the prognosis is guarded. If the implant diameter prevents replacement, particulate the bone segment and, with DFDB serving as an expander, apply it to the external surface of the defect. The patient's blood serves as a fibrinous grouting medium. Make the closure after placing a resorbable membrane over the entire graft complex. Although plate fracture often is difficult or impossible to avoid, leave it untreated if there is no displacement. On the other hand, do not permit the occurrence of perforations to go unacknowledged. Testing for perforations is simple: after completing each osteotomy (for all implant types, including the endodontic), test its integrity with a blunt, long, thin probe (such as the Kerr Dycal instrument or a 40-mm-long No. 50 endodontic reamer). If the tip falls through an inaccessible fault or perforation, it

would be wise to use a membrane (see the section in Chapter 8 on "Guided Tissue Regeneration Membranes," p. 116), tease a Colla Plug over it, or gently tap some synthetic or autogenous bone at the base of the defect. Then close the soft tissues, permit bone healing for 6 months, and reoperate. If the mandibular canal is involved, place a Colla Plug gently into the base of the defect to avoid forcing graft particles into the neurovascular bundle. If the perforation is in a visible and operable location such as the labial cortex, allow the implant to remain in position and cover its exposed portion with particulate bone, preferably autogenous, which may be harvested from the tuberosity. Complete the repair by covering the graft with laminar bone (Lambone) and a primary closure. If, while preparing an osteotomy beneath the antral floor, an unintentional perforation occurs but the tip of the drill has not penetrated or injured the sinus membrane, place the implant and allow it to extend beyond the cortex for up to 2 mm, thereby "tenting" the sinus lining. If the implant goes on to integration, it remains in successful equilibrium with its environment. If it fails to integrate, however, the extension into the cavity space (which had offered no additional bony retention) threatens the potential formation of an oroantral fistula (Fig. 28-7). Manage an unintentional perforation in a predictable and acceptable manner as recommended by the Summers technique (see Chapter 8).

Air bubbles emanating from the osteotomy denote perforation into the maxillary sinus (Fig. 28-8). In such instances, placement of a shorter implant after deep repair with a Colla Plug and graft material is an acceptable remedy. If this appears to be unsatisfactory, make a primary closure with a buccal (undermined) pedicle graft (see Chapter 7), suture the flap over intact bone, and prescribe the sinus regimen given in Appendix G. If osseointegration takes place, no treatment is necessary. If osseointegration fails to occur and a connective tissue interface results, anticipate the possibility of maxillary sinusitis. It is acceptable to tell the patient about the implant's proximity to the antral floor and describe the symptoms of sinusitis. If the symptoms occur at a later date, assess the implant's status and, if in a failing mode, remove it. Repair the communication between oral and antral cavities with either a buccal or palatal pedicle graft. These procedures, as well as nasal antrostomy, Caldwell-Luc operation, and antral lavage are described later in this chapter.

Significant bleeding characterizes perforation of the mandibular canal, which may be confirmed by a periapical radiograph with a probe or a gutta percha point in place. The best cure, in this case, is avoidance.

The following are the four most successful ways to prevent canal embarrassment:

- Measure carefully in the planning and operating stages.
- Use infiltration anesthesia rather than block (which may permit the patient to respond as an instrument approaches the canal).
- Employ tactile sense to inform yourself when contacting the cortical bone superior to the canal.
- Use undistorted intraoperative periapical films.

If the canal has been entered as indicated by inordinate bleeding, do not place an implant (Fig. 28-9). Simply close the incision, offering the possibility that the nerve will heal spontaneously. If signs of regeneration do not occur (tingling or formication) within several months, refer the patient to a specialist who performs mandibular neurorrhaphy procedures.

Refer to Chapter 4, "Surgical Anatomy," p. 55 for indication of the possible locations of the mental foramina and the peculiarities of route taken by their neurovascular bundles. When implanting in the region of the mental foramen, expose this structure so that its position is localized clearly as performing the osteotomies. Even while viewing, however, bear in mind that the bundle often courses forward, anterior to the foramen for 4 to 6 mm, before curving back to its exit (Fig. 28-10, A). Sometimes there may be two or more mental canals (Fig. 28-10, B). If the canal is entered or nerve is injured, do not place the implant. Close the wound in the hope that the resultant dysesthesia will correct with time. If symptoms persist unchanged for 6 weeks, consider microsurgical neurorrhaphy.

If the bone perforation occurs in an area without a vital structure (particularly in the vertical direction) and a decision is made to seat the implant, or if discovery of the overextension occurs postoperatively, treat the patient with antibiotics. After conditions appear to have stabilized (i.e., amelioration of postoperative ecchymosis, trismus, edema), evaluate the perforation.

If the perforation is through the mandibular inferior border, ascertain whether the implant can be palpated through the submandibular skin and whether it is sharp. If so, it may cause chronic injury to the overlying musculature. A small skin incision may be required (if "degloving" via the intraoral route cannot be done) to trim the extended segment of the implant with cooled diamond drills until it becomes level with the inferior border of the mandible. If it is not trimmed, inform the patient about the condition and ask him or her to await the first recurrent episode of pain or swelling before taking action (Fig. 28-11).

If the perforation occurred through the nasal floor, use a speculum with a source of good light to inspect the inferior nasal mucosa. If it has been penetrated and the implant can be seen, establish a method of trimming. Accomplish this intranasally with a diamond (Atwood 473) or a pear-shaped in a

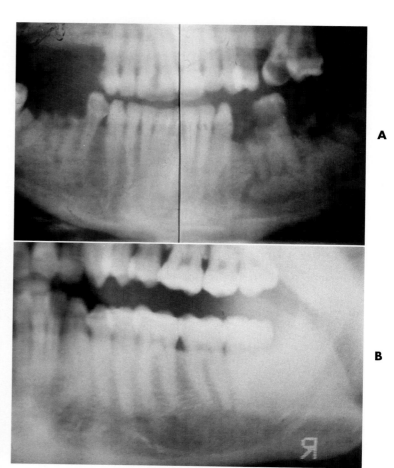

Fig. 28-10   **A,** The anterior mental loop can be very deceiving when the surgeon uses the clinical mental foramen as a guide. **B,** This panoramic view demonstrates an inferior alveolar nerve that bifurcates before exiting at two separate mental foramina.

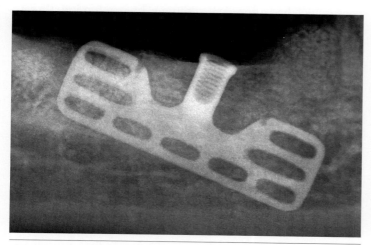

Fig. 28-9   If operative perforations of the mandibular canal are not recognized before implant seating, grievous accidents may occur. Retrieval of this implant becomes an invasive procedure.

water-cooled straight handpiece or Impactair. The abraded nasal mucosa will heal over the trimmed implant by secondary intention. This may be accomplished as well via an intraoral deep anterior vestibular incision, with exposure of the pyriform aperture and elevation of the nasal mucosa with a Freer elevator until the overextended implant can be visualized. Shorten it with the same diamond drill. If the nasal mucosa has not been penetrated and the patient does not complain of nasal soreness, keep the site under observation until such time as a symptom presents itself (Fig. 28-12).

Fractured Buccal or Lingual Cortical Plates

Fractured buccal or lingual cortical plates may be found with any kind of endosteal implant, but they are most frequently found while placing blades or when performing ridge expansion. If this occurs, the best choice is to discontinue the implant placement procedure. If the fractured plate appears to be attached to the mucoperiosteal flap, a good chance for its reattachment and subsequent healing may be expected. If the implant achieves firm seating, using a guided tissue regenerative membrane (GTRM) offers the possibility of salvaging the procedure along with a bone grafting material, precise tailoring and placing of the membrane, and an impeccable closure (see Chapter 8).

Inadequate Soft Tissue Flaps for Implant Coverage

Inadequate soft tissue flaps for implant coverage may occur after incision and flap reflection even if the tissues have been handled with great care. If the incision is not made directly on

the crest of the ridge through the linea alba, the tissue between the incision and this ubiquitous avascular white line of scar tissue may pull away. Novel or unique crestal incisions such as S-shaped or vestibular "visor" designs are discouraged. Recent research has indicated that lingual and facial flap capillaries do not anastomose at the ridge crest. Therefore, noncrestal incisions may result in a loss of vascularity to the tissues of the elevated flaps. In addition, when placing implants into sites immediately after tooth extraction or in cases of ridge expansion maneuvers, a paucity of the tissue required for primary closure exists. If the implant, either subperiosteal or endosteal, presents enough bulk so that the tissues from facial and lingual sides cannot be brought together, undermine the buccal or facial flap. This involves the elevation of the mucosa from the underlying buccinator or orbicularis oris muscle using a pair of sharp, curved scissors or a No. 15 BP blade (Fig. 28-13). In this fashion, release the mucosal flap from its un-

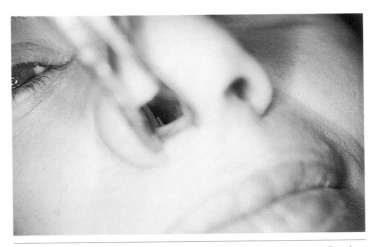

Fig. 28-12   The floor of the nose is another inviolate structure. If an implant pierces the nasal mucosa, immediate removal or repair by resection of the apex is mandated.

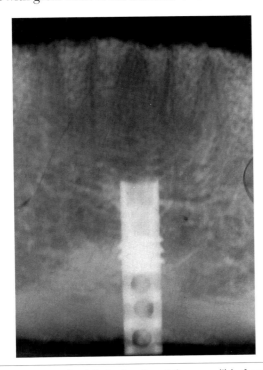

Fig. 28-11   Protect the inferior border of the mandible from penetration. Implants occupying such positions may require removal and Collaplug and HTR or HA repairs may need to be performed. As an alternative, trim an overextended but otherwise satisfactory implant via a submandibular skin approach or by degloving.

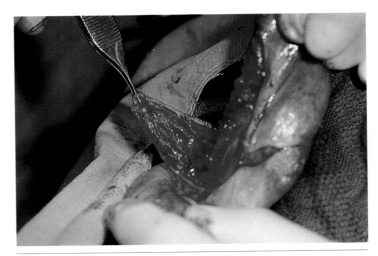

Fig. 28-13   When it is desirable to cover implants primarily and sufficient tissue is not available, undermining the mucosa from the adjacent buccal muscle surface offers the requisite flap, which is sutured without tension.

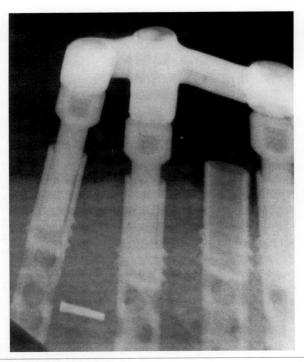

Fig. 28-14   Burs occasionally break in the bone if, when they are permitted to bind, the effort to remove them is made by wiggling the handpiece. A broken bur, if not in a critical location, is best left untouched.

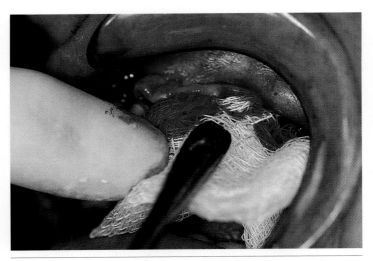

Fig. 28-15   Continued bleeding may be treated effectively by applying pressure with persistence and patience for a minimum of 5 minutes.

derlying muscle fibers, allowing it to be brought over the implant and ridge crest. This permits tension-free suturing. Perform closure with a continuous horizontal mattress configuration. Chapter 6, "Suturing," p. 76 and Chapter 7, "Soft Tissue Management," p. 94 outline this technique. Of course, vestibular integrity is lost, and a subsequent vestibuloplasty may be required.

Broken Burs

Broken burs may occur during the pilot osteotomy stage in preparing for placement of any type of endosteal implant. This unfortunate event occurs most frequently as a result of the bur (usually a fissure-type) binding in bone. The way to prevent bur fracture when binding occurs is to grasp the handpiece beneath its head at the point of bur emission with the thumb and forefinger and press the fingers together. Pinch the bur between its head and the bone, forcing it vertically upward and out of the bone in a non–torque-influenced movement. Do not remove the bur by wiggling the handpiece shank. This maneuver is the major contributing cause of bur breakage. A second technique is to release the bur from the handpiece, facilitating a trauma-free bur removal by rotating it in a counterclockwise direction with fingers or Howe pliers.

If a broken bur occurs, it usually is deep in the osteotomy and possibly close to a vital structure (Fig. 28-14). If simple probing and suction fail to dislodge it (after several technique-localizing radiographs have been taken), tell the patient of its presence (but only after completion of the procedure). He or she should be asked to sign a note acknowledging this information. If the patient is sedated, a complete recovery must

take place before he or she is informed and the signature obtained. Aggressive attempts to remove broken burs or instruments destroy potential host sites and may be responsible for injuries to adjacent vital structures. Burs in noncritical areas can remain safely in place for years. Attempt to remove them only if noting a local reaction on x-ray at some later date.

Inoperative Instrumentation

Occasionally, handpieces bind, internal irrigators fail, and suction becomes clogged. The key to solving each problem is to anticipate it, care for and check all equipment preoperatively, and, most important and despite the expense, have backup equipment, supplies, and implants on hand at all times.

Hemorrhage

Unusual amounts of bleeding may result from soft tissue dissection or intraosseous surgery. If a vessel is bleeding from within the soft tissues, clamp it with a fine hemostatic forceps and ligate or electrocoagulate it. Often, however, simple tamponade solves such problems (Fig. 28-15). After approximately 5 to 10 minutes of pressure, most small vessels embolize. Applying firm pressure for 5 or more minutes usually causes cessation of hemorrhage within bone as well. Use of bone wax forced into the bleeding site always offers satisfactory results (Fig. 28-16). In addition, Gelfoam, Surgicel, or Avitene (spun collagen) are effective hemostatic agents. Placement of the implant itself into the final prepared hemorrhaging osteotomy serves as an effective form of management.

If the hemorrhage is coming from deep within the soft tissues (e.g., the facial artery pulsating from within the buccal musculature), place a 2-0 Vicryl suture on a large half-round needle (40 to 65 mm) deeply posterior (proximal) to the bleeding site, and tie it in a figure-8 or circumferential configuration. This suture must encompass a mass of proximal tissue

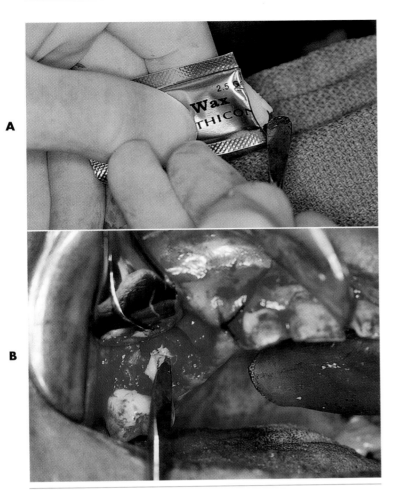

Fig. 28-16 A satisfactory technique for managing bone bleeding is to force bone wax into the errant osseous site. **A,** Sterile bone wax is available in individually wrapped packages. **B,** Small quantities are used effectively by burnishing them into the bleeding site with the tip of a periosteal elevator, which will create tamponade.

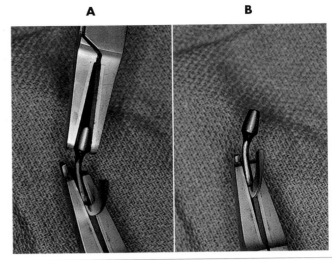

Fig. 28-17 One-stage blade implant abutments may be malaligned. **A,** Correction can be made by bending of the cervix using two titanium-tipped cone-socket pliers. **B,** Careful manipulation with controlled effort creates parallelism of the abutment to adjacent implants or teeth.

that contains the bleeding vessel within its loop. While tightening the knot, the surrounding drawn-in soft tissues obtund the bleeding artery.

The possibilities exist of life-threatening airway occlusion from hemorrhage or iatrogenic emphysema. All instances involving such a complication mandate careful intraoperative and postoperative observation. If there is any question of a compromised airway, consider endotracheal intubation or tracheostomy. To minimize edema from surgical trauma, give the patient dexamethasone, 20 mg IM or IV (for a 70-kg adult), and keep the patient posturally erect.

Poor Angulation or Position of an Implant

BLADE AND PLATE-FORM IMPLANTS   Poor angulation or position of an implant is rarely a problem if the implant is a one-piece device because blades are made of flexible, resilient, and compliant metals, and their abutments may be bent into positions of parallelism (Fig. 28-17). Bend the implant using titanium-tipped, cone-socket pliers so that foreign metals do not become deposited on the blade surfaces. Treat submergible blades with friction-fit abutment inserts in the same manner at the time of their insertion. Make the adjustment before seating of the implant, however, so that if the abutment fractures

and cannot be retrieved from its socket, a new blade may be selected. After bending the neck to achieve parallelism, remove the abutment and keep it until the second stage, when it may be inserted into the infrastructure socket. Since it is of the proper angulation, it is able to serve as a usable, parallel abutment.

In addition, some companies offer 15-, 25-, and even 30-degree angulated, threaded abutments. A number of trial seatings with different abutments, at the time of surgery, is necessary until achieving the proper angulation.

Straight, screw-in abutments present problems when making angulation corrections. Attempt gentle bending after the abutment has been placed into the implant but only before implantation. If angulation cannot be improved by bending (or by the use of an angled abutment), then an opportunity for a correction is available after integration by making a cast, telescopic, cementable coping in proper alignment.

ROOT FORM IMPLANTS   The guidelines used for blades may be applied in making angulation corrections for most root forms that have been placed in anatomically unacceptable positions. If using press-fit implants with internal threading and without antirotational devices (e.g., Integral) with angled one-piece abutments, insert the abutment into the implant before seating it. Rotate the implant to a position that makes the abutment parallel to the adjacent teeth, and tap it into its osteotomy (Fig. 28-18). Unscrew the abutment, replace it with a healing screw, and maintain it until integration when replacing it into the specific implant from which it had been taken. Another alternative for use after integration is making a direct impression for casting an angled, frictional-fit abutment that would require cementation. Sometimes placement of implants in the most appropriate position in bone (midway between facial and lingual cortices) causes their abutments to be located too far to the labial or lingual or emerging from unstable mucosa. If soreness or inflammation results, this problem can be solved by the use of free palatal grafting as described in Chapter 7. In addition, angled abutments are available that may be rotated on the implant's cervical platform and, when appropriately positioned in one of a half dozen fixed stops, fastened by its fixation screw into the implant's internal threading receptacle (see Chapter 22, "Abutments," p. 336).

As outlined in Chapter 4, the nature and dimensions of the patient's residual bone determines where, at what angle, and the number of root form implants that provide the best prognoses. Since the angulation of the ridge does not always permit ideal implant trajectories, a problem may exist that classic prosthetic procedures cannot solve. The implants may be canted in eccentric directions that would result in the retaining screws emerging from the labial surfaces of the completed prostheses or at other unacceptable sites when fixed-detachable techniques are the choice of reconstruction.

One possible and more frequently chosen approach to the difficulty of poor angulation is to ignore (within reason) the optimal intraosseous site for implant placement and to insert the implant at an angle that offers an optimal emergence posture. This, however, may result in a perforation of one of the cortical plates. Such a finding may be managed in accordance with the technique described earlier in the section on "Perforations," p. 406.

Prevention (i.e., not placing implants if their angulation problem appears to be insoluble), selecting blades or root forms that permit the use of significantly angled abutments, abutments with adjustable necks, angular corrections made with the use of bone-grafting materials, or using subperiosteal implants are all alternatives that assist in governing operative decisions. Despite the fact that accurately made surgical templates should prevent improper placement of implants, occasionally implants are placed too close to one another. The proper distance is a full implant width between each root form (i.e., 3.25 to 5.5 mm). In instances of closer proximity or poor angulation, permit the implants to remain buried and unused as "sleepers" (Fig. 28-19).

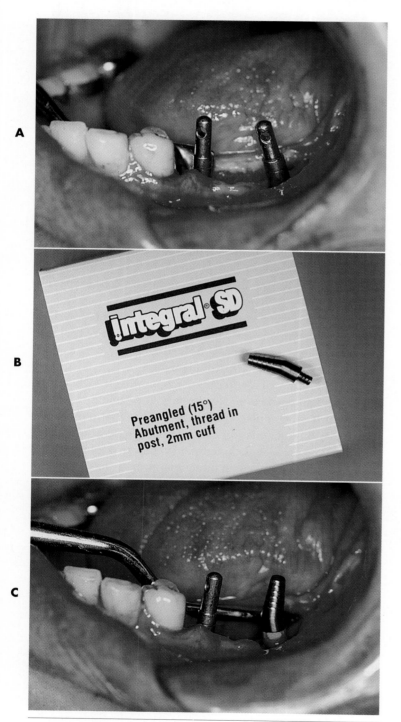

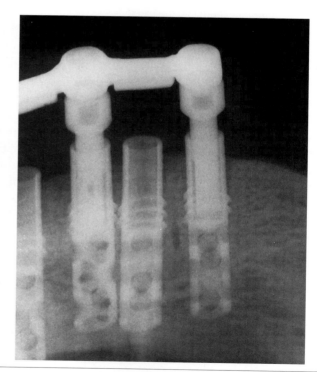

Fig. 28-18 **A,** Submergible (two-stage) implants may be placed in nonparallel posture as seen by the two trial-seating devices. **B,** Angled abutments are available in 15-degree and 25-degree inclinations. **C,** Alignment is ensured with use of correctly angled abutments, which must be placed into the implant before seating it.

Fig. 28-19 Implants that are placed in awkward positions may be left in position to "sleep" and possibly be put into future function.

Injuries to the Mandibular Neurovascular Bundle

In instances when an implant or instruments unintentionally penetrate the mandibular canal, remove the implant and inform the patient of the possibilities of dysesthesia. This is an event less frequently experienced, however, if employing infiltration anesthesia rather than nerve block.

If a nerve has been injured or cut and it is within the bony canal, time may permit healing. Less chance for healing exists if the injury occurs to a neurovascular bundle in soft tissues such as the mental branch.

If, after 6 weeks, the dysesthesia has not diminished or changed in depth, nature, or character, consider an exploration and possible repair. Although specially skilled oral and maxillofacial surgeons most often do these procedures, knowledge of this technique is important. If the mental or other soft tissue neurovascular bundle is totally or significantly torn or separated, perform a repair immediately. Carefully reflect the tissues, already opened, to below the foramen level, thereby exposing the entire nerve complex. The mental neurovascular bundle is moderately resistant to injury, and gentle reflection exposes it fully. Make the distal portion available, if any should be in evidence within the soft tissues lying lateral to the mandible. Perform this gentle, blunt dissection with ease using a pushing maneuver with a mosquito hemostat grasping a moistened 2 × 2-inch sponge.

If the proximal bundle offers insufficient length from within the foramen, elevate the periosteum adjacent and posterior to it to the mandibular inferior border. Insert a small, half-curved, blunted chisel or suitable elevator into the distal portion of the mental foramen to protect the bundle, and, using a saline-cooled Impactair or straight air turbine handpiece with a No. 4 L round surgical bur, brush the bone from behind the elevator (Fig. 28-20, A). The goal is to extend the mental foramen into the mandibular canal by removing its posterior lateral bony wall. With patience, care, and experience, this can be done with consistency. After 180 degrees of the canal has been removed (Fig. 28-20, B), slip a nerve hook beneath the neurovascular bundle so that it can be gently teased from its crypt. There are usually internal bony spicular attachments from which the sheath must be wrested carefully.

Once the portion of the nerve bundle that occupied the canal has been extricated, make it contiguous with the mental branch. After dissecting free the vascular elements, a generous additional lengthis presented to facilitate repair of the nerve that had been sectioned or compressed iatrogenically. If 1 cm of distal (tissue) bundle is available and another 2 cm of the proximal portion can be exposed, make an end-to-end anastomosis using 10-0 silk or Prolene. At least six sutures are required, and their placement must be guided by the use of four-power magnification. Enclosing the repaired segment in a polyethylene tube (made from a piece of slit IV catheter) offers additional stability and a mortise form to influence unobstructed healing (Fig. 28-20, C-E). Tuck the tube and its contents into the widened canal and close the wound primarily (Fig. 28-20, F). Positive results may not be forthcoming for 18 to 24 months.

If deficiency of length exists even after exposure of both ends, arrange a sural nerve graft.

Perform elective exposure of the intact bundle when requiring a deeper zone of usable bone for placement of a long endosteal implant or transosteal implant for the posterior mandible.

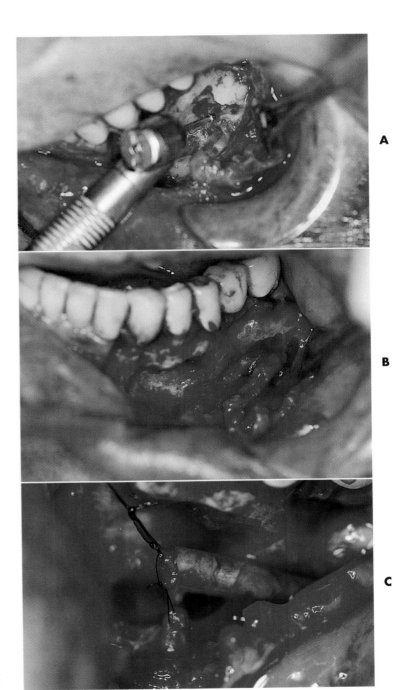

Fig. 28-20 Mentomandibular nerve repair requires careful tissue management. **A,** Use an Impactair with a round bur to brush away the bone overlying the canal. **B,** After exteriorization of the canal, the neurovascular bundle becomes visible. **C,** Separate the nerve sheath from the bundle, bring the two cut ends together in an end-to-end anastomosis, and make the neurorrhaphy with 10-0 black silk ophthalmic sutures. Magnification is essential for this operation.   *Continued*

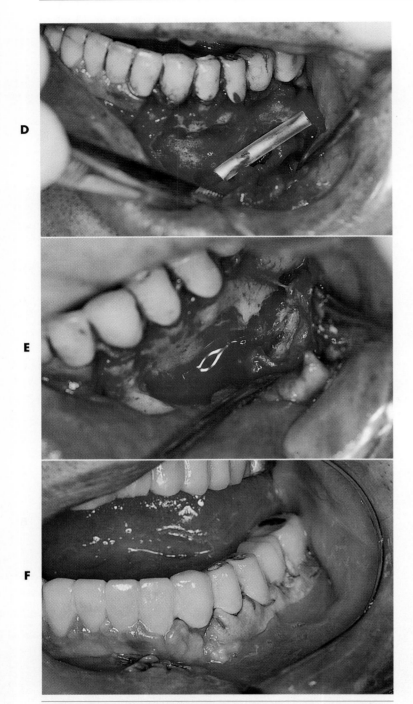

Fig. 28-20, cont'd **D,** Place a slit polyethylene sheath around the repaired nerve to protect it and to serve as a conduit for unobstructed healing. **E,** Replace the repaired nerve into the canal. **F,** Closure of the overlying soft tissue completes the operation.

Subperiosteal Implants

Loss of Anesthesia

Dissipation of regional anesthesia occurs occasionally during stage one if repeated impressions are required. If anesthesia begins to fade before completion, it becomes difficult to reinforce or reinstitute it because of the change in pH in the sur-

gically exposed tissues. Therefore, although attempts may be made to supplement anesthesia with additional doses, a possibility exists that the procedure may have to be terminated before its completion. Keep in mind that no more than eight anesthetic cartridges of 2% lidocaine (or less than 300 mg) should be given to an average weight (70 kg) adult at any one time. Additional amounts may be given with time, however, as the drug is hydrolyzed. Use of preoperative analgesics and intravenous sedatives also makes local anesthetics work more effectively. Probably the best way to prevent loss of anesthetic is to use bupivacaine (Marcaine) or ropivicaine (Naropin) along with lidocaine, at a ratio of 1:1. This grants three to four times longer anesthesia time. If anesthesia cannot be reestablished, even with the addition of IV sedation, discontinue the procedure, use sutures to close the wound margins, and make an attempt to complete the operation on another day. Allow a minimum of 1 week to pass before operating again. This interim allows a greater possibility of success because a more accurate tray can be made on the model that was derived from the failed impression.

Inability to Make an Accurate Impression

If, after three attempts, a satisfactory bone impression cannot be registered, seek help or, lacking that, close the wound.

Inability to Remove an Impression or to Seat a Tray Either for Full Upper (Pterygohamular Design) or for Full Lower (Lateral Rami Design) Subperiosteal Implants

Both pterygohamular and lateral rami designs present the possibilities of undercuts that may legitimately discourage a path of seating or removal. Sectioning the tray into halves or even in three parts for the mandible may solve this problem, with each of the parts fitting its own area of bone accurately (Fig. 28-21). After placing the tray segments into position and fitting them closely or even overlapping, remove them. Process a number of protruding copper tubes or similar retentive devices with heat or lute them to their exterior surfaces. Fill each segment with impression material and reseat it. After the impression material has set, take an index over the tubes, using additional tray material to engage them. These indices must be removable. After removing the tray segments, use the retention tubes to serve as guides for accurate reassembly with the indices. Suturing the wound completes the procedures. Using this technique, the surgeon may make the most complex impressions in sections and place them together for accurate completion of the casting by the laboratory.

Antral Perforations

While reflecting the mucoperiosteum in preparation for a maxillary subperiosteal implant impression, some eggshell thin maxillary cortical bone overlying the sinus might lift away attached to the flap. The intact antral membrane often is noted. It is bluish-gray in color and expands with every expiration of

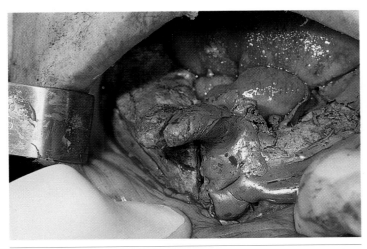

Fig. 28-21 When undercuts prevent placing or removal of a one-piece tray during the two-stage subperiosteal operation, the tray may be split into two or more sections, each seated separately, indexed, removed, and collated on the laboratory bench.

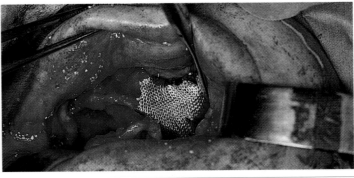

Fig. 28-22 Often during the tissue reflection phase of the maxillary or pterygohamular subperiosteal implant, the lateral sinus wall lifts away with the elevated mucoperiosteal flap. Before closure, perform a sinus elevation procedure, or if not appropriate, lay a sheet of Vicryl mesh or similar resorbable membrane over the defect.

the patient. If it is torn, bring the margins together gently with a nontoothed forceps and cover it with a square of Colla Cote (collagen sheet) or a resorbable membrane such as Surgicel or Vicryl mesh (Fig. 28-22) and permit the bone fragment to remain attached to the periosteum. Make the implant impression in the usual manner, replacing the Colla Cote as required at each step, and, on completion, bring the flaps together with the cortical bone still in place, position it anatomically, and suture it. The bone reattaches over the antrum in its proper location. The final casting design must not have struts placed over the repaired area or over any of the eggshell-type cortex overlying the antrum. If this design characteristic cannot be avoided, a need for a sinus floor elevation and graft procedure, as described in Chapter 8 is indicated. Perform these procedures at the first stage or just before implant placement at stage two.

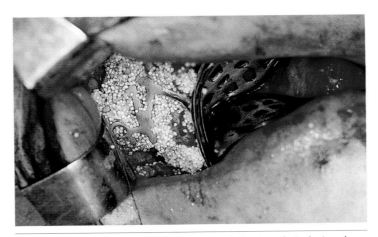

Fig. 28-23 Subperiosteal implants, particularly since their designs have become more complex, may not fit as accurately as is desired. CAD–CAM–generated castings are not as accurate as those made from direct bone impressions. For such discrepancies, particulate grafting materials serve as effective fillers.

Inaccurate Adaptation of Full or Unilateral Subperiosteal Implants

If an implant fails to go into place, particularly in maxillae, tap it with a mallet and orangewood stick. Often after tapping, the implant snuggles into place because of the compliance of the supporting bony structures. If, in either jaw, the implant has obviously been seated to its fullest extent and a rocking movement occurs when testing for stability, seek out the fulcrum and attempt to adjust it by eliminating a bony protrusion or by cutting away a strut (but only if that strut is a noncritical component of the casting). If the rocking cannot be eliminated, make a new impression. Simplify this procedure by fabricating a tray from the cast on which the discarded implant had been made. If, on the other hand, the implant does not go into place fully but there is no instability (i.e., it has at least three widely spaced points of simultaneous contact and the defects between struts and bone are not greater than 3 mm), fill them

and cover the entire infrastructure with a nonresorbable particulate synthetic bone grafting material (20-mesh HA) and follow with suturing (Fig. 28-23). HA coated implants cannot be seated by tapping.

Inaccurate Adaptation of Tripodal Subperiosteal Implants

The tripodal implant will not fit well if the two- or three-part impression segments had not been reassembled accurately. When feasible, it is best to remove the segments in one collated piece after intraoral assemblage. In most instances, however, each segment or islet of the casting will fit accurately on an independent basis. Make an assessment as to which of the islets is causing the rocking or inaccuracy. (It probably is only one of them.) After establishing this, section the Brookdale

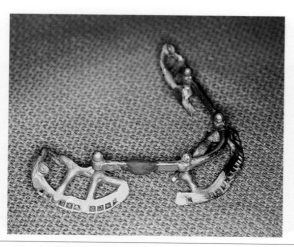

Fig. 28-24 Tripodal subperiosteal implants that had been produced from two- or three-part impressions may not fit the bone accurately. Separate the poorly adapted segment by cutting the Brookdale Bar, refitting the islets individually, and collating them using red Duralay or GC Pattern resin. The laboratory welds the bar, sometimes while the patient still is anesthetized.

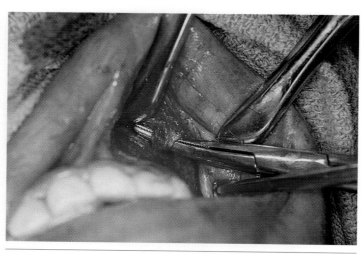

Fig. 28-25 The infraorbital nerve is encountered occasionally during maxillary implant surgery. Protect it carefully with a retractor.

bar, thus separating that component from the other two, and seat the infrastructural parts individually. If the two remaining connected segments still rock, separate them as well.

The surgical assistant stabilizes the separated components by finger pressure, or, if this is impractical, they may be screwed temporarily to their proper positions on the bone. Lute the disconnected bar segments using RC Prep, or GC Pattern, exercising care not to permit the exothermic reaction to injure the sensitive oral mucosa (Fig. 28-24). After polymerization, remove the newly assembled castings in one piece and send them to the laboratory for welding of the bar. Since the rejoined bar is supragingival, no adverse host-site effects will be experienced. It is not recommended, because of potential galvanism, that infrastructural components be welded. If inserting a one-stage implant and the laboratory is in close proximity to the operating theater, it is possible to pack the tissues with saline-moistened sponges while the implant bar is welded. If this can be done within 2 hours, complete the implant insertion period after once again defatting, passivating, and sterilizing it (see Appendix E).

Injury to the Infraorbital or Mental Nerves

When the mucoperiosteum is reflected in the canine fossa for purposes of impression making for the maxillary subperiosteal implant or in the premolar area for the mandibular type, exhibit great caution. Expose the most superficial portion of the adjacent foramen so that a protective periosteal elevator may be placed at its rim to shield the neurovascular bundle. If an injury to the infraorbital or mental bundle occurs and examination shows discontinuity of the segments, repair it immediately. However, if the sheath shows continuity, make closure after completion of the procedure. If the patient complains postoperatively of dysesthesia and there is no subjective change within 6 weeks, undertake repair as described earlier in this chapter or consult an expert (Fig. 28-25).

Careful planning and impeccable surgery generally prevent accidents to the mandibular or mental branches. On occasion, it may become desirable to mobilize and reposition a neurovascular bundle to facilitate impression making or permit a more rigid infrastructure.

Short-term Complications (First 6 Postoperative Months)

Endosteal Implants

Postoperative Infection

Infection may manifest itself by drainage, swollen tissues, or pain. The normal postoperative sequelae of edema, trismus, and pain, as distinguished from the presence of new symptoms representing a pathologic problem, must be established. If there is an abscess, incise and drain it (Fig. 28-26). Antibiotic

therapy (e.g., amoxicillin, 500 mg every 6 hours for nonallergic patients) is essential as well. When there is manifest drainage, perform a culture and testing for bacterial sensitivity. Early infections do not necessarily mean that the implant fails, but prompt and aggressive therapy is mandatory.

Intermediate drainage (i.e., 2 to 3 weeks) after surgery, particularly after a root form has been inserted, occurs occasionally. It is usually superficial; investigate it by taking a peri-

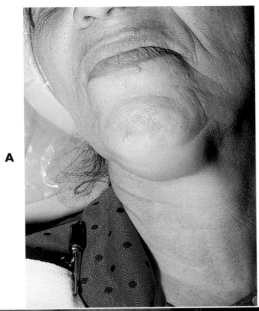

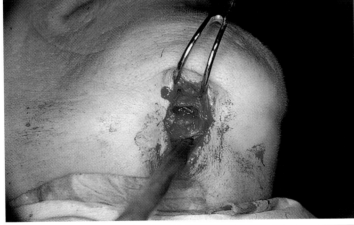

Fig. 28-26 **A,** A short-term postoperative abscess has occurred as a result of an overextended endodontic implant. The area is hot, inflamed, and fluctuant. **B,** Make an incision that permits drainage of the purulent material. After the acute phase has ended, perform a definitive corrective procedure. Reduce the extra length of implant, curette the bone, and make a primary closure via a submandibular approach.

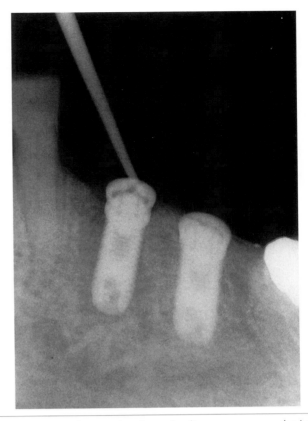

Fig. 28-27 Most frequently, a loose healing screw causes the inflammation noted over a submerged, recently placed implant. A radiograph taken with a gutta percha point placed into the fistula verifies this. Treatment consists of tightening the screw followed by light curettage.

apical radiograph with a gutta percha point inserted into the fistula or drainage site opening. It may indicate that the source of drainage is a bit of unresorbed or residual suture, a loose healing screw (Fig. 28-27), a speck of cement, or other debris. Such isolated areas do not respond to antibiotics but, rather, require opening and inspection to determine and eliminate the cause. Often the simple act of incising and irrigating with saline and povidone-iodine (50%), uncovering the site and packing with a ¼-inch iodoform gauze strip, or simply tightening a screw, solves the problem.

If, conversely, the radiograph indicates a more significant lucency or if pain or drainage persists, refer to paragraphs four and five of this section for suitable management advice.

Dysesthesia

The onset of dysesthesia during the postoperative period is most often a result of the patient failing to notice or report it immediately after surgery because he or she was unable to sort this symptom out among others, such as pain and swelling. If it is an accurate complaint after abatement of edema, suggest to the patient that the implant be removed immediately. If the symptoms do not seem to be abating in 6 weeks after implant retrieval, exploration and repair is indicated.

If paresthesia begins to develop during the long-range postoperative period, the chances are that subimplant resorptive influences are responsible because of the implant's close proximity to the mandibular nerve. Although paresthesia is most often a long-term complication, suggest removal of the implant as soon as symptoms become evident. Resect the implant with great care to avoid further insult to the bundle (Fig. 28-28).

If pain should occur after it had abated postoperatively or at any time during the period after healing, suspect infection as the cause. There may be other reasons, such as injury from an opposing tooth or pressure from a temporary superstructure or denture. A postoperative radiograph is indicated. Examine the overlying tissues and treat the problem as the pa-

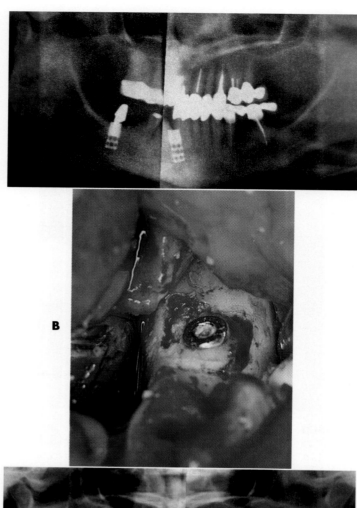

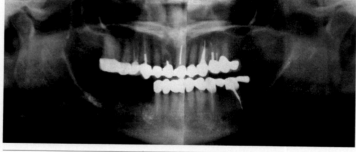

Fig. 28-28 A, If a postinsertion paresthesia persists, remove the implant. The panoramic radiograph suggests proximity of the implant to the neurovascular bundle. **B,** This Core-Vent resisted removal even with reverse use of the ratchet wrench. It required an *en-bloc* removal because of osseointegration. **C,** This postoperative radiograph shows the grafted host site. To ensure that no particles communicated with vital tissues, a barrier (Colla Cote) was used at the base of the osteotomy before placing the grafting material.

tient's symptoms dictate. Manage continuing insoluble pain by implant removal. If this fails to help, suspect an amputation neuroma. Such a phenomenon usually indicates surgical exploration and removal.

Dehiscent Wounds

In the immediate 10-day postoperative period, a wound sometimes breaks down and the underlying implants become exposed (Fig. 28-29, *A*). This results, most frequently, from visor

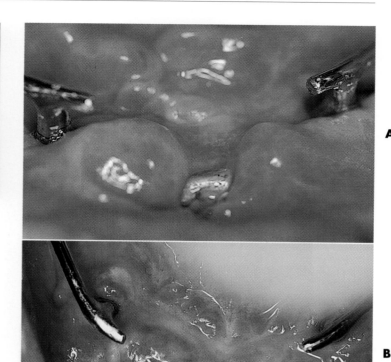

Fig. 28-29 A, Shortly after suture removal, some wound margins fail to heal by primary intention. Underlying struts of this subperiosteal implant and bone are dehiscent. **B,** Conservative treatment, which includes gentle rinsing, cleansing with cotton-tipped applicators, and good hygiene encourages secondary intention epithelization.

or other noncrestal incisions, by the presence of a GTRM, or by suturing the flaps under tension. At this point, it is impossible to regain primary closure, and if it is attempted, the tissues investing the implants recede even further, thereby exposing them to significant additional risk. Leave the wound untouched surgically and see the patient with frequency (every day or two) for irrigation. Gentamicin is a good choice. Make the solution by diluting 80 mg of the antibiotic in 50 ml of saline. Clean the exposed metal or membrane with a cotton-tipped applicator and instruct the patient to do the same at home using a rubber ear syringe and saline (one quart of boiled water to a level teaspoonful of salt). The use of Peridex is recommended as well. Usually, the wound fills in by secondary intention, either completely or at least adequately so that the bone becomes covered and the only remaining dehiscent structures are the implant healing screws or the membrane. With a strict hygienic regimen, such implants most often proceed to integration and even demonstrate reasonable epithelial recovery (Fig. 28-29, *B*). Remove membranes if they lose stability and appear to be the nidus of the problem. If their presence does not seem to be the responsible cause, however, maintain them for at least 3 months.

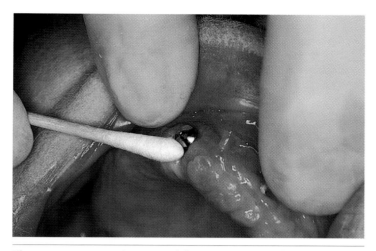

Fig. 28-30 In some instances, dehiscent root forms do not encourage reepithelization. This does not alter their prognosis, particularly if dry, wooden, cotton-tipped applicators followed by the application of Peridex are used conscientiously and with regularity.

Dehiscent Implants

From time to time, a two-stage blade or root form implant does not remain buried beneath the gingival tissues. There may not be signs of distress or infection, but a distinct implant component, usually the healing cap or screw, is seen. This does not indicate failure, nor is it necessarily portentous of loss of the implant. Do not attempt to close it surgically. Instead, keep it clean and teach the patient to use a dry cotton-tipped applicator to keep it free of material alba (Fig. 28-30). Follow this with applications with Peridex. A good chance of achieving osseointegration remains despite this complication. Evaluate the implant site at monthly intervals both clinically and occasionally with radiographs.

Radiolucencies

If, at the 4- or 8-week postoperative examination, the radiograph shows periimplant lucency, assume that osseointegration will not occur. In the case of a root form, it is appropriate to inform the patient that the implant may have to be removed (Fig. 28-31, A). If the lesion remains unchanged, continued observation may, on rare occasions, present evidence of idiopathic resolution. Occasionally, a small gingival fistula is seen without positive radiographic findings. However, a gutta percha point, if lodged deeply as shown by radiography, may dictate implant removal or at least an exploratory and repair procedure (Fig. 28-31, B). If a lucency appears at the apex of the implant only, it often represents a perforation of the cortical plate or the introduction of some epithelial cells, probably at the time of operation. An apicoectomy-like repair, using bone replacement materials to fill the defect, is often effective in managing this finding (Fig. 28-32).

Antral Complications

If during the insertion of an implant the surgeon enters the maxillary sinus, a postoperative infection may occur even if no

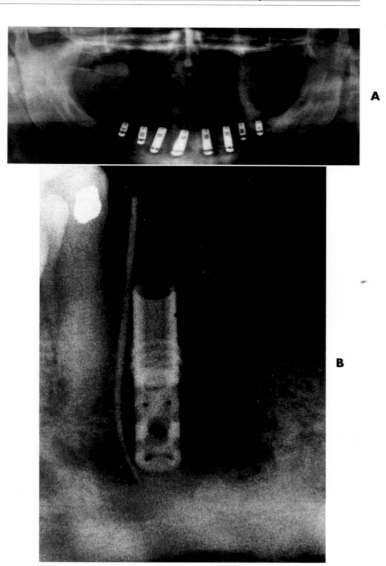

Fig. 28-31 **A,** A panoramic radiograph, taken of an asymptomatic patient during the eighth postoperative week, indicates significant periimplant lucencies. The prognosis for these implants is poor. Rarely will defects of this magnitude resolve spontaneously. **B,** Occasionally, a symptom-free implant presents with a tiny fistula or inflammatory lesion over it. A gutta percha point directed firmly can be very revealing using radiography.

portion of the implant appears to reside within the sinus cavity. Such a complication may result after sinus floor elevation or use of the Summers technique (see p. 162) as well, particularly if the integrity of the sinus membrane had been breached. Facial pain, purulent nasal drainage, foul smell or taste, fever, and sensitivity to palpation of the oral and facial tissues that overlie the antrum, which is exacerbated when lowering the head, characterize this problem. Confirm these findings by taking a Waters' view radiograph. If the antral area appears cloudy or opaque, institute active therapy (Fig. 28-33, A, B).

In addition to prescribing the sinus regimen in Appendix G, institution of surgical drainage may be indicated. The surgeon's adage that "penicillin doesn't cure pus" must serve as guidance. One method is antral lavage. Administer local anesthesia by blocking the infraorbital and greater palatine (second division) nerves. Place an 18-gauge, 1½-inch, disposable hypodermic needle against the maxilla through the areolar tissues high in the vestibule (never through fixed gingiva) in the

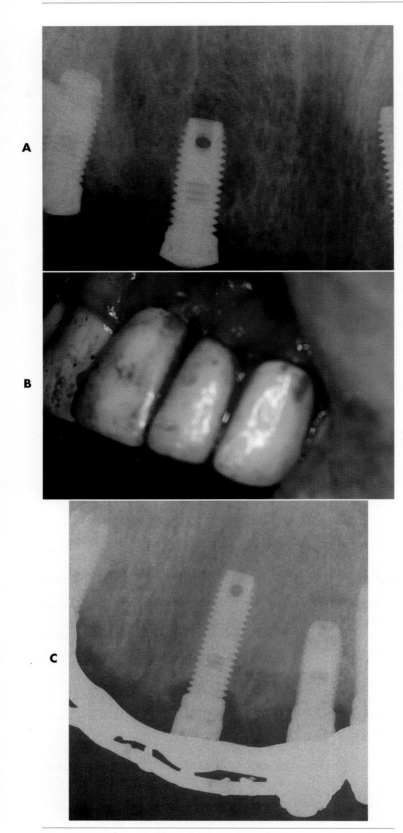

Fig. 28-32 **A,** A rare occurrence in relationship to an implant is an apical lesion. The cause probably is the introduction of epithelial cells at the time of osteotomy. **B,** A classic apicoectomy or apical repair procedure serves as the appropriate therapeutic approach. Synthetic grafting material (HA) is valuable. **C,** One year postoperatively, complete resolution of the area is noted on this radiograph.

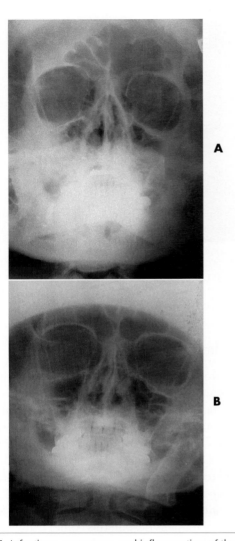

Fig. 28-33 **A,** Infections, empyema, and inflammation of the maxillary sinuses can accompany implant surgery. If the diagnosis is questionable, a Waters' view may be taken using a standard 70 kV 15 ma dental x-ray machine and a high-speed 8 × 10-inch cassette with intensifying screens. Place the patient's chin on the cassette, with the nose raised about 2 cm from it, and the tube at 0 degrees aimed through the head directly at the midface. The resulting film shows a cloudy antrum. **B,** After appropriate treatment, the antrum appears bilaterally clear.

region above the second premolar apex. The needle often pierces the cortical plate and its tip enters the antrum if its hub is tapped with a mallet. A resistant cortex requires a small incision at the site using a No. 15 BP blade. Insert the tips of a mosquito hemostatic forceps. Opening the instrument will permit the beaks to serve as retractors. With the assistant maintaining them, perform a microantrostomy through the lateral wall using a No. 2 round bur in the Impactair. Attach a short length of intravenous extension tubing to the needle and, at the other end of the tubing, a 20-ml syringe filled with warm saline (Fig. 28-34, *A*). Bend the patient's head down over his or her lap so that the forehead almost touches the knees, and place a kidney basin beneath the nostrils (Fig. 28-34, *B*).

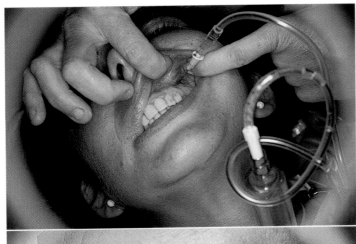

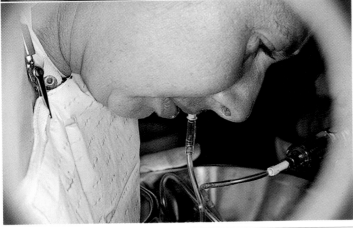

Fig. 28-34 **A,** Acute sinusitis and empyema require more aggressive therapy than antibiotics. Actual lavage must be done. This is accomplished by tapping an 18-gauge needle through the antral wall above the areolar tissue level with a mallet. Attach an intravenous extension tub to the hub. **B,** Position the patient's face forward so that the nose is lower than the mouth, and use a 20-ml syringe to introduce warm saline. The return from the nose first is purulent and then gets increasingly clear. It drips from the nose into a kidney basin. This is a simple but effective method for antral irrigation without the necessity of doing a Caldwell-Luc procedure or nasal antrostomy.

Inject the saline slowly and gently. With the needle tip in the antrum, the effect is a thorough irrigation. Wash out the purulent and infected matter through the natural ostium beneath the middle nasal turbinate and collect it in the kidney basin. Continue irrigation with four or more syringes full until the return is clear of purosanguinous material. Then bring the patient into an upright position and remove the needle. No dressings or sutures are required. Relief is almost instant. Order cultures and sensitivities from the washings and change the antibiotic if the result mandates it (Biaxin, 500 mg bid, is of particular benefit). The irrigation may have to be repeated daily for several days, but often a single treatment suffices.

If this should fail to ameliorate the symptoms and subsequent Water's views do not demonstrate a clearing sinus, Caldwell-Luc and nasal antrostomy procedures may be required.

The Caldwell-Luc operation, which is indicated for conditions of antral infection resistant to medical therapy, retrieval of foreign bodies (e.g., dental roots or implants), removal of polyps, or evacuation of purulence, requires a significant (at least 25-mm diameter) osteotomy through the maxillary wall in the canine fossa.

Make a curved, horizontal incision at least 5 mm above the attached gingival level through mucosa to bone (in several layers) with a scalpel or Bovie tip, starting at the canine and proceeding to the zygomatic buttress. After incising the periosteum with a blade, expose the canine fossa with an elevator. Take care not to injure the infraorbital neurovascular bundle. With the assistant retracting in an upward direction, enter the antrum using a Crane pick or if resistant, with bur holes. Enlarge the bone opening with backbiting Kerrison rongeur forceps (Fig. 28-35, *A*). When the opening is large enough to permit the insertion of an index finger to the first joint, inspect the internal environment (using a fiberoptic antroscope). Remove the foreign body, curette polyps, or perform whatever procedure is needed; then irrigate the antrum with warm saline. Often a lost implant is not readily visible but may be nestled beneath the sinus membrane, which requires incision and exploratory elevation. Once this procedure has been done and the internal environment is free of debris and gross infection, additional drainage may be required, particularly because of the preference for primary closure of the oral wound. To achieve this, place a nasal speculum into the nostril and, with a Freer elevator, lift the inferior turbinate. Punch through the thin nasal wall beneath the turbinate with the Crane pick at a level with the nasal floor. Enlarge the opening with increasing sizes of curved rasps and Kerrison rongeurs (Fig. 28-35, *B*) and then pass an opened, 4 × 4-inch, cotton-free sponge from the nose through the mouth by introducing it through the opening in the nasoantral wall with a tonsil forceps. Grasp the sponge through the Caldwell-Luc opening with a Kelly forceps, and release the tonsil clamp from the nasal end. Pull the sponge back and forth in shoeshine fashion to smooth irregular bone margins. Permit 2 inches of fenestrated ¼-inch Penrose drain to protrude from the sinus through the nasal antrostomy and out to the nostril rim. Stabilize it with a single 2-0 black silk suture that is passed through the nasal mucosa just inside the ala. Irrigate the antrum thoroughly and close the oral wound in two layers with 3-0 dyed Vicryl, using a continuous horizontal mattress suture. Closure is simple because the incision had been made in areolar tissues. Had it been made in fixed gingiva, suturing would be fraught with difficulties and the possibility of wound failure and antral fistulization would be amplified.

Use the drain, which is to be removed from the nose in 3 to 5 days, as a conduit for irrigation during this period.

If an oroantral fistula exists as a result of a failed implant, the techniques described in the "Soft Tissue Pedicle Grafting" section on p. 98 should be followed after completion of appropriate sinus manipulation as described in previous paragraphs of this chapter (Fig. 28-35, *C, D*).

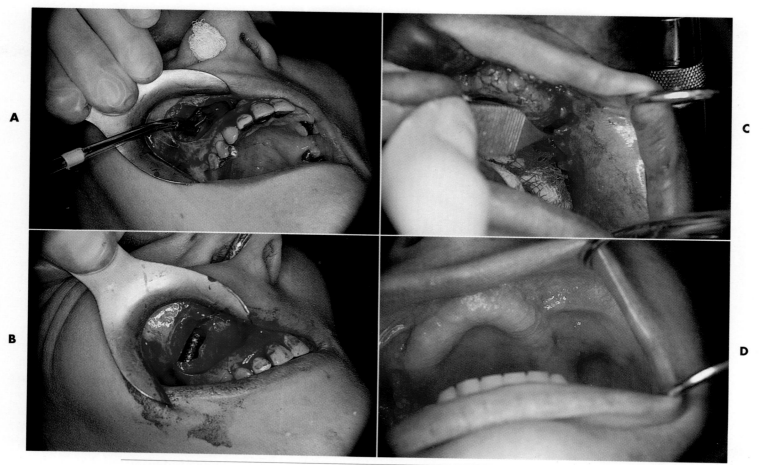

Fig. 28-35 **A,** In cases of chronic infection, foreign bodies (teeth or implants), or polyposis, a more aggressive approach (the Caldwell-Luc procedure) is undertaken. A window in the lateral wall of the maxilla, first opened by a puncture from the Crane pick, is enlarged using backbiting Kerrison forceps. The full size of the fenestration should permit comfortable entry of the first joint of the surgeon's forefinger. Corrective procedures may be done, foreign bodies removed, and a primary closure completed. **B,** If drainage is anticipated or sought, a nasal antrostomy should be done before oral closure. This is performed with curved rasps and Kerrison forceps beneath the inferior turbinate. A thin drain may be allowed to protrude from the nose. **C,** A buccal pedicle graft is fashioned by undermining and after fistula excision, is brought across the debrided bony defect host area. Interrupted sutures complete the graft procedure. **D,** Ten days after suture removal the well-vascularized graft has obtunded the fistulous area. A secondary vestibuloplasty may be required. For palatal graft description and vestibuloplasty, see Chapter 7.

An implant that is responsible for maxillary sinusitis, either endosteal or subperiosteal, and that does not respond to antibiotics and corrective irrigation or antrostomy, must be removed. These measures should lead eventually to a Waters' view radiograph that indicates a healthy maxillary sinus (Fig. 28-33, *B*). Recent advances in fiberoptic nasal antrostomy techniques may be indicated. In some cases, they simplify both the intraoperative and postoperative courses.

Implant Mobility

One-piece endosteal implants such as blades, the ramus group, or screws may become mobile before the initial healing phase comes to an end (3 to 6 months). If this finding is noted, the possibilities for reestablishing firmness are virtually nonex-

istent. It is advisable at this juncture to inform the patient of the finding and, with his or her permission, remove the implant. The less frequent occurrence of mobility with submergible implants also mandates removal (Fig. 28-36).

Postsurgical Scar Contracture

PTERYGOMANDIBULAR RAPHE   The pterygomandibular raphe may undergo scar contracture 4 to 6 weeks after performing surgery on the retromolar or post tuberosity areas (Fig. 28-37, *A* (P-R]). The patient may complain of being unable to open his or her mouth fully or of a feeling of tightness in the area. A technique designed to eliminate this linear contracture is called Z-plasty. In this operation, which may be completed with infiltration anesthesia, make two full-thickness horizontal incisions parallel to one another, below and above the scar and at right

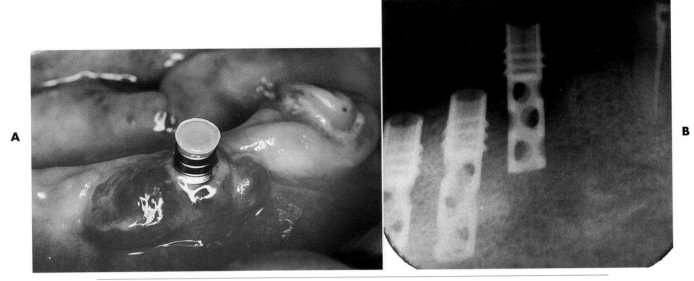

Fig. 28-36   A, Occasionally, a two-stage submergible implant becomes mobile, loosens, and begins to extrude. **B,** The radiograph confirms the hopeless prognosis of this root form device.

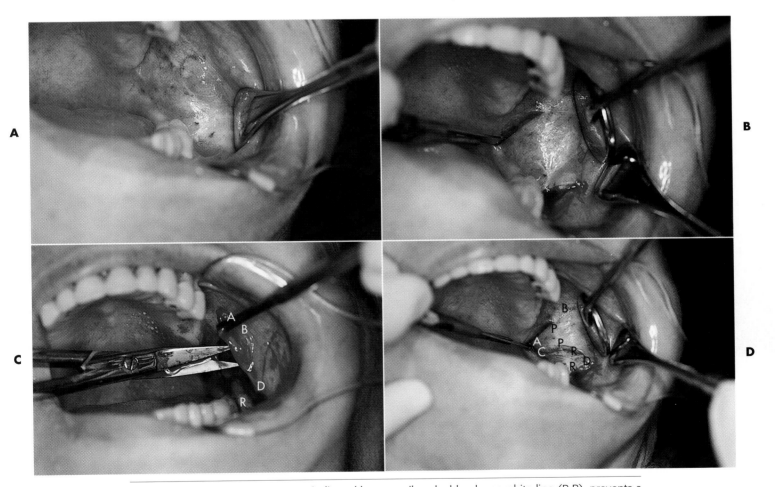

Fig. 28-37   A, Scar contracture, as indicated by an easily palpable, dense white line (P-R), prevents a patient from opening the mouth with ease. **B,** Corrective Z-plasty is begun by making incisions perpendicular to P-R, above it (A-B) and below it (C-D). **C,** Points A and D are connected by a diagonal incision and point A is immobilized with a Gerald forceps. Curved, sharp scissors are used to undermine flap BAD up to line BD. This is followed by creating flap CDA in a similar manner. **D,** Point A is grasped and moved to corner C. In the same fashion, point D is carried to corner B, thus transposing the two triangles. This creates a discontinuity of the newly sectioned scar (P-P and R-R may be noted).

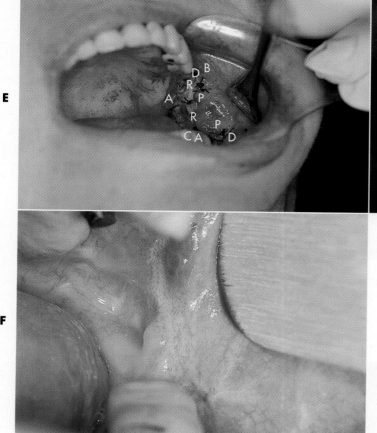

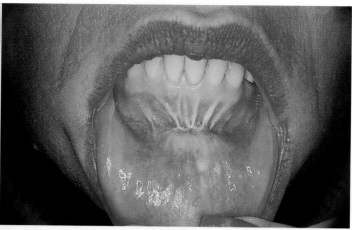

Fig. 28-37, cont'd   **E,** Closure of the transposed flaps makes *BAD* become *BCD* and makes *CDA* become *CBA.* They are sutured into their new positions, which causes corner reversal of the two scar halves: *R-R* acquires a position superior to *P-P.* **F,** Postoperative appearance shows elimination of original contracture. **G,** Poor incision location (e.g., in fixed gingivae), or suturing under tension can be responsible for severe scar contracture with consequent facial deformity and an inability to use the lips for labial seal, smiling and speaking. Vestibuloplasty is mandated (see Chapter 7).

angles to it (Fig. 28-37, *B*). Follow this by an incision made from the lateral end of the superior incision diagonally down to the medial end of the inferior one, thereby creating two triangles. The apex of each triangle is at the lateral end of the superior incision and the medial end of the inferior one. Grasp each apex with a Gerald forceps and, starting at that point, undermine it as a full-thickness flap to the fullest extent allowed (Fig. 28-37, *C*). Transpose each of the triangles, held by the forceps, moving the lower medial point up to the medial end of the upper horizontal incision and the upper lateral point downward to the lateral end of the lower incision (Fig. 28-37, *D, E*). Tack each into place and then fix them into their new relationships by suturing. The scar contracture will now have become so disoriented that it will seem to have disappeared. After the fifth postoperative day, initiate physiotherapy (jaw stretching). By the tenth day, the patient is able to open his or her jaw with increasing facility, and the appearance of the operative site indicates an ablation of the scar (Fig. 28-37, *F*).

ANTERIOR VESTIBULE   Anterior mandibular contracture occasionally occurs after placement of a root form, subperiosteal implant, or on the closure of the incision made for harvesting symphyseal bone for grafting. Symptoms are altered mobility of the lower lip, change in labial posture, or loss of labiomental fold. Should these symptoms occur, the completion of a vestibuloplasty as described in Chapter 7 offers therapeutic benefit (Fig. 28-37, *G*).

Subperiosteal Implants

Strut Exposure

Subperiosteal implant strut exposures occur as a result of wound breakdown, which often may be prevented by creating and properly suturing tension-free flaps. As stated in earlier paragraphs, secondary surgical closures should not be attempted. Keep the exposed strut clean and free of material alba with cotton-tipped applicators followed by Peridex; instruct the patient to do the same at home (Fig. 28-38). His or her skills in doing so should be ascertained, and if they are satisfactory, epithelial tissues may slowly grow over and even seal an exposed strut. If this does not occur, treat the dehiscent member just as if it were another permucosal component of the implant. Such exposed parts can survive for years without additional hard or soft tissue loss.

If soreness arises or persists and the strut is not a strategic one, it may be resected. Do this with the use of local anesthesia. The assistant should protect soft tissues with an elevator or retractor, and the mucosa pushed back 3 mm along that strut proximally and distally. This is followed by the removal of the exposed segment of strut by stroking each end, just beneath the overlying mucosa, with a well-cooled, high-speed tapered diamond drill. Cut metal ends require smoothing with the diamond, which also causes mucosal abrasion. The resultant bleeding initiates healing and coverage of the altered strut ends.

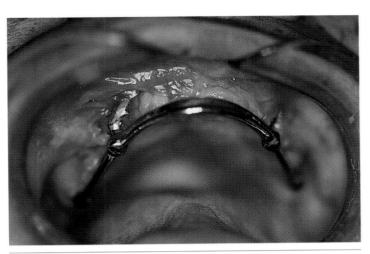

Fig. 28-38 Exposed struts of subperiosteal implants occur with some frequency. Good hygiene keeps such conditions stable for many years.

Postoperative Infection

Treatment of short-term postoperative infections of the tissues surrounding subperiosteal implants is essentially the same as that outlined for endosteal implants.

Scar Contracture, Pterygomandibular Raphe, or Anterior Mandibular Vestibule

Raphe and vestibular contractures are seen occasionally after insertion of mandibular subperiosteal implants. Management is the same as described in the section for "Endosteal Implants."

Long-Term Complications

Endosteal Implants

Ailing, Failing, or Failed Implants

Bone loss around implants often begins with gingival inflammation. The phenomenon of hyperemic decalcification is one of the contributing factors leading to demineralization of bone that lies beneath inflamed skin or mucosa. Other factors can be nutrition- or age-related, secondary to systemic disease (see Chapter 3), or caused by bruxism, traumatic occlusion, improperly designed superstructures, unacceptable oral hygiene, or physiologically incompetent implant design.

Most of the possible causes can be managed by the innovative practitioner who adds implants, corrects occlusion, revises superstructures, performs definitive periodontal therapy, and with persistence, trains and retrains the patient until he or she performs home care responsibilities at a satisfactory level.

Implant design has been questioned for over a decade as a cause of saucerization. Brånemark's initial 0.5 mm of bone loss was supposed to settle into a physiologic pattern of 100 μm per year thereafter. Acceptance of that concept appeared to be universal. No one could anticipate with validity, host sites that exhibited absolutely no change in bone level.

Therefore, implants that are manufactured with irregular exteriors (HA or titanium plasma spray [TPS] to produce greater surface area and retention) brought to their tops often portended failure. As the bone level drops, as predicted, the investing soft tissues become the interfacial components apposing the roughened implant surfaces. Professional and home care prophylactic measures become impossible to practice and the local problems exacerbate, introducing increasingly rapid bone loss. Some remedies are preventive, leading to machined titanium collars of from 1 to 2 mm in width, and, more recently, hybrid implant designs that show threads placed apically with superficial zones of smoothness.

Roland Meffert recognized the serious and self-promulgating nature of the host site problems adjacent to coated implants of both the press-fit and threaded variety and contributed some sound regimens for the management and maintenance of ailing, failing, and failed implants. His definition of *failed* was the presence of mobility. (This can be clinically determined by tapping and receiving a dull sound, by manipulating with two mirror handles and detecting movement, no matter how slight, and by use of the Periotest and eliciting a response of + 9 or higher.) All failed implants require instant removal with site repair by thorough debridement and grafting.

"Failing" implants are firm; osseointegration develops apically and is responsible for the implants' stability. Purulence is forthcoming from the pericervical gingival crevices. Bone loss is progressive. The "ailing" implant, however, demonstrates diminished but static levels of bone on follow-up radiographs.

THE FAILED IMPLANT In the event of the mobility of either a root form or blade implant, the only acceptable treatment is removal (Fig. 28-39). A major cause of loosening of a successful implant is cement failure on an adjacent natural abutment tooth. Castings should fit well, be cemented carefully, and checked with frequency for evidence of mobility or the telltale signs of fluid that appear at their margins when depressing them. An alternative, which discourages cement loosening, is the generous use of interlocks between the superstructural elements of natural and implant abutments. Bottomless female attachments lend additional benefit because they permit independent removal of either component.

If making a decision to remove an endosteal implant, remove all of the granulomatous and connective tissues lining the host-site walls. In order to retrieve an implant, even if it is mobile, make a full-thickness incision and reflection of the mucoperiosteum to reveal the entire host site. The benefits of

![Fig 28-39 radiograph]

Fig. 28-39 Many endosteal implants in less dire straits have to be removed. This 16-year-old implant rotated slowly into this unusual position. It was very firm and resistant to elevation.

x-rays and a clinical examination indicate any sites of bone bridging or similar impediments to removal, and, using a No. 2 L round bur in the high-speed handpiece, brush the bone away until the implant may be lifted out without undue force.

If there are deeper bony protrusions locking the implant to the host site, extra long, surgical No. 700 XXL fissure burs have to be used apically in a light brushing movement running directly against the implant. On occasion, in fact, an en bloc removal is required, as in cases of implants that are truly osseointegrated but have fractured or are causing dysesthesia, pain, or allergic symptoms (Fig. 28-40). Do this with extreme care, making the block outlines as close to the implant as possible because of the potentially highly destructive nature of such a procedure.

After implant removal, remove all debris and attached granulomas, and repair with DFDB and TCP or other alloplasts, followed by placement of a resorbable membrane (Fig. 28-41, A-C).

Nine or more months later, after maturation of the site, place root form implants (Fig. 28-41, D, E). After osseointegration, they are restorable in the classic manner (Fig. 28-41, F-H).

After removal of a mobile implant or one encased in soft tissue, use a scalpel with a No. 12 blade to incise the mucosa from the gingival margins in an oblique pattern downward directly to the bone that had surrounded the implant. Insert the back of a surgical curette from the incision down to the residual bony rim. From there, extend the curette carefully to the base of the recently vacated defect. Next, use a curved hemostat to grasp the tissue, now in a glovelike configuration, and, while elevating it, dissect it from its few remaining fibrous attachments to the bone with the No. 12 blade. If the incision was made efficiently, the soft tissue lining comes away cleanly in the form of a sac, leaving an unlined bony defect within the jaw. If an intact mandibular canal or antrum appears at the apex, place a resorbable bone substitute material (i.e., TCP) within the defect and, when full, tamp it gently to eliminate voids. After a resorbable GTRM has been placed, complete a continuous horizontal mattress suture with flap undermining, if necessary, to gain complete primary closure (Fig. 28-42, A-D). Allow 6 months for maturation of the area. At that time, after a clinical and radiographic analysis, consider the placement of a new implant (Fig. 28-42, E-I).

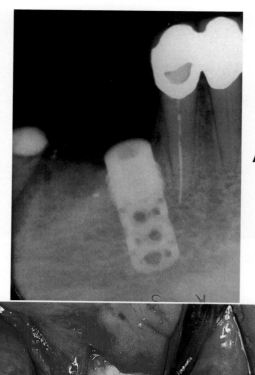

A

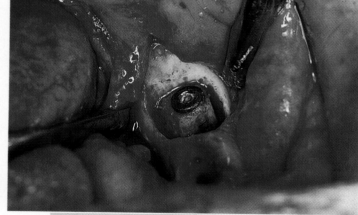

B

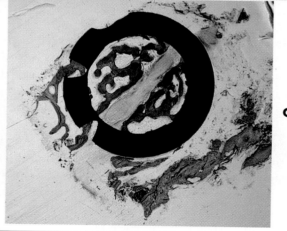

C

Fig. 28-40 **A,** This radiograph reveals a CoreVent implant at site No. 30 with virtually no change in the supporting bone after 4 years. It is osseointegrated, appears to extend into the mandibular canal, and has caused significant pain on chewing. **B,** Efforts to unscrew the implant failed and an en-bloc resection was required. The residual host site demonstrated the threads corresponding to the geometric outlines of the implant. **C,** Histologic appearance of the implant in situ presents evidence of true osseointegration. The inferior alveolar neurovascular bundle has been converted to a blue fibrous strand.

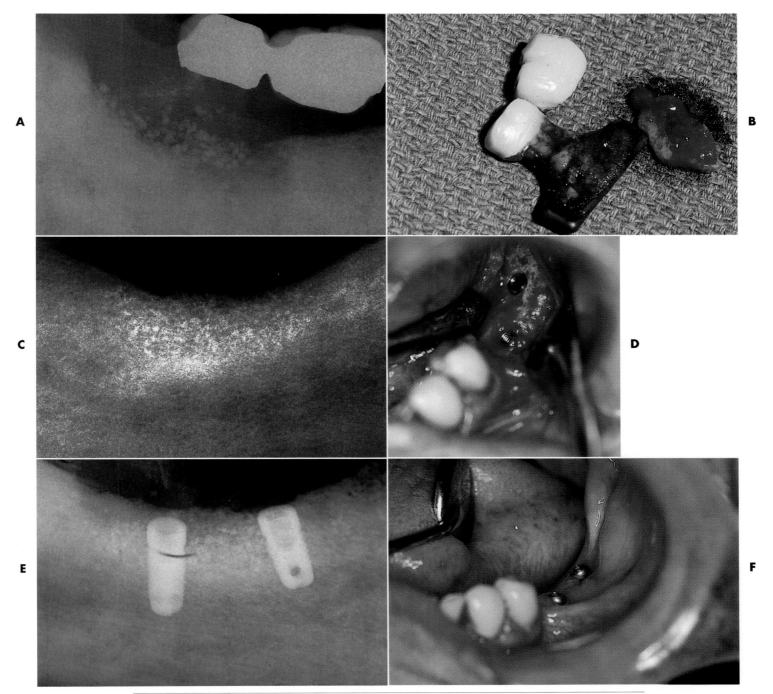

Fig. 28-41   A, A failing radiolucent carbon blade implant on radiography demonstrates a large rounded lytic host site. **B,** Granulomas are the most frequent lesions surrounding such failing endosteal implants. In order to restore the area, thorough curettage must be incorporated into the operative plan. **C,** The host site may be grafted (HTR and Osteogen) only after complete debridement. **D,** Nine months later, replacement root form implants may be inserted. **E,** A resulting well-ossified host site serves well to support the new implants, as may be noted on this radiograph. **F,** Six months are required to ensure osseointegration. At that time, second-stage surgery permits placement of healing collars. Periotest scores indicate true bony support.

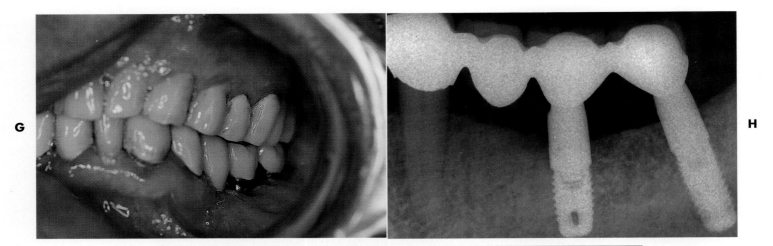

Fig. 28-41, cont'd **G** and **H,** The clinical and radiographic appearance of this restored mandibular left quadrant demonstrates a firm, fixed prosthesis, functioning satisfactorily in its seventh year.

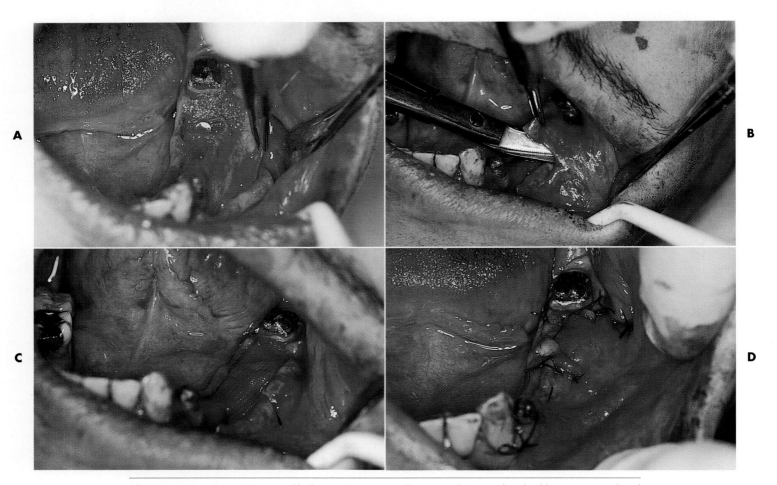

Fig. 28-42 **A,** A posterior mandibular operative area after a root form implant had been removed and grafting performed. **B,** In order to gain a tension-free closure, the buccal flap is undermined. **C,** Just before closure, a properly sized piece of membrane (Vicryl mesh) is tucked under the flaps. **D,** Tension-free closure is made with 4-0 dyed Vicryl suture material.

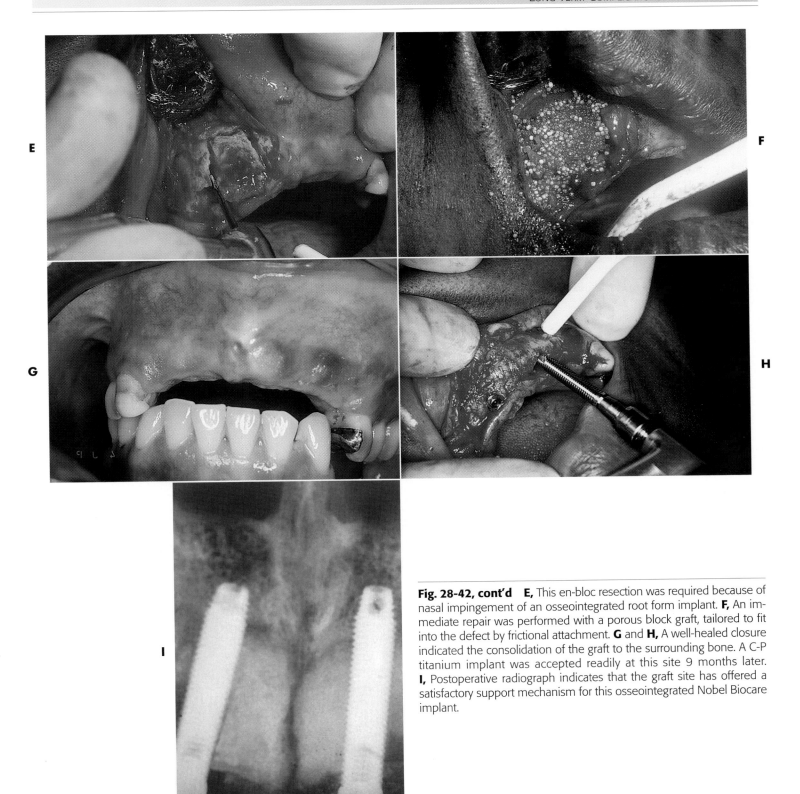

Fig. 28-42, cont'd   **E,** This en-bloc resection was required because of nasal impingement of an osseointegrated root form implant. **F,** An immediate repair was performed with a porous block graft, tailored to fit into the defect by frictional attachment. **G** and **H,** A well-healed closure indicated the consolidation of the graft to the surrounding bone. A C-P titanium implant was accepted readily at this site 9 months later. **I,** Postoperative radiograph indicates that the graft site has offered a satisfactory support mechanism for this osseointegrated Nobel Biocare implant.

If an antral communication has resulted, plan a closure after completion of the steps just listed for implant removal. Aggressively perform the excision of the intraosseous granulomas, or a primary closure of the antral defect will not be successful. On the excision of this soft tissue, a completely denuded ring of bone, 360 degrees around and with a 2-mm wide zone of exposed rim, should be evident. Then, depending on the location of the communication (palatal, buccal), design a pedicle graft and elevate it so that a primary closure can be performed. Instructions for these procedures are in the earlier paragraphs of this chapter and should become a part of every implant surgeon's skills. Prescribe the usual antral regimen as listed in Appendix G.

THE FAILING IMPLANT   If routine radiography demonstrates progressive bone loss around the cervical area of an implant (the

"failing" implant), seek the cause (e.g., traumatic occlusion, poor hygiene) and remedy it. Corrective surgery dictates the creation of full-thickness facial and palatal or lingual flaps as for periodontal operations. Curette the cervical granulomas down to bone, but take care not to scratch or injure the implant's surfaces (Figs. 28-43, 28-44). In cases of HA-coated implants, remove the particulate material. Thin, water-cooled, fine diamond stones are effective. If there is no sign of purulence, prime the area with an application of saturated citric acid for 5 minutes, followed by saline irrigation. Fresh bleeding should be evident. Tamp particulate TCP or DFDB into the defect to the highest level of the bone (Fig. 28-45). In cases where there had been purulence and after thorough preparation of the exposed portions of the implant, establish hemostasis and introduce tetracycline (100-mg soluble tablet in 5 ml of sterile saline) carried between the beaks of a col-

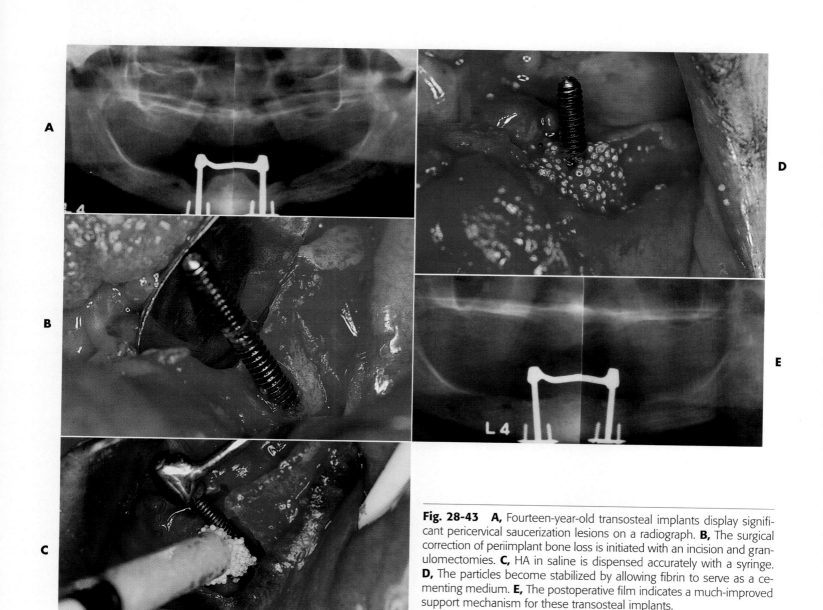

Fig. 28-43   **A,** Fourteen-year-old transosteal implants display significant pericervical saucerization lesions on a radiograph. **B,** The surgical correction of periimplant bone loss is initiated with an incision and granulomectomies. **C,** HA in saline is dispensed accurately with a syringe. **D,** The particles become stabilized by allowing fibrin to serve as a cementing medium. **E,** The postoperative film indicates a much-improved support mechanism for these transosteal implants.

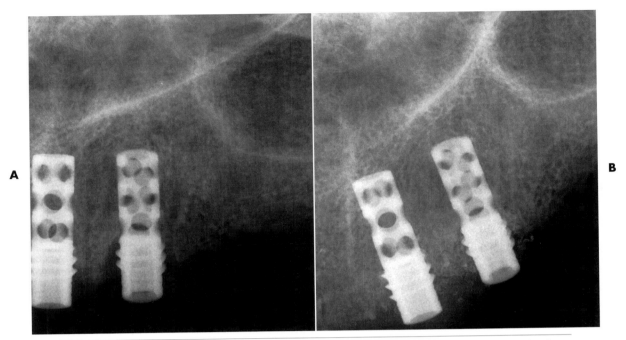

Fig. 28-44 The preoperative and postoperative radiographs of two Core-Vent implants repaired with HA in a classic periodontal manner.

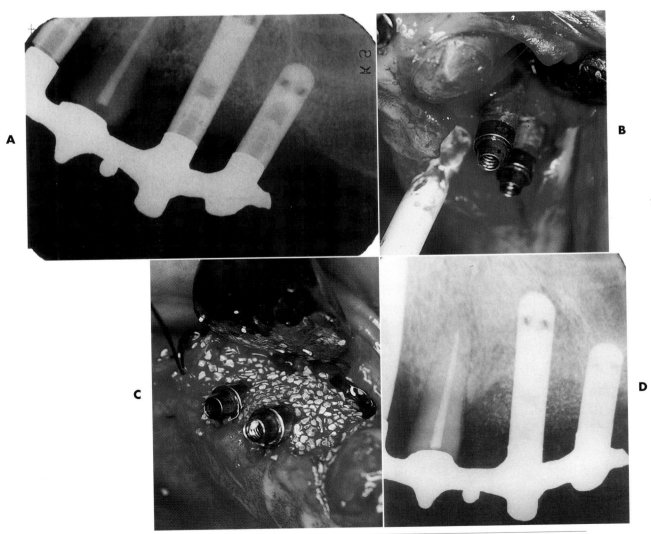

Fig. 28-45 **A,** This radiograph shows significant bone loss around HA coated Integral implants. **B,** A generous, well-vascularized flap is elevated as an introduction to treatment. The HA coating is removed using an ultrasonic tip. If there is no sign of active infection, citric acid treatment may be employed. **C,** Particulate HA, in an autogenous blood slurry, is used to serve as a graft material. **D,** Postoperatively, an improved environment is represented by this radiograph.

lege pliers into the defect for 5 minutes. Follow this by insertion of the graft material soaked in additional tetracycline. Apply pressure for several minutes to permit fibrin to serve as a grouting medium for the graft material, and, after placement of a resorbable membrane, complete the operation with a careful, tight, anatomic, primary closure. If there is a removable abutment, replace it with a healing screw. If not, prepare the GTRM as a poncho. Follow the patient carefully with clinical examinations and periapical films at intervals of 3 to 6 months (Fig. 28-46). Avoid probing.

THE AILING IMPLANT   The "ailing" implant is the least seriously affected of the three pathologic states. Nothing more than radiographic evidence of bone loss may direct the implantologist to be suspicious. Track down the problem, if minor, with the use of duplicable, serial periapical radiographs. If local conservative measures maintain the status quo, continued observation plus the use of the pocket watch system (see Chapter 29, "Maintenance and Hygiene,") for surveillance may be all that is required. On the other hand, if slow but consistent bone loss with deepening pockets is evident, make a flap, complete soft tissue correction, but do not remove the surface coating. Instead, expose the local environment to citric acid for 5 minutes and follow with irrigation, grafting, and closure. Again, take the treated implant out of function by removal of the abutment and substitution with a healing screw, which contributes to the stabilization of a mandatory membrane if managed in a poncho design.

Actisite

In cases of shallow pocketing, for which plastic or gold-plated curettes are used for debridement, the use of a tetracycline-impregnated copolymeric filament called *Actisite* is quite effective. Combine two polymers, ethylene and vinyl acetate, into a monofilament that is impregnated with 0.5 mg of tetracycline per centimeter of length.

Using this form of antibiotic therapy placed within the peri-implant pockets for 10-day periods can be responsible for a significant reversal of symptoms. After curetting the offending pockets, stop the bleeding (e.g., with racemic epinephrine cord), and isolate and dry the areas. Pack the Actisite into each pocket firmly and to their full depths using a cord packer or another instrument of choice. Two layers may be used for deeper pockets (greater than 8 mm), but do not allow them to protrude unless a shallow portion of a pocket forces this to occur.

After completing placement, apply cyanoacrylate (Crazy Glue) cement for stabilization with a tiny, disposable, plastic-tipped applicator. The therapeutic plastic filaments must remain in place for at least 7, and preferably 10, days at which time removal usually heralds a disease-free pocket. Reapplication every 3 to 9 months and maintenance of a state of oral health often solves the problem of chronic infection.

Prosthetic Management of Implant Loss

Losing one or several implants mandates a change in prosthetic strategy. Assess the status of the newly acquired support mechanism. The options are to shorten bars, eliminate cantilevers, change the locations of ERAs, O-rings, or other retentive devices from terminal bar positions to pier or intraimplant locations. If bars are retrievable, these changes can be done in the laboratory with the assistance of pickup impressions. Cemented bars may require the use of a pneumatic, reverse hammer, crown remover.

A viable alternative is to retrofit implants into existing coping or crowns. This may be a departure from the impeccable prosthodontic practices demanded by implantology, but experience has shown it to be an effective technique. Remove the coping-bar, hybrid prosthesis, or fixed bridge, lift the failed implant from its crypt, and completely resect the surrounding granulomata. If the residual site reveals healthy, bleeding bone and sufficient dimensions in width and length to satisfy the 40% rule in Chapter 12, "Immediate Placement of Blade

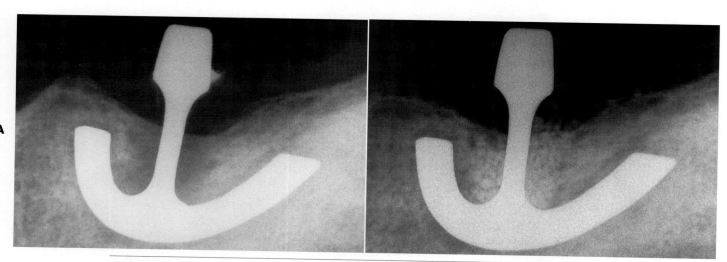

Fig. 28-46   A, A chrome-alloy anchor implant after 17 years, has undergone a saucerization defect. The shoulderless infrastructural design made maintenance and repair viable alternatives to removal. **B,** Postoperatively, the graft has served successfully to contribute to further function of this anchor implant.

Implants into Extraction Sites," p. 226, insert an immediate replacement implant, graft, and close. Such replacements should be threaded and of maximum height and length permitted by the host site. After allowing a 3 to 6 month hiatus to elapse in order to permit osseointegration, stage two surgery permits the fixation of an angled abutment of the three-piece variety (see Chapter 22). Collared abutments (e.g., Paragon) allow 18 different angulations, one of which should permit retrofitting into an existing crown or coping. Some diamond point alterations of the abutment may be required to bring it into conformation. Also a fixed-detachable unit made for it can be torqued into place after removing the old unit from the prosthesis and performing a classic dental floss or GC Pattern verification type assembly, leading to the soldering of a new superstructural component.

If immediate support is required after a tooth or implant is removed from beneath a conventional fixed bridge, cut away the occlusal surface of the crown completely, place the bridge into position, and use the crown as a surgical template for the accurate seating of a replacement implant. If 40% or more of the implant can be seated into freshly cut bone, graft the voids with autogenous bone (from the tuberosities or elsewhere) and place a straight or angled (if needed) tapered abutment, which, with adjustment, should fit into the existing crown. Complete the reconstruction with a composite lining and cementation with a filled composite resin.

Fractured Root Form Implants

The phenomenon of infrastructure fracture has been reported with all types of root form and blade implants.

The most frequent area of fracture occurs just below the abutment level (Fig. 28-47). Usually, the remaining apical por-

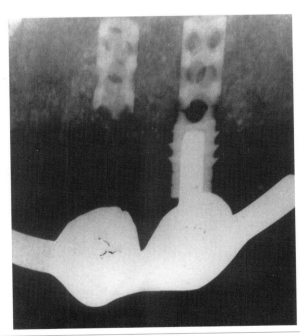

Fig. 28-47   Some root form implants may fracture because of design or manufacturing problems, poor prosthetic engineering, bruxism, or trauma.

tion is osseointegrated and should be left behind when removing the fractured elements. If replacing such an implant is the intention, removing the remaining apical implant segment requires an aggressive and traumatic *en bloc* osteotomy. Follow this by repair with a grafting material and a 6-month period of observation before undertaking the placement of a new implant.

Implants of Improper Angulation: The Double-bar Technique

Although the problem of angulation may have been anticipated at the time of surgery, it is usually not until the try-in stage of the prosthetic reconstruction that it becomes manifest (Fig. 28-48, A). This problem may be solved by the use of a double-bar technique. Instruct the laboratory to obtain three screw attachments from the European company Cendres & Metaux, S.A., Ors Dentaires, Biel Bienne, Switzerland. Each attachment is made in three parts: (1) an internally threaded cylinder or tube, (2) a smooth cylindrical collar, and (3) a fixation screw. Affix the three internally threaded cylinders (part 1) to the original malposed superstructure bar in positions that are angled lingually to permit esthetic placement of the fixation screws. In addition, place them as far apart from each other as possible and not in a straight line so that optimal support and stress distribution is encouraged. When the positions and angulations appear to be acceptable, solder these three threaded tubes to the bar (Fig. 28-48, B).

The next step is to have the laboratory transfer the location of these threaded tubes to the underside of an acrylic resin or cast metal second superstructure that is fitted onto the original bar, which now bears the threaded tubes. Make holes that pass through this second superstructure, each one directly over one of the threaded tubes. Into these holes, process the smooth cylindrical collars (part 2) with acrylic or solder, depending on whether the material chosen for the second bar is a polymer or a metal. At this point, seat the original cast bar onto the implant abutments in the normal manner and screw them into place, being sure that the screw heads are flush with the bar. Next, place the second superstructure bar over the first one and use the new fixation screws (part 3) to attach it through the three attached collars into the internally threaded cylinders now on the original bar. If the severe lingual angulations do not permit the use of a conventional screwdriver, make an offset driver by machining a No. 8 round, latch type bur and using it in a contra-angle. Turn it by rotating the spindle at the top of the handpiece.

If this technique is to be used with the Core-Vent system, select the titanium screw housings supplied by this company. Employ the technique for that system in precisely the same manner as described for the Swiss technique except that no cylindrical collars are required. The housings (TSFH), which should be soldered at correct angulations to the first bar, are available with fixative screws that have large enough heads to lock the secondary bar in place through simple holes made in it. If electing the second-bar option, acrylic is preferable to cast metal because it is lighter in weight,

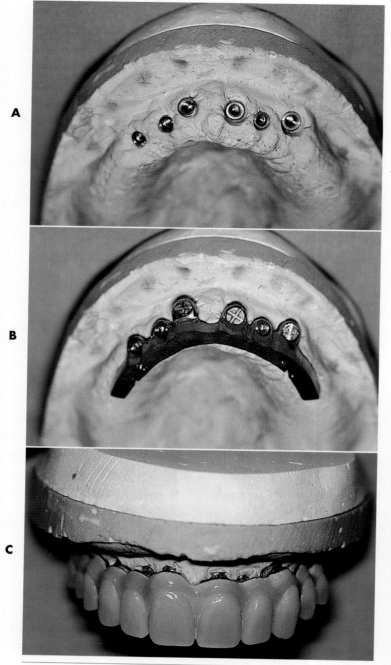

Fig. 28-48 **A,** Implants that diverge markedly, which cannot be brought into parallel configuration even by the use of angled abutments, need not be abandoned or removed. Even a mesostructural bar could have fixation screws in inaccessible positions or protruding from the labial surfaces of its hybrid's denture teeth. **B,** A classic mesostructure bar is constructed. Mill the bar to a 6-degree taper and position two female precision attachments to make a positive immobile seat for it. Then tap screw holes in it to retain a second prosthetic superstructure. This, the tooth-bearing component, may now have a minimum of three fixation screws placed at any appropriate angulation. **C,** The prosthetic superstructure is in place over the mesostructure bar. It shows an esthetic solution to malpositioned implants.

less costly, and more forgiving in regard to fabrication and repair (Fig. 28-48, C).

Broken Prosthetic Inserts

In root form and submergible blade implants, there are three types of abutments: threaded, cementable, and frictional. If, because of abuse (bending more than 20 degrees, overbending and straightening, or moving the pliers too sharply), an internal flaw in the cervix occurs or, because of metal fatigue, an abutment fractures at the implant body level, it may be necessary to retrieve the fractured insert so that another may be placed (Fig. 28-49). In the case of fracture of the threaded variety, which is, by far, less frequent, use a half-round bur to cut a groove into the superior surface for the use of a screwdriver. Machine an instrument handle into a screwdriver of the proper width and breadth, permitting the remaining broken portion of the insert to be backed out of the abutment receptacle. (Always use throat curtains when dealing with small parts intraorally in order to prevent their aspiration.) If the im-

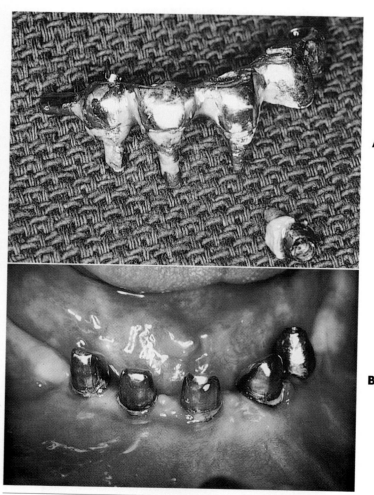

Fig. 28-49 **A,** Fracture of cemented prosthetic abutments insert is an occasional complication. **B,** After removal with cooled burs, direct Duralay patterns are made, cast in noble metal alloys, cemented, and the prosthetic reconstruction placed over them.

plant's angulation or position makes the use of a manual screwdriver difficult or impossible, machine a screwdriver from a large (No. 8) latch-type round bur, place it in the Implant Innovations contra-angle and use the wheel at the back to rotate it out of the implant (Fig. 28-50).

The cemented or frictional cold-weld (Morse taper) types present far greater problems. Drill out residual fragments bit by bit, carefully directing well-cooled 1/2 round and 700 dentate fissure burs in the long axis of the receptacle (Fig. 28-51). Follow use of these burs with thin, tapered diamonds. The components of the fractured post come out a bit at a time when flushed with irrigant, finally leaving the receptacle free of metal. The problem of lateral implant wall perforation is a major one, and if this should occur, a subsequent parietal ab-

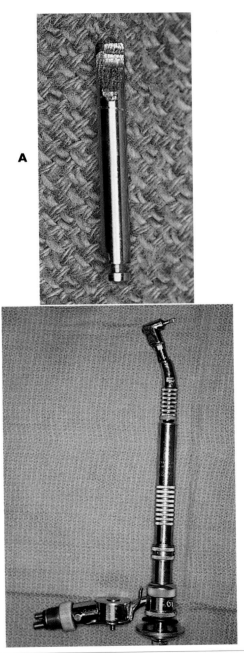

Fig. 28-50 **A,** Some fixation screws emerge at angles that make them inaccessible to a straight screwdriver. At No. 8 latch-type contra-angle round bur is machined into an offset screwdriver tip. **B,** When placed in the handpiece or contra-angle, it is used to engage the screw slot. Rotation is achieved by turning the wheel manually in a counterclockwise direction. In cases of a fractured threaded abutment, a one-half round bur is used to cut a slot in the screw's superior surface. The machined screwdriver is effective for backing such posts out of their implants.

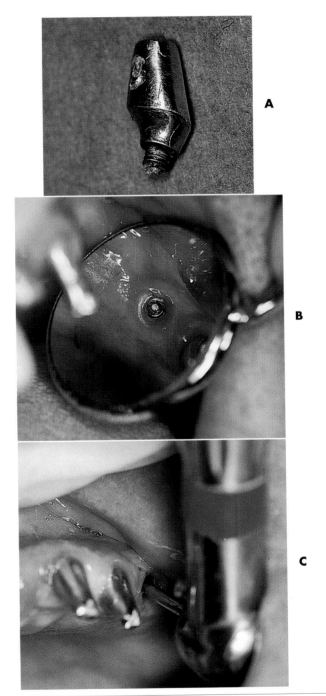

Fig. 28-51 **A,** Threaded abutments may be victims of fatigue. **B,** If their remnants cannot be backed out by screwdriver, they, like cemented abutments, must be drilled out. **C,** This may destroy the thread pattern and, if it does, cementable castings must be made using classic impression techniques.

scess or fistula may result. Should this happen, a flap with an HA/GTRM repair becomes necessary (see Chapter 8, "Bone Grafting," p. 136). After removing the broken component, perform standard impression-making procedures to allow the laboratory to cast a precious metal post-and-core replacement. Angulate it to a position of optimal prosthetic parallelism.

Screw Problems

One of the most frequent problems in the postoperative period is the fracture or stripping of screws or screw housings. This can occur during manipulation or simply while the prostheses is in function.

BREAKAGE OF RETENTION SCREWS IN FIXED-DETACHABLE BRIDGES
Breakage of retention screws in fixed-detachable bridges is a common problem that may occur when they have the addition of distal cantilevered segments. As stated in previous chapters, the maximum extension of the cantilever should be 15 mm in the mandible and none in the maxilla. If the posterior extensions are too long, the retention screws may loosen or break. This happens because posterior biting forces (especially if a balanced centric occlusion is not established properly) cause nonvertical loading, which affects the anterior segment. This places shearing forces on the retention screws, leading to loosening and, finally, to fracture. If the superstructure loosens repeatedly, a properly balanced centric occlusion must be established. Change the retention screws to new ones. Use Implaseal, a product available from Lifecore, to coat the fixation screws. It serves as an antibacterial sealant but does not interfere with screw placement or removal. The material peels away like rubber and must be reapplied with each reseating of the superstructure.

After completion of these corrective steps with balanced occlusal forces, the result will be lighter and more evenly applied stress to the retention screws.

BROKEN SCREWS   If a screw should fracture within the interior of an implant, remove the superstructure, and without creating damage to the internal threads, cut a groove cut into the top of the residual screw fragment. To retrieve the fragment, use a ¼-inch round, high-speed, water-cooled bur in the Impactair to scribe a horizontal groove into the top of the residual shaft. Then use a small compatible screwdriver to back off the fractured segment (Fig. 28-52).

STRIPPED IMPLANT THREADS   Excessive manual effort sometimes causes a stripping of a threaded interface. If this occurs, attempt to introduce a new screw. If this is successful, it indicates that the screw threads had failed. If the replacement screw fails to bite, the fault lies within the implant core. Each company manufactures a screw threader for purposes of recutting the internal threads within an implant. These tapping tools, made of hard carbon steel, are used manually and work efficiently and predictably. Screws of the same diameter as the tap are supplied to return the retention mechanism to its preincident condition.

When all else fails, the final alternative is to treat the implant as if it were a natural tooth, prepare it for a post-and-core, and fabricate one of precious metal. Casting cannot be done, however, until the abutment is retrofitted into the lubricated original crown using GC Pattern. After its completion, cement the new abutment into the implant, and cement the prosthesis resting over it as well.

Fabrication of Implant-Borne Temporary Prostheses

Occasionally, it may be necessary to send a fixed-detachable bridge to the laboratory for repair after it has been in use. A composite facing may have fractured, occlusal wear may have occurred, or a metal junction may need to be soldered. The temporary prosthesis that the patient wore during the fabrication of the fixed-detachable bridge should have been retained. If not, a new one has to be fabricated.

To do this, make a well-extended alginate impression of the arch with the prosthesis in place using a stock tray modified with periphery wax. Pour the impression with quick-setting stone. If sections of teeth are missing from the resultant model, restore them with wax or denture teeth. Place a two-sheet thickness of pink base-plate wax on all of the uncovered tissue surfaces of the model (e.g., palate, alveolar crest not covered by prosthesis), soak the model for 5 minutes in cold water, and make an impression of it in alginate. Pour the impression in quick-setting stone. When the stone has set, trim the model and make an Omnivac form over it using a 0.016-inch thick, clear sheet. Trim it so that the plastic just grasps the art border. Next, use a heatless stone on the first model to reduce the height of the teeth to 4 mm. Trim 2 mm from the facial surface of each tooth as well. Lubricate the model thoroughly with a separating medium. Fill the teeth in the Omnivac form to a three-fourths level with tooth-colored acrylic (or tooth-colored Triad material), and cover all other areas with pink denture base acrylic or Triad polymer. Seat the Omnivac onto the altered, lubricated model until the shell goes fully to place. The acrylic polymerizes by placing it into a curing unit. Remove the Omnivac form and newly fashioned denture from the model, trim it in the patient's mouth, and reline it with Coe Comfort or Viscogel to offer retention over the bar or implants (Fig. 28-53). As an alternative, screw it into place by opening two or three holes that correspond to the locations of strategically placed implants. Adjust the occlusion and instruct the patient to maintain a meticulous oral hygiene regimen.

Fractured Mesostructure Bars

Preinsertion bending, poor structural integrity, overly long spans, insufficient implant support, loss of integration of an abutting implant, or excessive occlusal trauma may cause a mesostructure bar to fracture.

If it is the fixed-detachable variety, remove it, take an index, and repair and reinforce the bar. If the etiology is known (i.e., long span, lost implant support, thin bar), take steps to institute correction. Reinsert the modified bar.

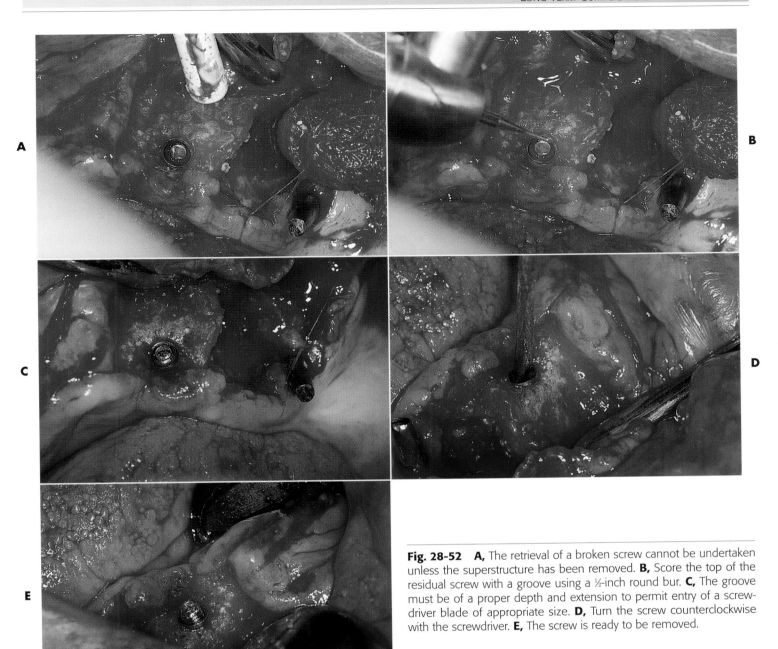

Fig. 28-52 **A,** The retrieval of a broken screw cannot be undertaken unless the superstructure has been removed. **B,** Score the top of the residual screw with a groove using a ½-inch round bur. **C,** The groove must be of a proper depth and extension to permit entry of a screwdriver blade of appropriate size. **D,** Turn the screw counterclockwise with the screwdriver. **E,** The screw is ready to be removed.

Fig. 28-53 A fixed prosthesis, if removed for repair, may be replicated with the Omnivac-Triad systems, in white and pink acrylic and used as a temporary denture. After its removal from the flask, it must be finished and polished and screw holes placed for transitional fixed-detachable application.

Manage cases of cemented coping-bars fractures or partial loss of cementation using a unique, simplified, chairside procedure.

Intraoral welding produces virtually no heat and creates firm, reliable unions on titanium and its alloys. Such welds resist the most significant challenges. Ingenuity, a welding machine (Hruska/Rome), and CP Titanium half-round rods of varying dimensions are the armamentaria required.

Remove the loosened or broken titanium copings by cutting the bar, thereby releasing them from the still cemented section, and bend a torque-free repair bar segment to the required contour of the fixed section. The Electrodex, which is handheld, serves as a clamp holding the bar to the titanium abutment. By the mere touch of a button on the console, a weld is achieved. The most successful welds are accomplished on broad, surface-to-surface relationships rather than by simple point contacts.

As the practitioner uses intraoral welding with greater frequency, a wider variety of uses becomes apparent.

Partial Loosening of Cemented Bars or Prostheses

Although the benefits of cementation are many, its major disadvantage is the difficulty of retrieval. If porcelain or composite material should fracture, if a solder joint breaks, or if a substructure problem such as implant infection or bone loss arises, bar removal must be possible.

The unswerving advocates of cementation argue that this was the accepted technique for affixing prostheses to natural teeth and served satisfactorily for decades. The worst solution to that scenario, if reverse hammer tapping failed, was to make bur cuts in the facial surfaces of the crowns and to use Weidelstadt chisels as levers to spring them off. Of course, a new prosthesis is then required.

Two possible remedies might be considered as substitutes for this draconian measure.

- Remove the loosened segment by sectioning with ultra-thin Carborundum disks, and prepare the crowns on either side of the removed segment with diamonds, to receive new crowns. Impression making is routine, and the newly constructed segment with its telescoping abutments may be cemented. Before doing this, seek the cause of the original cement failure. If the etiology was poor occlusion or a destructive patient habit, eliminate these before cementation of the replacement segment.
- An effective, pneumatic reverse hammer attached to the handpiece coupling has been shown to remove even the most recalcitrant cemented prostheses. Give thought to its use, however, in relationship to injury to support structures, fracturing abutments, or their screws or splitting implants. Once the practitioner becomes comfortable with its uses, it presents an additional tool of great benefit in the arena of trouble-shooting.

Inaccurate Fit of Castings

The number of complicated impression-making steps that must be completed at chairside, such as the fabrication of special trays, the dental floss/composite intraoral assembly of impression copings, the removal of implants by backing off screws followed by seating into an impression (further threatened by the pouring and separation processes), often results in inaccuracy of the fit of multiple unit castings. When designing these castings (either hybrid bars or crowns) to key into antirotational devices (spline or hex), the precision demanded for the creation of flawless interfaces virtually defies first-round acceptance.

It is a common event, therefore, to achieve passive fit by subsequent verification strategies. The technique, described in Chapter 22, involves the separation of the noncompliant units on the master cast, their transfer to the actual implants intraorally, and their reassembly with a stable polymer and a dental floss matrix. Achieving the demanding requirement of flawless fit requires patience and persistence.

Fractured Blade Abutments

One-piece blade implants are usually made of pure titanium and are designed to be bent (see Chapter 12). But overstressing, coupled with chewing forces and the galvanism caused by the dissimilar metals of a fixed prosthesis, may cause cervical fractures. Another common cause of fracture is related to cement loss beneath the abutment of a natural tooth in a bridge that shares natural and implant abutments. Attempts to tap the bridge from the still firmly cemented implant abutment often cause this. Use this maneuver only after great consideration. As a safe alternative, cut a slot in the cemented crown, permitting the bridge to be sprung free easily with the use of a small operative chisel. If, despite the most cautious approach, cervical fracture of a blade implant should occur but the infrastructure is firm and well imbedded in healthy bone (Fig. 28-54, *A, B*), it is possible to reconstruct and use the residual portion.

To replace a fractured abutment, make a crestal incision and expose the bone overlying the buried shoulder. Use a No. 2 L, round bur with coolant to brush the bone away, thus exposing the shoulder for a distance of 4 mm mesial and 4 mm distal from the fracture site. Make that portion of the shoulder accessible facially and lingually by removing bone from beneath it to a point 3 mm beneath its inferior border. A 9-mm-long segment of shoulder with a 3 mm opening beneath it should now be visualized (Fig. 28-54, *C*). Complete hemostasis must be achieved. Raccord is effective (but must be used with care in the hypertensive or epinephrine-labile individual), but tamponade works well, employing time and patience. When the area is dry, make an Impregum impression of the site using a syringe and sectional tray technique. A wax bite and counter impression are also necessary. Place periodontal packing (e.g., Coe Pak) beneath the exposed shoulder and press it into the bony cavity. Mold the excess material around the bar. Suture the remainder of the incision mesially and distally.

Instruct the laboratory to make a centrifuged epoxy model

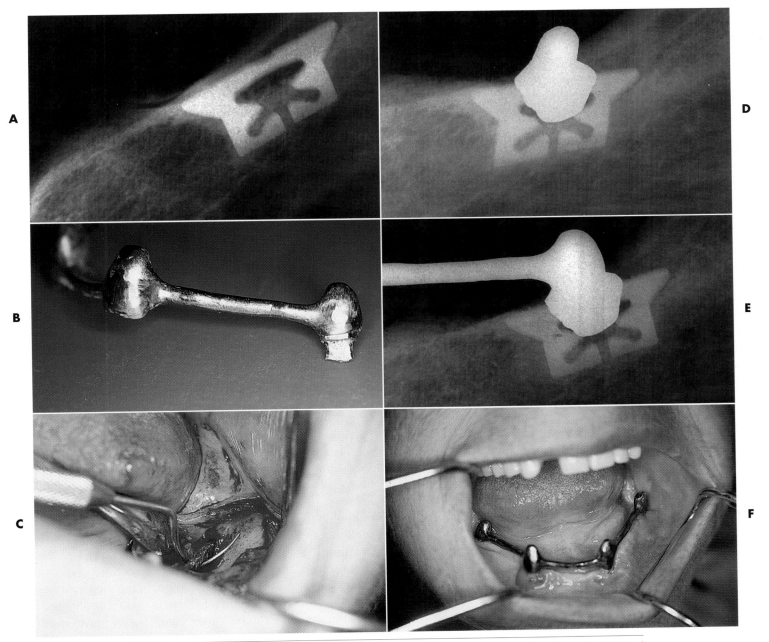

Fig. 28-54 **A,** A blade implant, placed 16 years before this radiograph, fractured at the cervix. **B,** It had served as the distal abutment for an all-important coping bar–overdenture reconstruction. The bar and fractured abutment are seen. **C,** The shoulder of this integrated blade had to be exteriorized. After this had been accomplished, an explorer could be passed beneath it. **D,** The new abutment consisting of twin, separtely cast leaves, was affixed with SMS screws. This radiograph shows the reconstruction. **E, F,** Six-year postoperative radiograph and photograph of the repaired implant with a functioning bar and overdenture.

(for strength and accuracy) and to cast a double-leaved abutment in gold using the Whaledent SMS (Splint-Mate), nonparallel, horizontal pin system, which can rivet the two leaves together. The two leaves, when pressed together, embrace the exposed bar accurately, with each having a concave depression designed to fit over its half of the bar. The threaded leaf component must be the lingual one, and the rivet head side must be the buccal. Ideally, four threaded pins should be used, two above and two below the bar.

At the second or insertion procedure, remove the Coe Pak, revealing the segment of shoulder now exteriorized. Healed epithelium will be seen beneath it. Place the newly cast abutment's two halves on each side of the bar, and with the assistant clamping them together using a heavy, curved Carmalt forceps, test the accuracy of alignment of the four holes using threaded SMS pins. Since the pins' handles are color coded, they should be aligned in the same order on the bracket table. Isolate and dry the field and join the two components with glass ionomer cement. Before the cement sets, fully thread into place all four pins, each covered with a swipe of cement, thereby locking and riveting the two leaves together. After setting, trim both protruding ends of each pin, and remove excess cement. The result is a new abutment that can serve as a fixed bridge retainer (Fig. 28-54, *D-F*).

Subperiosteal Implant

Bone Resorption

Problems with subperiosteal implants occur most often after a considerable period of time. Generally, they are related to bone loss beneath the primary struts in the posterior components, but on an unpredictable basis, particularly in women, resorption may take place almost anywhere even in time periods as short as 12 months (Fig. 28-55). If the involved areas are modest in size, inform the patient and track these areas with standardized radiographs. If the areas do not change significantly and remain symptom-free, keep them under observation. On the other hand, treat progressively enlarging lesions or those that cause pain, granulomatosis, or swelling, aggressively. Manage them by making crestal incisions and tissue reflections as if it were planned to remove the implant. The next step is arduous and requires great patience. Using a No. 12 BP blade on top of (or just alongside) the involved struts, incise the enveloping fibrous tissue. It is tough and, fortunately, avascular. It often camouflages the struts, so gentle stroking with sharp No. 12 blades must continue as if following a road map of struts. As they become revealed, it is possible to clarify the position and depth of the connective tissue that must be removed and to coordinate the radiographic components with those exposed surgically. Using a combination of sharp periodontal curettes and knives, fresh No. 12 blades, and fine (mosquito or tonsil) curved hemostats, the involved portions of the infrastructure eventually become completely stripped of its fibrous envelope. Do this to a part or an entire implant, one section at a time. After exposing the infrastructure, use a syringe of 20-mesh DFDB or HA, moistened with the patient's blood, to place the particles under each strut, filling in the voids over the bone. Cover the struts with additional material. Complete the operation with a closure, using 3-0 Polysorb or Biosyn in a continuous horizontal mattress suture configuration (Fig. 28-56).

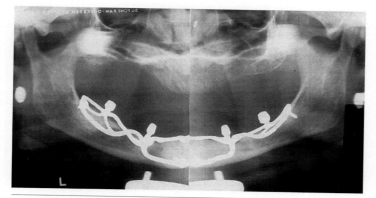

Fig. 28-55   Bone loss, on radiographs, is seen beneath the posterior abutments of mandibular subperiosteal implants more frequently in non–Brookdale bar designs.

Strut Dehiscence

Tissues sometimes shrink away from a strut after a considerable period of time. This occurs most frequently in the lingual posterior area of the mandible because of mylohyoid muscle activity and underlying bone resorption. The best cure is prevention, that is, by avoiding the placement of struts that lie in the mylohyoid region. When it does occur, if the patient has no symptoms, teach the patient to keep the strut clean with gentle abrasion using a firm wooden-stick, cotton-tipped applicator. In cases that do not respond to simple hygiene, perform strut resection after making a determination that a major structural component is not sacrificed. To resect a strut, use local anesthesia. Push the mucosa several millimeters back along the strut. Use a new, tapered diamond stone with gentle strokes and copious coolant to permit sectioning through the exposed metal. Smoothing the cut ends causes beneficial abrasion to the adjacent mucosa and encourages healing. Sutures need not be used and, after epithelization, the tissues will cover the remaining metallic stumps.

Recurrent Pericervical Granulomas

Buds of friable hemorrhagic tissue sometimes protrude from the pericervical gingival crevices of subperiosteal implants (Fig. 28-57). This occurs most frequently in the areas of the posterior abutments. Since the presence of this tissue is merely a symptom and not a disease, curetting does not make a valuable long-range contribution. Seek the etiology, which in all probability is that of subabutment bone resorption. If so, follow the previous paragraphs regarding curettage and synthetic bone implantation. If the problem fails to respond to such therapy, even though traumatic occlusion and bruxism (treated with a soft, protective occlusal appliance) have been eliminated, it may become necessary to reset the involved portion of the implant (Fig. 28-58). Do this in the same manner as described for strut resection. Instead of adding grafting material after exposing the offending components, however, transect a few strategic connecting struts with a fine diamond point so that the errant parts can be removed. If the implant is of the one-piece variety, perform the sectioning at the mental "bow-tie" configuration, being careful not to injure the neurovascular bundle. If the implant is of the tripodal design, cut the Brookdale bar just distal to the anterior or canine abutment so that a 5-mm cantilevered segment remains. Then dissect the posterior submandibular islet free and remove it. If any strut components are buried beneath bone, it is often preferable to permit them to remain rather than to injure the cortex needlessly. It is important to make an immediate postsurgical alteration of the superstructure. At the point where the denture no longer is bar supported, section the saddle and insert a DE hinge (Howmedica) or similar stress-breaking device, thereby permitting its independent movement in a more physiologic fashion (Fig. 28-59). Place a tissue-conditioning liner such as Coe-Soft beneath the newly hinged saddle. This may be changed to a permanent soft, silicone reline material after complete healing.

If acute infection and cellulitis precede the granulomas, treat the patient symptomatically before definitive surgery. Use incision and drainage as indicated; place drains; and use ice, saline rinses, and antibiotics as dictated by the clinical situation.

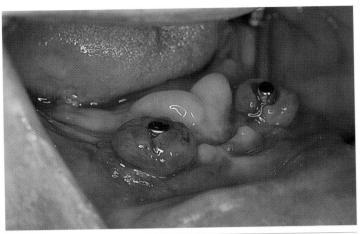

Fig. 28-57 Granulomatous pericervical lesions are a symptom of peri-implantitis. Their elimination without treatment of the underlying etiologic agent does not effect a cure.

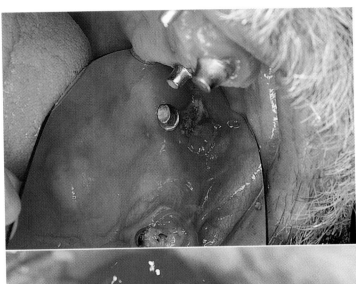

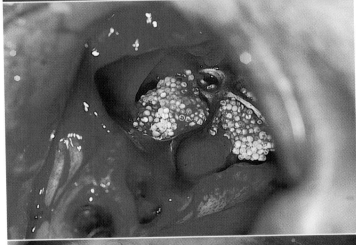

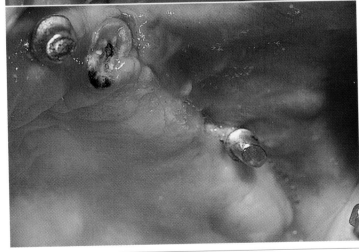

Fig. 28-56 **A,** A 24-year-old maxillary universal subperiosteal implant. Bleeding, soreness, and granulomas were found in the abutment areas. **B,** A complete and aggressive exposure of the infrastructure included curettage, bone grafting (HA), and a primary, tension-free closure. **C,** Postoperative healing was accompanied by firm, nontender, keratinized tissues.

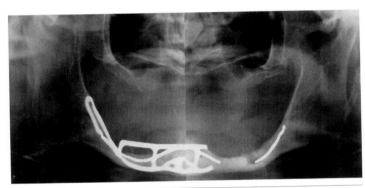

Fig. 28-58 Posterior subperiosteal segments that are troublesome may be resected. In this instance, the buccal peripheral strut had become integrated and was permitted to remain.

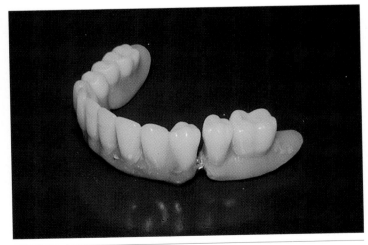

Fig. 28-59 A superstructure that rests on an altered implant distributes stresses more evenly if it is readapted to its new environment. In this case the tissue-borne distal end of the denture was transected and reattached with a DE hinge.

In instances when the continued maintenance of a subperiosteal implant is inimical to the patient's health because all efforts at repair have failed, the implant must be removed. Generally this applies only to subperiosteal implants that demonstrate mobility. This often is a difficult, complex, and time-consuming operation that may be performed using either local or general anesthesia.

Make a crestal incision from one posterior end of the infrastructure around to the other. Develop a facial flap using sharp dissection with a No. 12 BP blade. Take care to maintain this as a full-thickness flap and to avoid injuring the vital mental neurovascular bundles.

On the visualization of the most posterior peripheral strut, the assistant must retract firmly to make it accessible. Using a No. 12 blade, incise the dense fibrous envelope surrounding the metal. Continue this process with the scalpel, following the strut geometry. Inaccessible metal structure mandates more aggressive flap development and reflection. Finally, when all enveloping fibrous strands have been cut, thereby totally exposing the entire infrastructure, attempt to lift it out. There may be osseous impediments as well that re-quire removal with a cooled No. 6 round bur. Even after this, the implant usually requires sectioning in order to facilitate removal.

After removal and thorough debridement and irrigation, complete the procedure with a primary 3-0 Vicryl mattress suture closure. Reline the former superstructure with Coe Comfort and use it as a stent and temporary denture during healing.

Broken Abutments

Although subperiosteal implants rarely fracture, this can be prevented (with either chrome alloys or titanium) by taking metallurgic x-rays of all castings before surgical placement. Bubbles and casting defects show up easily with such views and indicate rejection of the casting (Fig. 28-60). If an abutment should break and enough cervix is left (which is unlikely), a casting may be made to telescope over it. If this is not possible, shave the protruding cervix down as much as possible, create some bleeding by abrasion with the diamond drill, and allow the epithelium to cover the altered stump by secondary intention. This is particularly applicable if the affected site is a posterior one. In such cases, make superstructural alterations by sectioning the saddle just distal to the anterior (canine) abutment and building in a DE hinge as a connector (see Fig. 28-59). This allows the posterior saddle to function on a stress-broken basis as described in the preceding paragraphs.

Other More Significant Symptoms

In cases of dysesthesia of recent or sudden onset or mobility of the slightest kind in a subperiosteal implant (usually as a result of settling), immediate removal is mandatory. Take care not to further injure the neurovascular bundle or other vital structures during the removal procedure. Facilitate this by sectioning the infrastructure into small segments, permitting

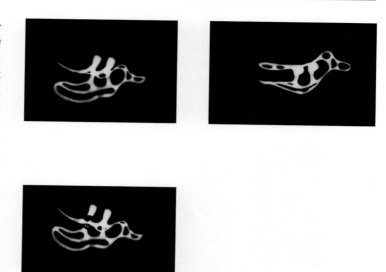

Fig. 28-60   Sound manufacturing quality control should include the use of industrial metallurgical radiographs.

some of the components to slide out from beneath the tissues and thereby minimizing trauma.

Postsubperiosteal Sublingual Floor Elevation

Flap elevation and replacement over a mandibular subperiosteal implant or repairs to endosteal implants in the anterior mandible sometimes cause sublingual elevation and malposture that places the anterior portion of the plicae sublingualis and the orifices of Wharton's ducts over the crest of the ridge (Fig. 28-61, A). As a result, when the patient places his or her superstructure or overdenture, they report pain and often experience salivary obstruction.

Perform surgical correction of this difficulty by repositioning the floor of the mouth. Under regional block anesthesia, make an incision at the crest of the edentulous ridge from one molar area to the other. Reflect the mucosa outlined by this introductory maneuver from the lingual surface of the anterior mandible, permitting the periosteum to remain in position (Fig. 28-61, B).

This permits the sublingual mucosa to be dissected free of the Wharton's ducts, the sublingual glands, and the fibers of the mylohyoid muscles. Bring the ducts, which had been cannulated with whalebone bougies, through the mucosa at sites made lingually to the ridge crest, where they are not obstructed by the overdenture flange. Suture the entire mucosal margin to the lingual periosteum 5 mm apically to the crest of the ridge (Fig. 28-61, C).

After ensuring the patency of the ducts, line the lingual flange of the overdenture with surgical cement and insert it as a stent.

The postoperative course is usually uneventful. Remove the stent on the fourteenth postoperative day. A zone of fixed gingiva epithelizes secondarily beneath the surgical cement over the exposed lingual periosteum. The structures of the floor of the mouth become stabilized in their newly placed, appropriate anatomic positions (Fig. 28-61, D).

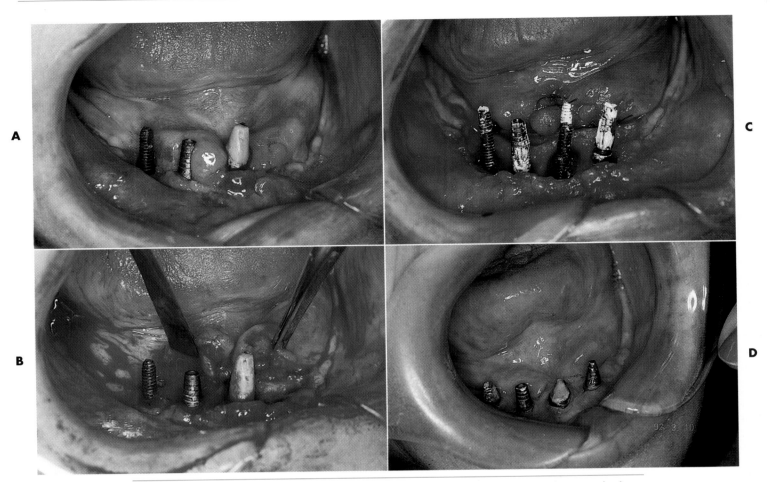

Fig. 28-61 **A,** This patient has an anteriorly displaced sublingual floor, which occurred as a result of previous surgery. **B,** Make a crestal incision from one retromolar pad to the other, which permits freeing and elevating the entire sublingual complex. **C,** Ensure the patency of Wharton's ducts before repositioning the wound margin and suturing it to the lingual periosteum at a point 5 mm below the ridge crest. **D,** One year postoperatively the sublingual anatomy is properly relocated without the possibilities of overdenture impingement.

Implantation in the Irradiated Jaw

Many patients who have received tumoricidal doses of radiation need implants in order to acquire improved levels of comfort, mastication, and esthetics. Current thought encourages the placement of multiple implants in numbers sufficient to permit the insertion of totally implant-borne prostheses. One of the principle causes of osteoradionecrosis is the pressure of saddles on the overlying mucosa; therefore their use is to be discouraged. Consensus favors the use of hyperbaric oxygen for preoperative and postoperative therapy.

A period of 9 to 12 months after radiation should elapse before implant surgery. At this point in time, considerable lev-els of revascularization have been reported. The patients should have undergone thorough oral prophylaxis, had all poorly prognosed teeth extracted before radiation, have given up smoking and the use of tobacco products, and be free of malignant disease. Before implant surgery, the patient should receive 20 hyperbaric oxygen treatments of 90 minutes each at 2 to 2.4 atmospheres. Three days before the surgery, institute an antibiotic regimen using Augmentin 500 mg every 12 hours.

The implant surgery should follow the guidelines presented in Chapter 9, with special considerations given to small incisions, preservation of periosteal attachments, the use of sharp, well-irrigated drills with small gradients of drill diameter change, and flawless soft tissue management and closure. Continue antibiotics for 10 postoperative days, and give the patient 10 more days of hyperbaric therapy. Double the time allowed for integration to give the implants optimal opportunity for success.

Suggested Readings

Ali A et al: Implant rehabilitation of irradiated jaws: a preliminary report, *Int J Oral Maxillofac Implants* 12(4):523-526, 1997.

Apse P et al: Microbiota and crevicular fluid collagenase activity in the osseointegrated dental implant sulcus: a comparison of sites in edentulous and partially edentulous patients, *J Periodontol Res* 24:96-105, 1989.

Asikainen P et al: Osseointegration of dental implants in bone irradiated with 40, 50, or 60 gy doses. An experimental study with beagle dogs, *Clin Oral Implants Res* 9(1):20-25, 1998.

Bain CA: Smoking and implant failure: benefits of a smoking cessation protocol, *Int J Oral Maxillofac Implant* 11:756-759, 1996.

Bain CA, Moy PK: The association between the failure of dental implants and cigarette smoking, *Int J Oral Maxillofac Implant* 8:609, 1993.

Balshi TJ: Hygiene maintenance procedures for patients with the tissue-integrated prosthesis, *Quintessence Int* 17:95-102, 1986.

Balshi TJ: Resolving aesthetic complications with osseointegration using a double-casting technique, *Quintessence* 17:281-287, 1986.

Bidez MW, Staphens BJ, Lemons JE: An investigation into the effect of blade dental implant length on interfacial tissue stress profiles. In Spilker RL, Simon MR, editors: *Computational methods in bioengineering*, Proceedings of the American Society of Mechanical Engineers Winter Annual Meeting, Chicago, November 17-December 2, 1988.

Branemark P-I et al: An experimental and clinical study of osseointegrated implant penetrating the nasal cavity and maxillary sinus, *J Oral Maxillofac Surg* 42:497-505, 1984.

Brogniez V et al: Prosthetic dental rehabilitation of osseointegrated implants placed in irradiated mandibular bone. Apropos of 50 implants in 17 patients treated over a period of 5 years, *Rev Stomatol Chir Maxillofac* 97(5):288-294, 1996. French.

Brygider RM, Bain CA: Custom stent fabrication for free gingival grafts around osseointegrated abutment fixtures, *J Prosthet Dent* 62:320-322, 1989.

Brygider RM: Precision attachment-retained gingival veneers for fixed implant prostheses, *J Prosthet Dent* 65:118-122, 1991.

Carlson B, Carlsson GE: Prosthodontic complications in osseointegrated dental implant treatment, *JOMI on CD-ROM, Quintessence* 9(1):90-94, 1994.

Carr AB, Papazoglou E, Lersen PE: The relationship of Periotest values, biomaterial, and torque to failure in adult baboons, *Int J Prosth* 8(1):15-20, 1995.

Chai JY, Yamada J, Pang IC: In vitro consistency of the Periotest instrument, *J Prosth* 2(1):9-12, 1993.

Chavez H et al: Assessment of oral implant mobility, *J Prosth Dent* 7(5):421-426, 1993.

Chiche G et al: Auxiliary substructure for screw-retained prostheses, *Int J Prosthodont* 2:407-412, 1989.

Christiansen RL: Latent infection involving a mandibular implant: a case report, *J Oral Maxillofac Implant* 6:481-484, 1991.

Cox JF, Pharoah M: An alternative holder for radiographic evaluation of tissue-integrated prostheses, *J Oral Maxillofac Implant* 56:338-341, 1986.

Dahlin C et al: Generation of new bone around titanium implants using a membrane technique: an experimental study in rabbits, *J Oral Maxillofac Implant* 4:19-25, 1989.

Davenport WL et al: Salvage of the mandibular staple bone plate following bone infection, *J Oral Maxillofac Surg* 43:981-986, 1985.

Davies JM, Campbell LA: Fatal air embolism during dental implant surgery: a report of three cases, *Can J Anaesth* 37:112-121, 1990.

Davis DM, Rogers SJ, Packer ME: The extent of maintenance required by implant-retained mandibular overdentures: a 3-year report, *Int J Oral Maxillofac Implant* 11:767-774, 1996.

Eckert SE et al: Endosseous implants in an irradiated tissue bed, *J Prosthet Dent* 76(1):45-49, 1996.

Esser E et al: Dental implants following radical oral cancer surgery and adjuvant radiotherapy, *Int J Oral Maxillofac Implant* 12(4):552-557, 1997.

Fisch M: Causes of failure with intraosseous implants, *Int Dent J* 33:379-382, 1983.

Fishel D et al: Roentgenologic study of the mental foramen, *Oral Surg Oral Med Oral Pathol* 41:682-686, 1976.

Fox SC, Moriarty JD, Kusy RP: The effects of scaling a titanium implant surface with metal and plastic instruments: an in vitro study, *J Periodontol* 61:485-490, 1990.

Franzen L et al: Oral implant rehabilitation of patients with oral malignancies treated with radiotherapy and surgery without adjunctive hyperbaric oxygen, *Int J Oral Maxillofac Implant* 10(2):183-187, 1995.

Gammage DD: Clinical management of failing dental implants: four case reports, *J Oral Implantol* 15:124-131, 1989.

Garfield RE: Implant prostheses for convertibility, stress control, esthetics, and hygiene, *J Prosthet Dent* 60:85-93, 1988.

Granstorm G et al: Titanium implants in irradiated tissue: benefits from hyperbaric oxygen, *Int J Oral Maxillofac Implant* 7(1):15-25, 1992. Review.

Hallman W et al: A comparative study of the effects of metallic, nonmetallic, and sonic instrumentation on titanium abutment surfaces, *Int J Oral Maxillofac Implant* 11:96-100, 1996.

Hass R et al: Examination of damping behavior of IMZ implants, *Int J Oral Maxillofac Implant* 10(4):410-414, 1995.

Heller AL: Blade implants, *Can Dent Assoc J* 16:78-86, 1988.

Hollender L: Radiographic techniques for precision analysis of bridges on osseointegrated fixtures, *Swed Dent J* 28(suppl):171-174, 1985.

Ibbott CG: In vivo fracture of a basket-type osseointegrating dental implant: a case report, *J Oral Maxillofac Implant* 4:255-256, 1989.

James RA: The connective tissue-dental implant interface, *J Oral Implantol* 13:607-621, 1988.

James RA, Kellin E: A histopathological report on the nature of the epithelium and underlining connective tissue which surrounds implant posts, *J Biomed Mat Res* 5:373-383, 1974.

James RA, Schultz RL: Hemidesmosomes and the adhesion of junctional epithelial cells to metal implants: a preliminary report, *J Oral Implantol* 4:294-302, 1974.

Jansen JA: Ultrastructural study of epithelial cell attachment to implant materials, *J Dent Res* 65:5, 1985.

Jensen O, Nock D: Inferior alveolar nerve repositioning in conjunction with placement of osseointegrated implants: a case report, *Oral Surg Oral Med Oral Path* 63:263-268, 1987.

Jisander S et al: Dental implant survival in the irradiated jaw: a preliminary report, *Int J Oral Maxillofac Implant* 12(5):643-648, 1997.

Kasten FH, Soileau K, Meffert RM: Quantitative evaluation of human gingival epithelial cell attachment to implant surfaces in vitro, *Int J Periodont Restor Dent* 10:69-79, 1990.

Keller EE et al: Mandibular endosseous implants and autogenous bone grafting in irradiated tissue: a 10-year retrospective study, *Int J Oral Maxillofac Implant* 12(6):800-813, 1997.

Keller EE: Placement of dental implants in the irradiated mandible: a protocol without adjunctive hyperbaric oxygen, *J Oral Maxillofac Surg* 55(9):972-980, 1997. Review. No Abstract available.

Koth DL, McKinney RV, Steflik DE: Microscopic study of hygiene effect on peri-implant gingival tissues, *J Dent Res* 66(special issue)186 (abstract 639), 1986.

Kwan JY, Zablotsky MH, Meffert RM: Implant maintenance using a modified ultrasonic instrument, *J Dent Hyg* 64:422-430, 1990.

Laboda G: Life-threatening hemorrhage after placement of an endosseous implant: report of a case, *J Am Dent Assoc* 121:599-600, 1990.

Larsen PE: Placement of dental implants in the irradiated mandible: a protocol involving adjunctive hyperbaric oxygen, *J Oral Maxillofac Surg* 55(9):967-971, 1997. Review. No abstract available.

Lavelle CLB: Mucosal seal around endosseous dental implants, *J Oral Implant* 9:357-371, 1981.

Lekholm U et al: The condition of soft tissue at tooth and fixture abutments supporting fixed bridges: a microbiological and histological study, *J Clin Periodontol* 13:558-562, 1986.

Levy D et al: A comparison of radiographic bone height and probing attachment level measurements adjacent to porous-coated dental implants in humans, *Int J Oral Maxillofac Implant* 12:544-546, 1997.

Lillard JF: Resolution of a complicated implant case using accepted multimodal guidelines, *J Oral Implantol* 17:146-151, 1991.

Lindhe J et al: Experimental breakdown of peri-implant and periodontal tissues: a study in the beagle dog, *Clin Oral Implant* Res 3:9-16, 1992.

Lindquist LW, Rockler B, Carlsson GE: Bone resorption around fixtures in edentulous patients treated with mandibular fixed tissue-integrated prostheses, *J Prosthet Dent* 59:59-63, 1988.

Linkow L: Mandibular implants: a dynamic approach to oral implantology, New Haven, Conn., 1978, Glarus, pp. 10-12.

Linkow L: The multipurpose Blade-Vent implant, *Dent Dig*, 1967.

Linkow LJ, Donath K, Lemons JE: Retrieval analysis of a blade implant after 231 months of clinical function, *Implant Dent* 1:37-43, 1992.

Manz MC, Morris HF, Ochi S: An evaluation of the Periotest system. Part II, *Implant Dent* 1(3):221-226, 1992.

Martin IC et al: Endosseous implants in the irradiated composite radial forearm free flap, *Int J Oral Maxillofac Surg* 21(5):266-270, 1992.

Meffert RM: Endosseous dental implantology from the periodontist's viewpoint, *J Periodontol* 57:531-536, 1986.

Meffert RM: The soft tissue interface in dental implantology, *J Dent Educ* 52:810-811, 1988.

Misch CE: Density of bone: effect of treatment plans, surgical approach, healing and progressive bone loading, *Int J Oral Implantol* 6:23-31, 1990.

Misch CE: Osseointegration and the submerged Blade implant, *J Hous Dist Dent Assoc* 1:12-16, 1988.

Misch CE, Crawford E: Predictable mandibular nerve location: a clinical zone of safety, *Int J Oral Implant* 7(1):37-40, 1990.

Misch CM et al: Post-operative maxillary cyst associated with a maxillary sinus elevation procedure: a case report, *J Oral Implantol* 17:432-437, 1991.

Mombelli A et al: The microbiota associated with successful or failing osseointegrated titanium implants, *Oral Microbiol Immunol* 2:145, 1987.

Newman MJ, Flemming FT: Periodontal considerations of implants and implant-associated microbiota, *J Dent Educ* 52:737, 1988.

Niedermeier W, Kublbeck K: Factors involved in endosseous implant function, *Deutsche Zahn Zeit* 46(9):589-594, 1991.

Niimi A et al: A Japanese multicenter study of osseointegrated implants paced in irradiated tissues: a preliminary report, *Int J Oral Maxillofac Implant* 12(2):259-264, 19XX.

Nyman S et al: Bone regeneration adjacent to titanium dental implants using guided tissue regeneration: a report of two cases, *J Oral Maxillofac Implant* 5:9-14, 1990.

Ochi S, Moris HF, Winkler S: The influence of implant type, material, coating, diameter, and length on Periotest values at second-stage surgery: DICRG interim report no. 4, *Implant Dent* 3(3):159-162, 1994.

Olive J, Aparicio C: The Periotest method as a measure of osseointegrated oral implant stability, *Int J Oral Maxillofac Implant* 5:390, 1990.

Orton GS et al: The dental professional's role in monitoring and maintenance of tissue-integrated prostheses, *J Oral Maxillofac Implant* 4:305-310, 1989.

Parham PL et al: Effects of an air powder abrasive system on plasma-sprayed titanium implant surfaces: an in vitro evaluation, *J Oral Implantol* 15:78-86, 1989.

Pietrokovski J: The bony residual ridge in man, *J Prosthet Dent* 34:456-462, 1975.

Quirynen M et al: The influence of titanium abutment surface roughness on plaque accumulation and gingivitis: short-term observations, *Int J Oral Maxillofac Implant* 11(2):169-178, 1996.

Rams T, Link C Jr: Microbiology of failing implants in humans: electron microscopic observations, *J Oral Implant* 11:93, 1983.

Rams T et al: The subgingival microbial flora associated with human dental implants, *J Prosthet Dent* 51:529-539, 1984.

Rapley JW et al: The surface characteristics produced by various oral hygiene instruments and materials on titanium implant abutments, *Int J Oral Maxillofac Implant* 5:47-52, 1990.

Roos J et al: A qualitative and quantitative method for evaluating implant success: a 5-year retrospective analysis of the Branemark implant, JOMI on CD-ROM, *Quintessence* 12(4):504-514, 1997.

Salonen MA et al: Failures in the osseointegration of endosseous implants, *Int J Oral Maxillofac Implant* 8(1):92-97, 1993.

Schnitman P et al: Three-year survival rates, blade implants versus cantilever clinical trials, *J Dent Res* 67(special issue):347, 1988.

Schon R et al: Peri-implant tissue reaction in bone irradiated the fifth day after implantation in rabbits: histologic and histomorphometric measurements, *Int J Oral Maxillofac Implant* 11(2):228-238, 1996.

Schulte W, Lukas D: Periotest to monitor osseointegration and to check the occlusion of oral implantology, *J Oral Implant* 19(1):23-32, 1993.

Sclaroff A et al: Immediate mandibular reconstruction and placement of dental implants at the time of ablative surgery, *Oral Surg Oral Med Oral Pathol* 78(6):711-717, 1994.

Smithlof M, Fritz ME: The use of blade implants in a selected population of partially edentulous adults: a 10-year report, *J Periodontol* 53:413-415, 1981.

Smithlof M, Fritz ME: The use of blade implants in a selected population of partially edentulous adults: a 15-year report, *J Periodontol* 58:589-593, 1987.

Stefani LA: The care and maintenance of the dental implant patient, *J Dent Hygiene* 447-466, 1988.

Taylor TD et al: Osseointegrated implant rehabilitation of the previously irradiated mandible: results of a limited trial at 3 to 7 years, *J Prosthet Dent* 69(I):60-69, 1993. Review.

Teerlinck J et al: Periotest: an objective clinical diagnosis of bone apposition toward implants, *Int J Oral Maxillofac Implant* 6(1):55-61, 1991.

Thomas-Neal D, Evans GH, Meffert RM: Effects of various prophylactic treatments on titanium, sapphire, and hydroxylapatite-coated implants: an SEM study, *Int J Periodont Restor Dent* 9:301-311, 1989.

Tolman DE, Keller EE: Management of mandibular fractures in patients with endosseous implants, *J Oral Maxillofac Implant* 6:427-436, 1991.

Tricia J et al: Mechanical state assessment of the implant-borne continuum: a better understanding of the Periotest method, *Int J Oral Maxillofac Implant* 10(1):43-49, 1995.

Truhlar RS et al: Assessment of implant mobility at second-stage surgery with the Periotest: DICRG interim report no. 3, *Implant Dent* 3(3):153-156, 1994.

Van Scotter DE, Wilson CJ: The Periotest method for determining implant success, *J Oral Implantol* 17:410-413, 1991.

Van Steenberghe D, Quirynen M: Reproducibility and detection threshold of peri-implant diagnosis, *Adv Dent Res* 7(2):191-195, 1993.

Viscido A: The submerged blade implant—a dog histologic study, *J Oral Implant* 5(2):195-209, 1974.

Walker L, Morris HF, Ochi S et al: Periotest values of dental implants in the first 2 years after second-stage surgery: DICRG interim report no. 8, *Implant Dent* 6:207, 1997.

Watzinger F et al: Endosteal implants in the irradiated lower jaw, *J Craniomaxillofac Surg* 24(4):237-244, 1996.

Weischer T et al: Concept of surgical and implant-supported prostheses in the rehabilitation of patients with oral cancer, *Int J Oral Maxillofac Implant* 11(6):775-781, 1996.

Whittaker JM et al: Implant-tissue interface: a case history, *J Oral Implantol* 15:137-140, 1990.

Zarb GA, Schmitt A: The longitudinal clinical effectiveness of osseointegrated dental implants: the Toronto study. Part III. Problems and complications, *J Prosthet Dent* 64:185-194, 1990.

29

Maintenance and Hygiene

All implant patients must carefully follow a regimen of postinsertion orders. The majority of patients who request implants lose their teeth because of decay or periodontal disease. By habit, they may be among the least conscientious of patients, and before implant surgery the surgeon must impress on them the importance of home care and maintenance. Implants suffer tissue breakdown and bone loss at a more rapid pace than natural teeth. Patients who undergo this form of therapy must exhibit a voluntary change in behavioral pattern. Follow them carefully to ensure that they continue to maintain their implants and prostheses. Instruct them to promptly report any problems to their physicians.

Following both implant surgery and prosthesis insertion, make appointments to see patients at 1, 2, 4, 12, and 24 weeks. (Because of the patient's oral hygiene or other prevailing circumstances, these time periods may be altered.) At recall appointments, evaluate the prostheses and their attachments for function, esthetics, and stability, and remove and replace them if necessary. Examine the implants radiographically for radiolucencies at a minimum of 1-year intervals using periapical and when needed, panoramic films. Use a standardized radiographic technique. Inspect the implants for mobility at each recall appointment. If the prosthesis is of the fixed-detachable type, either mesostructure bar or full superstructure prosthesis, remove it before assessing the implants. Use an instrument handle on the buccal and lingual surfaces of each implant abutment so that a gentle attempt may be made to rock it back and forth.

Periotest

An electronic mobilometer called the Periotest (Fig. 29-1) is available from Siemens, Germany. This instrument indicates levels of mobility of root form implants. Readings from -7 to $+18$ are representative of movement too imperceptible to be clinically detectable. When mobility readings are $+9$ and above, implants with even the best of radiographic findings must be evaluated and treated. The Periotest offers a more reliable method of diagnosing implant status by measuring levels of subclinical mobility in a reproducible manner. It is an electronic instrument that uses an ultrasonically vibrating probe to assess micromobility. The device has been used in a number of applications since its introduction in 1983 for determining the periodontal status of natural teeth. It has been an effective tool in evaluating implant stability from the time of second-stage surgery throughout all subsequent stages of management. Some have even claimed to use the instrument for balancing and fine-tuning the forces of occlusion. In vitro evaluations of the Periotest revealed that no statistically significant difference existed in measuring values (PTVs) from operator to operator. High levels of repeatability between different Periotest units have been shown as well.

Although the Periotest apparatus has been successful for assessing the stability of an implant, it often fails to detect saucerization of bone. Radiographs show the bone levels of implants more accurately. The Periotest does not detect the degree of bone loss until it is quite advanced. Based on these findings, the Periotest is a reliable tool for the diagnosis of the stability levels of implants. It may be used as well to evaluate the salvageability of an implant with advanced bone loss. The device, however, fails to diagnose an implant with progressive bone loss because its values remain the same until the bone loss is virtually complete. Because of this phenomenon, the information gained from application of the Periotest has to be combined with other clinically acquired information (e.g., periapical radiographs) to determine the true status of an implant. Record mobility as for natural teeth on a follow-up record form (see Appendix J). Inspect tissue color and tone and record it using the Löe and Silness Index. Muhlemann's Index is satisfactory for recording any bleeding.

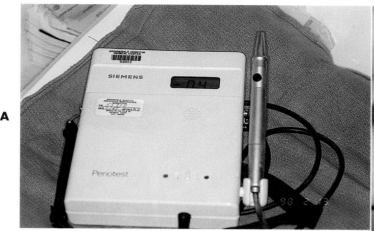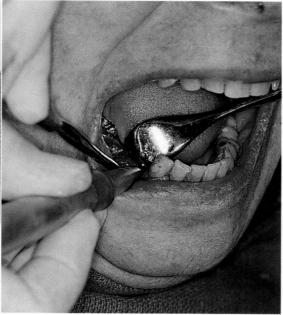

Fig. 29-1 A, The Siemens Periotest unit consists of a wand that is used intraorally and a console that gives readings digitally and by electronic voice. **B,** In order to use the Periotest properly, the wand must be parallel to the floor and placed at right angles to the implant or tooth in question.

Pocket Watch

The sulcular oral flora found in the mouths of those suffering from periodontal disease has been isolated from the periimplant environment. If saucerization or other bone loss is suspected of affecting implant host sites, and the problems of traumatic occlusion, bruxism, or inappropriately designed crown margins and pontic ridge laps have been eliminated, using a simple chemical test may be valuable.

Steri-Oss markets a product called *Pocket Watch* (Fig. 29-2), which consists of chemically treated strips, reagents, and testing trays. It assesses the presence and quantity of aspartate aminotransferase (AST) in gingival crevicular fluid (GCF). To gain results, test the crevices in question by inserting paper strips for 30 seconds. Then use the four reagents with which the strips are interacting to assess the presence of the enzyme by comparing the various shades of pink with a standard. The test is of value not only to the clinician but also to the patient because it presents tangible evidence of a need for improved oral hygiene efforts.

Measurements

Evaluate pocket depths and chart them in the normal manner. Probe gently with plastic instruments because of the tentativeness of the cervical epithelial adhesion (Fig. 29-3). Palpate the periimplant tissues to assess for exudate or pain. Record these findings on the follow-up form. If radiographs indicate saucerization phenomena or other signs of bone loss, make decisions in regard to bone substitute, guided tissue membrane repairs, or even implant removal with subsequent prosthesis alteration.

Patient Skills

Finally, and of great importance, take note of the patient's home care skills. After using a disclosing agent, there should

be a response to the presence and quantity of plaque. Record this on the follow-up chart for all surfaces of each implant, abutment, and areas of bars, mesostructures, or superstructures. For comparisons, when possible, use the patient's natural teeth to serve as longitudinal parameters. This information permits decisions as to whether any corrective procedures are required. If so, Chapter 28 contributes to the therapeutic approaches that may be required.

Recall Visit

At recall appointments, clean the implant abutments using plastic scalers, curettes, wooden-tipped porte polishers, or automated instruments (Figs. 29-4, 29-5). Teflon-coated or gold-plated tips are necessary to protect the highly polished transepithelial (cervical) surfaces of the abutments. Manual and mechanical scaler tips (Cavitron, Titan) can be obtained with Teflon coatings. E.A. Beck and Company of Costa Mesa, California, supplies these services. Implant Innovations makes handheld gold-plated and rigid plastic scalers (Fig. 29-6). Exercise extreme care to protect epithelial adhesion at the cervices.

Home Care

Instruct patients painstakingly in home care procedures, which should be performed two to three times per day. The use of a toothbrush, plastic-coated Proxibrush (Fig. 29-7), rubber tips (Fig. 29-8), stimulators, rotary brush (Fig. 29-9), Rotadent, Rotobrush, Interplak, or WaterPik (at ultra–low settings) is recommended. In addition, depending on the size, shape, and location of the prosthesis, Superfloss (Fig. 29-10), Implant Innovation's G-floss (Fig. 29-11), Butler's Post Care Floss (Fig. 29-12), pipe cleaners, and even 2 × 2-inch gauze sponges opened to full length and used as shoeshine cloths may be useful (Fig. 29-13). If the prosthesis is an overdenture, instruct

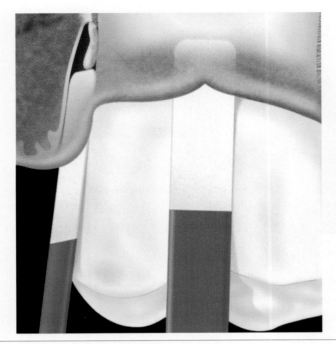

Fig. 29-2   Pocket Watch is a strip that, when placed into a periimplant pocket, detects the presence of pathogens.

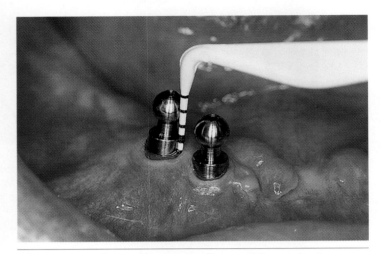

Fig. 29-3   If pocket probing is to be done at all, it must be done gently and with a plastic probe.

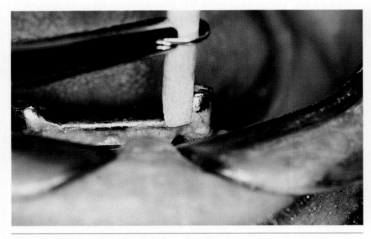

Fig. 29-4   The use of a wooden porte polisher with pumice is a gentle but effective method of professional plaque removal.

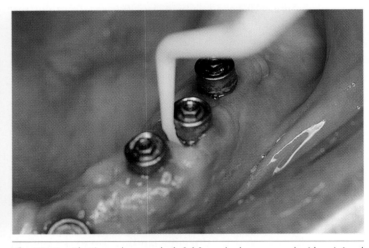

Fig. 29-5   Plastic scalers are helpful for calculus removal with minimal abrasion to polished implant surfaces.

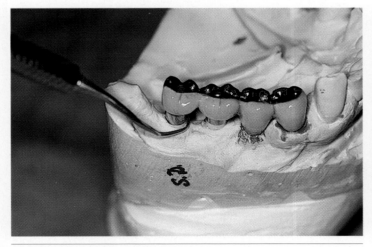

Fig. 29-6   The gold-plated scaler (Implant Innovations) causes less injury to delicate implant cervices than steel instruments.

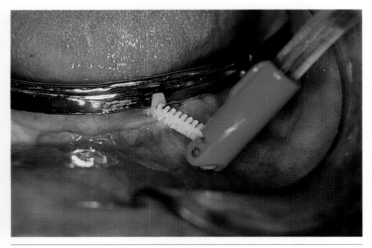

Fig. 29-7   A simple but efficient interproximal hygienic device is the new, plastic coated Proxibrush.

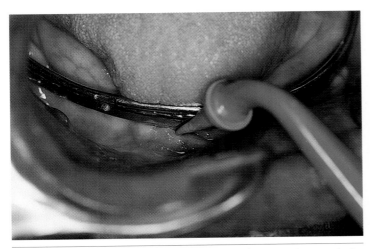

Fig. 29-8 A requisite for all patients seeking high-levels of hygiene is the tapered rubber tip, which may be used with toothpaste or chlorhexidine.

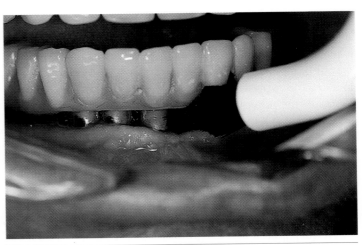

Fig. 29-9 An electrically powered, handheld, rechargeable, home-care product called Rotadent is effective for plaque reduction. Its handle presents an angle that permits a high level of patient compliance.

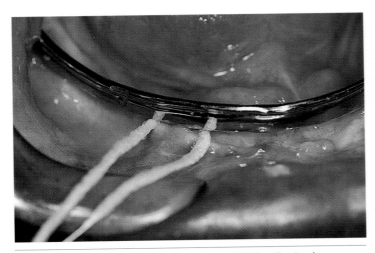

Fig. 29-10 Superfloss, a fuzzy, gentle but highly effective home-care material, may be difficult to introduce, but it is very efficient.

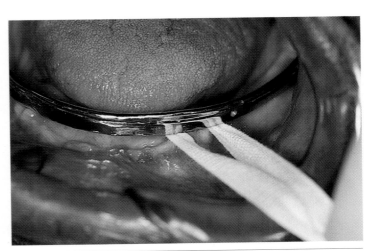

Fig. 29-11 G-floss, which is slightly greater in diameter than Superfloss, performs with predictive capability as a plaque remover.

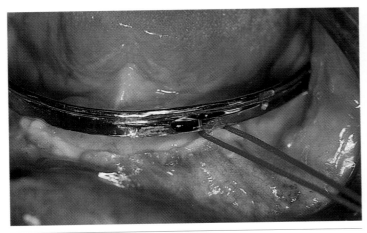

Fig. 29-12 The Butler Company makes Post Care, which is self-threading and somewhat less compliant than ordinary floss, but its pleasant color and ease of application make it a popular product. Patients require careful instruction in the proper manipulation of such materials.

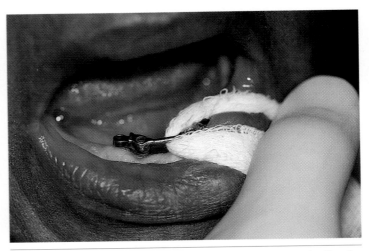

Fig. 29-13 A simple but practical approach to hygiene embodies the use of an opened 2 × 2-inch gauze pad. When passed successfully (which may be thwarted by small embrasures), it offers great benefit. It should be used in a shoeshine cloth manner.

the patient to remove it three times daily so that the superstructure and abutments may be cleaned thoroughly. If and when possible, the patient should leave the denture out of the mouth (kept in water) at night or at least for 4 hours or more to allow the supporting tissues to recover. The patient should practice the home-care regimen of the practitioner's choice for 2 weeks, at which time the prescriber should evaluate the patient's efficiency levels and institute any necessary corrections. Place the patient on a chlorhexidine mouth rinse (Peridex or PerioGard) twice daily if periimplant inflammation occurs or fails to resolve despite oral hygiene practices or other undetermined causes.

Note the hygiene measures recommended on the chart, and if the patient's manual dexterity or other inability prevents him or her from performing them with good results, institute changes that simplify the procedures. If an effective home care program cannot be introduced, schedule more frequent hygiene maintenance appointments.

Careful evaluation at the indicated time intervals is mandatory. This allows the notation of any departures from acceptable form and function and the institution of corrections before the occurrence of irreversible damage. If an implant's status indicates removal, do this promptly to spare bone loss or injury to adjacent implant host sites. Proper maintenance by both patient and clinician helps ensure the health and longevity of the implants and the prostheses supported by them.

Suggested Readings

Balshi T: Hygiene maintenance procedures for patients with the tissue-integrated prosthesis, *Quintessence Int* 17:95-102, 1986.

Carr AB, Papazoglou E, Lersen PE: The relationship of periotest values, biomaterial, and torque to failure in adult baboons, *Int J Prosth* 8(1):15-20, 1995.

Chai JY, Yamada J, Pang IC: In vitro consistency of the periotest instrument, *J Prosth* 2(1):9-12, 1993.

Chavez H et al: Assessment of oral implant mobility, *J Prosthet Dent* 7(5):421-426, 1993.

Cox JF, Pharoah M: An alternative holder for radiographic evaluation of tissue-integrated prosthesis, *J Prosthet Dent* 56:338-341, 1986.

Fox SC, Moriarty JD, Kusy RP: The effects of scaling a titanium implant surface with metal and plastic instruments: an in vitro study, *J Periodontol* 61:485-490, 1990.

Hass R et al: Examination of damping behavior of IMZ implants, *Int J Oral Maxillofac Implant* 10(4):410-414, 1995.

Hollender L: Radiographic techniques for precision analysis of bridge on osseointegrated fixtures, *Swed Dent J* 28(suppl):171-174, 1985.

James RA, Keller EE: A histophathological report on the nature of the epithelium and underlying connective tissue which surrounds oral implants, *J Biomed Mater Res* 8:373-383, 1974.

James RA: The connective tissue-dental implant interface, *J Oral Implantol* 13:607-621, 1988.

Manz MC, Morris HF, Ochi S: An evaluation of the periotest system. Part II. *Implant Dent* 1(3):221-226, 1992.

Meffert RM: Endosseous dental implantology from the periodontist's viewpoint, *J Periodontol* 57:531-536, 1986.

Meffert RM: The soft tissue interface in dental implantology, *J Dent Educ* 52:810-811, 1988.

Newman MJ, Flemming FT: Periodontal considerations of implants and implant associated microbiota, *J Dent Educ* 52:737, 1988.

Niedermeier W, Kublbeck K: Factors involved in endosseous implant function, *Deutsche Zahnarztleche Zeitschrift* 46(9):589-594, 1991.

Ochi S, Morris HF, Winkler S: The influence of implant type, material, coating, diameter, and length on periotest values at second-stage surgery, DICRG interim report no. 4, *Implant Dent* 3(3):159-162, 1994.

Orton GS et al: The dental professional's role in monitoring and maintenance of tissue-integrated prostheses, *J Oral Maxillofac Implant* 4:305-310, 1989.

Rams TE et al: The subgingival microbial flora associated with human dental implants, *J Prosthet Dent* 51:529-533, 1984.

Rapley JW et al: The surface characteristics produced by various oral hygiene instruments and materials on titanium implant abutments, *J Oral Maxillofac Implant* 5:47-52, 1990.

Salonen MA et al: Failures in the osseointegration of endosseous implants, *Int J Oral Maxillofac Implant* 8(1):92-97, 1993.

Schulte W, Lukas D: Periotest to monitor osseointegration and to check the occlusion of oral implantology, *J Oral Implantol* 19(1):23-32, 1993.

Teerlinck J et al: Periotest: an objective clinical diagnosis of bone apposition toward implants, *Int J Oral Maxillofac Implant* 6(1):55-61, 1991.

Tricia J et al: Mechanical state assessment of the implant-bone continuum: a better understanding of the periotest method, *Int J Oral Maxillofac Implant* 10(1):43-49, 1995.

Truhlar RS et al: Assessment of implant mobility at second-stage surgery with the periotest. DICRG interim report no. 3, *Implant Dent* 3(3):153-156, 1994.

Van Scotter DE, Wilson CJ: The periotest method for determining implant success, *J Oral Implantol* 17:410-413, 1991.

Van Steenberghe D, Quirynen M: Reproducibility and detection threshold in peri-implant diagnosis, *Adv Dent Res* 7(2):191-195, 1993.

Whittaker JM et al: Implant-tissue interface: a case history, *J Oral Implantol* 15:137-140, 1989.

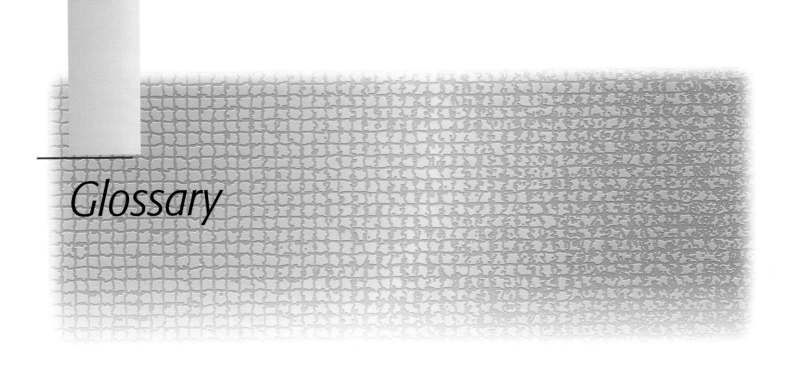

Glossary

Abscess   a localized collection of purulence in a cavity formed by disintegration of tissues.

Abutment   that portion of an implant above the neck utilized to provide support for a fixed, fixed-detachable, or removable dental prosthesis.

Adhesion   the sticking together of dissimilar materials.

Adnexae   adjunct parts or structures adjacent to a tooth or other structure.

Allograft   see alloplast.

Alloplast   a relatively inert synthetic biomaterial; generally metal, ceramic or polymeric material.

Alloys   strong and relatively ductile substances that provide electropositive ions to a corrosive environment and can be polished to a high luster; characterized by metallic atomic bonding; most often used for surgical implants because of a combination of favorable properties and the long-term experience for the construction of surgical implants, primarily titanium-, cobalt-, or iron-based systems.

Alterable blade implants   a blade type of implant that can be changed and reshaped to conform to the given clinical situation.

Aluminum oxide (alpha single crystal)   an inert, highly biocompatible, strong ceramic material from which endosseous implants are fabricated.

Aluminum oxide (polycrystal)   a fused Al_2O_3 biocompatible material.

Alveolar   pertaining to an alveolus.

   Alveolar crest   the most coronal portion of the alveolar bone.

   Alveolar process   that portion of the maxillae or mandible that forms the dental arch and serves as a bony investment for the teeth.

   Alveolar ridge   the bony ridge of the maxillae or mandible that contains the alveoli (sockets of the teeth); the remainder of the alveolar process after the teeth are removed.

Alveolar mucosa   the mucous membrane covering the basal part of the alveolar process and continuing without demarcation into the vestibular fornix and the floor of the mouth. It is loosely attached to the periosteum and is movable.

Alveoloplasty   conservative contouring of the alveolar process to achieve an acceptable contour.

Ambulate   to move about, walk.

Anastomosis   communication between vessels by collateral channels

Anchor   an endosteal metal implant in the shape of a ship's anchor.

Anesthesia   absence of sensation to stimuli.

Anneal   to heat and then cool slowly to prevent brittleness.

Anterior nasal spine   see nasal spine.

Anteromedially   forward and toward the midline.

Antrum   a cavity or chamber within the maxillary bone.

Arc   a bowlike curved line.

Areolar   pertaining to the areolae; any minute space or interstice in a tissue; loose mucosa adjacent to alveolar mucosa.

Armamentarium   the total store of available resources; the equipment, such as instruments, drugs, and other items, used in a technique.

Articulation (artificial)   the use of a mechanical device that simulates the movements of the temporomandibular joint, permitting the orientation of casts in a manner duplicating or simulating various positions or movements of the patient.

Asepsis   prevention from contact with microorganisms; the state of the surgical field desirable for implant surgery.

Atrophy   a decrease in the size of the ridge due to resorption of the bone.

Attached gingiva   the portion of the gingiva extending from the marginal gingiva to the alveolar mucosa; the attached gingiva is fairly dense and tightly bound down to the underlying periosteum, tooth, and bone.

Attachment   a mechanical device for the fixation, retention, and stabilization of a dental prosthesis.

Auger   a tool for boring a hole.

Augmentation   the placement of autogenous or alloplastic materials to correct bony insufficiencies.

Autogenous   self-generated.

Autograft   a graft taken from one part of the patient's body and transplanted to another part.

Available bone   the quantity and quality of residual bone that the patient has accessible for implantation.

Avascular   without blood.

Bacteremia   presence of bacteria in the blood.

Bacteriostatic   inhibiting or retarding the growth or multiplication of bacteria without actually destroying them.

Biodegradable   susceptible to degradation by biologic processes.

Biointegration   implies that a contact is established without interposition of nonbony tissue between implant surface coating and host-remodeled bone, forming a biochemical bond at the light microscopic level.

Biomaterial   a relatively inert, naturally occurring, or man-made material that can be used to implant in or interface with living tissues or biologic fluids without resulting in untoward reactions with those tissues or fluids; can be used to fabricate devices designed to replace body parts or functions.

Blade (implant)   a thin, wedge-shaped metal implant that is placed into the bone to provide an abutment. (See metal plate implants.)

Blanching   to make white or pale.

Block form   any large solid piece; bulk.

Bone   the material of the skeleton of most vertebrate animals; the tissue constituting bones.

   Bone, alveolar   the specialized bone structure that contains the alveoli or sockets of the teeth and supports the teeth.

   Bone, basal   that part of the mandible and maxillae from which the alveolar process develops.

   Bone, bundle   the bone that forms the immediate attachment of the numerous bundles of collagen fibers incorporated into bone.

   Bone, cancellous (spongiosa, spongy bone, supporting bone, medullary bone, trabecular bone)   the bone that forms a trabecular network, surrounds marrow spaces that may contain either fatty or hematopoietic tissue, lies subjacent to the cortical bone, and makes up the main portion (bulk) of a bone.

   Bone, compact   hard, dense bone constituting the outer, cortical layer and consisting of an infinite variety of periosteal bone, endosteal bone, and Haversian systems.

Bone curretage   gentle moving of medullary bone, by use of hand instruments, to create an implant receptor site or to remove diseased intraosseous tissue.

Bovine   of or like an ox or a cow.

Brookdale bar   a one-piece, continuous mesostructure bar design for use with subperiosteal implants.

Buried   placing an implant below the soft tissue without being in function.

Buttressed   supported or reinforced.

CAD-CAM   computer-assisted design–computer assisted manufacturing. Milled by computer control.

Calibrate   to correct the gradations of an instrument.

Cancellous bone   see Bone.

Carbons   vitreous (polycrystalline or glassy) or pyrolitic graphitic structures of relatively hard, inert, and stable compounds that are conductors of thermal and electrical energy; characterized by ionic and Van der Waals-type atomic bonding; primarily carbon or carbon-silicon compounds; once used in endosseous dental implant systems and as an implant coating.

Caveat   a warning.

Cellulitis   purulent inflammation of loose connective tissue.

Centric   pertaining to or situated at the center.

Centric occlusion   maximum intercuspation of the teeth.

Centric relationship   the most posterior relationship of the mandible to the maxilla when the condyles are in their most posterior positions in the glenoid fossa.

Ceramics   compounds of a metal and oxygen formed of chemically and biochemically stable substances that are strong, hard, brittle, and inert nonconductors of thermal and electrical energy; characterized by ionic bonding.

Cervix   the neck of the implant; connects the infrastructure with the abutment.

Cessation   a ceasing; stop; pause.

Circummandibular   around the mandible.

Circumosseous   around the bone.

Circumzygomatic   around the zygoma.

Coagulate   to cause to clot.

Coagulum   the clot that closes the gap made in the vessel or between the wound margins.

Coaptation   to approximate the edges of a wound.

Coated   an outer covering; a layer of some substance over a surface.

Coherent   sticking together of the same material, having cohesion.

Cold-weld   a frictional or press-fit.

Collate   to put into proper order.

Compliant   yielding, submissive.

Connecting bar   a fixed bar that connects two or more permucosal extensions; in the case of the ramus frame or subperiosteal implant, it can be an integral part of the substructure.

Connective tissue   the binding and supportive tissue of the body; it is composed of fibroblasts, primitive mesenchymal cells, collagen fibers, and elastic fibers, with associated blood and lymphatic vessels, nerve fibers, etc.

Contralateral   the opposite side.

Conventional blade implant   a one-stage implant design; does not incorporate buried healing.

Conversion appliance   a temporary fixed-detachable prosthesis.

Cornua   a horn.

Corrosion (biomaterials)   where the elemental constituents of metals are lost to the adjacent environment due to corrosion mechanisms; the same types of phenomena exist for carbons (conductors) and ceramics (nonconductors), although at reduced magnitudes. The polymers undergo biodegradation due to preferential leaching of lower molecular weight fractions and polymeric chain breakdown by enzymatic cleavage and/or hydration and/or oxidation-reduction processes.

Cortical bone   a peripheral layer of compact osseous tissue; the average thickness of the cortex of alveolar bone is 2 mm (See also Bone, compact.)

Counterbore   the slight enlargement at the superior aspect of the osteotomy that allows the next gradual enlargement to take place.

Countersink   to enlarge the top part so that it will accept or receive the head or cervix.

Countertorque   that force used to act against or in the opposite direction from the rotating motion being produced.

Crevicular   referring to the gingival crevice.

Crossbite   malocclusion in which the mandibular teeth are in buccal version to the maxillary teeth.

Cross-sectional slice   a computed tomographic scan slice that is vertical.

Cruciform   shaped like a cross.

Custom-cast blade implant   an implant that is specifically designed and made to the unique specifications of the patient's available bone.

Cyst   any closed epithelial-lined cavity or sac, usually containing liquid or semisolid material.

Debridement   the removal of foreign material and contaminated or devitalized tissue from or adjacent to a traumatic or infected lesion until surrounding healthy tissue is exposed.

Defatting   to remove the fat from the surface of a metal.

Deglove   to expose the bone by dissecting and reflecting all soft tissue.

Degreaser   a chemical for the purpose of removing organic contaminants from implant surfaces.

Dehiscence   implant dehiscence, a splitting open, a break in the covering epithelium leaving an isolated area of an implant or bone exposed to the oral cavity. Mandibular dehiscence: exposure of inferior alveolar nerve caused by extreme resorption of the mandible to the point that the roof of the mandibular canal is no longer covered with bone, leaving only soft tissue separating the contents of the canal from the oral cavity.

Dehydration   removal of water from a substance, excessive loss of water.

Delaminate   to remove a layer.

Demarcated   separate, well-marked limits or boundaries.

Demineralize   to remove the mineral content.

Dental implant   a permucosal device that is biocompatible and biofunctional and is placed on or within the bone associated with the oral cavity to provide support for fixed or removable prostheses.

Dentoalveolar   pertaining to a tooth and its alveolus.

Depassivation   when local conditions produce an acidic environment at the metallic interface, the metallic oxide is broken down.

Disclosing agent (or solution)   dye used to allow visualization of dental plaque through staining with a selective medium.

Dissection   the act of cutting apart and disclosing the individual tissues; the separation of tissues in surgical procedures.

Dorsum   the posterior or superior surface of a body part.

Dysesthesia   a disturbance or impairment in sensory nerve transmission.

Ecchymosis   hemorrhagic area in the skin or mucous membrane forming a nonelevated, rounded blue or purplish patch.

Edema   an abnormal accumulation of fluid in intercellular spaces of the body.

Elastomeric   rubber-like.

Electrocoagulation   coagulation of tissue by means of an electric current.

Endodontic endosteal implant   a smooth and/or threaded pin implant that extends through the root canal of a tooth into periapical bone, to stabilize a mobile tooth.

Endodontic stabilizer implant   see endodontic endosteal implant.

Endosteal (endosseous)   occurring or located within a bone.

Endosteal (endosseous) implant   a device placed within alveolar and/or basal bone.

Epithelial attachment   the continuation of the sulcular epithelium that is joined to the tooth or implant structure and is located at the base of the sulcus, or pocket.

Epithelial cuff, implant   the band of tissue that is constricted around an implant cervix.

Epithelium   the outer layer covering the underlying connective tissue stroma.

Epithelium, gingival   a stratified squamous epithelium consisting of a basal layer; it is keratinized or parakeratinized when comprising the attached gingiva.

Epithelium, sulcular   the stratified squamous epithelium forming the covering ot the soft tissue wall of the gingival sulcus, or crevice.

Evert   to turn inside out; to turn outward.

Exploratory surgery   surgery performed for the purpose of examining, studying, or diagnosing.

Exteriorization   to cause to be on the outside.

External oblique ridge   a smooth ridge on the buccal surface of the body of the mandible that extends from the anterior border of the ramus, with diminishing prominence, downward and forward to the region of the mental foramen. This ridge changes very little in size and direction throughout life and is an important landmark in the design of a subperiosteal implant.

Exudate   a fluid with a high content of protein that has escaped from blood vessels and has been deposited in tissues as a result of inflammation; pus.

Fenestrations   any window-like openings.

Fibro-osteal (fibro-osseous) integration   see fibrous integration.

Fibrosis   formation of fibrous tissue.

Fibrous   composed of or containing fibers.

Fibrous integration   soft tissue to implant contact: interposition of healthy, dense, collagenous ligament tissue between implant and bone that transmits loads from the implant to the bone.

First-stage surgery   this refers to the preparatory stage for an implant procedure. In the case of the subperiosteal implant, it refers to the surgical bone impression and bone bite, which is done in order to construct the implant. For endosteal implants, it refers to the placement of the implant that is to be submerged for a healing period prior to being placed into function.

Fistula   an abnormal tract connecting two body cavities or organs or leading from a pathologic or natural internal cavity to the surface.

Oroantral an opening between the maxillary sinus and the oral cavity.

Oronasal an opening between the nasal cavity and the oral cavity.

Fixed bridge   a prosthetic dental appliance that replaces lost teeth, being supported and held in position by attachments to natural teeth and/or implants in a nonremovable manner.

Fixed-detachable   a fixed bridge that cannot be removed by the patient but can be removed by the practitioner.

Follicle   a sac or pouchlike depression or cavity.

Foramen   a natural opening or passage out of or through bone containing a neurovascular bundle or nerve.

Free-standing implant   an implant that can withstand functional forces without being splinted to any adjacent abutments.

Freeze-dried   damaged or attenuated by the exposure to cold and dehydration.

Frenulum   a small fold of integument or mucous membrane that checks, limits, or curbs the movements of an organ or part.

Friable   easily crumbled, pulverized.

Functional occlusion   that contact of the teeth that will provide the highest efficiency in the centric position and during all excursive movements of the jaw that are essential to mastication without producing trauma.

Galvanism   electropotential difference of dissimilar metals that can occur in dental implant metallurgy.

General anesthesia   a state of unconsciousness and insusceptibility to pain, produced by administration of anesthetic agents by inhalation, intravenously, intramuscularly, rectally, or via the gastrointestinal tract.

Generic   referring to a kind, class or group; general as opposed to specific.

Genial tubercles   mental spines, small round elevations (usually two pairs) clustered around the midline on the lingual surface of the lower portion of the mandibular symphysis. These tubercles serve as attachments for the genioglossus and geniohyoid muscles and are critical landmarks for the subperiosteal implant.

Graft   material used to replace a defect in the body; anything that is inserted into something else for it to become an integral part of the latter; in the case of bone, either artificial or synthetic bone, usually for the purpose of increasing its strength and/or dimension.

Granuloma   a tumorlike mass or nodule of granulation tissue due to a chronic inflammatory process.

Guarded   cautious, questionable, needing supervision.

Habituating   to make used to, accustom, familiarize.

Harvest   the gathering or collecting of material (bone).

Head   see Abutment.

Healing abutment   a temporary cuff used after uncovering so that the soft tissues can heal in the permucosal areas.

Hemisection   the process of dividing or cutting a tooth or structure into two parts.

Hemostasis   the arrest of bleeding, interruption of blood flow.

Heterograft   a graft taken from one species and placed in another.

Hollow grind   to tunnel or make concave; producing a cavity within the appliance or substance being used.

Homograft   a graft taken from one human subject and transplanted to another.

Host site   see receptor site.

Hydrophilic   capable of absorbing water.

Hydroxyapatite   a mineral compound of the general formula $3Ca^3(PO^4) + Ca(OH)^2$, which is the principal inorganic component of bone, teeth, and dental calculus.

Hydroxyapatite ceramic   a dense, nonresorbable ceramic, which, when implanted into bone, displays a highly attractive generic profile, which features a lack of local or systemic toxicity.

Hyperesthesia   Abnormally increased sensitivity of the skin, mucosa, or other organ of special sense.

Hyperostotic   hypertrophy of the bone.

Hyperplasia   the abnormal multiplication or increase in the number of normal cells in normal arrangement in a tissue.

Hypertrophy   an increase in bulk of tissue beyond normal limits, caused by an increase in size but not number of cellular elements.

Hypoplasia   defective or incomplete development.

Iatrogenic resulting from the activity of the doctor.

Impaction the condition in which a tooth or other structure or material is blocked by a physical barrier.

Implant see Oral implant.

Implant dentist one who practices the art and science of implant dentistry.

Implant dentistry that area of dentistry concerned with the diagnosis, design, and insertion of implant devices and implant restorations that provide adequate function, comfort, and aesthetics for the edentulous or partially edentulous patient.

Implant denture a denture that receives its stability and retention from a dental implant.

Implant integration tissue-to-implant contact.

> *Fibrous integration* interposition of healthy, dense, collagenous tissue between implant and bone.

> *Osseointegration* implies that a contact is established without interposition of nonbone tissue between normal remodeled bone and an implant, entailing a sustained transfer and distribution of load from the implant to and within the bone tissue.

Implant interstices the small spaces or pores within and on the surface of the implant infrastructure.

Implantologist one who practices the art and science of implant dentistry.

Implantology the study of the art and science concerned with the surgical insertion and restoration of materials and devices restoring the partially or totally edentulous patient to function.

Implant prosthodontics that portion of implant dentistry that concerns itself with the construction and placement of fixed or removable prosthesis on any implant device.

Implant prosthodontist one who practices the art and science of diagnosis, surgical placement of implant, construction of superstructure restoring occlusion, and postoperative maintenance of oral implants.

Implant surgery that portion of implant dentistry that concerns itself with the placement, surgical repair, and removal of implant devices.

Incision a cut or wound produced by cutting with a sharp instrument, laser, or electrosurgical scalpel.

Incisive foramen the incisive foramen is located in the midline on the anterior extreme of the hard palate; it transmits the left (more anterior) and right (more posterior) nasopalatine (scarpa's) (long sphenopalatine) nerves and vessels; a critical landmark for implant surgery.

Infection invasion and multiplication of microorganisms in body tissues, especially those causing local cell injury.

Inflammation a protective tissue response to injury or destruction of tissues that serves to wall off both the injurious agent and the injured tissues.

Infraosseous below the bone.

Infrastructure implant substructure below the soft tissue.

Insert that part that goes into the opening in the implant; abutment, cervix.

Integration period that time in which the bone grows to and surrounds the implant surface and makes it a part of the whole.

Interdental implant implant used between natural tooth abutments (Pier abutment).

Internally threaded having thread pattern within the housing of the implant.

Interocclusal distance situated between the occlusal surfaces of opposing teeth of the mandibular and maxillary arches.

Interposed in between.

Intramucosal insert (syn: subdermal implant) alloplastic devices placed into the tissue-bearing surface of a removable prosthesis to mechanically maintain the mucostatic seal; generally made of titanium, surgical stainless steel, or aluminum oxide and shaped with a narrow permucosal neck, a wider retentive head, and a broad, flat, denture attaching base; general utilization: maxillary complete denture or mandibular and maxillary removable partial dentures.

Intraosseous within bone.

Involuted rolled or turned inward.

Ishemia loss of blood supply to a tissue due to mechanical obstruction that may result in cell death.

Islet a very small island.

Isometric maintaining the same length; of equal dimensions.

Isthmus narrow strip.

Keratinized gingiva the portion of the mucosa that is covered by keratinized epithelium.

Knife-edged very sharp, very narrow morphology (ridge).

Ligate to tie or bind with a ligature.

Ligature a wire or suture used to bind or tie, to secure, stabilize, or immobilize.

Linea alba a white line or narrow white scar, such as at the crest of the residual ridge after tooth loss.

Locking taper see cold-weld.

Lumen the cavity or channel within a tube or needle.

Mandibular basal bone that portion of the body of the mandible that supports and underlies the alveolar bone; that portion of the body of the mandible that remains after resorption of the alveolar process.

Mandibular nerve the third division of the trigeminal nerve. This nerve leaves the skull through the foramen ovale and provides motor innervation to the muscles of mastication, to the tensor palati, the tensor tympani, the anterior belly of the digastric, and the mylohyoid muscles. It provides general sensory innervation to the teeth and gingivae, the mucosa of the cheek and floor of the mouth, the epithelium of the anterior two thirds of the tongue, the meninges, and the skin of the lower portion of the face.

Mandibular staple (bone plate) a form of a transosseous implant in which a plate is placed at the inferior border, and a series of retentive pins is placed partially into the inferior border with two continuous screws going transcortically and penetrating the mouth in the canine areas to be used as abutments.

Master cast the final model that represents the exact positioning of the abutments, on which the prosthesis is fabricated.

Matte finish a nonglossy or dull surface finish.

Maxillary sinus the anatomic space located superior to the posterior maxillary alveolus that limits the volume of alveolar bone in this area; a landmark in maxillary implant surgery.

Medullary Pertaining to the bone marrow.

Mental foramen Opening in the lateral surface of the mandible, which allows the exit of the third division of the trigeminal nerve and vessels; considered one of the five anatomic landmarks for the subperiosteal implant.

Mesostructure that part that couples the implant complex (infrastructure) to the superstructure.

Metal plate implants flat, blade-shaped implants of various thicknesses that derive their support from a horizontal length of bone. They can be perforated, smooth, fluted, textured, coated, vented, multiheaded, and submerged or nonsubmerged forms in a variety of biocompatible materials. (See blade implants.)

Monomer the liquid portion of acrylic (polymethyl methacrylate) resin.

Morbidity the condition of being diseased, unhealthy.

Mucobuccal fold the cul-de-sac formed by the mucous membrane as it turns from the upper or lower gingivae to the cheek.

Mucogingival junction the scalloped linear area denoting the approximation or separation of the gingiva and the areolar mucosa.

Mucoperiosteum a layer of mucosa, connective tissue, and periosteum that covers bone in the oral cavity. It sometimes gives rise to muscle attachments.

Mucosa (mucous membrane) a membrane, composed of epithelium and lamina propria, that lines the oral cavity and other organs and cavities of the body.

Muscle mold, border mold   the shaping of a material by the manipulation or action of the tissues adjacent to the border sof an impression.

Mylohyoid ridge   an oblique ridge on the lingual surface of the mandible that extends from the level of the roots of the last molar as a bony attachment for the mylohyoid muscles, which form the floor of the mouth; determines the lingual boundary of the mandibular subperiosteal implant.

Nasal spine   a median, sharp process formed by the forward prolongation of two maxillae at the lower margin of the anterior aperture of the nose; used to support a maxillary subperiosteal implant.

Necrosis   death of tissue.

Neoplastic   pertaining to new or abnormal growth.

Neuropathy   any functional disturbance or change to a nerve.

Neurovascular   pertaining to blood vessels and nerves.

Noninvasive   does not actively destroy surrounding tissue.

Nonresorbable   substances that show relatively limited in vivo degradation.

Obtundant   a material used to obturate.

Obturate   the act of closing or occluding.

Occlusal equilibration   the achievement of a balance between opposing element sof the masticatory apparatus.

One-piece implant   abutment and implant infrastructure constructed of the same continuous piece of metal.

Oral implant   a biomaterial or device made of one or more biomaterials, biologic or alloplastic, that is surgically inserted into soft or hard tissues, to be used for functional or cosmetic purposes.

Osseointegration   implies that a contact is established without interposition or nonbony tissue between normal remodeled bone and an implant at the light microscopic level, entailing a sustained transfer and distribution of load from the implant to and within the bone tissue.

Osseous   of the nature or quality of bone.

Osteoconduction   a process in which bone is stimulated to grow from a host bone surface in a predictable fashion.

Osteoconductive   a material that supports but does not stimulate bone growth.

Osteogenesis   the development of bony tissue; ossification; the histogenesis of bone.

Osteoinduction   a process that involves cellular change or cellular interaction. The cells are made to differentiate and do something they normally would not do. This technique is used when large bone grafts are performed.

Osteoinductive   a material that stimulates new bone growth that would not be expected in routine healing.

Osteointegration   see Osseointegration.

Osteoodontotomy (odonto-osteotomy)   a single osteotomy made through both a tooth and its supporting bone for endodontic implant placement.

Osteophilic response   a condition in which the bone "likes" to grow on the surface of a biomaterial.

Osteosynthesis   see Osteogenesis.

Osteotomy   the cutting of a bone.

Ostium   opening in the bone from sinus to nasal cavity.

Overdenture, overlay denture   a removable partial or complete denture whose built-in secondary copings overlay or telescope over the primary copings fitting over the prepared natural crowns, posts, or studs.

Parafrenular   around the frenulum.

Parallel pin   a directional guide used to assess the line of implant placement.

Parasymphyseal   around, associated with, or pertaining to the symphysis.

Paresthesia   the onset of dysesthesia during the immediate postoperative period.

Parietal   of or pertaining to the walls of a cavity; a bone of the skull.

Particulate   a process wherein metals are treated to eliminate or reduce local surface areas of positive and negative ionic charges; a process whereby the thickness of the oxide layer of a metal is increased.

Passive   without resistance, inert.

Patent   open, unobstructed, not closed.

Pedicle graft   a full thickness of the skin or periodontal tissue attached to the donor site by a stalk with a nutrient blood supply.

Pedunculated   having a stemlike connecting part.

Penultimate   next to the last.

Perforate   to pierce or make a hole.

Periapical   around or about the apex of the tooth.

Pericervical   about or around the cervix.

Peri-implant   around the implant.

Peri-implantitis   general term defining an inflammatory disease process surrounding or involving implanted foreign materials; can be traumatic, ulcerative, resorptive, exfoliative (as periodontitis).

Periodontoplasty   the surgical repair and reconstruction of the periodontium (as peri-implantoplasty).

Periosteum   specialized connective tissue that covers all bones of the body except the cartilaginous extremities.

Peripheral struts   those supports of a subperiosteal implant casting that are at the outermost area or farthest extent of the implant.

Permucosal   through the mucosa.

Permucosal pin implants   endosseous dental implants, shafts of which are threaded or smooth, used in bipodal or tripodal configurations as abutments.

Phlebotomy   incision of or entry into a vein.

Pier abutment   intermediate abutment, see interdental implant.

Plaque   a soft thin film of food debris, materia alba, and dead epithelial cells deposited on a surface (teeth, prosthesis) providing the medium for the growth of various microorganisms.

Polyhema, polyhydroxylethylmethacrylate   a synthetic hydrophilic polymeric material used in the body alone or in combination with other materials (contact lenses).

Polymer   a naturally occurring or synthetic substance consisting of giant molecules formed from smaller molecules of the same substance.

Polymer tooth replica   polymethylmethacrylate (PMMA) alone or in combination with other polymers (e.g., pHema) used to form an implant, shaped like a tooth root recently extracted, and immediately placed into the tooth's alveolus.

Porosity   the condition of having minute openings or pores.

Posterior palatal seal, postdam   postpalatal seal, the seal at the posterior border of a denture.

Postoperative   occurring after the operation.

Press-fit   retention of an implant from close proximity of the bone without the use of threads or tapping.

Primary healing   a process of cure: the restoration of wounded parts by first intention union.

Primary retention   that fixation in the initial period after implant placement before integration occurs.

Primary struts   those supports of a subperiosteal implant casting that cross the ridge crest and to which the abutments are affixed.

Procumbent   excessive labioaxial inclination of the incisors; protruding.

Prolapse   to slip out of place.

Prosthetic   serving as a substitute.

Protocol   the established methods.

Provisional restorations   prosthesis made for temporary purposes.

Pterygoid notch   a groove located at the pyramidal process of the palatine bone between the pteygoid plates and the maxillary tuberosity.

Pterygomandibular space   a part of the infratemporal space that lies between the medial pterygoid muscle and the ramus of the mandible.

Pulley   a small wheel with a groove in which a rope runs as to raise weights by being pulled down, the hamulus for the levator veli; palatinus tendon.

Punctate   resembling or marked with points or dots.

Purulence   the formation of presence of pus.

Pus   a protein-rich liquid inflammation product made up of cells.

Pyriform aperture   the pear-shaped anterior nasal cavity opening.

Radiopaque the quality of appearing light or white on exposed x-ray film; capable of blocking x-rays.

Ramus frame full-arch implant of tripodal design that consists of a horizontal supragingival connecting bar with endosteal segments placed into the two rami and symphyseal areas.

Ramus implant a type of endosteal blade implant placed in the ramus.

Reamer a sharp-edged tool for enlarging or shaping holes.

Receptor site former a duplicate form of a root-shaped or blade-shaped body of an implant; designed to form an osseous implant receptor site for implant shapes that cannot be prepared with rotating instruments; utilized for compression of intramedullary trabeculation or expansion of intramedullary space; a "try-in."

Receptor sites areas in bone or soft tissue that are prepared to receive an implant or an intramucosal insert.

Reepithelization the process by which connective or osseous tissue recovers its epithelial surface.

Reflection the elevation or folding back of the mucoperiosteum to expose the underlying bone.

Rehabilitation to restore, to put back into good condition.

Reimplantation act of reinserting a tooth into the alveolar socket from which it had been avulsed.

Resect to excise part or all of a structure surgically.

Residual ridge a remnant of the alveolar process and soft tissue covering after the teeth are removed.

Resilient springing back into shape or position.

Resorbable capable of assimilation or dissolution of a substance or material after it has been implanted into the body.

Resorption (of bone) a loss of bone substance by physiologic or pathologic means considered to be associated with the natural aging process, metabolic disturbances, and trauma.

Retainer any type of clasp, attachment, or device used for the fixation or stabilization of a prosthesis.

Retraction the holding back of the tissue to maintain operative site exposure and protect the tissues from trauma.

Retromolar pad a mass of tissue frequently pear-shaped that is located at the distal termination of the mandibular residual ridge, made up of the retromolar papilla and the retromolar glandular prominence.

Rhytidectomy excision of skin for elimination of wrinkles.

Ridge (alveolar) the alveolar process and its soft tissue covering that remain after teeth are removed.

Ridge augmentation adding to, increasing the dimensions of the existing ridge morphology.

Ridge crest the highest continuos surface of the alveolar ridge.

Ridge maintenance the process of keeping the ridge in an existing state.

Root form endosteal implants root-shaped implants that derive their support from a vertical expanse of bone; implants are in the form of spirals, cones, rhomboids, and cylinders. They can be smooth, fluted, finned, threaded, perforated, solid, hollow, or vented. They can be coated or textured and are available in submergible and nonsubmergible forms in a variety of biocompatible materials.

Rudiment an incompletely developed or vestigial part.

Saddle that part of a complete or partial denture that rests on the ridge and to which the teeth are attached.

Salutary conducive to health.

Saucerization (pericervical) the circular bone resorption that occurs about the necks of endosteal implants shortly after their insertion and continues slowly during the time of the implant's biologic presence.

Schneiderian membrane the membrane that lines the antrum.

Scout film the primary film in a computed tomography scan series that dictates the scan parameters.

Screw implant see Root form endosteal implant.

Secondary epithelization healing by the growth of epithelium over a denuded area.

secondary struts those supports of a subperiosteal implant casting that build in strength and rigidity.

Second-stage surgery in relation to the subperiosteal implant, this refers to the reopening of the tissue, and placement of the infrastructure that was constructed, after the first-stage surgery. For endosteal submerged implants, this refers to the reexposure of that portion of the implant that receives the attachment or abutment.

Semiadjustable articulator a device simulating jaw movements that may be adjusted so that it conforms with the mandibular functions of a patient.

Semilunar resembling a crescent or half-moon.

Sequela coming as a result of something else; follows as a result.

Serosanguineous composed of serum and blood.

Sessile attached by a broad base.

Settling to sink, to move downward; caused through bone resorption under primary struts.

Shoulder the flat horizontal projection connecting the infrastructure to the cervix.

Single crystal sapphire a material for implantation composed of a single crystalline alpha aluminum oxide that is identical in crystalline structure to a gem sapphire.

Sinusitis inflammation of a sinus.

Sinus lift augmentation with bone substitutes to the antral floor for the purpose of creating a host site for implant placement; antroplasty.

Site former see Receptor site former.

Speculum an instrument for opening or extending an orifice or cavity to permit visual inspection and entry for manipulation.

Spinous pertaining to or like a spine.

Spiral implant see Root form endosteal implant.

Splint a prosthetic device used to stabilize hard tissues (bone and teeth) during periods of healing.

Splinting the joining of two or more abutments into a unit.

Staple see Transosteal design.

Stent a prosthetic device used to influence and guide the healing of soft tissues.

Sterile technique a standard technique in which an aseptic area is established and maintained to a specific conclusion (e.g., the proper sterilization of instruments, drapes, gowns, gloves, and surgical area); and the systematic maintenance of asepsis throughout an implant insertion procedure.

Sterilization complete elimination of microbial viability. Caution must be exercised to ensure the preservation or the integrity and properties of the implant.

Stress normally defined in terms of mechanical tensile stress, which is the form divided by perpendicular cross-sectional area over which the force is applied.

Stress broken use of devices that relieve the abutment teeth of all or part of the occlusal forces.

Stripping to break or jam the threads.

Stylus a pointed, needlelike marking device.

Subapical below the apex of the tooth.

Subcuticular situated or occurring beneath the skin.

Submandibular below the mandible.

Submental below the chin.

Submerged implant an endosseous implant with a removable head and neck to permit healing and maturation of the osteotomy and allow intraimplant trabeculation isolated from the oral cavity without a permucosal opening; a buried endosteal implant.

Subperiosteal implant a framework specifically fabricated to fit the supporting areas of the mandible or maxilla with permucosal extensions for support and attachments of a prosthesis; the framework consists of: permucosal extensions with or without connecting bars and struts. Struts are classified as peripheral, primary, and secondary. The subperiosteal implant can be complete-arch, unilateral, or universal.

Superstructure the prosthesis that attaches to the mesostructure.

Surgery treatment by manual or operative methods.

Surgical jaw relationship (subperiosteal)   a registration of the vertical dimension in centric relationship of the exposed superior surface of the mandibular or maxillary bone with the opposing arch to provide intermaxillary registration for determination of abutment height of a subperiosteal implant framework.

Surgical occlusion rim (subperiosteal)   a conventional occlusion rim with a base that has been adapted to provide an accurate recording of the surgical vertical-centric relations.

Surgical template   a device designed to guide the location and direction of osteotomies preparatory to implant placement.

Suspensory ligament   the ligament arising from a bone surface that surrounds and supports an endosseous or subperiosteal implant.

Suture   the act of joining together as by sewing.

Symphysis   the immovable dense midline articulation of the right and left halves of the adult mandible.

Tamponade   the use of compression to control hemorrhage.

Tapping   cutting threads for a screw-type implant into medullary bone.

Telescopic coping   thin metal covering or cap that is fitted over the prepared tooth or implant abutment to accept a secondary or overlay crown or prosthesis.

Template   a guide.

Tendinous   like or having the characteristics of a tendon, inelastic cords of tough, fibrous connective tissue by which muscles are attached to bones.

Threaded   spiral or helical surface of an implant.

Three-dimensional implant   an endosteal implant that is placed from the lateral aspect of the alveolar ridge and supplies support in both the horizontal and vertical dimension.

Tissue-borne overdenture   supported by the tissue and retained by the implant.

Torque   a force or combination of forces that produce a twisting or rotating motion.

Toxicity   the adverse reactions (dose-response time relationships) of tissues to selected foreign substances resulting in unacceptable in vivo interactions. The toxicity can be at the local or systemic level depending upon the amount, rate of release and specific type of substance available to the tissues.

Transaxial slice   a computed tomography scan slice that is horizontal.

Transcortical   across the cortex of the bone.

Transect   to divide by cutting across.

Transepithelial   going through or across the epithelium.

Transepithelial abutment   that part of an implant that attaches directly to the infrastructure and passes through the soft issues into the oral cavity (permucosal) and acts as a platform for either a mesostructure bar or a prosthetic superstructure.

Transillumination   the passage of light through an examined object for the purpose of examination of its internal structures.

Transitional   temporary.

Transosteal   this refers to the penetration of both the internal and external cortical plate by a dental implant.

Transosteal design   a type of implant designed to penetrate the mandible from the inferior border to the alveolar crest and to protrude sufficiently into the oral cavity through mucous membrane to provide retention and stability for a dental prosthesis.

Trephine   surgical method of creating a circular opening.

Trial inserts   implant replica to test a receptor site; modified intramucosal inserts worn during the healing phase at "try-in."

Tricalcium phosphate   an inorganic, particulate or solid form of relatively biodegradable ceramic, which is used as a scaffold for bone regeneration; it can act as a matrix for new bone growth.

Tripodal   three legged.

Trismus   motor disturbance of the trigeminal nerve, especially spasm of the masticatory muscles, limited opening of the mouth.

Truncated   having a square or broad end; truncated bone.

Try-in implant   a replica, usually made of stainless teel, of the actual implant, used to check osteotomy for shape and size of the osteotomy before placing the actual implant.

Tuberosity, maxillary   the most distal portal of the maxillary alveolar ridge that is applicable for implant support.

Uncovering   to unroof; after healing of a buried two-stage implant, the act of going through the soft tissue to relocate the implant.

Undermine   to incise beneath, to form as a tunnel to separate mucosa or skin from underlying stroma.

Unaesthetic   without improvement of appearance, without beauty.

Unilateral subperiosteal implant   a partial subperiosteal implant usually located in the posterior area of the mandible or maxilla.

Unit-built pontic   a hollow coping-shaped casting designed to permit the placement of individual telescopic porcelain jacket crowns.

Universal subperiosteal implant   a full arch subperiosteal implant that circumvents the remaining natural teeth.

Vertical dimension   the superinferior dimension of facial height, it can be altered by depressing or elevating the occlusal plane.

Vestibuloplasty   the surgical modification of the gingival mucous membrane relationships in the vestibule of the mouth, including deepening of the vestibular trough.

Wolff's law   every change in the use of static relationships of a bone leads not only to a change in its internal structure and architecture, but also to a change in its external form and function.

Xenograft   see Heterograft.

Zygoma   the area formed by the union of the zygomatic bone and the zygomatic process of the temporal and maxillary bones, used for support of the subperiosteal implant.

Sources for Glossary

1. Yablonski S: *Illustrated dictionary of dentistry*, Philadelphia, 1982, WB Saunders.
2. *Glossary of prosthodontic terms*, ed 5, St. Louis, 1987, Mosby.
3. Cranin AN: *Oral implantology*, Springfield, Ill., 1970, Charles C Thomas.
4. *Dorland's Medical Dictionary*, ed 27, Philadelphia, 1988, WB Saunders.
5. *Webster's 2nd Concise Edition*, New York, 1982, Simon and Schuster.
6. *American Academy of Implant Dentistry Glossary*, (with thanks to Dr. Robert James, Dr. Carl Misch, and Dr. T. Whicker [Chmn]).
7. Dr. A. Norman Cranin.

Appendix A *Past Medical and Dental History*

Name_____ Sex_____ Age____ Date of Birth_____
Address_____
Telephone (Res.)_____ (Bus.)_____ Height____Weight___

Directions
Please circle Yes or No and answer all questions:

1. Are you in good health?... YES NO
   a. Has there been any change in your general health
      within the past year?... YES NO
   b. If so, please explain_____
      _____

2. My last physical examination was on_____
   My last dental examination was on_____

3. Are you now under the care of a physician?................ YES NO
   If so, what is the condition being treated?_____
   _____

4. My physician's name and address is_____
   _____

5. Have you had any serious illness or operations?.............. YES NO
   If so, what was the illness or operation?_____

6. Have you been hospitalized or had a serious illness
   within the past five (5) years................................... YES NO
   If so, what was the problem?_____

7. Do you have, or have you had, any of the following
   diseases or problems?
   a. Rheumatic fever or rheumatic heart disease   YES NO
   b. Congenital heart lesions   YES NO
   c. Cardiovascular disease (heart trouble, heart attack,
      coronary insufficiency, coronary occlusion, high
      blood pressure, arteriosclerosis, stroke)................. YES NO
      1) Do you have pain in your chest upon exertion?....... YES NO
      2) Are you ever short of breath after mild exercise?.... YES NO
      3) Do your ankles swell?................................ YES NO
      4) Do you get short of breath when you lie down,
         or do you require extra pillows when you sleep?.... YES NO
   d. Allergy.. YES NO
   e. Asthma or hay fever... YES NO
   f. Hives or skin rash.. YES NO
   g. Fainting spells or seizures.................................. YES NO
   h. Diabetes... YES NO
      1) Do you have to urinate (pass water) more than
         six times a day?.. YES NO
      2) Are you thirsty much of the time?.................... YES NO
      3) Does your mouth frequently become dry?........... YES NO
   i. Hepatitis, jaundice, or liver disease...................... YES NO
   j. Arthritis (painful, swollen joints)........................ YES NO
   k. Stomach ulcers.. YES NO
   l. Kidney trouble... YES NO
   m. Tuberculosis... YES NO
   n. A persistent cough or a cough that brings up blood.... YES NO
   o. Low blood pressure... YES NO
   p. Venereal disease.. YES NO
   q. Other_____

8. Have you had abnormal bleeding associated with
   previous extractions, surgery or trauma?................... YES NO
   a. Do you bruise easily?....................................... YES NO
   b. Have you ever required a blood transfusion?............ YES NO
      If so, explain the circumstances_____
      _____

9. Do you have any blood disorder, such as anemia?............ YES NO
10. Have you had surgery or x-ray treatment for a tumor,
    growth, or other condition?................................... YES NO
11. Are you taking any drugs or medicine?...................... YES NO
    If so, what?_____
12. Are you taking any of the following?........................ YES NO
    a. Antibiotics or sulfa drugs................................. YES NO
    b. Anticoagulants (blood thinner)........................... YES NO
    c. Medicine for high blood pressure........................ YES NO
    d. Cortisone (steroids).. YES NO
    e. Tranquilizers.. YES NO
    f. Aspirin... YES NO
    g. Insulin, tolbutamide (Orinase), or a similar drug........... YES NO
    h. Digitalis or drugs for heart trouble...................... YES NO
    i. Nitroglycerin.. YES NO
    j. Other_____
13. Are you allergic to or have you reacted adversely to
    any of the following?
    a. Local anesthetics... YES NO
    b. Penicillin or other antibiotics............................ YES NO
    c. Sulfa drugs.. YES NO
    d. Barbiturates, sedatives, or sleeping pills................ YES NO
    e. Aspirin.. YES NO
    f. Other_____
14. Have you had any serious trouble associated with any
    previous dental treatment?................................... YES NO
    a. Are you having dental pain?.............................. YES NO
    b. Does food pack between your teeth?.................... YES NO
    c. Do your gums bleed when you brush your teeth?....... YES NO
    d. Do you grind your teeth during the night?.............. YES NO
    e. Do you have any pain in or near your ears?.............. YES NO
    f. Have you ever had periodontal (pyorrhea) treatment? YES NO
    g. Have you ever been instructed on proper home
       care of your teeth?... YES NO
    h. Do you have any sores or lumps in your mouth?......... YES NO
    i. Do you want to keep your teeth?......................... YES NO
15. Do you have any disease, condition, or problem not listed
    above that you think I should know about?................... YES NO
    If so, please explain_____
    _____

Questions for Women

16. Are you pregnant?.. YES NO
17. Do you have any problems associated with your
    menstrual period?... YES NO
18. Date of the onset of your last menstrual period
    _____

Remarks:

Signature of Patient:

Date:

Appendix B *Laboratory Values*

Normal Complete Blood Count

			Differential	Segmented neutrophils	41-71%
WBC (cells/μl)	4.800-10.800			Stab neutrophils	5-10%
RBC (cells/μl)	M: 4.7-6.1 × 10⁶			Eosinophils	1-3%
	F: 4.2-5.4 × 10⁶			Basophils	0-1%
Hemoglobin	M: 14-18			Lymphocytes	24-44%
(g/dl)	F: 12-16			Monocytes	3-7%
Hematocrit	M: 40-54				
(%)	F: 37-47				
MCH (pg)	27-31				
MCHC (%)	33-37				
MCV (fl)	M: 80-94				
	F: 81-99				
RDW	11.5-14.5				
Platelets (μl)	150-450				

F = female; M = male; WBC = white blood cells; RBC = red blood cells; RDW = red blood cell distribution width. See the section on Differential Diagnosis of mean corpuscular volume (MCV), mean corpuscular hemoglobin (MCH), mean corpuscular hemoglobin concentration (MCHC) to calculate these values.

Normal Urine Values

Appearance: "yellow, clear," "straw colored, clear"
Specific gravity:
Neonate: 1.012
Infant: 1.002-1.006
Child and adult: 1.001-1.035
pH:
Newborn/neonate 5-7
Child and adult 4.6-8.0

Negative for: Bilirubin, blood, acetone, glucose, protein, nitrite, leukocyte esterase
RBC: 0-3 per high-power field (HPF)
WBC: 0-4 per HPF
Epithelial cells: Occasional
Hyaline casts: Occasional
Bacteria: None

Chemistry Values (μgdl)

Glucose	75-110		Calcium	8.5-10.5
Urea	7-24		Phosphorus	2.5-4.5
Creatinine	0.6-1.6		Total protein	5.7-8.0
Sodium	133-145		Albumin	3.67-5.0
Potassium	3.5-5.5		Alkaline phosphatase	28-120
Chloride	94-108		Total bilirubin	0.2-1.0
Carbon dioxide	22-28		Cholesterol	150-250
Uric acid	2.0-7.0			

Prothrombin Time (PT) Range

11.5-13.5 seconds (within 4.0 seconds of control)

Partial Thromboplastin Time (PTT) Range

27-38 seconds (within 5.0 seconds of control)

Appendix C   *CAD-CAM Computed Tomography*

Subject: Tape-handling requirements for all bone modeling exams sent to Techmedica.

The image data from the exam must be stored using the standard GE archiving program and copied onto a new, unused magnetic tape. The raw or scan data should be saved for 3 months as back up. If the scan is performed on the GE 9800 scanner, the image data *must* be converted to the 8800 low-density format.

The magnetic tape must be clearly labeled as follows:

Scanner site, name, and address
Telephone number
Scan technician's name
Scanner type (8800/9800/9800 Quick/9800)
Tape density (low or high)

Patient's name
Patient's side (left or right)
Run number
Scan protocol number
Referring physician's name

Film the scout view with the slice locations posted (post every other or every third slice location if the scan interval is small) and the sagittal and coronal arrange cuts through the plastic rod. Do not film the axial images for Techmedica.

The tape, along with the film of the scout view and arrange cuts, should be immediately sent Federal Express to Techmedica, Inc., 1380 Flynn Road, Camarillo, CA 93010.

Mandible Modeling for Subperiosteal Implant

CT Scan Protocols	Data Transmission
Patient Movement	Scanner Maintenance Check
Anatomical Feature for Study:	Mandible
Patient Positioning:	With the patient lying supine, place the head as far as possible into the GE coronal head holder so that the mandible is behind the metal in the forward part of the head holder. Place a pillow under the patient's knees for comfort. Wedge sponges between the head and head holder if space is available, to prevent patient movement. Strap the chin and forehead.
Plastic Rod Location:	Tape the ⅜-inch diameter plastic rod to the patient's face, down the midline, from the end of the nose to past the end of the chin so that the rod is approximately perpendicular to the scan plane.
Scout View:	Lateral
Scan Thickness:	1.5 mm
Scan Interval:	1.0 mm (entire body of mandible)
	1.5 mm (rami of mandible)
Prospective Target:	Center target half the distance between mentum and anterior aspect of body of vertebra
Calibration File:	Head
Target Factor (GE 8800 Scanner):	1.25 (key in all three digits)
Field of View: (GE 9800 Scanner):	20 cm
Algorithm:	0 (bone)
mA (GE 8800 Scanner):	320 mA at 2 pulse width, KV = 120 (Note: If fast tube cooling is available, use dynamic scan at 320 mA, 2 pulse width with interscan delay of 7 seconds for first 20 slices.)
mA (GE 9800 Scanner):	200 mA at 2 seconds scan time, KV =120
Raw/Scan Data Save:	Yes (save for 3 months at your facility. Do not send Raw/Scan Data to Techmedica)
First Slice Location:	1.5 mm below inferior border of the body of the mandible.

Procedure:

Remove all metal from patient's head and neck (jewelry, hairpins, etc.)

Position the patient with the head as far into the head holder as possible. Wear gloves.

Wet intraoral jig and shake off excess moisture. Sprinkle gum areas of jig with Rigident powder and shake off excess. Insert jig in patient's mouth. Lubrication of the lips with lubricating jelly may be necessary.

Attach vacuum line to jib tube and set for lowest possible setting that still evacuates saliva. If vacuum "grabs" tongue, reduce vacuum further.

Palpate inferior border of anterior body of mandible and position parallel to scan plane. Secure patient's head in head holder.

Position ⅜ inch plastic rod on patient's face and tape in place.

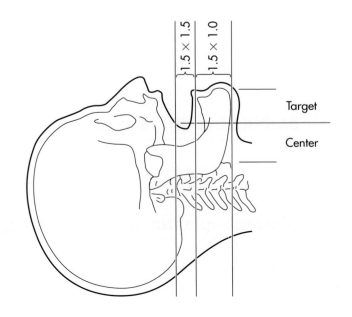

Take a lateral scout. Center target half the distance between mentum and anterior aspect of body of vertebra.

Locate first slice position and scan at 1.0 mm intervals until just past the crest of the ridge of the body of the mandible anteriorly. Continue the scan at 1.5 mm intervals until 5 mm below the sigmoid notch.

Note: Check first slice to ensure you are below bone and within target area. If adjustment is necessary, do so before starting run.

Under no circumstances should the gantry be angled.

After the exam is completed and the images have been reformatted, hold the patient and perform both a sagittal and a coronal reconstruction of the plastic rod, using the "arrange" program. These reconstructed images of the rod should appear straight with no "jogs" or bends. Perform a screen save of the reconstructed images of the rod. Only after this movement check is complete may the patient leave.

Patient Positioning and Scanning Range: Anatomical Modeling of Mandible and Maxilla

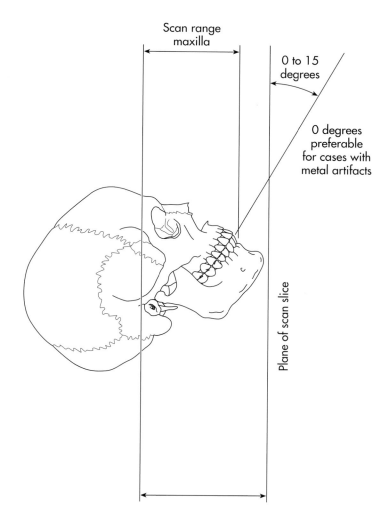

Scan range maxilla

0 to 15 degrees

0 degrees preferable for cases with metal artifacts

Plane of scan slice

Scanner Settings for Maxillofacial and Mandibular Regions

GE 9800 QUICK
120kV, 100mA, Dynamic Scan
(6 sec. delay)
512 × 512 Matrix
1.0 to 2.0 mm thickness/1.0 mm spacing
(13 or 14 cm Field of View)
0.4 mm pixel
Gantry angle—zero
Bone Algorithm

GE 8800
120 kV, 200 mA 9 or 3 sec. Dynamic Scan
320 × 320 Matrix, 576 views
1.0 to 2.0 mm thickness/1.0 mm spacing
Target 2, (0.4 mm pixel size)
Gantry angle—zero
Bone Algorithm

Siemens—DR Series
120 kV, 200-280 MAS, Dynamic Scan
480, 720, or 960 Projection
1.5 mm thickness/1.0 mm spacing
Zoom Factor
Avg. head 3.7 = 0.29 mm pixel
    (13.78 cm)
Small head 4.5 = 0.24 mm pixel
    (11.3 cm)
Large head 2.7 = 0.4 mm pixel
    (18.9 cm)
Archive images *in view from below* form
Gantry angle—zero
Bone detail, Kernel 8

Philips (310, 350, T60, TX60)
120 kV, 100 mA, Dynamic Scan
(4.5 to 7 sec.)
512×512 Matrix
1.5 mm thickness/1.0 mm spacing
Zoom Factor
320 matrix = 13 cm
512 matrix = 14 cm
Gantry angle—zero
Bone Algorithm, Filter 4C

Picker 1200
120 kV, 200 MAS, Dynamic Scan
(2 to 3.4 sec.)
512 × 512 Matrix
1.0 to 2.0 mm thickness/1.0 mm spacing
14 cm Field of View = 0.4 mm pixel
Gantry angle—zero
Bone Algorithm no. 4

Technicare 2000 Series
120 kV, 100 mA, Dynamic Scan
(2 sec. scan)
512×512 Matrix
1.0 to 2.0 mm thickness/1.0 mm spacing
0.4 mm or less pixel size (mag 2)
Gantry Angle—zero
Normal Head Filter

- Archive the *image* data to a new magnetic tape in the *uncompressed* (800 or 1600 bpi) form. (GE 9800 compressed data is the only exception.) No gantry tilt.
- Only one case should be loaded on each new magnetic tape. Please label the tape with patient name, scanner type, and physician's name.
- Area of interest must completely fill the screen using the smallest field of view, which provides for a smaller pixel size.
- A cold-cure bite jig placed in the mouth is highly recommended. If one is not available, a non-opaque article, such as a tongue depressor wrapped in gauze, should be placed between the teeth.

- Absence of motion artifacts is essential. The patient's head should be taped securely, and dynamic scanning should be used to eliminate motion.
- To aid in determining patient motion, an acrylic rod or ball point pen (with the insides taken out) should be taped vertically on the lateral portion of the patient's face.

- An interscan delay of 7 to 10 seconds is recommended to keep tube cooling time to a minimum.
- Metal braces, fillings, and dentures should be removed before scanning.

Appendix D *Stereolithographic Reproduction of Anatomic Structures Using C-T Scan*

How to Order an Anatomic Model

1. Call scan facility for appointment.
2. Find out if the facility has ever used the scanning protocol required for anatomical model generation before.
3. Fill out the patient information sheet.
4. Send a scan protocol to the scanning facility. More importantly, send it to the technologist doing the scan. To prevent any mistakes, send a copy of the scan protocol with the patient.
5. It is important to fill out the patient information sheet and send it directly to the facility generating the anatomical model via fax, or it can be sent with the electronic CT data. Since there is necessary scanner data on the patient info sheet, ask the scanning technologist to fill out that portion.
6. To prevent any misunderstandings with regard to the anatomy to be scanned, mark on the skeletal work sheet the area to be scanned, and send it with the patient to the scan facility.
7. Whether the data is being sent from the hospital or the doctors office, include the necessary patient information sheet and Skeletal Worksheet.
8. Send the data overnight delivery. This will help prevent any delays or damage to the electronic data.
9. If you are concerned with the scan facility or with the scan quality, call your model generating facility and they will call the scan facility immediately before the scan. They should go step by step through the protocol to obtain a quality scan.
10. Inform your office staff of modeling activities so the modeling facility can contact them in case of your absence.

Scan Protocol for Technologist

- *Always use 0° gantry tilt*
- When scanning patient, please proceed three slices above and below area of interest.
- Choose appropriate field of view for area of interest.
- Field of view, patient position, and table height must not be changed during scan!
- Please scan patients with appropriate technical factors for the anatomy.
- Monitor the patient closely for any motion during the scan. If motion is detected during the scan, rescan the patient.
- It is not necessary to use bone algorithm or edge enhancement. Simply use combination of bone and soft tissue if possible.

- Please send files to modeling facility on 4 or 8 mm DAT tape or Optical Disk (contact modeling facility to confirm data delivery mode). One study per tape, or multiple on Optical Disk.
- Place patient on supine table. Position head so that the nasomeatal line is perpendicular to the table. 1 mm by 1 mm slice interval is recommended for individual bony facial anatomy, including the mandible. For complete skull, 2 mm by 2 mm interval is acceptable. It might be wise to use radioopaque positioning rods during the scan. A rod can be reconstructed in 3D on the scanner to check for motion.

*The above was adapted from Innova International.

Anatomic Modeling Facilities

Innova International
850 S. Greenville Ave. Suite 114
Richardson, Texas 75081
Tel: 972-761-0491
Fax: 972-761-0495
Innova@dallas.net

3D Systems, Inc.
26081 Avenue Hall
Valencia, CA 91355
1-888-3dsystem
www.3dsystems.com

Medical Modeling Corp.
17301 West Colfax Ave.
Suite 300
Golden, Colorado 80401
1-888-273-5344
Tel: 303-273-5344
Fax: 303-277-9472

Questionnaire

ANATOMICAL MODELS ARE NOT FOR DIRECT IMPLANTING

Patient Name:_____Date of Scan:_____Time:_____

Check all that apply:
Patient-Specific Bone Model: _____
Patient-Specific Soft Tissue Model: _____
Selectively Colored Model: _____
3-Dimensional .stl File Only: _____
Custom Implant Design: _____
Computer-Aided Design for Custom instruments: _____

Circle One:

CT SCAN

OR

MRI

Patient History/Diagnosis: _____

Physician Information:

Dr._____

Add:_____

_____

City/St.:_____ _____

Zip:_____

Tel: (_____) _____-_____

Fax: (_____) _____-_____

Scan Information:

Hospital/Clinic:_____

_____

Technologist:_____

Phone:_____

Scanner Model:_____

Technical Factors: KV_____ MA_____ S_____

Slice/Slice Spacing:_____

Gantry Tilt:

Physician Signature Required:

Dr._____

If billing other than to Physician, please contact modeling facility for assistance.

*Adapted from Innova patient information sheet

Appendix E *Treatment of Metals*

Metals that require special treatment are nontitanium castings (e.g., Vitallium subperiosteal or blade implants). By following the instructions that follow, the practitioner will be assured of passivated (oxide-coated), fat-free, clean, and wettable surfaces. They will require autoclaving after such treatment has been completed. Autoclaving is done best in a nonmetallic container, such as a porcelain coffee cup.

ARMAMENTARIUM

Half dozen glass laboratory beakers

Two porcelain coffee cups

Arm and Hammer bicarbonate of soda

Triple distilled water (that can be released from a spout, spigot, or petcock for rinsing)

Special filter for compressed air systems to eliminate oil and other lubricants

10% phosphoric acid

30% nitric acid

Acetone

An autoclave and autoclaving bags

Respect and follow this seemingly complicated series of steps. They may make the difference between success and failure of your implant.

Do not handle castings with bare fingers. Use new talc-free rubber gloves. Talcum powder can cause serious tissue reactions.

1. The casting must be degreased in an organic solvent. Acetone is an excellent choice. Use a porcelain cup for these solutions. Immerse the casting for 10 minutes.
2. The next step in the sequence is to dry the casting using an air syringe. The compressor must be equipped with a filter to eliminate oil and other contaminants.
3. Then place the casting in a beaker filled with 1 heaping tablespoon of bicarbonate of soda in distilled water and boil it for 5 minutes.
4. Rinse the casting in cold, triple-distilled water using a gloved finger to scour every exposed part.
5. Next, dip the casting in 10% phosphoric acid, which should be placed in a second cup or beaker.
6. Again, thoroughly rinse the casting in cold, triple-distilled water using a gloved finger.
7. Passivation is done by immersing the casting in 30% nitric acid at 130° F for 30 minutes. A third porcelain or glass vessel is required.
8. Use cold triple-distilled water for rinsing.
9. Next, rinse the casting in hot triple-distilled water.
10. Dry the casting using clean air.
11. Autoclaving the casting is the final step. This must be done at 270° F for 15 minutes in a porcelain or glass beaker or, if immediate implantation is not planned, it should be bagged for dating and storage.

Radiofrequency and Plasma Glow Discharge: Cleaning, Treating, and Sterilization

The use of a radiofrequency glow discharge (RFGD) unit will prepare an implant for insertion without subjecting it to the arduous steps just listed.

A goal in placing implants is to achieve the greatest adhesive strength to host tissues by promoting excellent tissue bonding to their surfaces. In addition, that portion of each implant that protrudes into the oral cavity needs to resist bacterial colonization and discourage the formation of plaque and the production of endotoxins; this encourages primary healing around the abutments and contributes to good oral hygiene. Useful tools available to help reach these goals are the Picotron plasma glow discharge system (Surgical Innovators of America, Park Dental Research

Implant Center) and A RFGD unit as designed by Dr. Robert Baier (Herricks, Inc., Ossining, NY). With these units, the surface of an implant can be cleaned, sterilized, and conditioned. These techniques will increase the wettability of an implant and thereby enhance its surface energy, which promotes bioadhesion. The cycle time of these units is approximately 5 minutes, and their use requires no technical skills. Simply insert the implant, close the door, create a vacuum in the chamber, release the argon gas, and set the timer. On removal, the casting is to be placed in a sterile beaker or sealable vessel containing triple-distilled water until it is ready for use.

The implant surgery procedure has been explained to me and I understand what is necessary to accomplish the placement of the implant under the gum or in the bone. The Dr./s have carefully examined me. To my knowledge, I have given an accurate report of my health history. Any prior allergic or unusual reactions to drugs, foods, insect bites, anesthetics, pollen, dusts, blood or body disease, gum or skin reactions, abnormal bleeding, or any other conditions concerning my health are included.

I was informed of other methods that would replace missing teeth. I have tried or considered these methods and I prefer an implant(s) to help secure the replaced missing teeth. I understand that any of the following may occur: bone disease, loss of bone and/or gum tissue, inflammation, swelling, infection, sensitivity, looseness of teeth, followed by necessity of extraction. Also possible are temporomandibular joint problems, headaches, referred pains to the back of the neck and facial muscles, and tired muscles when chewing. I also understand that if conventional removable dentures are used, I may suffer injury to and/or loss of teeth and bone as well.

The Dr./s have explained to me that there is no method to accurately predict the gum and bone healing capabilities in each patient following the placement of an implant. I understand that smoking, alcohol, or departures from acceptable dietary practices may affect gum healing and may limit the success of the implant(s). I agree to follow home care and diet recommendations per his/her instructions. I agree to report for check-ups as instructed. A reasonable fee will be made for these examinations after the first year of implant placement. If for any reason, at the discretion of the Dr./s, it is deemed that the implant is not serving properly, it is agreed that the implant will be removed. It will be replaced with conventional prosthesis or another implant, depending on the decision of the Dr./s.

I have been informed and understand that occasionally there are complications of surgery, drugs, and/or anesthesia. Pain, swelling, infection, discoloration, and numbness of the lip, chin, face, tongue, cheek, or teeth may occur, the exact duration of which may not be determined. The numbness may be irreversible. Also possible are inflammation of a vein, injury to teeth if present, bone fractures, nasal or sinus penetration, delayed healing and allergic reactions. It has been explained to me that implants may fail and must be removed.

With full understanding, I authorize the Dr./s to perform dental services for me, including implants and other surgery. I agree to the type of anesthesia chosen. I agree not to operate a motor vehicle or other hazardous devices for 24 hours or until fully recovered from the effects of the anesthesia or drugs given for my care, whichever is longer.

I authorize photos, slides, videos, x-rays, or any other viewing of my care and treatment during its progress to be used for the advancement of dentistry. I approve any modification in designs, materials, or care if in the professional judgment of the Dr./s it is in my best interests.

I understand that there is no warranty or guarantee as to any result. I am further advised that I can get additional explanations of risks before or during the progress of my treatment merely by asking.

The procedure and its risks have been explained to me by

_____

_____	_____	_____
Date	Patient	Witness
_____	_____	_____
Date	Patient	Witness

Appendix G *Postoperative Guidelines for the Surgeon*

Routine

Antibiotics. Use preoperative antibiotics routinely. Double the therapeutic level or greater, or the recommended AHA prophylaxis dose. Administration should provide maximum blood levels at time of incision.

Analgesics. Depending on the severity of the procedure and an assessment of the patient's level of pain tolerance. Ibuprofen (Motrin) 400 to 600 mg every 6 hours is effective. More potent are the codeine drugs, with aspirin or Tylenol, 30 to 60 mg. In further ascending order of effectiveness is hydrocodone (Vicodin) or Extra Strength Vicodin or oxycodone (Percodan [with aspirin] or Percocet [with acetaminophen]). These last two may be quite habituating. For those patients who are sensitive to codeines, Demerol 100 mg is effective. Gastritis, if it occurs can be handled with an antacid such as Maalox or by administrating the analgesic with yogurt.

Edema. Generally, nature should be allowed to take its course. If the patient or doctor is concerned, and it has been established that the edema is not related to infection, use steroids both intraoperatively and postoperatively. During the procedure, 20 mg intravenous of dexamethasone may be given. This can be followed postoperatively for several days with 5-mg tablets four times daily. (Do not prescribe medications every 6 hours because it often confuses patients who forget to take the fourth pill because of the hours of sleep). When anti-inflammatory drugs are used, it is wise to keep patients covered with antibiotics. Ice is of importance only for the first 48 hours and should be used, wrapped in a towel, over the facial tissues apposing the operative site, 20 minutes on and 20 minutes off.

Local Care

1. *Chlorhexidine (Peridex, Perioguard) rinses,* should be done gently three to four times daily for 2 weeks.
2. *Hygiene.* Discourage brushing at the operative site for the first 3 to 4 days. Then a very soft brush (i.e. Oral B-20 or 30) can be used carefully for cleansing. Any dentifrice is satisfactory.

Diet. For the first 2 days, only a liquid or blender-produced pureed diet is acceptable. The mastication of food of challenging texture that might cause injury to the operative site should be avoided. Plan a reasonable diet for each patient. It should not cause physical or local injury. It should be high in protein and moderate in texture. A sample diet day by day for the immediate postoperative period can be found in Appendix I.

Postoperative Problems. Instruct patients to call immediately if any difficulty arises about which they may have a question. If, after an examination, some unanticipated complication is noted, refer to Chapter 28, "Diagnosis and Treatment of Complications" for guidance.

Postoperative Regimens: Special - Antral

Place an implant into the sinus after cortical penetration. The treatment of such complications should be reviewed in Chapters 18 and 23. HTR and hydroxyapatite repairs are always of benefit, and routine antibiotic regimens should accompany their use. In these conditions, initiate a special plan. Instruct the patient in the following manner:

1. Do not blow your nose.
2. Try not to sneeze.
3. Take a decongestant for 10 days: Ornade spansules, one every 12 hours; or for hypertensives, pseudoephedrine (Sudafed) 60 mg, one every 6 hours.

4. Recommended Antibiotics:
   Ampicillin 500 mg four times daily
   or
   Augmentin 500 mg three times daily
   or
   Ceftin or cefazolin 500 mg twice daily
   °If patient is allergic to penicillin:
   Biaxin 500 mg twice daily
   or
   Zithromax 500 mg first day then 250 mg once daily to complete 5 days
   All above are oral administration
5. Afrin 12-hour nasal spray (Oxymetazolin), or a steroid such as Beconase, Flonase, or Vancenase two puffs in each nostril twice daily for 3 days.

Appendix H *Postoperative Instructions for the Patient*

1. Fill the prescription(s) and follow the instructions on the label(s).
2. Apply ice in a cloth to your face 10 minutes on, 20 minutes off, for 48 hours.
3. Make the following solution: To 1 quart of tap water, add 1 level teaspoon of table salt. Mix. Bring to boil. Store in a covered container. Use as a gentle irrigant 8 ounces each hour. Do not use vigorously. Start tomorrow and continue until your sutures are removed.
4. Eat very soft foods as tolerated. They should be of a high protein nature. Soft boiled eggs, milk, ice cream, malts, boiled chicken and soup, cheeses, junior foods, etc. are good.
5. For the first 24 postoperative hours, drink plenty of fluids: juice, soda, water, milk.
6. Take 2 tablespoons of milk of magnesia tonight.
7. EXPECT A GOOD AMOUNT OF SWELLING AND SOME DISCOLORATION. These findings are common and do not indicate infection or other problems. Sleep with your head well elevated; even so, you will find swelling to be most marked on arising tomorrow morning.
8. In case of severe bleeding, elevate head, apply ice to the back of your neck, and bite on a piece of gauze for 25 minutes. If the bleeding persists, bite on a wet teabag.
9. Do not hesitate to telephone if any question regarding your condition or operation arises. In an emergency, you should call us at (telephone number).

Appendix I *Recommended Diet Following Implant Surgery*

Day 1:	Liquid diet: soups, Jell-O, high protein drinks (e.g., Sustacal, Ensure). Patients should not wear prostheses for eating and should wear them only for esthetics for the first postoperative 2 weeks.
Day 2:	Same as day 1.
Day 3:	Puree diet, any food that can be blenderized well; applesauce; mashed potatoes; soft boiled eggs.
Day 4:	Same as day 3.
Day 5:	Same as day 4.
Days 6-14:	Soft diet: salisbury steak, tuna fish, boiled chicken, soup, cheeses.
after day 14:	Return to normal diet.

Appendix J *Implant Patient Follow-up Form*

Patient Name_____ Follow-up Date_____
Address_____
Age_____ Sex_____ Telephone_____
Dentist_____Surgical Implantation Date_____
Prosthetic Loading Date_____

1. Check mobility (at each abutment/implant junction) | Periotest
     Less than 0.5 mm laterally   _____
     More than 0.5 mm laterally   _____
     Depressable with finger pressure yes_____
                                                  no_____
2. Intaoral color photograph taken_____
3. Condition of gingival tissue (at each abutment/implant junction)
   Normal_____Hyperplastic_____Suppuration_____Gingivitis_____
   Inflamed_____
4. Intraoral radiograph taken_____
   Appearance: Normal   _____
                  Bone Resorption 0.5-1.0 mm _____
                                   1.0-2.0 mm _____
                                   2.0-3.0 mm _____
                                   3.0-4.0 mm _____

5. Pain:
   None_____Nocturnal_____Upon Function_____Intermittent_____
6. Prosthesis:
                       Mobility: yes_____ no_____
                       Plaque: yes_____ no_____
                       Occlusion: normal _____
                                            needed adjustment_____

7. Treatment needs:
   Soft tissue procedure   _____
   Osseous graft   _____
   Replacement of prosthetic componentry   _____
   Tightening of prosthetic screws

   _____

Examiner's Signature_____

Date_____

Use a form for each implant.

Appendix K   *Equipment Manufacturers*

ACE Dental Implant
ACE Dental Implant System
1034 Pearl Street
P.O. Box 1710
Brockton, MA 02403
infor@acesurgical.com

Actisite
Proctor & Gamble

AlloDerm Acellular Dermal Graft
Lifecore (q.v.)

Anchor Implant
Vancouver Implant
  Resources Inc.
2370 Maple St.
Vancouver, BC, V6J 3T6
  Canada
AnchorSimpler@MSN.com

Aseptico
Aseptico
P.O. Box 3209
Kirkland, WA 98083

Astra Tech Implants
Astra Tech Inc.
1000 Winter Street, Site 2700
Waltham, MA 02154

Attachments
Attachments International Inc.
600 S. Amphlett Blvd.
San Mateo, CA 94402-1325

Atwood 347 Diamond Bur
Atwood Industries
P.O. Box 531
Cardiff by the sea, CA 92007

Autostaple Skin Closure
U.S. Surgical Corp.
150 Glover Avenue
Norwalk, CT 06856

Avetine
Surgical Product Division
Alcon Laboratories Inc.
Fort Worth, TX 76134

Bard Parker
Becton & Dickinson & CO.
Lincoln Park, NJ 07035

Basic Implant
Dental Implant Systems Inc.

Bell International
Bell International
133 North Amphlett Boulevard
San Mateo, CA 94401

Bicon Implants
Bicon Dental Implants
1153 Center Street
Boston, MA 02130
bicon@bicon.com

Bioceram Kyocera Implant
Kyocera America Inc.
8611 Balboa Ave.
San Diego, CA 92123

BioHorizon/Maestro system
BioHorizons Implant System, Inc.
2129 Montgomery Highway
Birmingham, Alabama 35209

Bosker TMI Implant
Walter Lorenz Surgical
P.O. Box 18009
1520 Tradeport Drive
Jacksonville, FL 32229

Branemark Implant
Nobel Biocare
777 Oakmont Lane, Suite 100
Chicago, IL 60559

**Brasseler Burs
Internally Irrigated
Pilot & Spade**
Brasseler USA
800 King George Blvd.
Savannah, GA 31419

C-R Syringe
Centrix Inc.
30 Stan Rd.
Milford, CT 06460

Calcitite HA
Sulzer-Cacitek
2320 Faraday Ave.
Carlsbad, CA 92008

CAPSET
Lifecore (q.v.)

**Cendres & Metaux
S.A. Ors Dentaires**
Biel Bienne, Switzerland

**Coe Comfort
Coe Pak
Coe Soft**
Coe Laboratories Inc.
Chicago, IL 60658

**Colla Cote
Colla Plug**
Sulzer-Cacitek (q.v.)

Collagen Biomedical
3i
2500 Farber Place
Palo Alto, CA 94303

Crete Mince Pins
Bauer Co. (Chercheve)
14 Elleonorehring
6350 Bad Nauheim, Germany
or Megeve, France

**Cytoplast Regenetex
GBR200**
Innova (q.v.)

**Dalla Bona Abutment
O-Ring Abutment
Snap Abutment
UCLA Gold/Plastic combo**
Lifecore (q.v.)

**Dalla Bona, Dalbo,
Dolder, ERA, Hader,
Octolink, Rothermann,
Tube-lock, Tube & Screw,
Zest, ZAAG**
APM Sterngold
23 Frank Mossberg Dr.
Box 839A
Attleboro, MA 02703

**Demineralized Bone
Irradiated Bone**
See Bone Bank Appendix

Dental Eye II/III
Yashica, Inc.

Disposaboots
Cabot Medical Corporation
2021 Cabot Boulevard West
Langhorn, PA 19047

Duo-Dent Implant
Duo-Dent Implant
Systems, LLC
340 West Butterfield Road
Elmhurst, IL 60126

Dura Base
Relliance Dental Mfg. Co.
Worth, IL 60482

Duralay
Relliance Dental Mfg. Co.
(q.v.)

Durapatite
Cook Waite (q.v.)

DVA Abutment
Dental Ventures of America
100 Chaparral Court
Anaheim Hills, CA 92808

Dycal
L.D. Caulk Company, Division
  of Dentsply International
  Industries
Milford, DE 19963-0359

Dynadent
Dynadent
151 East Columbine Ave.
Santa Ana, CA 92707

DynaSurg
Lifecore (q.v.)

**Endodontic Stabilizer
Implants**
Park Dental Research Corp.
19 West 34 Street - Suite 301
New York, NY 10001

Endopore Implant
Innova
525 University Avenue,
  Suite 777
Toronto, Ontario
M5G 2L3, Canada

Fibermesh
Pulpdent Corp. of America
2301 Rt. 70
Cherry Hill, NJ 03002

Flexiroot
Dr. Andras Haris
Bala, Cynwood, PA

Frialit-2 Implant
FRIATEC Dental, Inc.
16261 Laguna Canyon Road,
  Suite 100
Irving, CA 92618

GC Pattern Resin
G.C. International
7830 E. Redfield Rd., Suite 12
Scottsdale, AZ 85260

**Gore - Tex Augmentation
  Material**
W.L. Gore & Assoc., Inc.
P.O. Box 5260
3773 Kaspar Ave.
Flagstaff, AZ 86003

**HA Coating for Subperiosteal
  Implants**
Biointerface
11095 Flintkote Ave.
San Diego, CA 92121

Artech Corp.
14554 Lee Rd
Chantilly, VA 22021

Quintron, Inc.
Driskell Bioengineering
5229 Cheshirine Road
Glena, OH 43201

Sulzer - Calcitek (q.v.)

Hall Implant
Hall Reconstruction Systems
1055 Cindy Lane
Carpinterra, CA 93013

Hapset
Lifecore (q.v.)

Hi Tech Consoles
Hi Tech Co.
4532 Telephone Rd.
Ventura, CA 93003

Howmedica - Vitallium
Howmedica
359 Veteran's Boulevard
Rutherford, NJ 07070

HTR
HTR Sciences
US Surgical Corporation (q.v.)

Park Dental Research Corp.
  (q.v.)

**Hygiene and Maintenance
  Instruments**
Implant Innovations, Inc.
1897 Palm Beach Lakes Blvd.
West Palm Beach, FL 33409

Johnson & Johnson
  Professional Care
10040 N. 25th Ave. Suite 110
Phoenix, AZ 85021

Oral-B Laboratories
Redwood City, CA 94065

IMCOR Implant
IMCOR
74 Northeastern Blvd
Bldg. 19
Nashua, NH 03062

Impac Abutment
Vident
5130 Commerce Drive
Baldwin Park, CA 91706

Impactair handpiece
Pallisades Dental
1 New England Av.
Piscataway, NJ 08855

Impla-Med Implant
Impla-Med Inc.
13794 N.W. 4th Street
  Suite 207
Saw Grass International
  Corporate Park
Sunrise, FL 33325

Implant Innovations, Inc.
Implant innovations, (1.v.)

Implant Support Systems
Lifecore (q.v.)

Implants Support Systems
Implants Support Systems,
  Inc. (q.v.)

Implaseal
Lifecore
3515 Lyman Blvd
Chaska, MN 55318

Impregum
ESPE Premier Sales Corp.
Norristown, PA 19401

IMTEC
IMTEC
2401 North Commerce
Ardmore, OK 73401

IMZ Implant
Steri-Oss
22895 East Park Drive
Yorba Linda, CA 92887

IMZ Membrane Tack System
Steri-Oss

Integral Implant
Sulzer - Calcitek (q.v.)

Interpore/HA
Steri-Oss
22895 Eastpark Drive
Yorba Linda, CA 92887

Interpore 200 HA
Steri-Oss

Interpore Implant
Steri-Oss

Interpore/HA
Steri-Oss (q.v.)

Intramucosal Inserts
Park Dental Research (q.v.)

ITI Implant
Straumann Co.
Reservoir Place
1601 Trapelo Road
Waltham, MA 02154

Kentosil
Kent Dental Supply Co. Inc.
25 Commerce Drive
Aston, PA 19014

Lambone
Pacific Coast Tissue Bank
2500-19 South Flower St.
Los Angeles, CA 90007

Lambone
Pacific Coast Tissue Bank
2500-19 South Flower St.
Los Angeles, CA 90007

LaminOss Implant
Impladent Inc.
19845 Foothill Ave.
Holliswood, NY 11423

Lew Attachment
Park Dental Research (q.v.)

Linkow Blades
Ultimatics, Inc.
P.O. Box 400
Springdale, AK 72726

Medidenta
Medidenta International Inc.
39-23 62 Street
Woodside, NY 11377

Minidriver
Hall International
3M Surgical Products Division
P.O. Box 4307
Santa Barbara, CA 93103

Monitoring Equipment
Criticare Systems, Inc.
20900 Swensin Drive
Waukesha, WI 53186

Monitoring Unlimited, Inc.
3010 South Tech Blvd.
Miamisburg, OH 45342

Neoplex
Columbus Dental Inc.
1000 Chouteau Ave.
P.O. Box 620
St. Louis, MO 63188

Nobel Biocare Implant
Nobel Biocare
5010 S. Keeler Ave.
Chicago, IL 60632

Omniloc Implant
Sulzer - Calcitek (q.v.)

Optosil C
Columbus Dental Miles Inc. (q.v.)

Orangewood Sticks
Any local dental supply house

**Oratronics
Blade Implants
Spiral**
Implants International
Suite 5600 The Chrysler Bldg.
New York, NY 10017

Orthomatrix HA
Orthomatrix Inc.
1055 10th Ave, S.E.
Minneapolis, MN 54140

Orthomatrix HA
Lifecore (q.v.)

Osada Consoles
Osada Electric Co. Inc.
8242 West 3rd Street, Suite 150
Los Angeles, CA 90048

Osseotite Implant
3i Implant Innovations
4555 Riverside Drive
Palm Beach Gardens, FL 33410

Osteo Implant
Osteo-Implant Corporation
2415 Wilmington Road
New Castle, PA 16105

**Osteogen
Linkow Blades**
Ultimatics Inc.
P.O. Box 400
Springdale, AK 72765

**Osteogen
(HA resorb)
Osteograft**
Impladent Inc.
CeraMed Corp.
12860 West Cedar Drive
Lakewood, CO 80228

Osteomed Implant
Osteomed Corporation
3150 Premier Drive, Suite 110
Irving, Texas 75063

Panavia
J. Morita, USA Inc.
Tustin, CA 92680

Paragon Implants
Paragon Implant Company
15821 Ventura Blvd
Suite 420
Encino, CA 91436

Peridex
Proctor & Gamble
Two Proctor & Gamble Plaza
Cincinnati, OH 45202

Periograf
Cook Waite (q.v.)

Periotest
Siemens

Permaridge
CeraMed Corp. (q.v.)

Physiotron
Picotron
PocketWatch
Polygel
Park Dental Research (q.v.)

Steri-Oss
L.D. Caulk Company (q.v.)

RA1-RA2
Ramus Frame
Pacific Implant, Inc.
920 Rio Dell Ave.
Rio Dell, CA 95562

Racord
Pascal Co. Inc.
P.O. Box 1478
Bellevue, WA 98009-1478

Radiofrequency Glow
Discharge Unit
Park Dental Research (q.v.)

Replace Implants
Steri-Oss (q.v.)

Reprosil
Dentsply-Caulk (q.v.)

Restore Implants
Lifecore (q.v.)

Ross TR Implant
Dr. Stanley Ross
240 W. Palmetto Park Rd.
Boca Raton, FL 33433

Rotary Brushes
Braun Oral-B Plaque Remover
Braun Inc.
66 Broadway Route 1
Lynnfield, MA 01940

Sargon Dental Implants
Sargon Enterprises, Inc.
260 South Beverly Dr.
2nd Floor
Beverly Hills, CA 90212

Sendex Abutments
Preat Corp.
1120 7th Ave.
San Mateo, CA 94402

Sendex Mini Implants
Sendex Minidental Implant
　Center
30 Central Park South;
　Suite 14B
New York, NY 10019

Simpler Implant
Vancouver Implant
　Resources Inc.
2370 Maple St.
Vancouver, BC, V6J 3T6
　Canada
AnchorSimpler@MSN.com

Smooth Staple Implant
Steri-Oss (q.v.)

Sphero Flex
Preat Corporation
1120 Seventh Ave.
San Mateo, CA 94402

Standardized Stainless
Steel Marking Spheres
Implant Innovations (q.v.)

Ace Surgical (q.v.)

Startanius Implant
Starvent Implant
Steri-Oss
Park Dental Research (q.v.)

Steri-Oss (q.v.)

Stryker hand pieces
Stryker Instruments
4100 East Milham
Kalamazoo, MI 49001

Super Bite
Harry J Bosworth Co.
Chicago, IL 60605

Surgical Instruments
Ace Surgical Supply Co.
1034 Pearl Street
Brockton, MA 02403

Salvin Dental Specialists
6723 Colony Rd.
Charlotte, NC 28226

Schein
5 Harbor Park Drive
Port Washington, NY 11050

Walter Lorenz Surgical
Instruments (q.v.)

Sustain Implants
Lifecore (q.v.)

Sustain Implants
Lifecore (q.v.)

Synthograph
Synthograph, Johnson
　& Johnson
Dental Products Co.
CN 7060
East Winsor, NJ 08520

TCP Augment
Miter, Inc.
P.O. Box 1133
600 E. Winona Av.
Warsaw, IN 46580

TefGen Regenerative
Membrane
Lifecore (q.v.)

Teflon Coating for Scalers
E.A. Beck & Co.
657 West 19th Street
Costa Mesa, CA 92627

Thermometry
North Pacific Dental Inc.
P.O. Box 3209
Kirkland, WA 98083

Three Dimentional
Radiology
CT-Scanners
CT-Reformation
Software Programs
CAD-CAM Technology
Columbia Scientific Co.
3D-Dental
8940 Old Annapolis Rd.
Columbia, MD 21046

General Electric Company
Medical Systems Group
New Berlin, WI 53151

MPDI-Dental - Scan
General Electric Co. (q.v.)

Techmedica
1380 Flynn Rd.
Camarillo, CA 93010

Titanium Mesh
Techmedica (q.v.)

Torque Wrench
See appendix

Transosteal Implants
Anchor (Blade) Implants
Dr. A. Norman Cranin
Dept. of Dental and Oral Surgery
Brookdale University Hospital
　and Medical Center
Linden Blvd at Brookdale Plaza
Brooklyn, NY 11212

Tubingen Implant
Friedrichsfeld
Division of Mdizinaltechnic
P.O. Box 7 D-6800
Mannheim, Germany

UCLA Abutment
Currently available from most
　implant support companies.
Available in plastic and gold

Ultimatics
Ultimatics (q.v.)

Velmix Stone
Kerr Manufacturing Co.
Romulus, MI 48174

Ventplant Implant
Ventplant Corp.
1829 JFK Boulevard
Philadelphia, PA 19103

Viscogel
Dentsply
15821 Ventura Blvd.
Encino, CA 91436

W&H elcomed Hand
Piece
BioHorizons (q.v.)

W&H elcomed

Whaledent
Whaledent Inc.
236 15th Ave.
New York, NY 1001

Zest
Zest Anchors, INC
2061 Wineridge Place #100
Escondido, CA 92029

Appendix L *Distributors of Musculoskeletal Tissue*

Alabama Tissue Center
855 THT, 1900 University Blvd
Birmingham, AL 35294
Ph: 205-934-4314
Fx: 205-934-9219
Ms. Sandra Phiilips

American Red Cross Tissue Services
Central States Area (Peoria)
405 West John Gwynn Ave
Peoria, IL 51605
Ph: 309-674-7171
Fx: 309-674-7692
Mr. Jeff Testin

American Red Cross Tissue Services
Southeastern Area
2751 Bull Street
Columbia, SC 29201
Ph: 803-251-6150
Fx: 803-251-6105
Ms. Beverly Bliss CTBS
(800-922-5986)

Central California Blood Center Tissue Service
3445 N. First Street
Fresno, CA 93726
Ph: 209-224-1168
Fx: 209-225-1602
Ms. Frances Cordova
(800-201-8477)

Central Texas Regional Blood and Tissue Center
4300 North Lamar Boulevard
Austin, TX 78765
Ph: 512-451-2222
Fx: 512-206-1363
Ms. M. Tracy Martin CTBS
800-580-1121

AlloSource
8085 E. Harvard Ave
Denver, CO 8023
Ph: 303-755-7775
Fx: 303-337-4100
(800-447-3587)
Mr. Jeffrey Sandlet

American Red Cross Tissue Services
Greater Northeast Region
636 South Warren Street
Syracuse, NY 13202
Ph: 315-464-1300
Fx: 315-425-0471
Dr. Nancy Dock, PhD

American Red Cross Tissue Services
Southern Plains Area
601 NE 6th Street
Oklahoma City, OK 73104
Ph: 405-232-7121
Fx: 405-236-6819
Ms. Linda Belcher
(800-343-6667)

Central Florida Tissue Bank
32 West Gore Street
Orlando, FL 32806
Ph: 407-849-6100 x422
Fx: 407-649-8517
(800-753-9109)
Ms. Tammy Franz CTBS

Community Tissue Services
(Dayton)
349 South Main Street
Dayton, OH 45402
Ph: 800-684-7783
Fx: 937-461-4237
Ms. Diane Wilson CTBS

Intermountain Tissue Center
University of Utah Medical Center
50 North Medical Dr.
Salt Lake City, UT 84132
Ph: 801-581-4299
Fx: 801-581-3271
Mr. Jan L. Pierce CTBS

LifeShare of the Carolinas
Charlotte Mecklenburg Hospital Authority
101 W. T Harris Blvd., Suite 5302,
PO Box 3286
Charlotte, NC 28232
Ph: 704-548-6850
Fx: 704-548-6851
Mr. William J. Faircloth
(800-932-4483)

LifeLink Tissue Bank
8510 Sunstate Street
Tampa, FL 33634
Ph: 813-886-8111
Fx: 813-888-9419
(800-683-2400)
Mr. Dana L. Shires III

Lions Doheny Eye and Tissue Bank
1450 San Pablo Street, Suite 3600
Los Angeles, CA 90033
Ph: 213-223-0333
Fx: 213-342-7155
Mr. Jeffrey Thomas

American Red Cross Tissue Services
Central States Area (Ft. Wayne)
1000 C Airport North Office Park
Fort Wayne, IN 46825
Ph: 219-497-7159
Fx: 219-489-6994
Mr. Jeffery Testin
(888-272-2787)

American Red Cross Tissue Services
North Central Region
100 South Robert St.
St. Paul, MN 55107
Ph: 800-847-7838
Fx: 612-290-8925
Ms. Ann Naas
612-291-3858

American Red Cross Tissue Services
Western Area
3535 Hyland Avenue
Costa Mesa, CA 92626
Ph: 714-708-1300
Fx: 714-708-1331
Ms. Caroline Kiam
(800-272-5287)

Central Indiana Regional Blood Center
Tissue Bank
3450 North Meridian Street
Indianapolis, IN 46208
Ph: 317-927-1692
Fx: 317-927-1763
Dr. Linda Griffith MD, PhD

Community Tissue Services
(Fort Worth)
708 South Henderson Street
Suite A
Fort Worth, TX 76104
Ph: 817-882-2556
Fx: 817-882-2557
(800-905-2556)
Mr. Richard Jordan

LifeNet
5809 Ward Court
Virginia Beach, VA 23455
Ph: 757-464-4761
Fx: 757-464-5721
(800-847-7831)
Mr. Scott Bottenfield, RN

Methodist Hospital of Indiana Eye and Tissue Bank
1701 North Senate Boulevard,
BG 54
Indianapolis, IN 46206
Ph: 317-929-2333
Fx: 317-929-8216
Mr. Anthony Burnett CTBS

Michigan Tissue Bank
1215 E Michigan Ave.
P.O. Box 30480
Lansing MI 48909-7980
Ph: 517-483-2929
Fx: 517-483-2190
Ms. Kathleen A. Pearson CTBS
(800-968-5005)

Musculoskeletal Transplant Foundation
Edison Corporate Center
125 May Street, Suite 300
Edison, NJ 08837
Ph: 732-661-0202
Fx: 732-661-2297
Mr. Joel C. Osborne CTBS
(800-433-6576)
(800) 946-9008

Northern California Transplant Bank
2593 Kemer Blvd.
San IL~fael, CA 94901
Ph: 415-455-9000
Fx: 415-455-9015
(800-922-3100)
Dr. James Forsell, PhD

Ohio Valley Tissue and Skin Center
2939 Vernon Place
Cincinnati, OH 45219
Ph: 513-558-6442
Fx: 513-558-6440
(800-558-5004)
Mr. Ronald Plessinger CTBS

Pacific Coast Tissue Bank
2500-19 S. Flower St.
Los Angeles, CA 90007
(800-745-0034)
Tel (213) 745-560
Fax (213)745-3031

Rubinoff Bone and Tissue Bank
Mount Sinai Hospital
600 University Ave., 6th Floor
Toronto, Ontario, CANADA
M5G IX5
Ph: 416-586-8870
Fx: 416-586-8628
Ms. Madeleine Beauad-Clouatre CTBS

Tennessee Donor Services, Tissue Services
1714 Hayes Street
Nashville, TN 37203
Ph: 615-327-2247
Fx: 615-320-1655
Mr. John Lee CTBS

UCSF Tissue Bank
150 B South Autumn Street
San Jose, CA 95110
Ph: 408-975-2080
Fx: 408-275-1724
(800-444-2663)
Mr. Jason Tufts

US Navy Tissue Bank
Naval Medical Center San Diego
34800 Bob Wilson Drive
   (Code KM)
San Diego, CA 92134-500
Ph: 619-532-8124
Fx: 619-532-8137
Lt. Christine C. Rivera, MSC, USNR, CTBS

Mid-America Tissue Center, Inc
2860 Lincoln Way East
Massillon, OH 44646
Ph: 800-451-3587
Fx: 216-830-0628
Ms. Karen A. Baer CTBS

National Tissue Bank Network
Georgia Tissue Bank, Inc.
126 Hammond Drive
Atlanta, GA 30328
Ph: 404-252-5051
Fx: 404-252-1712
Mr. Jesus Hernandez, CTBS

Northwest Ohio Tissue Bank
2736 N. Holland-Sylvania Rd
Toledo, OH 43615-1823
Ph: 419-534-6930
Fx: 419-534-6928
Ms. Cheryl Martin CTBS

Pennsylvania Regional Tissue Bank
814 Cedar Avenue
Scranton, PA 18505
Ph: 717-343-5433
Fx: 717-343-6993
(800-344-7782)
Dr. Hans Burchardt, PhD

Sierra Regional Eye and Tissue Bank
1700 Alhambra Blvd., Suite 112
Sacramento, CA 95816
Ph: 916-734-2298
Fx: 916-456-3731
Ms. Kathy Howard

Transplant Services Center
University of Texas SW
Medical Center
5323 Harry Hines Blvd.
Dallas, TX 75235-9074
Ph: 214-648-2609
Fx: 214-648-2086
Ms. Ellen Heck

University of Miami
Dept. of Ortho Rehab,
   Tissue Bank
P.O. Box 06969
1600 N.W. 10th Ave
Miami, FL 33136
Ph: 305-243-6786
Fx: 305-548-4622
Mr. Alvato Flores CTBS

UTMB Tissue Bank
301 University Blvd.
Galveston, TX 77555-1080
Ph: 409-772-4958
Fx: 409-772-6302
(800-772-3938)
Ms. Kathleen Sheridan

Mid-America Transplant Services
1139 Olivette Executive Parkway
St. Louis, MO 63132
Ph: 314-991-8655
Fx: 314-991-5171
Ms. S. Diane Chandler

New England Organ Bank
Tissue Banking Services
One Gateway Center,
Washington Street
Newton, MA 02158
Ph: 617-244-8000
Fx: 617-244-8755
Mr. Larry Sussman CTBS

Northwest Tissue Center
921 Terry Ave
Seattle, WA 98104
Ph: 206-292-1879
Fx: 206-343-5043
(800-858-2282)
Ms. Margery Moogk

Rocky Mountain Tissue Bank
2993 South Peoria Street,
   Suite 390
Aurora, CO 80014
Ph: 303-337-3330
Fx: 303-337-9383
Ms. Deborah Spillman CTBS

South Texas Blood and Tissue Center
6211 I-H 10 West
San Antonio, TX 78201
Ph: 210-731-5555
Fx: 210-731-5505
Mr. Tim Harris

UCSD Regional Tissue Bank
200 West Arbor Drive, MC 8778
San Diego, CA 92103-8778
Ph: 619-294-6034
Fx: 619-297-0849
(800-648-4560 CA; 800-358-8273)
Ms. Judy K. Perkins

University of Pennsylvania Medical Center
Bone and Tissue Bank
3508 Market Street, Suite 490
Philadelphia, PA 19104-4283
Ph: 215-662-7488
Fx: 215-349-5083
Mr. Darren Ebesutani CTBS

Distributes Skin Only

Firefighters' Skin Bank
University of Alberta
8440 12 Street
Edmonton, Alberta, CANADA
   T6G 2R8
Ph: 403-431-0202
Fx: 403-431-0461
Dr. Locksley McGann, PhD

Regional Skin Bank
The Regional Medical Center
   at Memphis
877 Jefferson Ave
Memphis, TN 38103
Ph: 901-545-8313
Fx: 901-545-8005
Mr. Randy Butler

Life Cell, Corp
3606 Research Forest Drive
The Woodlands, TX 77381
Ph: 281-367-5368
Fx: 281-363-3360
Mr. Glenn Greenleaf, CTBS

University of Michigan Skin Bank
1500 E. Medical Center Dr.
Rm IC435-UH, Box 0033
Ann Arbor, MI 48109
Ph: 313-936-9673
Fx: 313-936-9657
Mr. Tom Taddonio CTBS

New York Firefighters Skin Bank
New York Hospital/Cornell
   Medical Center
525 East 68th Street
New York, NY 10021
Ph: 212-746-7546
Fx: 212-746-8177
Ms. Nancy M. Gallo, RN

Distributes Reproductive Tissue Only

BioGenetics Corporation
1130 Rte. 22W, P.O. Box 1290
Mountainside, NJ 07092
Ph: 800-637-7776
Fx: 908-232-2114
Mr. Albert Anouna

California Cryobank, Inc.
(Mass)
955 Massachusetts Ave.
Cambridge, MA 02139
Ph: 617-497-8646
Fx: 617-497-6531
Ms. Kelley Fitzgerald

California Cryobank
1019 Gaycy Ave
Los Angeles, CA 90024
Ph: 310-443-5244
Fx: 310-443-5258
(800-231-3373)
Dr. Charles Sims, MD

Cryogenie Laboratories, Inc
1944 Lexington Avenue North
Roseville, MN 55113
Ph: 612-489-8000
Fx: 612-489-8989
Mr. John H. Olson

California Cryobank
770 Welch Road
Palo Alto, CA 94304
Ph: 415-324-1900
Fx: 415-324-1946
Ms. Holly R. Preece

Idant Laboratories
350 5th Ave., Suite 7120
New York City, NY 10118
Ph: 212-244-0555
Fx: 212-244-081
Dr. Joseph Feldschuh MD

Reproductive Resources, Inc
4720 1-10 Service Road, Ste 509
Mewtairie, LA 70001
Ph: 504-454-7973
Fx: 504-885-3932
(800-227-4561)
Dr. Brenda Bordson, PhD

Sperm & Embryo Bank of New Jersey
1130 Rte. 22W, P.O. Box 1290
Mountainside, NJ 07092
Ph: 800-637-7776
Fx: 908-232-2114
Mr. Albert Anouna

Appendix M *Antibiotic Prophylactic Regimens*

Prophylactic regimens adapted from *Prevention of Bacterial Endocarditis: Recommendations by the American Heart Association by the Committee on Rheumatic Fever, Endocarditis, and Kawasaki Disease* (endorsed by the American Dental Association)

Prophylactic Regimen for Dental and Oral Surgical Procedures (Follow-up Dose No Longer Recommended)

1. **Standard general prophylaxis for patients at risk:**
   Amoxicillin: Adults, 2.0 g given orally 1 hour before procedure
2. **Unable to take oral medications:**
   Ampicillin: Adults, 2.0 g given IM or IV within 30 minutes before procedure
3. **Penicillin allergic patients:**
   Clindamycin: Adults, 600 mg given orally 1 hour before procedure,

   OR -

   Cephalexin or Cefadroxil (Cephalosporins should not be used in patients with immediate-type hypersensitivity reaction to penicillins): Adults, 2.0 g orally 1 hour before the procedure.

   OR -

   Azithromax or Clarithromycin: Adults, 500 mg orally 1 hour before procedure

4. **Penicillin allergic patients unable to take oral medications:**
   Clindamycin: Adults, 600 mg IV within 30 minutes before procedure.

   OR -

   Cefazolin: Adults 1.0 g IM or IV within 30 minutes before procedure.

NOTE: For patients already taking antibiotics, please refer to JAMA 1997, 227:1794-1801. Circulation 1997, 96:358-366. Also in JADA, August 1997.

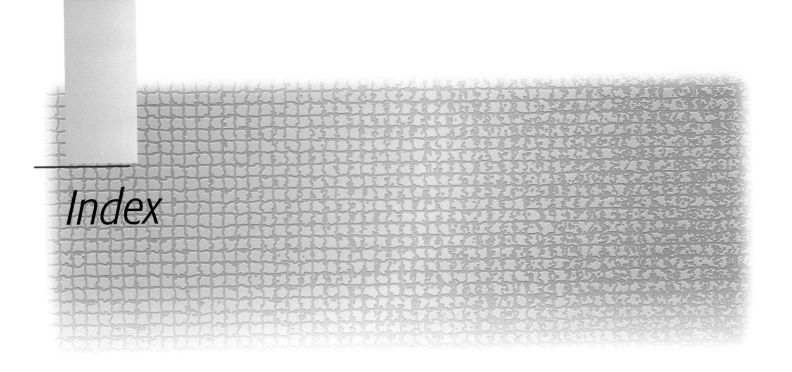

Index

A

Abbreviations, 17
Abscess after implant, 416-417
Abutment
  in blade implant surgery, 219
  in Bosker transmandibular reconstruction
    system, 294, 295
  broken, 442
  casting for accurate placement, 374
  cleaning of, 447
  in computer assisted design-computer as-
    sisted manufacture technology, 254
  fracture of, 434
  for hybrid bridge fixed-detachable pros-
    thesis, 362, 363
  overdenture, 385
  in partially edentulous implant, 246, 247
  poor angulation or position, 411-412
  in ramus blade implant, 235, 236
  root form implant, 188, 320-340
    angled, 331-332, 333
    angled variants, 332-334, 335
    bypass of antirotational component,
      327, 329
    for cement retention, 330-331
    cement *versus* screw retention, 322-323
    custom made, 327, 328
    direct gold copings, 336, 338
    for flat-surfaced implants, 323-324
    flat-topped, 336-339
    immediate impression implants, 337-339
    for implants that engage antirotational
      component, 326-327
    for implants with antirotational features,
      324-326
    for implants with Morse-taper interface,
      327-330
    one-stage two-piece implants, 339
    for overdentures, 337, 338
    requiring crown or coping cementation,
      330
    requiring screws for crown or coping re-
      tention, 334
    tapered shouldered, 336, 337
  in single tooth implant restoration, 343-
    344, 345-346

Abutment—cont'd
  in Smooth Staple Implant System, 293
  for submergible implant, 221, 349
  for subperiosteal implant, 247, 248
  for transitional denture, 313
  for transosteal implant, 381-382
Ace implant, 48
Ace torque wrench, 327
Acquired immunodeficiency syndrome, 13, 25
Acromegaly, 20
Acrylic in fixed and fixed-detachable
    prostheses, 357
Actisite, 432
Acute lymphocytic leukemia, 24
Acute myeloid leukemia, 24
Addison's disease, 20
Adrenal insufficiency, 20
Adson forceps, 96
Ailing implant, 432
Air-powered systems, 74
Albright's disease, 23
Albumin, 459
Alcoholism, 13
Alkaline phosphatase, 13, 459
Allergic asthma, 22
Allergic eczema, 22
Allergic purpura, 23
Alloderm, 105-106
Allogenic mucosal grafting, 105-106
Allograft, 112
Alloplast, 113
Alterable blade implant, 221, 222
Alveolar ridge
  augmentation of, 124-125
  maintenance after dental extraction, 123
Alveoplasty, 80, 89
  for anterior mandibular width deficiencies,
    147
  for posterior mandibular width
    deficiencies, 153
Amalgam carrier, 124, 125
Amalgam powder and acrylic powder, 37
American Society of Anesthesiology, 11
Ametycin, 15

Amoxicillin
  postoperative, 416
  preoperative, 75
  prophylactic regimen, 474
Ampicillin, 75, 474
Analgesics, 466
Anaphylaxis, 22
Anatomic fixed-detachable prosthesis,
    352-356
Anatomic model, 462
Anatomy, surgical, 55-56
Anchor implant, 432
Anesthesia
  in blade and plate-form implant surgery,
    216
  in Crête Mince implant, 297
  injury to mandibular neurovascular bun-
    dle, 413
  loss during subperiosteal implant surgery,
    414
  in maxillary pterygohamular subperiosteal
    implant, 257
  methods of, 75-76
  for postsubperiosteal sublingual floor ele-
    vation, 442
  for ramus blade implant, 235
  for ramus frame implant, 230
  in single-unit transosteal implant, 285
Anesthetic syringe, 110
Angioneurotic edema, 22
Angle of mandible, 55
Angled root form implant abutment, 331-
    334, 335
Angulation problems
  double-bar technique, 433-434
  endosteal implants, 411-412
Anterior blade and plate-form implants, 226
Anterior border of mandibular ramus, 55, 56
Anterior iliac crest graft, 137-140
  inferior border augmentation, 149, 150
Anterior mandibular contracture, 424
Anterior mandibular width deficiency, 147,
    148
Anterior maxillary height deficiency, 160, 161
Anterior maxillary width deficiency, 157-160

Anterior mental loop, 408
Anterior nasal spine, 55, 56
Anterior vestibule scar contracture, 424, 425
Antibiotics
  postoperative guidelines, 466
  preoperative, 75
  prophylactic regimens, 474
Antirotational root form implant abutments,
    324-327
Antral cavity, 56
Antral complications
  endosteal implant, 419-422
  perforation, 414-415
  postoperative guidelines, 466
Antral floor perforation, 407-408
Antroplasty, 168-169
Aortic insufficiency, 22
Apical lesion, 419, 420
Apicoectomy, 420
Arteriosclerosis, 21
Arteriovenous fistula, 21
Articulator, 397, 400
Artifact, metallic, 41, 42
Ascending ramus graft, 111
Aseptico handpiece, 73
Astra implant, 48, 213
Atherosclerosis, 21
Ativan; *see* Lorazepam
Atopic dermatitis, 22
Atopic diseases, 22
Atrisorb membrane, 114
Atrophy, mandibular, 239
Atwood 473 diamond drill, 287
Augmentation of chin, 134
Autoclavable motor, 72
Autogenous bone graft, 137-140
Autograft, 111

B

B-Series blade, 53
Bacteremia after heart valve surgery, 12
Balanced occlusal scheme, 397-402
  creation of, 397-400
  functional adjustment for, 400-402
Ball-bearing evaluation, 30-32
Ball castings, 66
Bar fixation, 64
Base-preparing bur, 267, 268
BASIC implant, 49
Beaver tail retractor, 97, 216
Bicon handpiece, 73
Bicon implant, 48, 206-207, 208
  angled abutments, 331-332, 333
  antirotational features of, 324-326
Bilateral mandibular lingual flap, 97
Bilirubin
  testing for hepatic disease, 13
  total, 459
Bio Gide membrane, 114
Bio-Mend membrane, 114
Bio-Oss, 112
Bio-Vent implant system, 196
Bioactive glass-alloplast, 113
Bioblade blade, 53
Bioceram Alumina Anchor, 282
Bioceram No.2 threaded endodontic Anchor
    Pin Implant, 282
BioHorizons implant, 48-49
BioHorizons/Maestro system, 206, 207
BioHorizons torque wrench, 327
Biologic bone augmentation materials, 8
Biologic glue, 131-135
Bispade drill, 74

Blade abutment fracture, 438-439
Blade implant, 5, 6, 215-229, 422, 423
  alterable blade implants, 221, 222
  anterior implants, 226
  burs used for, 74
  closure in, 220-221
  coated implants, 222-225
  conventional single-stage implants, 216-217
  cortical plate perforation, 406-409
  custom-cast implants, 225
  dehiscent, 419
  failed, 425-430
  fractured, 438-439
  immediate placement into extraction site,
    226-228
  maxillary posterior implants, 225-226
  osteotomy in, 217-218, 220
  oversized osteotomy and, 406
  particulate bone grafting with, 136
  periimplant support and repair, 135-136
  placement of implant, 219-220
  poor angulation or position, 411
  submergible implants, 221-222, 224
Blade selection, 53
Bleeding
  in perforated mandibular canal, 408
  in periodontal defect correction, 113
Bleeding time, 18
Bleomycin, 15
Block bone graft, 126, 127, 128, 131, 134, 135
  for anterior maxillary height deficiencies,
    160, 161
Blood dyscrasias, 23
Blood sugar examination, 17
Blunt rake, 216
Blunt-toothed rake, 97
Boley gauge, 27, 28, 180
Bone
  augmentation materials, 8
  Boley gauge measurements of, 27, 28
  disorders contraindicating implant
    surgery, 22
  implant selection chart, 47
  resorption after subperiosteal implant, 440
Bone density, 47
Bone graft, 109-174
  general guidelines, 110-136
    alveolar ridge maintenance, 123
    block form, 131, 134, 135
    bone management, 110-112, 113, 114
    maxillofacial reconstruction, 130-131
    particulate grafts, 131, 132, 133
    periimplant support and repair, 135-136
    periodontal defect correction, 112-116
    platelet-rich gel, 131-135
    technique, 123-130
    use of guided tissue regeneration mem-
      branes, 114, 116-123
  to improve ridge dimension for accommo-
    dation of implant, 147-172
    anterior mandibular height deficiencies,
      147-153, 147-172
    anterior mandibular width deficiencies,
      147, 148
    anterior maxillary height deficiencies,
      160, 161
    anterior maxillary width deficiencies,
      157-160
    mandibular neuroplasty and nerve
      management, 154-156
    posterior mandibular height
      deficiencies, 154
    posterior mandibular width deficiencies,
      153

Bone graft—cont'd
  to improve ridge dimension for accommo-
    dation of implant—cont'd
    posterior maxillary deficiency and mini-
      plate, 170-172
    posterior maxillary height deficiencies,
      162-170
    posterior maxillary width deficiencies,
      160-162
  for root form implant host sites of inade-
    quate dimension, 136-146
    anterior border of mandibular ramus,
      140-142
    lateral border of mandibular ramus,
      142, 143
    mandibular symphysis, 142-146
    techniques for obtaining autogenous
      bone, 137-140
Bone loss
  ailing implant and, 432
  around implants, 425
  detection of, 446
  in mandibular subperiosteal implant, 440
Bone wax, 411
Bosker transmandibular reconstruction
    system, 294-295
Bovine graft, 112
Box-lock suture, 78, 79, 80
Bracket table, 69
Brånemark implant, 367-371
  exposed cervical collars, 338
  flat-topped abutments, 336
  straight abutments, 330, 331
Brasseler spade drill, 178
Brassler fluted bone drill, 74
Bridge
  in Crête Mince implant, 297-300
  fixed provisional prosthesis, 315-316, 317
  hybrid, 362-373
    fully edentulous arch, 362-371
    partially edentulous arch, 371-373
Brookdale bar
  bilateral, 64
  casting for accurate placement, 374
  overdenture, 63
  recurrent pericervical granuloma and, 440
  in subperiosteal implant, 59
    mandibular, 242, 244-246
    maxillary pterygohamular, 260, 261, 263
    tripodal, 416
Bruxism, 433
Buccal cortical plate fracture, 409-410
Buccal flap, 97, 99
Buccal papilla, 81
Buccinator muscle, 99
Buccopharyngeal tumor, 14
Buerger's disease, 21
Bullous erosive lichen planus, 22
Bupivacaine, 414
Bur, 73-74
  in alveoplasty, 147
  for anterior maxillary width deficiencies,
    157
  in blade implant surgery, 217
  in bone harvesting
    anterior border of mandibular ramus,
      140
    mandibular symphysis, 142-143, 144-145
  broken, 410
  in intramucosal insert surgery, 267, 268
  for mandibular tori removal, 87
  in ramus blade implant, 236
  in ramus frame implant, 234
  to remove palatal torus, 86

Burkitt's lymphoma, 25
Butler's post care floss, 447, 449
Button implant with intraoral bar welding, 300-303
Buttressed anchor, 225, 226

C

C-clamp, 285-286
CAD-CAM; *see* Computer assisted design-computer assisted manufacture technique
Calcitek blade, 53
Calcitek implant, 52
    angled abutments, 331-332, 333
    antirotational features of, 324
    for oversized osteotomy, 405
    press-fit, 195
Calcium
    metabolism of, 12
    normal values, 459
Calculus removal, 448
Caldwell-Luc operation, 421, 422
Caliper, 44
Calvarium graft, 111
Canine fossa, 55
Cantilevering, 359
Capset membrane, 114
Carbocaine; *see* Mepivacaine
Carbon dioxide values, 459
Cardiovascular diseases, 21
Cartilage in rib graft, 140, 141
Casting
    for accurate placement of abutment, 374
    in computer assisted design-computer assisted manufacture technique, 251
    design in tripodal implant, 246
    in fabrication of superstructure, 357
    for fixed provisional prosthesis, 315
    inaccurate fit of, 438
    partially edentulous unilateral maxillary pterygohamular
        unilateral design, 265-266
        universal design, 263-264
    in single tooth implant restoration, 343
Cefadroxil, 474
Cefazolin, 474
Ceka attachment, 65
Cement
    in fixed and fixed-detachable prostheses, 350-352, 360
    in implant abutments, 60
    in matte-finished tapered implants, 278-280
    partial loosening of, 438
    platelet-rich gel, 131-135
    in provisional prosthesis, 318, 319
    in root form implant abutment, 330-331
        options for cement retained prostheses, 321
        screw retention *versus*, 322-323
    in unilateral and universal subperiosteal implants, 247, 248
Cementable crown, 345-347
Centric recording
    in functional adjustment for balanced occlusion, 400, 401
    in mandibular subperiosteal implant surgery, 241, 374
Centric relationship
    in balanced occlusal scheme, 397
    in mandibular subperiosteal implant surgery, 251-255, 378
    in maxillary pterygohamular subperiosteal implant surgery, 259-263
    in overdentures, 387-388

Centrifuge, 135
Cephalexin, 474
Cephalosporins, 474
CerAdapt system, 332-334, 335
Ceradent Call ceramic abutment, 335
Ceramic alloplast, 113
Ceramic bone augmentation materials, 8
Ceramic-coated implant, 282
CeraOne system, 332, 335
Chemistry values, 459
Chemotherapy, 14-15
Chin augmentation, 134
Chlorhexidine mouth rinse, 450
Chloride, 459
Cholesterol, 459
Christensen's phenomenon, 395, 396
Chromic gut suture, 77
Chronic lymphocytic leukemia, 24
Chronic myeloid leukemia, 24
Circummandibular ligation procedure, 82, 83
Circumosseus ligation, 82
Circumzygomatic ligation procedure, 82-85
Clarithromycin, 474
Cleaning of implant, 464
Clindamycin
    preoperative, 75
    prophylactic regimen, 474
Closed tray technique for fixed-detachable prosthesis, 352-355
Closure
    in blade and plate-form implant surgery, 220-221
    in mandibular subperiosteal implant surgery, 241, 242, 243
    in maxillary pterygohamular subperiosteal implant, 259-260
    methods of, 77-81
    of mucoperiosteal flap, 120
    in periodontal defect correction, 115
    in root form implant surgery, 185
    in single-unit transosteal implant, 288
    in soft tissue grafting vestibuloplasty and pedicle grafting, 98-103
Clotting time, 17, 18
Coagulation disorders, 24
Coated blade and plate-form implants, 222-225
Cold-weld attachment, 324-326
    for fixed-cementable prosthesis, 350
Colla plug, 407
Collagen disease, 25
Columbia Scientific software, 42-46, 47, 48
Combination syndrome, 396
Complete blood count, 459
Completely edentulous site template, 177
Composite resins, 357
Composite retained fixed provisional bridge, 315-316, 317
Composite retained provisional restoration of single tooth, 341
Computed tomography
    computer assisted design-computer assisted manufacture and, 249-250
    denture as radiographic guide, 307
    in implant choice, 32-33, 34, 35
    metallic artifacts and, 41-42
    scanner settings for maxillofacial and mandibular regions, 461
    scout view, 39
    stereolithographic reproduction of anatomic structures, 462-463
Computed tomography scan intraoral stabilizing device, 249, 250

Computer assisted design-computer assisted manufacture technique, 249-251
    casting for accurate placement of abutment, 374-375
    discrepancy in fit, 415
    in inferior border augmentation, 151
    particulate bone grafting with, 136
    protocol, 460-462
    in unilateral maxillary pterygohamular subperiosteal implant, 266
Condylar guidance, 396
Congenital deficient malar prominence, 134
Congestive heart failure, 21
Connective tissue disease, 25
Connective tissue grafting, 106-108
Consent form, 465
Console in electrical delivery system, 70
Continuous bar, 63-64
Continuous box-lock suture, 78, 79, 80
Contra-angle handpiece, 72
Contracture, scar
    endosteal implant, 422-424
    subperiosteal implant, 425
Conversion prosthesis, 350
Coping
    impression making for overdentures, 385
    in mandibular staple implant, 293
    root form implant abutment and, 330, 334
    in single tooth implant restoration, 342
    transfer, 390, 391
    with transosteal implants, 289
    in universal subperiosteal implant, 379
Coping bar splint, 59
    after transepithelial abutment placement, 329
    fixed-detachable prosthesis, 384
    in transosteal implant, 382
Core-Vent blade, 53
Core-Vent system, 433
Cortical plate perforation, 406-409
Corticosteroids, 13-14
Coumadin; *see* Warfarin
Counterbore, 180
Crash cart, 69
Creatinemia, 15
Creatinine, 459
Crête Mince implant, 4-5, 296-303
    mini subperiosteal button implants with intraoral bar welding, 300-303
    mini transitional implants, 300, 301
    surgical and prosthodontic techniques, 297-300
Cross-sectional view
    in judging operative sites, 44, 45
    of maxillae, 43
    of radiopaque markers, 39, 40
Crown
    cementable, 345-347
    implant-supported, 394, 395
    in matte-finished tapered implants, 280
    to retrofit implant, 432-433
    root form implant abutment and, 330, 334
    single, 62, 343-344
Curette, 185, 186
Cushing's syndrome, 20
Cusp-balanced occlusion, 396
Custom-cast blade implant, 225
Custom-cast root form implant abutment, 327, 328, 334
Custom tray, 376
Cutting needle, 76
Cyst, repair with graft material, 132

Filleting soft tissue flaps, 98
Finishing stage drill, 74
Fistula
 arteriovenous, 21
 gingival, 419
 oroantral, 101, 421
 submandibular, 131, 149
Fixed bridge, 60-61
 buttressed anchor and, 226
Fixed-detachable bar, 58
 maxillary root form implant and, 329
Fixed-detachable prosthesis, 61, 348-361
 breakage of retention screws in, 436
 coping bar splint, 384
 hybrid bridge, 362-373
  fully edentulous arch, 362-371
  partially edentulous arch, 371-373
 impression making, 350-356
 preparatory phases, 349-350
 superstructure fabrication, 357-360
 support requirements, 348-349
Fixed prosthesis, 348-361
 impression making, 350-356
 preparatory phases, 349-350
 superstructure fabrication, 357-360
 support requirements, 348-349
Fixed provisional prosthesis, 314-317
Flap
 in blade implant surgery, 217
 design, elevation, and retraction, 96-98
 inadequate implant coverage, 409-410
 in mandibular subperiosteal implant, 239-240
 in periodontal defect correction, 112-113
 in Z-plasty, 424
 in ramus blade implant, 235
 in ramus frame implant surgery, 230, 231
 in root form implant surgery, 185, 186
Flat-topped root form implant abutment, 323-324, 336-339
Flexiguard, 293, 294
Flurazepam, 75
Foramina for cervical colli branches, 56
Fosfestrol, 15
Fossa-balanced occlusion, 396
Fracture
 blade abutment, 438-439
 buccal or lingual cortical plates, 409-410
 of mandibular body, 132
 mesostructure bar, 436-438
Free-end saddle template, 176
Free-floating central retaining screw, 327
Free grafting mucosa and connective tissue, 103-104
Freeze-dried bone matrix graft, 112
Frenulectomy, 91
Fresh frozen bone graft, 112
Frialit-2 implant, 49, 211
Friatec implant, 49, 211
Full arch alginate impression, 29
Full-thickness mucoperiosteal flap, 123, 124

G

G-floss, 449
Gall stones, 15
γ-glutamyl-transpeptidase, 13
General anesthesia
 in maxillary pterygohamular subperiosteal implant, 257
 in single-unit transosteal implant, 285
Gentamicin, 418
Gerald forceps, 96

Gingiva
 fistula of, 419
 metal hybrid bridge and, 367
 soft gingival prostheses in single tooth restoration, 346
 submerged root form implant and, 188, 189
 transepithelial abutment and, 321, 322
Gingivomucosal pedicle, 94
Glucose, 459
Gold copings, 336, 337, 338
 in fixed-detachable prosthesis, 354, 355
 in overdenture, 388
Gold-plated scaler, 448
Gortex membrane, 114
Gow-Gates technique, 76
Grafting
 bone, 109-174; see also Bone graft
  alveolar ridge maintenance, 123
  block form, 131, 134, 135
  bone management, 110-112, 113, 114
  to improve ridge dimension for accommodation of implant, 147-172
  maxillofacial reconstruction, 130-131
  particulate grafts, 131, 132, 133
  periimplant support and repair, 135-136
  periodontal defect correction, 112-116
  platelet-rich gel for, 131-135
  for root form implant host sites of inadequate dimension, 136-146
  technique for, 123-130
  use of guided tissue regeneration membranes, 114, 116-123
 soft tissue, 94-108
  allogenic mucosal grafting, 105-106
  connective tissue grafting, 106-108
  flap design, elevation, and retraction, 96-98
  free grafting mucosa and connective tissue, 103-104
  incision in, 95
  vestibuloplasty and pedicle grafting, 98-103
Granulocytopenia, 24
Granuloma
 failing endosteal implants and, 427
 recurrent pericervical, 440-442
Granulomatous disease, 20-21
Greater palatine foramen, 55
Greater palatine neurovascular bundle, 55
Groove and slot abutment connection system, 195
Guidance appliance with radiopaque teeth, 41
Guided tissue regeneration membrane, 8
 in blade and plate-form implant surgery, 228
 in bone grafting, 114, 116-123
 for fractured buccal or lingual cortical plates, 409
 in miniplate for posterior maxillary deficiency, 171, 172
 in root form implant surgery, 184-185
Guidor membrane, 114
Gutta percha
 in splint fabrication, 33, 36-39
 in trial dentures for edentulous arch, 37

H

Hader bar, 64
Hader clip, 65
 in mandibular subperiosteal implant, 242, 380
 in maxillary pterygohamular subperiosteal implant, 260
Hamulus, 55

Hanau Quint, 396
Hand-Schüller-Christian disease, 22
Handpiece, 72, 73
Handpiece power zone, 72
Hard tissue surgery; see Bone graft
Hay fever, 22
Healing cap, 183
Healing collar
 failing endosteal implants and, 427
 hybrid bridge and, 363-364
 in root form implant surgery, 188, 189, 190
 for transitional denture, 313
Healing screw, 417
Height deficiency
 anterior mandibular, 147-153
 anterior maxillary, 160, 161
 posterior mandibular, 154
 posterior maxillary, 162-170
Hematocrit, 17, 459
Hematologic disorders, 23
Hematopoietic disorders, 14
Hemoglobin, 459
Hemophilia, 23
Hemorrhage during endosteal implant surgery, 410-411
Hemostasis, 113
Hemovac, 138, 140
Henahan retractor, 97
Henoch-Schönlein disease, 23
Heparin, 75
Hereditary coagulation disorders, 23-24
Hereditary hemorrhagic telangiectasia, 23
Hexed implant, 51
High-tension steel clips, 63
High-water fixed-detachable prosthesis, 359
Histiocytosis X, 22
Hodgkin's disease, 24
Hollow cylinder, 202, 203
Home care, 446-450
Homograft, 112
Horizontal mattress suture, 78, 80
 for guided tissue regeneration membranes, 122
 in mandibular subperiosteal implant surgery, 243
 in maxillary pterygohamular subperiosteal implant, 261
 in miniplate for posterior maxillary deficiency, 171, 172
 in ramus frame implant surgery, 235
 in submergible blade implant, 221
Hormone deficiencies, 17
Hruska titanium welder, 300, 302, 303
Human bone ash graft, 112
Human immunodeficiency virus infection, 13, 25
Hybrid bridge, 359, 362-373
 fully edentulous arch, 362-371
 partially edentulous arch, 371-373
Hydroxyapatite-coated blade implants, 225
Hydroxyapatite-collagen block, 130
Hypaque, 41
Hyperadrenal cortical syndrome, 20
Hyperbaric oxygen, 443
Hyperparathyroidism, 20
Hyperpituitarism, 20
Hyperplasia, 86-92
Hypersensitivity reactions, 22
Hypersplenism, 23
Hypertensive vascular disease, 21
Hyperthyroidism, 20
Hypertrophic muscle attachments, 89, 91
Hypoparathyroidism, 20
Hypothyroidism, 20

R

RA-1 ramus frame, 234-235
RA-2 ramus, 230-234
Radiofrequency and plasma glow discharge
  unit, 464
Radiographic ball-bearing template, 30-32
Radiographic template, 307
Radiography
  of augmented mandible, 152
  in crown insertion for single tooth
    restoration, 346
  of failed blade in right maxilla, 163
  intraoperative, 111
  of mandibular subperiosteal implant, 244
  in miniplate for posterior maxillary
    deficiency, 171, 172
  of mixed tooth and implant-supported
    prosthesis, 307
  of neurovascular bundle variations, 408
  panoramic, 30, 31
  of periimplant radiolucencies, 419
  in periodontal defect correction, 115, 116
  of postinsertion paresthesia, 418
  of radiolucencies, 419, 420
  in ramus frame implant surgery, 231, 234
  of severely atrophied mandible, 150
  in uncovering submergible implants, 187
Radiolucencies after endosteal implant,
  419, 420
Radiotherapy
  contraindication for implant surgery, 13
  implantation in irradiated jaw, 443-444
Ramus blade implant, 6, 235-237
Ramus frame implant, 6, 230-237, 381
  inability to remove impression, 414, 415
  RA-1 ramus frame model, 234-235
  RA-2 ramus model, 230-234
  ramus blade, 235-237
Ratchet, 405
Reamer
  in endodontic stabilizer implant surgery, 276
  in matte-finished tapered implants, 277-280
Reconstruction of blade implants, 221
Recurrent pericervical granuloma, 440-442
Red blood cell count, 459
Red blood cell distribution width, 459
Reduced diameter implant, 52
Reduction handpiece, 72, 73
Reflection
  in blade and plate-form implant surgery,
    216-217
  in edentulous tripodal design, 244-245
  in mandibular subperiosteal implant,
    239-240
  in maxillary pterygohamular subperiosteal
    implant, 257-258
  in periodontal defect correction, 113
Regenetex membrane, 114
Remount procedures using articulator, 400
Removable provisional prosthesis, 316-317,
  319
Renal disorders, 12, 15
Replace implant, 51-52
Resolute membrane, 114
Resolute XT membrane, 114
Resorbable membrane, 116
Restoration
  multiple teeth, 314-319
  single tooth, 341-347
    provisional prosthesis in, 314, 315
    template for, 176, 177
Restore design, 200

Reticulum cell sarcoma, 24
Retractor, 97
Rheumatoid arthritis, 25
Rib graft, 111, 140, 141
Rickets, 13
Ridge augmentation, 177
Ridge splitting in posterior maxillary width
  deficiencies, 160
Rigid bone block, 126-127
Roferon-A, 15
Root form implant, 4-7, 175-214
  abutments, 320-340
    angled, 331-332, 333
    angled variants, 332-334, 335
    bypass of antirotational component,
      327, 329
    for cement retention, 330-331
    cement *versus* screw retention, 322-323
    custom made, 327, 328
    direct gold copings, 336, 338
    for flat-surfaced implants, 323-324
    flat-topped, 336-339
    immediate impression implants, 337-339
    for implants that engage antirotational
      component, 326-327
    for implants with antirotational features,
      324-326
    for implants with Morse-taper interface,
      327-330
    one-stage two-piece implants, 339
    for overdentures, 337, 338
    requiring crown or coping cementation,
      330
    requiring screws for crown or coping
      retention, 334
    tapered shouldered, 336, 337
  bone grafting in host sites of inadequate
    dimension, 136-146
    anterior border of mandibular ramus,
      140-142
    lateral border of mandibular ramus,
      142, 143
    mandibular symphysis, 142-146
    techniques for obtaining autogenous
      bone, 137-140
  burs and drills for, 74
  cortical plate perforation, 406-409
  dehiscent, 419
  failed, 425-430
  fractured, 433
  generic, 175-191
    armamentarium for, 175
    immediate placement of implant into
      extraction site, 184-186, 187
    nonthreaded press-fit implants in, 182,
      183, 184
    surgical techniques, 177-181
    surgical templates in, 176-177
    threaded pre-tapping implants, 181-182
    uncovering submergible implants,
      187-190
  in maxillary sinus floor elevation, 167-168
  mobility of, 446
  osseointegrated implant, 61
  overdenture, 382-383
    abutments for, 337, 338
  for oversized osteotomy, 405-406
  particulate bone grafting with, 136
  periimplant support and repair, 135-136
  poor angulation or position of, 411-412
  proprietary I, 192-205
    Implant Innovations Incorporated, 202

Root form implant—cont'd
  proprietary I—cont'd
    Lifecore Biomedical threaded implants,
      200-201
    Nobel Biocare and 3i systems, 193-194
    Paragon implant systems, 196
    Steri-Oss system, 197-199
    Straumann ITI system, 202-204
    Sulzer-Calcitek implant system, 195
    types of implants, 192, 193
  proprietary II, 206-214
    Astra Tech Dental implant, 213
    Bicon implant, 206-207, 208
    BioHorizons Maestro system, 206, 207
    Friatec and Frialit 2 implants, 211
    Innova Endopore implant, 210-211
    Kyocera Bioceram implant, 210
    Omni-R implant, 209
    Oratronics Spiral implant, 209
    Osteomed Hextrac fixture, 214
    Park Dental Startanius, Starvent, 207-208
    Sargon implant, 212
  selection chart, 48-52, 53
  single tooth implant restoration, 341-347
Ropivicaine, 414
Rotadent, 449
Rotherman attachment, 65
Round root form osteotome, 159
Rubber apron dam, 299, 300
Rubber tip, 449

S

Saddle drill, 74
Sagittal view of facial skeleton, 56
Sampson titanium inferior border mortise-
  form mesh, 151
Sarcoidosis, 21
Sargon implant, 51, 212
Saucerization phenomenon, 216, 430
Scalpel, 95
Scar contracture
  endosteal implant, 422-424
  subperiosteal implant, 425
Scleroderma, 25
Scout film, 42-43
  in computed tomography, 39
  preimplant, 250
Screening of patient, 10-16
Screw
  in Bosker transmandibular reconstruction
    system, 294, 295
  cause of inflammation, 417
  for coping in single tooth implant
    restoration, 342
  for crown or coping retention, 334
  in fixed-detachable bridge, 359-360
  in hybrid bridge, 367
  in mandibular subperiosteal implant
    surgery, 241-242, 243
  in maxillary pterygohamular subperiosteal
    implant, 261
  in miniplate for posterior maxillary
    deficiency, 171
  mobility of, 422, 423
  in monocortical block grafting, 147, 148
  postoperative problems, 435, 436, 437
  in provisional prosthesis, 318, 319
  in root form implant surgery, 183, 321, 323
  for single tooth restoration, 62, 343
  in single-unit transosteal implant, 288
  in Smooth Staple Implant System, 293
  for transepithelial abutment, 67